TEXTBOOK OF ANATOMY

VOLUME 1

FOUNDATIONS OF HUMAN STRUCTURAL ANATOMY

José Adán Amaya Duarte and Kareling Alexandra Lopez Sandoval

ALLIED HEALTH PRESS

Textbook of Anatomy

Volume 1: Foundations of Human Structural Anatomy

Authors: **José Adán Amaya Duarte and Kareling Alexandra Lopez Sandoval**

Allied Health Press
4164 Lakeshore Road
Burlington ON L7L 1A4
Canada
www.alliedhealthpress.com
Email: orders@arclereducation.com

ISBN: 978-1-77956-770-3

ABOUT THE AUTHORS

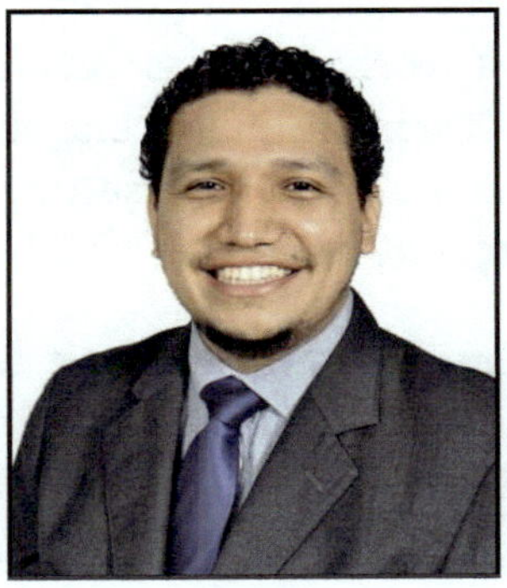

José Adán Amaya Duarte is a medical doctor, academic consultant, and entrepreneur with extensive experience in the industrial, educational, and public health sectors. He currently serves as General Manager (CEO) and co-founder of INVALA S.A., a manufacturing company in Nicaragua, where he has led operational and financial development since 2019.

With a medical degree from UNAN-León, where he also worked as a university professor and research assistant, his profile combines scientific rigor with advanced managerial skills. He also has worked as a medical academic content consultant on global platforms such as Upwork and as a technical advisor and instructional designer for the Pan American Health Organization (PAHO/WHO), participating in multiple virtual training projects, course design, and the updating of pedagogical health content.

In the academic field, he has served as an online tutor, academic coordinator, and designer of educational materials, including audiovisual media, for the Virtual Campus of Public Health. He has also conducted workshops and collaborated in international seminars on topics such as Biofabrication, anatomy, environmental toxicology, educational innovation, and human resource management.

Adán is fluent in English (advanced level) and has basic knowledge of German. In addition, he possesses strong skills in digital tools, ERP/CRM systems, data analysis (SPSS), audiovisual editing, and basic programming (AS3, Swift, Java). His multidisciplinary approach and leadership capacity position him as an influential figure at the intersection of medicine, virtual education, and business management.

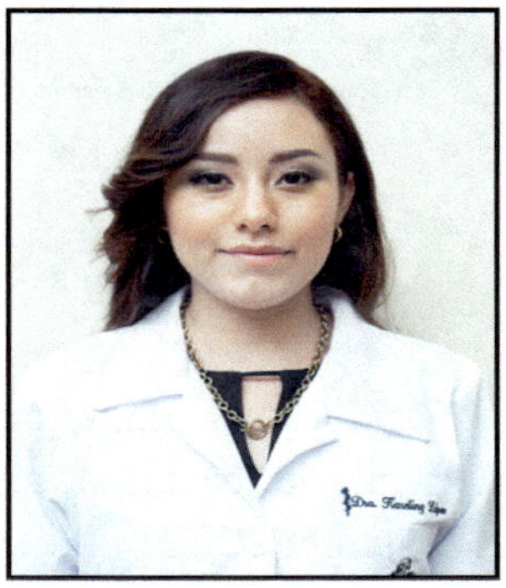

Kareling Alexandra López Sandoval is a medical doctor with experience in clinical care, healthcare operations supervision, and medical translation. She currently serves as Clinical Operations Supervisor at Oclinicals/GI Alliance, coordinating remote teams and maintaining direct communication with clinics in the United States to ensure high standards of patient care.

Graduated as a Doctor of Medicine and Surgery from the National Autonomous University of Nicaragua (UNAN-León), Kareling has worked across various medical areas, developing solid skills in patient assessment, diagnosis, and education. Her career includes roles in both hospital and remote settings, allowing her to adapt to diverse healthcare environments.

In the academic and scientific communication field, she has worked as a medical content reviewer for academic texts, medical article writer based on scientific evidence, and translator of medical documents (Spanish English) with technical accuracy. Her C2-level English proficiency has enabled her to collaborate on international projects, ensuring terminological precision and effective communication with global healthcare teams.

With a combination of clinical training, operational expertise, and medical communication skills, Kareling stands out for her commitment to quality, self-discipline, and continuous improvement in the healthcare sector.

Brief Table of Contents

Getting Started with This Book

Chapter Openers

A list of Chapter Outline is presented providing a brief Introduction to what will be covered in the chapter.

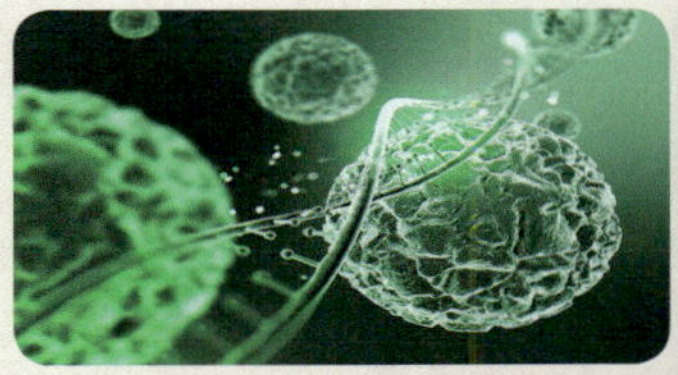

Introduction

Often referred to as the science of life, biology is a broad field of study aimed at comprehending the several kinds of life on Earth, from tiny creatures to sophisticated multicellular entities. Comprising several subfields, including molecular biology, ecology, and evolutionary biology, each of which advances our knowledge of living systems, this field clarifies the mechanisms controlling life events, including development, reproduction, and interaction with the surroundings, which is the central goal of biology. Moreover, biology fills in the void between the natural sciences and medicine by offering a necessary understanding of health, illness, and the interactions between organisms and their environments. Dealing with urgent global issues such as climate change, biodiversity loss, and new diseases depends on an awareness of these complex biological interactions, therefore highlighting the critical part biology plays in modern civilization. Fundamentally, biology explores and tests ideas about the living world using the scientific method. Through methodical observation and experimentation,

LEARNING OBJECTIVES

After studying this chapter, you will be able to:

1. Discuss the scientific method in biology;
2. Explain the cell theory;
3. Discuss the genetics and heredity;
4. Evolution and natural selection;
5. Focus on ecology and ecosystems;
6. Learn about human biology;
7. Evaluate the plant biology;
8. Explain the microbiology;
9. Focus on current trends in biology.

1.1. The Scientific Method in Biology

Learning Outcome

1. Describe the steps of the scientific method;
2. Focus on hypothesis formation;
3. Learn about experimental design.

Learning Outcomes

The beginning of each section of every chapter contains a set of Learning Outcomes that inform students of concepts they should understand. These outcomes help students understand what they should be able to do if they have mastered the material in that section.

Test Your Knowledge

Throughout each chapter, Test Your Knowledge cues you to note which topics have been covered and to self-test your understanding of the material presented.

Test Your Knowledge

1. Explain why correlation does not imply causation in scientific experiments.
2. How does the scientific method help reduce the influence of personal opinions in research?

Chapter Summary

The Summary Section appear at the end of each chapter and summarize main concepts covered throughout the chapter. These points provide key concepts in an engaging and meaningful way.

Summary

The investigation of biological principles highlights the importance of a comprehensive view of life by reflecting the intricate interactions that occur within living systems. The complexity of biology goes beyond individual species or systems, as this essay highlights; it also includes the interactions that mold ecosystems and affect biodiversity. Researchers can conduct in-depth analyses of metabolomic data using sophisticated technologies like MetaboAnalyst, which offer insights into the molecular mechanisms underlying these interactions. As demonstrated by the developments in MetaboAnalyst, for example, the integration of diverse omics data promotes a thorough understanding of metabolic pathways and helps identify important biological markers necessary for research on development and disease (Chong et al., 2018). Additionally, the phenomenon of ecological invasions is a key component of biological research and a vital field of study. The introduction of non-native species into unfamiliar habitats has significant ramifications and calls for multidisciplinary management strategies. Examining the origins and effects of these biological incursions, invasion science has become a crucial field that highlights the need to comprehend ecological dynamics and community interactions. As interest in biological invasions increases, new findings are emerging that put conventional ecological theories and practices to the test. The importance of incorporating various scientific viewpoints is shown by this developing discipline, which also highlights how invasive species shape ecosystems and advances our knowledge of ecological resilience (David et al., 2013). When taken as a whole, these discoveries from invasion science and metabolomics highlight the value of multidisciplinary biology research. Fostering cross-disciplinary collaboration and utilizing technological breakthroughs to improve our comprehension of intricate biological interactions are crucial as we look to the future of biological research. In addition to deepening our understanding of the complexities of life, this method lays the groundwork for tackling urgent environmental issues. Future studies can ensure the continued relevance of biology in a world that is constantly changing by acknowledging the interconnection of biological systems and opening the door to creative solutions that support sustainability and biodiversity conservation. We might imagine a thorough comprehension of life that serves both academia and society at large through ongoing investigation and integration of scientific knowledge.

Knowledge Assessment

The chapter includes material designed to review and reinforce each content. It includes Critical Thinking Questions to help test of your understanding of information presented in the chapter and Short answer Questions to review your understanding of the key concepts presented in the chapter.

Critical Thinking Questions

1. **Who is known as the "Father of Modern Biology"?**
   a. Aristotle
   b. Charles Darwin
   c. Gregor Mendel
   d. Louis Pasteur
2. **What is the basic unit of life?**
   a. Atom
   b. Molecule
   c. Cell
   d. Organism
3. **Which branch of biology studies the interaction of organisms with their environment?**
   a. Genetics
   b. Ecology
   c. Physiology
   d. Botany
4. **Which macromolecule is the main source of energy for living organisms?**
   a. Proteins
   b. Lipids
   c. Carbohydrates
   d. Nucleic acids
5. **DNA is primarily responsible for which function in living organisms?**
   a. Energy production
   b. Protein synthesis
   c. Storing genetic information
   d. Regulating body temperature

Short Answer Questions

1. What is biology, and why is it important to study biology?
2. What are the three main domains of life, and how are they different from one another?
3. Define homeostasis and give an example of how it works in living organisms.
4. What is the cell theory, and why is it fundamental to biology?
5. How do autotrophs and heterotrophs differ in the way they obtain energy?
6. What is the scientific method, and how is it applied in biological research?
7. Discuss how biology helps address global challenges such as climate change, disease, and food security.
8. Explain the levels of biological organization from the smallest unit to the largest. Provide examples at each level.
9. Describe the relationship between structure and function in biology, giving specific examples from cells or organs.
10. How has the discovery of genetics shaped our understanding of inheritance and variation among organisms?

Supplementary Materials

Key Terms: A list of key terms is given for quick reference

KEY TERMS FROM THIS CHAPTER

Annotation enrichment analysis	Biological structure	Cell
Cell theory	Cellular structure	Ecology
Ecosystems	Genetics	Human biology
Microbiology	Natural selection	Organism
Plant biology		

Further Resources: Recommendations for additional readings, websites, and multimedia resources.

References

1. Argelaguet, R., Velten, B., Arnol, D., Dietrich, S., Zenz, T., Marioni, J. C., Buettner, F., et al. (2018). Multi-omics factor analysis—A framework for unsupervised integration of multi-omics data sets. *Molecular Systems Biology, 14*. https://doi.org/10.15252/msb.20178124.
2. Bacher, S., Blackburn, T. M., Essl, F., & Genovesi, P. (2017). *Socio-Economic Impact Classification of Alien Taxa (SEICAT)*. https://core.ac.uk/download/286567949.pdf (accessed on 8th March 2025).
3. Barnett, R., Brace, S., Cucchi, T., & Dobney, K. (2013). *Divergent Evolutionary Processes Associated with Colonization of Offshore Islands*. https://core.ac.uk/download/20664364.pdf (accessed on 8th March 2025).

Detailed Table of Contents

CHAPTER 3

The Skeletal System: Overview 73

CHAPTER 4

Axial Skeleton 109

CHAPTER 5

Appendicular Skeleton 143

CHAPTER 8

Muscles of the Head and Neck 243

CHAPTER 9

Muscles of the Thorax and Abdomen 279

CHAPTER 10

Muscles of the Lower Limb 311

CHAPTER 11

Muscles of the Upper Limb 345

Index 379

LIST OF FIGURES

PREFACE

The human body is an evolutionary marvel of functional integration, with an astonishing array of components all working together harmoniously to create the movements we often take for granted. At the most basic level, isolated cells group together to form distinct tissues—epithelial coverings that cover our organs, connective strands that support them, contractile fibers that exert force, and networks of neurons that carry information. These tissues subsequently condense into organs with specific functions, such as the heart, which pumps blood through miles of tubing, and the lungs, which transport gases. Systems that span several parts of the body exist outside of the organs. For example, the musculoskeletal (MSK) system provides both the skeleton and the machinery for movement. In contrast, the nervous and endocrine systems organize communication and regulation. hese levels of structure and function together form a continuum of complexity, and modifications made at one level often have an impact on the others. Knowledge of how cells aggregate to form tissues, how tissues aggregate to form organs, and how organs aggregate to form systems is pertinent to anyone who wants to understand health, diagnose illnesses, or develop treatments that enable the body's incredible capacity for self-repair.

As we learn about how the various parts of the body work together, a yet more astonishing tale unfolds about resilience and flexibility. Tissues withstand mechanical loads, bending or compressing under stress, and then spring back to their original shape as the pressure relaxes. Joints offer a lovely compromise between strength and flexibility: cartilage cushions impact, ligaments restrict destructive motion, and synovial fluid lubricates, enabling bones to glide smoothly past one another. Muscle layers—superficial fibers that power gross movements and deeper ones that maintain posture—function in coordinated patterns, converting chemical energy into precise mechanical work. When any point in this sequence is interrupted by trauma, disease, or wear—our understanding of standard architecture guides the choice of corrective measures, ranging from physical therapies that rebuild strength to surgical interventions that reposition. By tracing the ladder of organization from microscopic histology to the organization of whole limbs, students develop an understanding that accounts for both how the body functions optimally and how it can be guided back toward health when something goes awry. This bird's-eye perspective enables effective practice in medicine, rehabilitation, sport science, and beyond.

In this volume, *Textbook of Anatomy: Volume 1*, readers will find an organized, step-by-step guided tour of the basic fields of tissues, skin, skeleton, joints, and muscles. In this volume, detailed descriptions and clear diagrams are brought together to complement the learning process. The presentation strikes a judicious balance between depth of information and clarity, allowing learners to develop a clear mental picture and a satisfactory factual basis.

Chapter 1 provides a general introduction to histology, including information on how cells are organized to form the four primary tissue types: epithelial, connective, muscle, and nervous. It highlights significant staining methods and general microscopic appearances. Chapter 2 deals with the integumentary system, which describes the layers of the skin, its accessory organs, and the functions of protection and temperature regulation.

Chapter 3 is an overview of the skeletal system, introducing bone classification, structure, and development. Chapter 4 describes the axial skeleton, including the skull, vertebral column, and thoracic cage.

Chapter 5 examines the appendicular skeleton, such as limb bones, and how they are attached to the trunk. Chapter 6 discusses joints and ligaments, where types of joint articulations and mechanisms of stability are described.

Chapter 7 recapitulates the overall concept of the muscular system, covering the concepts of muscle contraction and muscle anatomy terminology. It becomes more specific about the head and neck muscles in Chapter 8, illustrating their attachments and functions.

Chapter 9 concerns the muscles of the thorax and abdomen and how these muscles are employed for respiration, posture, and core stability. Chapter 10 focuses on the muscles of the lower limb, highlighting the muscle groups involved in locomotion, balance, and weight support. Chapter 11 concludes with an examination of the muscles of the upper limb and the movements of the shoulder, elbow, wrist, and hand.

This text is designed for health sciences and medical students who require a solid base in anatomy as a stepping stone to clinical procedures. It will also serve allied health practitioners, such as occupational therapists, physical therapists, and those working in biomechanical studies. Its uncluttered structure, together with appropriately chosen illustrations and concise summaries, renders it an indispensable reference for gaining a deep and lasting understanding of the body's structural foundation.

HISTOLOGY: THE STUDY OF TISSUES

1

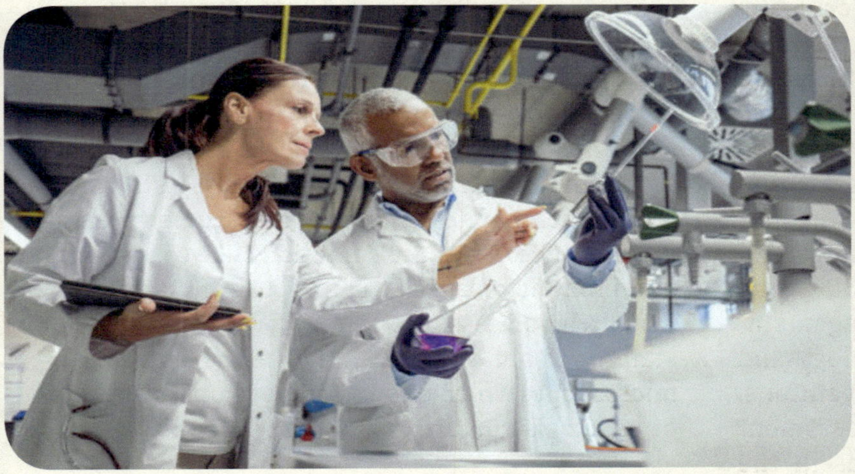

LEARNING OBJECTIVES

After studying this chapter, you will be able to:

1. Discuss the types of human tissues
2. Discuss the techniques in histological analysis
3. Discuss the epithelial tissue: structure and function
4. Define connective tissue: diversity and functions
5. Understand the muscle tissue: types and characteristics
6. Discuss the nervous tissue: structure and function

Introduction

Histology, the microscopic study of the human tissues, is one of the central foundations for an understanding and appreciation of the complex architecture of the body's organ systems. It bridges the gap between medicine and biology, giving special significance to tissue structure about function. By studying tissues microscopically, histologists can identify pathological changes that are often predictive of disease processes. The method generally involves sophisticated methods, e.g., staining and microscopy, that allow for the view of cell ultrastructure and cell interactions. Histology knowledge not only increases the potential to appreciate normal physiology better but also offers a superior ability for recording abnormalities reflective of underlying disease. For this reason, histology provides critical aid for clinical diagnosis, research, and treatment, creating a dynamic system for the study of human biology. With progressive tissue research, it is realized that histology education cannot be handled with the typical lecture techniques alone. It requires innovative pedagogical methods to engage the students' participation. Only through self-discovery learning is focus on an active engagement of the students in the learning process. Practical histology textbooks incorporating visual materials, pictures, and sketches are designed to enhance student interest and comprehension. Further, the use of interactive components, such as self-testing questions and areas for note-taking, allows students to manage time and learning objectives efficiently. These methods are found to be advantageous in formulating the skill of thinking critically and enjoying the intricate relationship between structure and function of the tissue, therefore making histology education more effective as a whole (Alaminos et al., 2013). Moreover, the application of histology extends beyond academia to encompass a wide range of medical branches, including pathology, immunology, and regenerative medicine. Histological study has broad implications in patient management, yielding data on disease pathophysiology and the effectiveness of treatment interventions. For instance, histological sample assessment can reveal foreign body reactions, as in the case of some orthopedic interventions involving implants (Bric et al., 2019). Furthermore, advancements in technology are continuously improving histological methods, allowing for more precise and efficient tissue examination. These developments not only expand the understanding of human disease and health but also pave the way for new therapeutic strategies, exemplifying the interplaying dynamic between clinical practice and histological research. In conclusion, a review of histology establishes the basis for an understanding of human tissues required for future advances in medical science.

Definition of Histology

Histology is the study of tissues under the microscope, that is, groups of cells that work together to perform specific functions in the body. It is essential for the appreciation of the shape and function of human tissues at the cellular level. Histology is a multi-disciplinary field that involves anatomy, pathology, and physiology. By studying the intricacies of cell, fiber, and interstitial element organization, histologists can uncover the invisible workings of disease and health. This knowledge is most critical for doctors because it helps them in diagnosis, in treatment planning, and in developing therapeutic strategies. The value of histology does not lie in merely identifying tissue types, as it can also correlate function with tissue structure, provide insight into evolutionary biology, and offer a deeper understanding of the developmental process. The importance of histology also extends to its practical applications in the field of medicine, particularly in pathology. By examining tissue samples, histologists can identify cellular abnormalities that would reveal the presence of disease conditions like cancer or autoimmune diseases. The process of diagnosis usually involves tissue sample preparation and staining to obtain maximum contrast under the microscope, which allows for close observation of cellular structure (Figure 1.1).

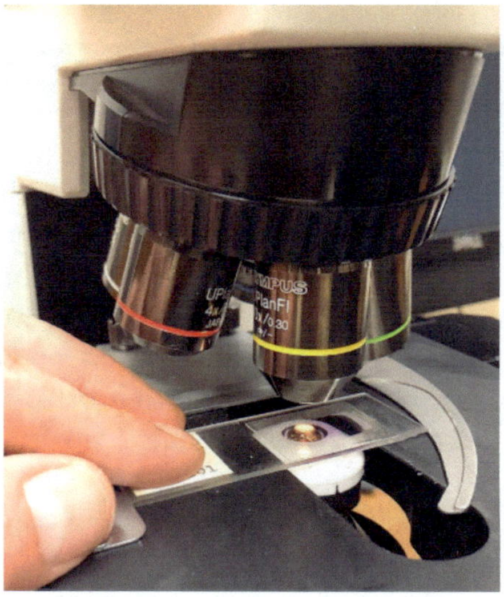

Figure 1.1. Histologic specimen being placed on the stage of an optical microscope.

Source: https://en.wikipedia.org/wiki/Histology#/media/File:Slide_under_a_microscope.jpg.

Further, the application of advanced imaging technologies such as magnetic resonance imaging (MRI) continues to enhance histological studies, giving insights into tissue metabolism and health. For instance, studies employing oxygen challenge techniques have enlightened the metabolic status of brain tissues and provided valuable information, which is applied in guiding clinical practice regarding ischemic incidents and therapeutic modalities (Condon et al., 2008). In addition, histology training is evolving, stressing the need for quality-based teaching practices. Experiential learning is now positioned at the forefront of histology training, with students taking part in active and self-directed learning processes. New practice sessions and didactic textbooks have been shown to significantly improve students' knowledge of complex histological structures since it has been demonstrated through various studies that active content like clinical cases, self-test exercises, and visual materials are highly beneficial when it comes to understanding and remembering (Alaminos et al., 2013). By creating a learning environment that allows students to explore histological structures and their significance to human health, teachers can instill a comprehensive understanding of the field, ultimately enabling future practitioners to contribute to the advancement of medical science and patient care.

Importance of Histology in Medicine

Histology is an essential element of the medical practice, predominantly in providing vital information concerning the human tissue structure and function. Microscopic examination allows for the identification of both standard and pathological conditions, serving as a foundation for accurate diagnosis. Based on tissue specimen examination, doctors can discern cellular changes that may signify diseases such as cancer, infections, and inflammation. The dense visual information yielded by histological techniques, particularly with advanced imaging modalities, offers more insight into cell-to-cell relations and tissue structure. The saying that "a picture is worth a thousand words" is significantly applicable here, since the histological images reveal complex biological processes that are hard to convey with verbal or textual descriptions. Therefore, histology is an essential bridge linking clinical presentation and the disease-related underlying biological processes to enable specific interventions and therapeutic strategies (Andrén et al., 2018). Additionally, histological analysis has also become a critical component of cancer diagnosis and treatment. Through assessment of specimens derived from tumors, histopathologists assess malignancy levels, the presence of specific biomarkers, and the tissue microenvironment in general. For example, studies have identified that crosstalk between cancer cells and pancreatic stellate cells is a critical factor in the pathogenesis of PDAC and drug resistance (Antal et al., 2019). By analyzing interactions at the histological level, researchers can identify potential therapeutic targets and enhance treatment strategies. Therefore, histology not only teaches diagnosis but also informs the formulation of personalized medicine, where the patterns of therapy are formulated based on the specific histopathological features of the individual tumor. The integration of histological and clinical data improves patient outcomes and makes oncological management more accurate. In addition, the advancement in histological techniques has been instrumental in promoting the linkage of genomics and metabolomics into practice. One such technique is imaging mass spectrometry (IMS) that can provide tissue analysis at a molecular level, thereby enabling the linking of phenotypic characteristics with the underlying genomic information. This strategy represents an evolution towards an integrated view of disease where structural and molecular data are combined, yielding an integrated vision of pathological processes (Andrén et al., 2018).

Profiling for molecular constituents of the tissue allows not only for the identification of disease mechanisms but also facilitates the definition of new therapeutic opportunities, most notably in the case of multifactorial diseases such as cancer. The significance of histology to medicine cannot be overemphasized since it continues to form the basis of understanding human health and illness, opening the way to innovations that will redefine future medicine.

Historical Background of Histological Studies

The development of histological investigation in the past is closely related to advances in the microscope and anatomical science. Human tissue observation began years ago, beginning in ancient times when philosophers such as Hippocrates and Galen established the basis of knowledge regarding the way organs and their systems operate. But it wasn't until the compound microscope was invented in the 17th century that scientists could view tissues closely on a cellular level. Visionaries like Robert Hooke, who famously observed cells in a piece of cork, and Antonie van Leeuwenhoek, who first reported observing living cells, advanced the field. By the 19th century, histology had evolved as a distinct science because of the refinement in the techniques of staining and the emergence of cellular theory. This provided a basis for the study of complex tissue structures and understanding their roles in anatomy and physiology. With the passage of the 19th century, the integration of histological investigation with emerging sciences such as pathology and embryology gained greater importance. Histologists like Rudolf Virchow pioneered the explanation of disease processes by attributing changes in cells to disease conditions, thereby applying the principle of Omnis cellula e cellula, which reiterates that all cells are derived from already existing cells. This revolution provided valuable insights into the mechanism of diseases and stimulated the development of contemporary medical sciences. Secondly, histological techniques were used to understand various conditions, such as cancer, where the examination of tissue samples became a central part of diagnosis and therapy. The ability to classify and ascertain abnormalities in tissues not only revolutionized medicine but also reinforced histology's status as a core subject that commingles with clinical practice. Today, the traditional course of histology has led the way to novel methodologies and techniques that more and more facilitate further research and medical diagnostics. Immunohistochemistry and molecular biology have allowed histologists to analyze tissue samples with hitherto unknown specificity and depth, revealing the molecular mechanisms of numerous diseases. In addition, technical advancements in high-resolution imaging have significantly improved tissue visualizations, and cellular multifaceted interactions have been greatly understood. Histology's own history, from simple observation to complex analysis, has enabled spectacular advancements in fields such as regenerative medicine and individualized therapeutics. With the progression of histological research, its fundamental concepts remain core in characterizing human tissues and exploring the laws of disease and health, constituting the backbone of the pivotal role of histology in medicine today.

1.1. Types of Human Tissues

Learning Outcome

1. Define epithelial tissue and connective tissue
2. Explain the muscle and nervous tissue

It is required to know the types of human tissues in order to comprehend the complexity of the biological functions as are necessary for life. Typically classified into four basic categories—epithelial, connective, muscular, and nervous tissue—each one of them has its unique structure and function. Protective by nature, epithelial tissue is not just responsible for lining the organ surfaces but also the body cavities, thus playing a significant role in absorption, secretion, and sensation. Connective tissue, the most heterogeneous tissue type, holds other organs and tissues together, supports, and defends them. Consisting of a variety of subtypes such as adipose, bone, and blood, these are all needed for homeostasis and structural support to the body. Special arrangement and composition of specific tissue types enable them to perform their respective functions within the many systems that comprise human physiology. Muscle tissue, comprising skeletal, cardiac, and smooth muscle, is essential for contraction and movement, which are necessary for both voluntary and involuntary functions. Skeletal muscle, which is connected to bones, accommodates orderly motion, and cardiac muscle, in the heart, supplies the pumping motion required in the circulation of blood. Smooth muscle, within most hollow organs, is responsible for involuntary movements such as digestion and respiration. The arrangement of the muscle fibers is considerably different in these three types, with substantial variation in contractile characteristics and responsiveness to stimulation. Awareness of such differences is significant in the diagnosis and treatment of muscle disease. Moreover, the presence of specialized structures such as intercalated discs in cardiac muscle enhances the functional efficiency of such tissues, making coordinated contractions possible for the survival of organisms. Finally, nervous tissue is also accountable for receiving and conducting signals in the body and, therefore, critical to the operation of the central and peripheral nervous system. Nervous tissue consists mainly of neurons and glial cells and facilitates information transmission between different parts of the body and the external world. Neurons, with their intricate structures, allow for the transmission of electrical impulses at a rapid rate, enabling reflexes as well as responses to stimuli. Glial cells, on the other hand, support and provide protection so that neurons can function optimally. The complexity within nervous tissue allows even high coordination and integration of activity to take place, which is necessary for cognitive function and sensory perception. Advanced research has shown evidence of protein expression differences in nervous tissue, which reflects the complex regulation and specialization that happens behind its superior abilities (Asplund et al., 2025). Besides, novel technologies create novel opportunities to decipher the tissue specificities, and the door is thus opened for new diagnostic and therapeutic methods (Aguilera et al., 2019) (Figure 1.2).

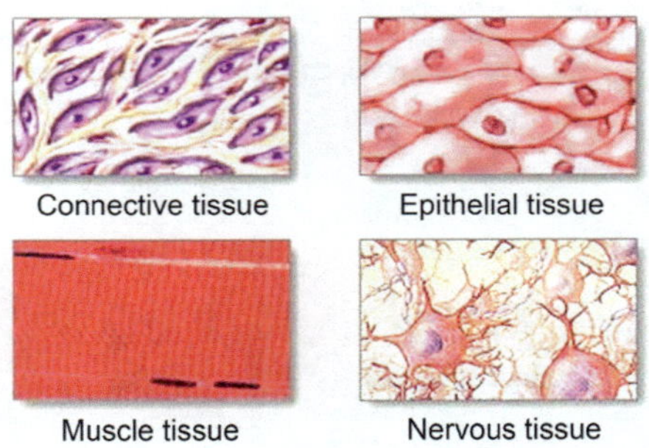

Figure 1.2. Types of tissue.

Source: https://medlineplus.gov/ency/images/ency/fullsize/8682.jpg.

1.1.1. Epithelial Tissue

Epithelial tissue, a fundamental element of histology, plays several vital roles in the human body. With tightly packed cells and little extracellular matrix (ECM), this tissue type creates protective coverings while enabling absorption, secretion, and sensation. Epithelial cells are rooted to the underlying connective tissue through a basement membrane, enabling complex communication and nutrient exchange. Although epithelial tissue can be separated into various shapes—such as squamous, cuboidal, and columnar—it also exists in layer structures, which can be simple or stratified depending on its region and function. Simple squamous epithelium, for instance, is found in areas that require efficient diffusion, like alveoli in the lungs, whereas stratified squamous epithelium serves to protect from abrasion, like in the skin. This variation illustrates the important role that epithelial tissue plays in controlling homeostasis and responding to environmental stimuli. Epithelial tissue actively contributes to the maintenance of physiological processes rather than only acting as a barrier to react. For instance, hormones, enzymes, and other secretions necessary for bodily functions are released by glandular epithelial cells (Figure 1.3).

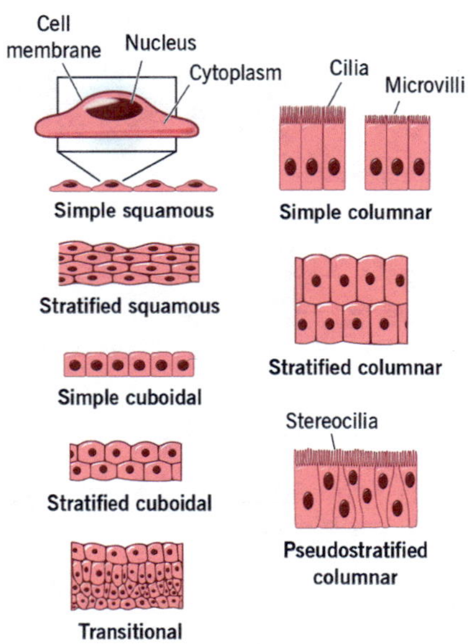

Figure 1.3. There are several different types of epithelial cells based on their shape and arrangement.

Source: https://my.clevelandclinic.org/-/scassets/images/org/health/articles/22062-epithelium-illustration.

Glandular epithelium is classified into endocrine and exocrine glands based on the method of secretion. Endocrine glands secrete hormones into the blood, which play significant roles in growth and metabolism regulation, while exocrine glands secrete their products through ducts to the epithelial surface. Functional diversity is also emphasized by the involvement of epithelial tissues in activities like intestinal absorption, where microvilli are employed to enhance surface area for increased nutrient absorption. Therefore, the histology of epithelial tissue goes beyond its structure to encompass its general functional implications in disease and human health. Histologists have been interested in how sensitive epithelial tissues are to chemicals, environmental stimuli, and infectious agents. For instance, environmental pollutants with estrogenic effects can interfere with critical developmental processes and affect the form and function of epithelium. This has been shown in studies to have a negative impact on the development of reproductive organs in animal models, as evidenced by observations with domestic hens under the influence of endocrine disruptors, leading to eggshell thinning and reproductive competence disruption. The experiments draw attention to the importance of epithelial tissue sensitivity to environmental signals, as they play a controlling role in tissue homeostasis and health in general. Exploring these interactions not only builds the field of histology but also enlightens public health policies regarding lessening the dangerous effects of environmental toxins on human tissue and organ systems, thereby focusing on the integrative function of histological studies in determining human health.

1.1.2. Connective Tissue

Connective tissue is a critical component of the structural framework of the human body, supporting the body and binding organs and tissues in place. It is recognized for the large variety of elements that are found in its composition, which varies from fibers such as collagen and elastin to cells such as fibroblasts, macrophages, and adipocytes. All these have been classified into six primary types, which are loose connective tissue, dense connective tissue, cartilage, bone, blood, and lymph. Every category of classification has specific functions, such as elasticity, tensile strength, and the ability to carry waste and nutrients.

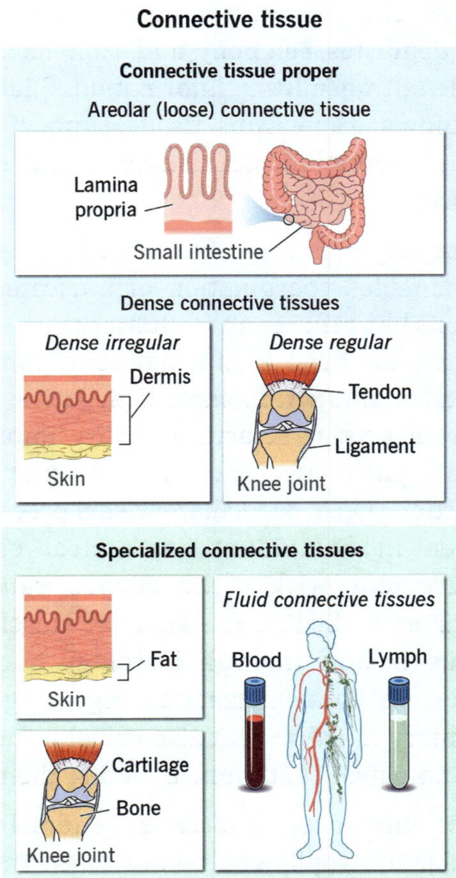

Figure 1.4. Connective tissue can take many forms and do many jobs, depending on its structure and location.

Source: https://my.clevelandclinic.org/-/scassets/images/org/health/articles/connective-tissue.

The ECM richness in the connective tissue not only permits these activities but also provides it with mechanical features that are intrinsic to tissue integrity and health. Therefore, an understanding of the histological characteristics of connective tissue is required to understand how they contribute to homeostasis and general body function. The mechanical characteristics of connective tissue are of great importance in physiological contexts. One such example is the study of hyperelastic tissues, which include most forms of connective tissues, since it emphasizes the predominance of collagen structure and composition in dictating these mechanical characteristics. In research involving human coronary arteries, methods have been developed that correlate microscopic histological data with macroscopic predictions of tissue response to stress. These analyses provide insights into how connective tissues resist and respond to biomechanical loading, delineating the importance of achieving structural composition in disease and health. The development of models to include histological data through micromechanical approaches allows for advanced predictive capabilities in medical studies and treatments, further clarifying our understanding of connective tissue functions within the cardiovascular system (Menzel et al., 2012) (Figure 1.4).

Moreover, the interaction of connective tissue with implantable materials, such as dental restorative materials, stresses its role in healing and response to tissue. Studies of mineral trioxide aggregate (MTA) subcutaneously implanted in animal models indicate significant observations regarding connective tissue response to materials. The chronic inflammatory reaction profile relative to the histological examination does provide valuable information on biocompatibility and healing via tissue remodeling processes. It indicates that connective tissue is integral not only to structural support but also to responses to injury and implants. These studies highlight the importance of histological examination in disclosing the dynamics of connective tissue, ultimately culminating in clinical practice in tissue engineering and regenerative medicine (Camilleri et al., 2016). In revealing such connections, scientists can enhance therapeutic strategies using or mimicking the native dynamics of connective tissue.

1.1.3. Muscle and Nervous Tissue

Muscle and nerve tissue are two integral components of the body responsible for movement and signal transmission, functions critical to survival and interaction with the environment. Muscle tissue is a type of contracted tissue and comes in three forms: skeletal, cardiac, and smooth. Voluntary skeletal muscle is striated and attached to bones and facilitates locomotion. Cardiac muscle, found only in the heart, is involuntary and possesses particular structural features such as intercalated discs that promote synchronized contractions.

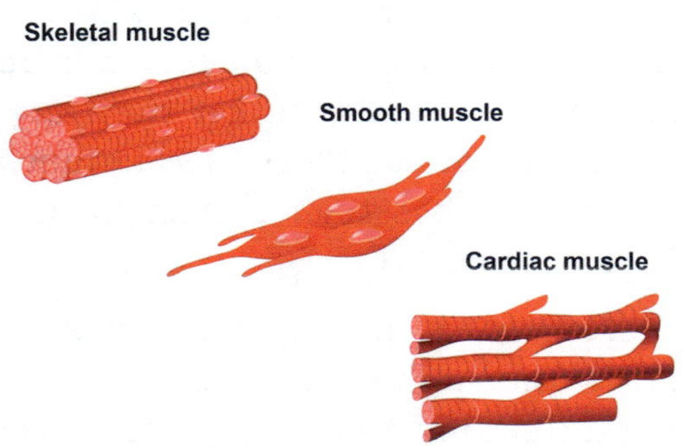

Figure 1.5. Types of muscle tissue.

Source: https://www.sciencelearn.org.nz/images/2357-types-of-muscle-tissue.

Smooth muscle, found in hollow organ walls, facilitates involuntary movement such as peristalsis and the contraction of blood vessels. Information regarding these classes of muscle through histological techniques is essential to both anatomy and physiology and facilitates understanding the way these tissues react under varying physiological conditions (Figure 1.5).

Contrary to muscle tissue, nervous tissue plays a role in the body's communication and consists predominantly of neurons and glial cells. The neurons, which are carriers of information in the nervous system, conduct electrical impulses efficiently, allowing quick communication between the various sections of the body. The organization of the neuron, such as the dendrites, cell body, and axon, facilitates the role of transmitting information. Glial cells, also known as nervous tissue support cells, provide protection, nourishment, and repair to neurons.

The very organized structure of the nervous tissue enables coordination of intricate body functions like reflexes and voluntary movement. Evidence has been found that conditions like prenatal malnutrition have a negative effect on nervous tissue structure quality, impacting central pathways like interhemispheric conduction speed, particularly visual processing, as seen in studies of anatomical change measurement within the corpus callosum (Aboitiz et al., 2012). The study of muscle and nervous tissues through histology not only provides us with information regarding their elementary functions but also valuable insights on pathological conditions affecting them.

For instance, muscle degeneration in muscular dystrophy can be described through a histological study, demonstrating changes in the size and shape of muscle fibers. Similarly, neurodegenerative ailments like Alzheimer's disease (AD) need a close understanding of the changes at the neuronal level and glial response. Histological techniques, including the use of stains to examine certain cell types and structures, are essential to these investigations. Microscopically, through examination of these tissues, researchers can tune into early disease biomarkers and develop targeted therapies, at last bridging the gap between basic sciences and clinical practice, rendering histology today more relevant in medicine (Cozart et al., 2017).

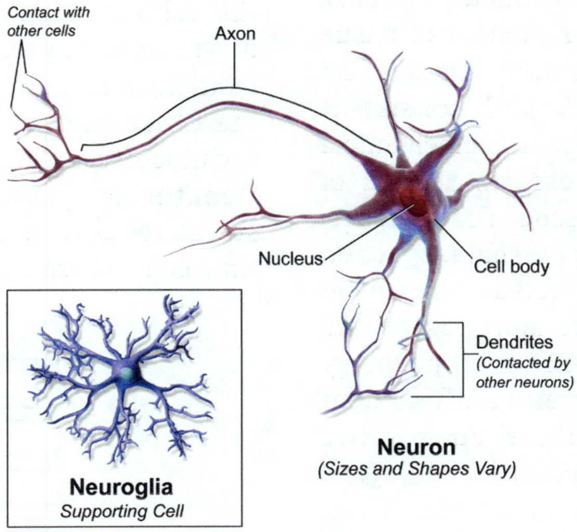

Figure 1.6. Neural tissue.

Source: https://en.wikipedia.org/wiki/Nervous_tissue#/media/File:Blausen_0672_NeuralTissue.png.

Test Your Knowledge

1. How does connective tissue differ from epithelial tissue in structure and function?
2. What roles do muscle and nervous tissues play in the coordination and movement of the body? D

1.2. Techniques in Histological Analysis

Learning Outcome

1. Define tissue preparation methods
2. Understand the staining techniques
3. Discuss the microscopy in histology

Histological examination consists of numerous techniques through which scientists and medical professionals can view tissues from humans at the microscopic level. Some of the necessary steps include tissue fixation, embedding, sectioning, and staining. Fixation is required to preserve tissue morphology and prevent enzymatic degradation, most commonly done using formaldehyde-based fixatives. Fixed tissues are then usually embedded in paraffin, from which thin sections can be cut for microscopic examination. These pieces must then be accurately cut with a microtome with caution to ensure that they are of uniform size, allowing for detailed study of cellular structures. Further staining enhances the observation of certain cell components using various stains such as hematoxylin and eosin or more specialized procedures such as immunohistochemistry, depending on the recognition of particular antigens. This precise order of procedure enables histologists to obtain high-quality samples, which are very important in disease diagnosis and a lot of research in histology. One of the crucial advancements in histological procedure is the utilization of computer-assisted histomorphometry systems, which enable objective measurement of tissue samples. These systems quantify histological properties, allowing quick and consistent measurement that often augments biochemical analysis, as has been the case in studies of engineered cartilaginous tissue. For instance, a candidate for an innovative visual inspection system graded engineered tissues based on uniformity of staining, tissue morphology, and matrix deposition. The correlation of histology scores with glycosaminoglycan (GAG) content accentuates the value of these quantitative systems in augmenting standard histological inspection with objective measures. Thus, blending conventional approaches with high-technology imaging and analysis tools is a significant step in histological processes to enhance the appreciation of tissue integrity and disease. Virtual microscopy is another revolutionary technique that has transformed histological training as well as research. By digitizing tissue samples and using software such as Zoomify®, teachers can create rich, interactive learning environments that enhance students' familiarity with tissue pathology and morphology. This new methodology is illustrated by the DMU e-Parasitology and DMU e-Biology packages, incorporating extensive libraries of digitized images, clinical slides, and mini-videos. This also enhances educational processes through 3D imaging methods, instilling in students a deeper understanding of the spatial organization of tissues and cells. This kind of instruction is particularly worth it in the training of health science, as it allows students to see complex structures that are fundamental to the understanding of a variety of diseases. Thus, virtual microscopy not only facilitates a deeper understanding of histological techniques but also fosters enhanced engagement in the complex world of human tissues (Barbero et al., 2006; Acosta et al., 2019).

1.2.1. Tissue Preparation Methods

The histological process of tissue sample preparation is a step-wise process that decides the caliber of analysis and interpretation of diagnosis to be performed. Typical steps involve fixation, embedding, sectioning, and staining of the tissue, each designed to preserve cellular architecture and highlight specific components. Denaturing proteins and stabilizing cell structures against degeneration over a period of time is the function of fixatives such as formalin.

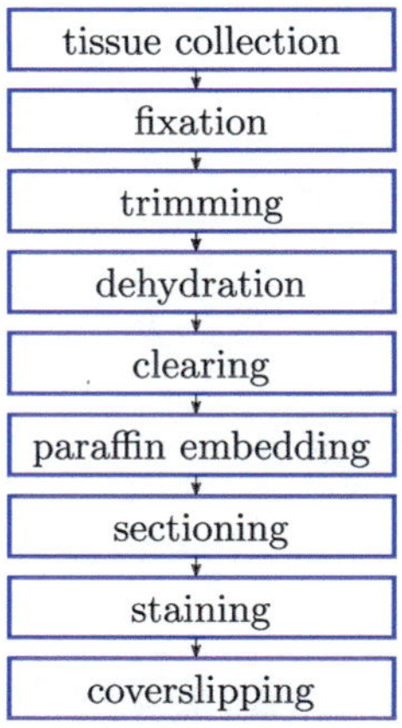

Figure 1.7. The steps of tissue processing for microscopy slides.

Source: https://www.researchgate.net/profile/Marc-Aubreville/publication/341881925/figure/fig39/AS:898407698796544@1591208495144/The-steps-of-tissue-processing-for-microscopy-slides.png.

Following correction, tissues are usually embedded in paraffin wax to enable them to be thinly and accurately cut. This precise preparation yields micrometer-thin slices which may be fixed to glass slides for microscopic study. This even age-old technique can sometimes be time-consuming, and rapid and effective tissue preparation methods are thus essential in both clinical diagnosis and research. The most recent developments in tissue preparation have witnessed techniques that enhance the efficiency and speed of histological inspection without compromising on quality (Figure 1.7).

One of the methods used in accomplishing this is microscopy with ultraviolet surface excitation (MUSE), which can deliver high-resolution imaging of tissue surfaces without needing traditional slide preparation. MUSE utilizes ~280-nm ultraviolet light to excite fluorescent stains, focusing on tissue surface characteristics. The time required to obtain diagnostic histological information can be reduced from days to minutes by using MUSE. In addition to delivering excellent visualizations as their traditional counterparts, MUSE also maintains the integrity of downstream molecular assays, a capability particularly valuable in high-resource and low-resource settings. The continuous advancement of these alternatives is a step in the direction of more accessible and integrated tissue analysis methods in histology. Apart from conventional techniques, the tissue characterization framework is being reorganized by developments in imaging technology. Quantitative ultrasound (QUS) techniques, for instance, offer a new way to study tissue structural properties, e.g., in fascicles of nerves. By correlating ultrasound images and histological sections, one is able to unravel correlations between tissue composition, e.g., the levels of collagen and myelin, and acoustic parameters. This interrelating technique makes it possible to find significant correlations that enhance our knowledge about tissue organization and function. The conjoining of QUS with histological techniques not only complements traditional preparation methods but also aids in a better understanding of tissue dynamics in disease and health. As technology improves, diagnostic potential increases, and better insight is anticipated within the scope of histology and tissue studies, symbolizing the importance of methodological progress within the field (Figure 1.8).

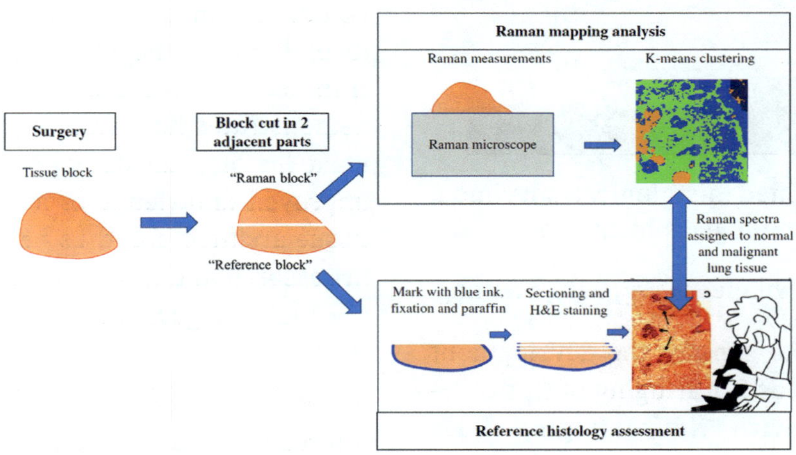

Figure 1.8. Schematic description of the tissue preparation steps and study protocol.

Source: https://www.researchgate.net/profile/Irshad-Soomro/publication/335080084/figure/fig1/AS:790043769708545@1565372521475/Schematic-description-of-the-tissue-preparation-steps-and-study-protocol.png.

1.2.2. Staining Techniques

Staining techniques are the foundation of histology because they make the various cell components in human tissue more observable. The staining techniques employ specific dyes or stains, which selectively bind to cellular structures, making their features visible that were not observable using a regular light microscope. The most frequently used staining methods are Hematoxylin and Eosin (H&E), which stain nuclear and cytoplasmic structures against the background, and special stains like Masson's trichrome or Gomori's silver stain, which stain definite tissue components like collagen fibers or nervous tissue. The choice of staining method depends on the specific structures to be studied by researchers, and thus, the option is still crucial in histological research because the result can significantly influence the evaluation of tissue morphology and pathology.

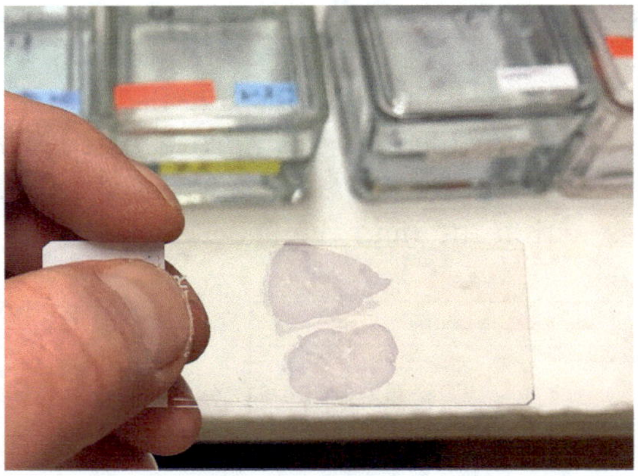

Figure 1.9. A stained histological specimen, sandwiched between a glass microscope slide.

Source: https://en.wikipedia.org/wiki/Staining.

Also closing the gap are the development of techniques such as 3D Bridging of Optically-clear histology with Neuroimaging Data (3D-BOND). Providing precise correspondence between imaging information and histological characteristics, these techniques pave the way for improved diagnostic capability. The ability to bring together high-resolution histological images and diffusion-MRI data enhances knowledge of tissue microstructures at the cellular level. It reveals correlations among various histological parameters and imaging metrics. Thus, the staining techniques are not just histological procedural processes; they are indispensable mediators connecting the microanatomy of tissues to their functional properties, emphasizing the importance of such methods towards expanding our understanding of human tissues and their roles in disease and health (Erturk et al., 2018).

Emerging staining techniques are continuously being developed to address the requirements for higher specificity and resolution for tissue analysis. Techniques such as immunohistochemistry and in situ hybridization enable the identification of particular proteins or nucleic acids in tissues, providing us with information about the functioning of cells and disease mechanisms. Combining these with imaging tools such as confocal microscopy has revolutionized the way scientists perceive the structure of tissue and cell-to-cell communication. Moreover, new techniques, i.e., the biphasic hydrogel technique, allow volumetric measurement of irregular tissues to offer more insight compared to traditional thin-section histology. This development demonstrates how staining protocols not only make histological study possible but also allow improved knowledge of normal and abnormal tissue architecture, thus being of greater value in research and in the clinical context (Arda et al., 2017) (Figure 1.9).

1.2.3. Microscopy in Histology

Microscopy is a vital discipline used in histology to allow the detailed examination of human tissue at subcellular and cellular levels. Microscopes are essential instruments that enable heightened visualization to allow researchers and clinicians to identify specific structures and pathology in tissue. Traditional techniques, such as light microscopy, appreciably improved tissue studies using techniques such as hematoxylin and eosin staining. This age-old technique makes differentiation between cell types and tissue architecture possible. Microscopy improvements have also made it possible to utilize advanced techniques like fluorescence and electron microscopy, which offer unmatched resolution and quality, making it possible to study intricate cellular structures. Besides enhancing diagnostics, these innovations also make it possible to gain more insight into the disease pathology that lies beneath, thus making microscopy a very important discipline of histology. Remarkably, the most recent developments in virtual microscopy are redefining the learning process in histology. Virtual platforms facilitate a repository of digitized tissue images and virtual slides that researchers and experts can remotely access. Remarkably, the DMU e-Parasitology package includes a virtual microscope to facilitate an interactive learning process, showcase digitized slides that unveil healthy and pathogenic tissues. With the help of digital technologies, students can access a vast library containing various staining techniques, further enriching their understanding of tissue morphology and parasite identification (Acosta et al., 2019). This shift towards e-learning not only makes high-quality histological training universal but also prepares students for modern clinical and research environments, where digital skills are increasingly vital. Advanced imaging tools, such as optical coherence microscopy (OCM), represent the state of the art for histological examination, offering the capability to visualize tissues with unprecedented precision. OCM, for example, relies on backscattered illumination to define the microstructure of brain tissue, permitting cellular arrays and density within individual cortical layers to be examined. Current studies have evidenced that OCM is capable of attaining notable rates of colocalization when put into perspective with classical histological techniques such as Nissl staining, thereby highlighting its potential as a semi-high-throughput instrument for brain tissue examination (Augustinack et al., 2018). With the development of microscopy, the adaptation of such sophisticated techniques into everyday histological practice promises greater diagnostic specificity and new insights into human tissue pathology, supporting microscopy's position in histology and its vital role in medical science and education (Figure 1.10).

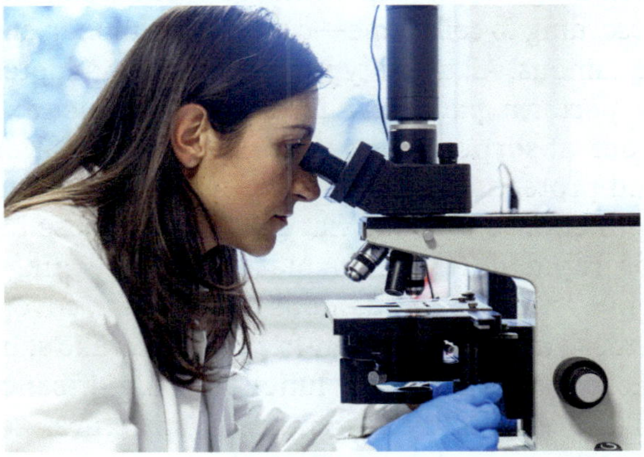

Figure 1.10. Microscopy used in histology.

Source: https://www.laemmegroup.it/wp-content/uploads/2022/07/leamme-histologymicroscopy-header-technician-reading-the-slides-2799x1891.jpg.

Test Your Knowledge

1. What are the basic steps involved in the preparation of tissue samples for histological examination?
2. Name two common staining techniques used in histology and explain their purposes.

1.3. Epithelial Tissue: Structure and Function

Learning Outcome

1. Discuss the classification of epithelial tissue
2. Explain the functions of epithelial tissue
3. Identify the role in protection and absorption

Epithelial tissue is one of the four significant tissue categories in the human body, distinguished by its unique structure and extensive array of functions and composed of closely bound cells with minimal ECM, epithelial tissue forms protective interfaces and barriers between body compartments. This tissue can be classified into many types based on the layers of cells, including simple and stratified epithelium, and according to cell shape—cuboidal, columnar, and squamous. All these types are specially adapted to perform particular physiological functions, from absorption and secretion to sensation and protection. For instance, simple squamous epithelium's thin and flat cells make it possible for rapid diffusion in places like the lungs, while stratified squamous epithelium covers underlying tissue in high-friction areas like skin, thereby showing the functional significance of the variability of epithelial structure. Yet another essential attribute of epithelial tissue is its functional specialization, which closely correlates with its various forms. For example, the presence of microvilli in specific epithelial cells enhances absorbent capability, particularly in the intestines, and ciliated respiratory epithelium aids in mucus and debris removal. The rapid regenerative capacity of epithelial tissue also illustrates the necessary role in maintaining homeostasis and responding to extrinsic stresses. This regenerating capacity is crucial in the case of damage or injury, wherein the epithelial cells multiply quickly to re-establish integrity. The complex interplay of structure and function of epithelial tissue reflects its significance in many bodily processes, rendering an understanding of its histological characteristics increasingly crucial in terms of overall health (Figure 1.11).

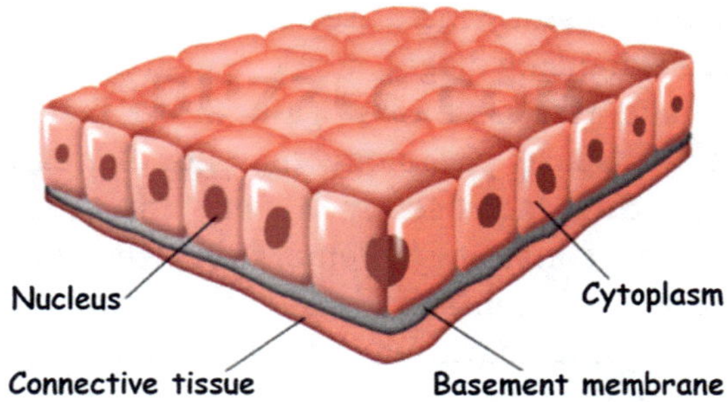

Figure 1.11. Epithelial tissues cover and protect body surfaces.

Source: https://www.careerpower.in/school/biology/epithelial-tissue.

Besides, the epithelial tissue is centrally involved in the operation of numerous organs and systems, being not only a barrier but also contributing to physiological functions like secretion and absorption. For instance, glandular epithelium adapted for secretion can be further divided into exocrine and endocrine glands, which are both individually crucial for the achievement of homeostasis. Exocrine glands secrete substances like enzymes and mucus onto epithelial surfaces, but endocrine glands release hormones into the circulatory system directly, thus influencing several metabolic processes. Further, the innervation of epithelial tissues by senses, as observed in specific systems like dental pulp, indicates that they are implicated in sensation and response to stimuli (Bécavin et al., 2014). Understanding structural heterogeneity and the functional roles of epithelial tissue is essential to explaining numerous pathologies, highlighting the importance of histological findings in the development of successful treatment strategies (Bochsler et al., 2007).

1.3.1. Classification of Epithelial Tissue

The classification of epithelial tissue is key to an understanding of the broad array of functions played by the epithelial cells in human physiology. Epithelial tissues are primarily differentiated based on the number of cell layers and cell shape within them. Stratifying these results in two primary classes: stratified and simple epithelia. Single-layered epithelia comprise a straightforward layer for processes such as diffusion, absorption, and secretion. In contrast, multi-layered epithelia consist of various layers capable of offering protection against physical and chemical damage. This layering is particularly important in areas that experience abrasive forces, such as the skin and lining of the mouth. In addition, epithelial cell variations like transitional and ciliated epithelia are present to facilitate specific functions, such as motion and adaptation to changing volumes, highlighting the versatility of epithelial tissues to keep up with physiological demands. Delving deeper into the classification based on cell shape, epithelial tissues are categorized into the three principal types: cuboidal, squamous, and columnar. Squamous epithelial cells are flat and facilitate rapid diffusion of substances, which is critically necessary in lung alveoli. Cuboidal epithelial cells, however, with their cubic nature, preferentially line glands and are involved in secretion and absorption functions, as seen in kidney tubules. Columnar epithelial cells, which are column-like and heightened, are typically found in the gastrointestinal tract and carry out tasks that include absorption and secretion of enzymes and mucus (Figure 1.12).

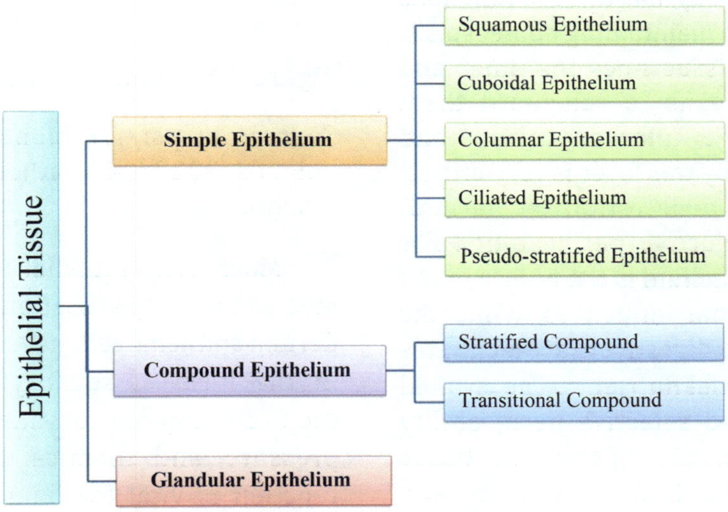

Figure 1.12. Classification of epithelial tissue.

Source: https://easybiologyclass.com/wp-content/uploads/2017/01/different-types-of-epithelial-cells.jpg.

Diversity in these cell forms and organization allows epithelial tissues to perform specific tasks within various organs and systems of the body, reflecting their significant role in maintaining homeostasis and responding to environmental stress. Apart from structural classification, the significance of epithelial tissue also extends to clinical pathology, where an understanding of these classifications aids in the diagnosis of many diseases. Epithelial cells can undergo pathologic changes that express underlying disease and must be recognized to achieve therapeutic success. For instance, changes in normal epithelial cell architecture indicate carcinogenic change, e.g., the progression of normal squamous epithelium to dysplastic or neoplastic tissue in squamous cell carcinoma. Computer-based diagnostic tools have also advanced this field by allowing pathologists to benefit from high-tech image analysis technology in the investigation of epithelial tissue, facilitating increased accuracy in prognosis and diagnosis of diseases in such vital tissues (Boucheron et al., 2009; Hedley et al., 2018). This integration of technology and histological evaluation demonstrates the evolving nature of histology as it regards the classification and clinical relevance of epithelial tissues.

1.3.2. Functions of Epithelial Tissue

Epithelial tissue, being one of the four primary tissues of the human body, has diverse functions that are most crucial in maintaining homeostasis. Primarily, epithelial tissue lines the inner and outer surfaces of organs to safeguard them from physical damage, microorganisms, and chemicals. Protection by this layer is very critical because it prevents penetration by harmful agents but allows selective permeability. For instance, the skin epithelium is the body's initial barrier against external influences, while the epithelial lining of the digestive tract facilitates the ingestion of essential nutrients. The twofold role of protection and selective permeability underscores the importance of epithelial tissue as a protector of the body's integrity and overall function. As demonstrated by glandular epithelium, epithelial tissue plays a crucial role in secretion and absorption in addition to its protective function. Glands, composed of epithelial cells, are specialized to secrete and produce chemicals such as hormones, enzymes, and mucus. To give an example, within the respiratory system, epithelial tissue contains goblet cells that secrete mucus utilized in trapping foreign particles, a reflection of the function of the tissues in ensuring respiratory function. Moreover, microvilli present in the intestinal epithelium enhance surface area for nutrient absorption so that the body's capability to obtain energy and vital components from food becomes simpler. As such, functional specialization of the cells of the epithelium reveals their key functions in metabolic activities and homeostasis control within the human body (Figure 1.13).

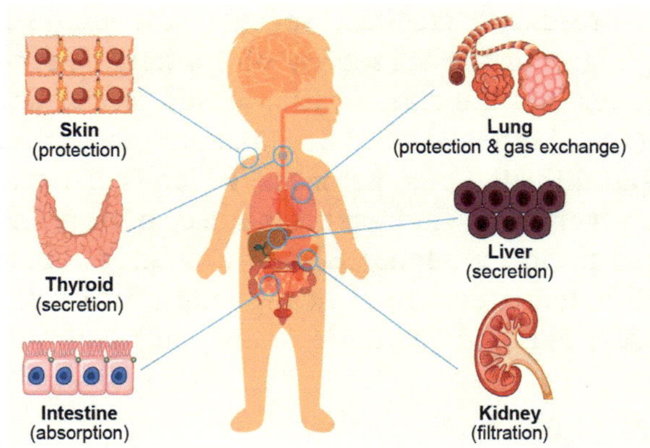

Figure 1.13. Epithelial tissue and their function.

Source: https://rsscience.com/wp-content/uploads/2022/04/epithelial-tissue-and-their-function.jpg.

Moreover, epithelial tissue is also heavily involved in body sensation and communication. Certain epithelial cells have specialized structures in the form of sensory receptors whereby they can respond to stimuli like temperature, pressure, and chemical changes. This sense function is vital for homeostatic mechanisms since it enables the body to react appropriately to internal and external changes. As an example, olfactory epithelium's sensory receptors detect airborne chemicals contributing to the sensation of smell. This ability to sense environmental change and provide information is essential for survival, and the functions of epithelial tissue are thus not merely passive but actively involved in the body's adaptive processes. Therefore, the realization of epithelial tissue extends beyond its structural and shielding role to encompass dynamic activity in total function and well-being in the human body.

1.3.3. Role in Protection and Absorption

Epithelial tissues protect and absorb, and the process is central to the health and homeostasis of the human body. Epithelial tissues are involved in the production of barriers that protect the inner structures from physical damage, pathogenic organisms, and chemicals. For example, the outer skin layer's stratified squamous epithelium serves as the body's first line of defense against environmental harm while permitting controlled absorption of certain chemicals, such as water and electrolytes. This dual function shows how histological structures engage in both protective and absorptive functions and how tissue type and physiological function are closely related. More than that, characteristics of epithelia may vary significantly in various areas of the body, with specializations to specific environmental stresses and substrate requirements. In absorptive capacity, certain epithelial cells, and most especially those that line the gastrointestinal tract, have specialized adaptations in the way of microvilli, which serve the purpose of significantly increasing surface area and allowing for the uptake of nutrients. This histological adaptation is critical to facilitating the best possible uptake of essential nutrients and water and thus contributing significantly to human nutrition and metabolic processes. The presence of tight junctions between epithelial cells also contributes to their complex functioning by regulating paracellular transport and allowing selective permeability. Such structural enhancements allow for proper absorption while simultaneously protecting potentially harmful substances absorbed through the intake of food or fluids. This balance between safety and absorption illustrates the diversity of functions carried out by epithelial tissues for the effective functioning of biological systems. Furthermore, subsequent studies have begun exploring the impacts of exogenous factors such as the consumption of aluminum-containing antiperspirants on tissue integrity. Information shows that long-term application may lead to the absorption of aluminum in breast tissues, thereby causing pathologies such as breast cysts as well as raising the question of breast cancer risk. Most particularly, the relationship between aluminum deposition and disruption of normal epithelial function puts a spotlight on the significance of preserving unaltered protective and absorptive tissue functions. If indeed antiperspirants cause a change in tissue, as some research has suggested, this raises questions about the balance among protective applications and overall tissue health. Thus, quantifying the influence of prevalent substances on histological integrity in epithelial tissue will become pivotal to developing disease prevention and health maintenance measures, thus illustrating the core position of tissue histology in expanding human health knowledge.

Test Your Knowledge

1. How is epithelial tissue classified based on cell shape and number of layers?
2. How does epithelial tissue contribute to protection and absorption in organs like the skin and intestines?

1.4. Connective Tissue: Diversity and Roles

Learning Outcome

1. Discuss the types of connective tissue
2. Understand the functions of connective tissue
3. Discuss the importance in supporting organs

In the body of a human, connective tissues are characterized by their diversity and adaptability in function and are responsible for basic functions in many organ systems. The tissues, among which types such as loose connective tissue, dense connective tissue, adipose tissue, cartilage, bone, and blood exist, provide structural support and facilitate interaction among different types of cells. There are two classes of connective tissues based on the proportion of cellular content to ECM: loose and dense. Loose connective tissue, composed of a gel-like matrix, provides flexibility and support to organs that require cushioning. In contrast, dense connective tissue, rich in collagen fibers, gives tensile strength to bodies such as tendons and ligaments. Such heterogeneity accentuates the inherent role of connective tissues in maintaining homeostasis along with growth and repair in the human body. Connective tissue is not merely reserved for structural needs; it is intimately involved in phenomena such as inflammation, healing, and pathological development of diseases. Increased fibrotic activity in connective tissues can result in various pathological processes, such as chronic pain and stiffness of tissues, which seriously impair functionality. For example, research indicated that fibrotic connective tissue stiffness is crucial in drug-resistant chronic pain mechanisms (Langevin and Sherman, 2007). The interaction of extracellular nucleotides and fibroblasts also influences collagen production, which plays a significant role in tissue remodeling and repair. These findings reveal the significance of understanding the dynamics of connective tissue in terms of normal physiology and the development of pathologies, in which the significance is further underlined for focused therapeutic intervention in the treatment of these diseases. The active role of connective tissues in the body's response to injury and degeneration is also supported by the information known about tendon pathology. Tendon injury, often associated with chronic pain, is characterized by a complex interaction of cellular processes leading to modifications in the ECM. Degeneration, which is cell-mediated, involves increased turnover and remodeling of the tendon ECM by matrix metalloproteinases and other enzymes that degrade the tendon matrix, opening up spaces for therapeutic interventions (Riley et al., 2005). Understanding these mechanisms not only illuminates the challenges faced in the therapy of tendon diseases but also encourages the introduction of innovative methods of therapy that will maximize healing and restore function. Thus, comprehensive knowledge regarding connective tissue functions and their pathological impacts is imperative to the advancement of therapeutic approaches in histology and clinical practice.

1.4.1. Types of Connective Tissue

Connective tissue is a general group of tissues that are required for the support and integrity of organs in the whole human body. This group of tissues can be divided into various types of tissues, including loose connective tissue, dense connective tissue, adipose tissue, cartilage, bone, and blood. Loose connective tissue, an elastic matrix with several types of cells, provides support and cushioning for organs. It is the most prevalent type of connective tissue, a route for support and nourishment. Dense connective tissue, similarly rich in collagen fibers, has immense strength and resistance to elongation, which qualifies it for use in tendons and ligaments. The unique properties of these connective tissues point to their specific roles, reinforcing the significant roles they play in the general structure of the human body (Figure 1.14).

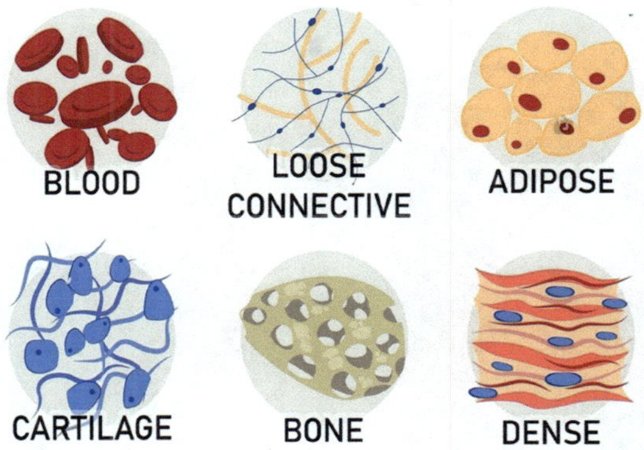

Figure 1.14. Types of connective tissue.

Source: https://www.shutterstock.com/image-vector/types-connective-tissue-medical-vector-600nw-2180225021.jpg.

Adipose tissue, which is itself a loose connective tissue, consists principally of adipocytes, which store energy in the form of fat. Apart from serving as an energy storage area, adipose tissue provides insulation and padding to the internal organs. As a dynamic tissue, adipose tissue is involved in the modulation of metabolism, with a function in endocrine activity by producing hormones such as leptin and adiponectin. Furthermore, because mesenchymal stem cells (MSCs) can differentiate into a variety of cell types, such as chondrocytes and osteoblasts, their discovery in adipose tissue has drawn attention to their potential use in regenerative medicine. Fat tissue's metabolic and protective roles highlight its contribution to the homeostasis of the body and its response to injury, thereby highlighting the intricate relationship between connective tissue types and health. Cartilage, a second type of connective tissue, is a strong yet pliable support structure within the body. Subdivided into hyaline, elastic, and fibrocartilage, each type possesses unique properties permitting specialized function. Hyaline cartilage, the most prevalent, covers joint surfaces and facilitates smooth articulation, while elastic cartilage, in structures like the ear, allows flexibility. The highly populated fibrocartilage found in intervertebral discs (IVDs) and tendons provides tensile strength and shock absorption. The participation of growth factors such as TGF-ß in cartilage repair and cartilage remodeling, particularly in a case like chronic tendon lesion, where healing is blocked because of the absence of signaling pathways, has been noticed in the expression of TGF-ß in disease tissue. Such complexity mirrors the importance of understanding different kinds of connective tissue in histology and their applicability for therapeutic purposes.

1.4.2. Functions of Connective Tissue

Connective tissue has a vast array of critical roles to play within the human body, performing the all-important role of supporting organs and systems both structurally and functionally. This highly adaptable group of tissue includes such subgroups as loose connective tissue, dense connective tissue, adipose tissue, blood, and cartilage, each serving a unique array of functions. One of the principal roles is to provide stability and coherence; organs are brought together by connective tissue and stabilized in their position against one another, so that the body maintains its integrity. In order for structures to endure compressional and tensile pressures, connective tissue also gives them flexibility and resistance. Their mechanical characteristics are under constant investigation to improve our understanding and management of many diseases, as borne out by the new techniques that use micromechanics to investigate tissue behavior in healthy and diseased states (Menzel et al., 2012). Another vital function of connective tissue is energy storage, particularly in adipose tissue, and as a reservoir of nutrients and metabolic wastes. Adipocytes, or fat cells, are a crucial component of energy homeostasis due to their ability to store calories in excess for future use and to release fatty acids during periods of increased energy requirement (Figure 1.15).

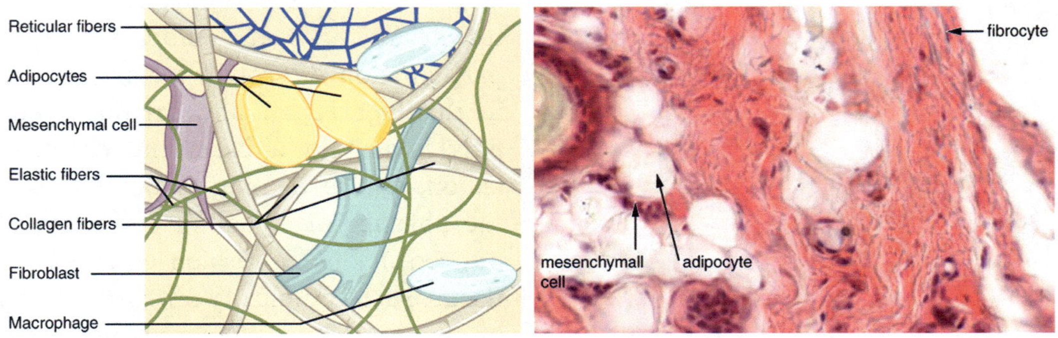

Figure 1.15. Connective tissue proper. Fibroblasts produce this fibrous tissue. Connective tissue proper includes the fixed cells fibrocytes, adipocytes, and mesenchymal cells. LM × 400.

Source: https://courses.lumenlearning.com/suny-ap1/chapter/connective-tissue-supports-and-protects/.

Furthermore, the highly ECM material-containing connective tissues, such as collagen and elastin, permit nutrients and waste products to be transported into and out of the vascular system. This interplay between connective tissue and blood supply is central to tissue health and function.

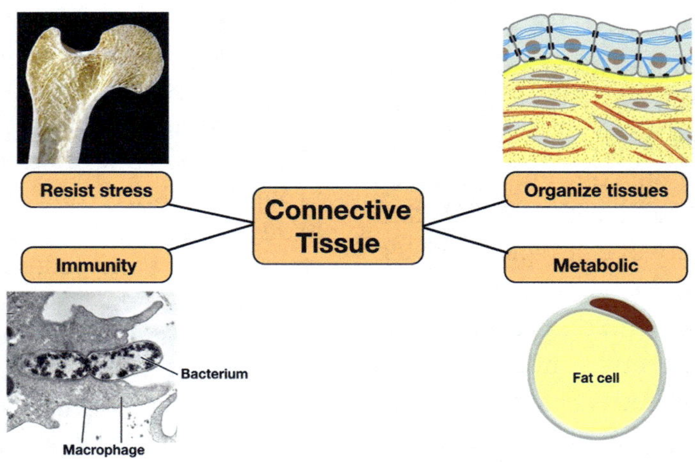

Figure 1.16. Connective tissue serves a variety of functions throughout the body.

Source: https://www.medcell.org/tbl/structure_and_function_of_connective_tissue_and_bone/reading.php.

The role played by growth factors, such as TGF-β, in the process of connective tissue repair and remodeling further bears witness to the fine balance that takes place in such structures. TGF-β signaling pathways have also been extensively investigated in the context of tendinopathy and chronic injury and found to display a complex interaction between cell behavior and matrix structure in the repair of connective tissue (Curry et al., 2001). Lastly, immune response and defense are provided by connective tissues through being part of the body's overall homeostasis. They carry various kinds of cells, such as fibroblasts, macrophages, and mast cells, that facilitate immune surveillance and response. For instance, macrophages are extensively engaged in phagocytosis, responding to pathogens and debris, while mast cells release histamine in inflammatory responses, contributing to the body's defense mechanisms. The ability of connective tissues to synthesize multiple signaling molecules also allows them to communicate with other tissues as well as immune cells, proving their ability to coordinate complex biological responses. While exploring the multifunctional roles that the connective tissue plays in the human body, it is evident that this tissue is not just a support structure but is vital in ensuring health and facilitating recovery processes across a broad range of physiological contexts (Figure 1.16).

1.4.3. Importance in Supporting Organs

The position of histology within the support of organs cannot be overstated, given that the intricate structure of the cell is necessary to ensure the viability of tissues.

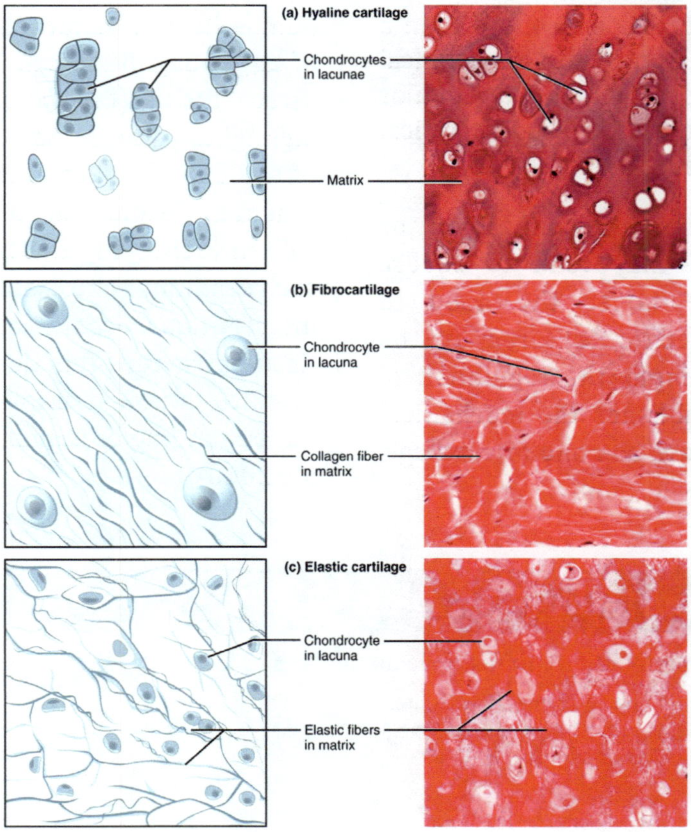

Figure 1.17. Types of cartilage.

Source: https://s3-us-west-2.amazonaws.com/courses-images-archive-read-only/wp-content/uploads/sites/18/2014/07/19181054/412_Types_of_Cartilage-new.jpg.

All organs of the body are composed of specialized cells that play specialized roles, which, in themselves, facilitate the occurrence of complex physiological activity. The ability to study histology allows scientists to examine the organization, morphology, and cellular pattern of organs and understand how these equate to organ vitality. By understanding the interactions among different cell types, extracellular matrices, and derived signals, researchers can describe the mechanisms of organ support and function, necessary in healthy physiology as well as in disease states. This study demonstrates the intrinsic dynamism of histology as a field that goes beyond static observation and instead enables us to comprehend organ function through structural integrity and cellular interactions. In this case, the ECM comes into prominence in maintaining organ function as more than a passive scaffold. The ECM provides biochemical and mechanical support, influencing cellular behavior and differentiation through physical signals such as stiffness (Figure 1.17).

Abnormalities in the organization or composition of ECM may lead to severe pathologies and emphasize the need to investigate tissue-specific features at the cellular level. For example, the regulation of ECM components establishes the mechanical properties of tissues such as bone or cartilage, which are directly involved in weight-bearing functions. Experiments have shown that the mechanisms governing ECM properties can also govern cellular organization, and consequently, learning how such correlations work is at the core of histology science as well as its practice in regenerative medicine and tissue engineering (Matusch et al., 2013). The interaction between cell communication and biochemical signals within the ECM necessitates comprehensive histological investigations to reverse-engineer the complexity of organ support. For instance, pathways such as TGF-beta have been shown to regulate both cell differentiation and ECM material properties, suggesting that the matrix composition of tissues is at the heart of their function in human health. Disturbances of these pathways of large magnitude can lead to conditions like osteoarthritis (OA) or cardiovascular disease, highlighting the importance of the regulation of the ECM for preserving organ integrity and function. Histological studies thus occupy a key role in identifying the molecular pathology of such conditions and examining potential therapy interventions. From a long-term exploration of tissue structure-function, histology opens up avenues to new therapies as well as increased understanding of human disease (Alexandra et al., 2010).

Test Your Knowledge

1. What are the main types of connective tissue found in the human body?
2. List three primary functions of connective tissue.

1.5. Muscle Tissue: Types and Characteristics

Learning Outcome

1. Define skeletal muscle and cardiac muscle
2. Explain the smooth muscle

Muscle tissue is a vital component of the human body, which makes movement and posture possible. There exist three major classes of muscle tissue: skeletal, cardiac, and smooth muscle, each possessing distinctive structure and function. Skeletal muscle is under voluntary control and maintains a striated appearance as well as multinucleate fibers. It serves to provide a significant portion of locomotion and is attached to bone through tendons. Cardiac muscle, found exclusively in the heart, is striated but involuntary, with intercalated discs permitting regulated contractions for efficient blood pumping. Smooth muscle, found lining hollow organs such as the digestive tract and blood vessels, is non-striated and involuntary, allowing regulation of internal processes such as digestion and blood flow. Knowledge of such differences in muscle tissue is crucial to comprehending their specific roles in the human body. Histological examination of muscle tissue offers excellent information regarding its structure and character. Skeletal muscle possesses, in its constitution, myofibrils organized in the form of sarcomeres, allowing for contraction through a sliding filament mechanism. This structure forms a part of the muscles' overall strength and function. Cardiac muscle has features such as branching fibers and the previously described intercalated discs that are required for the rapid transmission of electrical impulses, ensuring heart contractions occur in a coordinated manner. Simultaneously, smooth muscle has a fusiform shape with no striations like those observed in skeletal and cardiac muscle because it performs a different function in involuntary movement. The systematic examination of such structural characteristics provides valuable information regarding muscle tissues' reaction to physiological demands and their conditioning under various situations, thereby influencing the general well-being and mobility. The advances in histological techniques over the recent past have significantly enhanced our comprehension of the muscle tissues at both macroscopic and microscopic levels. Technologies such as three-dimensional tissue visualization techniques allow for closer inspection of the muscle structure, and the inspection that can be performed through them may not be achievable under traditional thin-section histology. By way of illustration, application of biphasic hydrogel methods allows researchers to investigate the spatial organization of the muscle fibers more closely, revealing patterns of growth, repair, and degeneration of staggering significance in the investigation of muscle pathology (Arda et al., 2017). Moreover, ongoing research on the role played by MSCs in the healing of muscle demonstrates the enormous therapeutic scope to repair muscle damage (Grange et al., 2011). These developments highlight the critical intersection of histology and clinical practice in improving human welfare since they not only demonstrate our understanding of muscle tissues but also open the door to the development of targeted medications for a variety of muscular illnesses.

1.5.1. Skeletal Muscle

Skeletal muscle is one of the three major types of muscle tissue in the human body, and its specific histological characteristics distinguish it from cardiac and smooth muscles. Composed of long, cylindrical muscle fibers, skeletal muscle is voluntary, with the capability to have conscious control over movements. Every multinucleated and striated fiber has a distinctive pattern that arises from the organization of actin and myosin filaments within sarcomeres. In addition to facilitating muscle contraction, the complex organization enables the generation of force and motion necessary for different aspects of physical activity. The differentiation of skeletal muscle fibers into slow-twitch and fast-twitch fibers further contributes to its functional adaptability by making it adaptable to various physiological demands, which is crucial in athletic training and the exercise of rehabilitation. The microarchitectural properties of skeletal muscle tissue significantly contribute to its overall functionality and flexibility. Histologically, muscle fibers of skeletal muscle are surrounded by sheaths of connective tissue, i.e., endomysium, perimysium, and epimysium, which provide structural support and allow transmission of forces generated during contraction. Satellite cells between the basal lamina and the plasma membrane of muscle fibers are also important in the repair and regeneration of muscle after damage or stress.

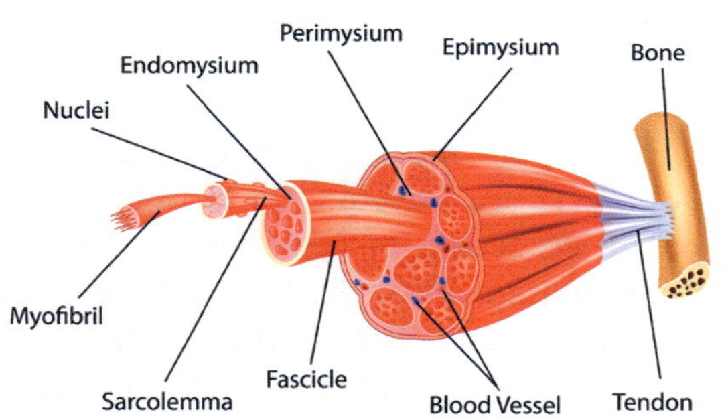

Figure 1.18. Structure of skeletal muscle.

Source: https://external-content.duckduckgo.com/iu/?u=https%3A%2F%2Fcdn.dribbble.com%2Fusers%2F3988742%2Fscreenshots%2F7149810%2Fmedia%2F51505a89f3a348709d03d55e28bdd4e0.jpg&f=1&nofb=1&ipt=cc609b8fc7f0fdfd7da9062fafba4a530c1582bc34ff8104365ca5c544cfd4c4.

This regenerative capacity suggests the importance of skeletal muscle to maintain overall well-being and functionality of the organism. Appreciation of these histological features is significant for clinicians and researchers as these are directly related to muscle performance, fatigue resistance, and the recovery mechanism, all of which are of extreme significance in exercise physiology and rehabilitation programs (Figure 1.18).

The recent development in the area of skeletal muscle histology has broadened our view of its function in disease and health, revealing promising avenues for therapeutic intervention. New evidence has begun to link skeletal muscle pathology with many systemic pathologies, including obesity, diabetes, and cardiovascular disease. Investigation of the cellular and molecular mechanisms that regulate muscle adaptation has gained momentum, a sign of the expansion of the field's importance and clinical significance. As the scientific community continues to explore the significance of skeletal muscle health, there has been an increasing acknowledgement of its role in enhancing human mobility and general welfare. Integration of evidence from disciplines such as myology and translational medicine reflects the varied methodologies involved in comprehending the complexities of skeletal muscle function and its application to more universal considerations for health (Bochsler et al., 2007; Adamo et al., 2018).

1.5.2. Cardiac Muscle

The cardiac muscle, or myocardium, is a unique muscle tissue with distinctive functions and structural properties. Unlike skeletal muscle, cardiac muscle cells or cardiomyocytes are involuntary striated without the voluntary control of skeletal muscles. Cardiac muscle cells are linked through intercalated discs containing gap junctions, allowing rapid electrical conduction so that the heart can function as an organ. This structural organization is fundamental to providing rhythmic contractions significant in blood circulation. An understanding of these histological features not only provides us with information regarding the mechanical function of the heart but also helps cardiac disease studies, which can occur due to anomalies in these cells or their interactions. The intricacy of cardiac muscle structure is made possible by a diffuse spread system of mitochondria, an indication of the tissue's high energy demand. Cardiomyocytes require enormous amounts of adenosine triphosphate (ATP) to sustain continuous cycles of contraction and relaxation. Because cardiac muscle relies to a great extent on aerobic metabolism to provide its energy requirements, the existence and function of mitochondria become critical in deciding its status and activity. The fact that it relies on aerobic pathways also signifies the importance of comprehending the functions of mitochondria in relation to cardiac pathologies. It has been noted that techniques like electron paramagnetic resonance spectroscopy help evaluate mitochondrial function and can reveal signs of respiratory chain failure in several cardiac disorders. (Bennett et al., 2016) (Figure 1.19).

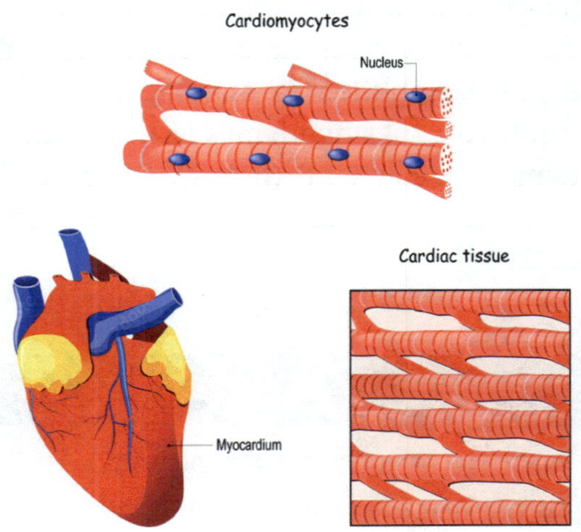

Figure 1.19. Cardiac muscle.

Source: https://as1.ftcdn.net/v2/jpg/03/04/84/72/1000_F_304847289_qpy4qscAN0c62uf6J6kMOqBUdBpyC7Mt.jpg.

This indicates the importance of histological research in explaining normal and pathological functions of cardiac muscle. Ultimately, cardiac muscle research via histology yields critical information regarding cardiovascular disease and health. Histological assessment enables researchers and clinicians to identify structural defects predisposing individuals to heart disease. Understanding of cellular architecture, like that concerning myocyte hypertrophy or fibrosis, can influence diagnosis and treatment approaches. Additionally, as cardiology has grown as a specialty, a better knowledge of the pathophysiology of cardiac disease depends on the incorporation of cutting-edge histological tools in molecular diagnosis. There is increasing space for innovative therapy paradigms that target particular histopathological alterations as more knowledge about the intricate interactions between cardiac tissues is generated, which will improve cardiovascular medicine outcomes (Leveson-Gower et al., 2025).

1.5.3. Smooth Muscle

Human tissue research reveals that smooth muscle is of paramount significance in various physiological functions, particularly in hollow organ walls such as blood vessels, the gastrointestinal tract, and the respiratory tract. Smooth muscle fibers are unlike striated muscle, as they are not striated, involuntary, and spindle-shaped to be able to sustain a more prolonged contraction without inducing the fatigue commonly observed in skeletal muscle. This one-muscle organization enables the smooth muscle to successfully contribute to involuntary movements, which are important for the maintenance of such body functions as peristalsis in the intestine and regulation of blood pressure through vasodilation and vasoconstriction. Histological characteristics of smooth muscle are studied to unravel its many functions in different organ systems, whose significance in health and disease is underlined. In organogenesis, smooth muscle plays a crucial role in human development, for example, in the development of the reproductive and pancreas systems. Research highlights the centrality of smooth muscle to the anatomy and function of these organs and to the formation of critical structures such as the blood vessels and lymphatics (Figure 1.20).

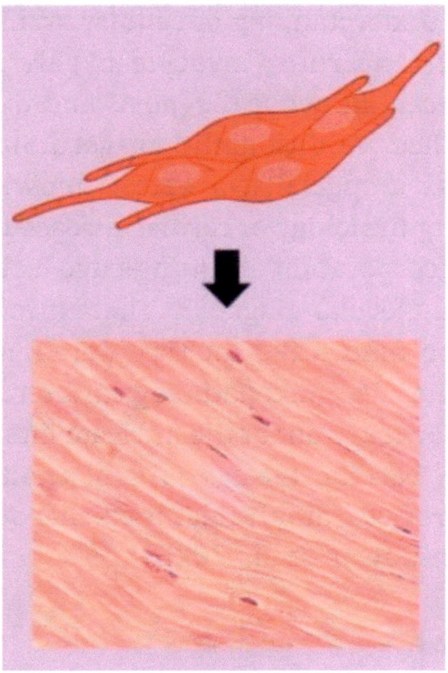

Figure 1.20. Smooth muscle.

Source: https://old-ib.bioninja.com.au/_Media/muscle-tissues_med.jpeg.

For instance, during pancreas development, smooth muscle cells begin to fill up blood vessels by the 14.5-week stage, demonstrating their significant role in the formation of vascular networks responsible for efficient nutrient delivery to islets of Langerhans. This function integration is crucial for higher studies in smooth muscle function across all types of tissues, particularly in understanding the pathologies that arise from smooth muscle dysfunction in its layers, such as hypertension or gastrointestinal motility disturbances. Moreover, knowledge of smooth muscle is crucial in the design of therapeutic approaches in regenerative medicine. As research continues to grow, an understanding of the intricacies of smooth muscle functioning and behavior can lead to advances in the treatment of diseases such as diabetes and blood vessel integrity disorders. Smooth muscle development, along with that of the blood and lymphatic system, offers the foundation for creating effective cell-replacement therapy and surgical interventions. For example, integration of histological information on smooth muscle will guide bioengineered tissue design mimicking the native organ system, thus improving the quality of outcome for patients in repair and transplant scenarios. These advances underscore the interdisciplinarity of histological studies and their relevance across biomedical fields, as exemplified by ongoing work on the multirole roles of smooth muscle in human body systems, as dealt with through topics such as those explored in (Carlotti et al., 2014; Baskin et al., 2019).

Test Your Knowledge

1. What are the key structural features of skeletal muscle, and where is it typically found in the body?
2. How does cardiac muscle differ from skeletal and smooth muscle in terms of function and location?

1.6. Nervous Tissue: Structure and Function

Learning Outcome

1. Discuss the neurons and their components
2. Define glial cells and their roles
3. Understand the importance in signal transmission

Nervous tissue is a critical component of the human body, facilitating the different areas to communicate with one another through a highly complex arrangement of cells. The nervous tissue consists of neurons and glial cells, which carry out specialized but dependent functions. Neurons are specialized cells responsible for transmitting electrical impulses throughout the body to facilitate sensory perception, movement, and thought processes. On the contrary, glial cells provide neurons with structural support, nutrition, and protection to enable them to work at their best. The intricate relation between glial cells and neurons makes homeostasis and response to the environment possible, which testifies to the sophistication of nervous tissue in coordinating the workings of the body. The arrangement of nervous tissue is specially designed in accordance with its functions. Neurons possess specialized morphology in the shape of dendrites to accept the signal, an axon to carry the impulse, and synapses through which they exchange information with other neurons or target cells. Specialized morphology allows neurons to receive and transmit information efficiently. Glial cells such as astrocytes and oligodendrocytes further enhance the nervous tissue's functional capability by performing metabolic support, sheathing their myelin around axons, and regulating the extracellular medium. Given the significance of nervous tissue to the overall operation of the nervous system, the integrated form of glial cells and neurons enables intricate integration and processing of information. Our knowledge of the structure and function of nerve tissue has improved because to recent developments in histology techniques, such as biphasic hydrogel approaches. Compared to classical thin-section histology, which does not maintain the three-dimensional topology intrinsic to nervous tissue, these new techniques can perform quantitative high-throughput analysis of tissue architecture in a less disturbed state. This shift in approach is significant, particularly in neural structure studies of disease, as it reveals the dynamics of neuronal pathology and development in an integrative way. The ability to study spatially-irregular and friable tissue has significant potential to advance research in neurology and other domains, potentially leading to groundbreaking progress in the study and treatment of nervous system diseases (Leveson-Gower et al., 2025; Arda et al., 2017).

1.6.1. Neurons and Their Components

Neurons, the functional elements of the nervous system, are specialized to receive and conduct nerve impulses. Each neuron has a few basic components: the cell body (soma), dendrites, and axon. The nucleus and cellular functioning organelles are located within the soma, while dendrites are receiving areas for synaptic signals with which neurons interact. The axon, which is typically long and sheathed in a myelin covering, is responsible for the fast transmission of electrical signals from the cell body. This specialized form not only underscores neuronal specialization in information handling but also their essential role in maintaining the general functioning of human tissues through complex signal pathways. The histological examination of neurons and their components is key to understanding various neurological diseases as well as the underlying tissue structure. Traditional histological techniques, such as formalin fixation, have been found to influence immunostaining integrity and preservation of neuronal morphology. As highlighted in recent work, fixation protocol modifications, for example, the proposed mixture of formic acid and formalin, enhance immunolabeling of long-stored tissues, like the critical marker NeuN, which is essential to neuron mapping in many pathologies. These innovations not only improve the consistency of histological analysis but also enable researchers to delineate neuronal changes associated with various pathologies, e.g., epilepsy and sudden infant death syndrome (SIDS) (Lavezzi et al., 2018) (Figure 1.21).

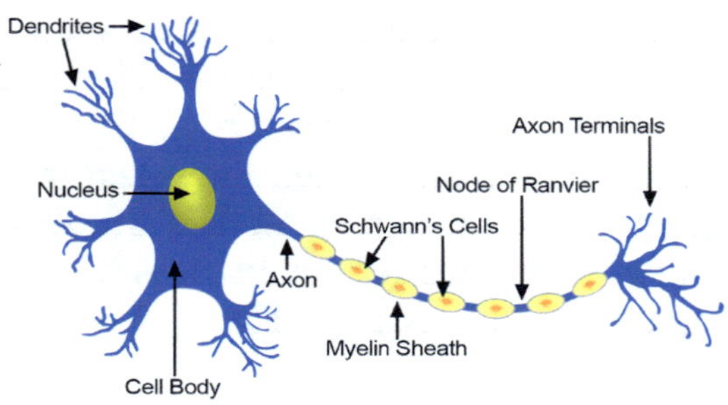

Figure 1.21. Structure of nerve tissue.

Source: https://training.seer.cancer.gov/images/anatomy/nervous/neuron-structure.jpg.

New histological technologies, particularly those aimed at three-dimensional tissue structure, have continued to revolutionize the study of neurons. Conventional thin-section histology does not readily preserve the complex, irregular surface anatomy of nervous tissue, and thus, our access to its physiology and disease is limited. New technologies such as biphasic hydrogel approaches allow for volumetric, high-throughput imaging of tissue, permitting finer-scale investigations of neuronal organization and interaction in disease. This approach provides a new avenue for examining how neuronal elements alter or degrade during disease conditions, substantially improving our capacity to study complex tissue dynamics compared to traditional methods (Arda et al., 2017). As these techniques continue to be refined, they have the possibility of improving our comprehension of the histological complexity of human neurons and their role in disease and health.

1.6.2. Glial Cells and Their Roles

Glial cells, often overshadowed by neurons in discussions of the central nervous system, play a critical role in maintaining homeostasis, supporting neuron function, and promoting overall brain health. Non-neuronal glial cells are made up of astrocytes, oligodendrocytes, and microglia, all serving unique roles within the neural environment. Astrocytes, for instance, help regulate ion balance and provide metabolic support to neurons, maintaining them at optimal functioning. Oligodendrocytes form the myelin sheaths that enwrap axons, allowing for rapid electrical conduction. Microglia are also the central nervous system's immune defenders, constantly scanning for potential damage and responding to disease or injury. A comprehension of the complexity and interactions between the glial cells is necessary to understand the intrinsic function of the glial cells in normal physiology and disease, with a focus on their relevance to histological analysis of human tissue. In contemporary histological studies, glial cells are also increasingly being seen to have a role in various neurological conditions. Glial cells, for example, show a highly intricate response during neuroinflammation with consequences for diseases such as multiple sclerosis and AD. A lack of regulation of glial cell activity can result in adverse effects like neuronal damage and persistent dysfunction. Studies have established some markers and pathways that are involved in glial activation, with therapeutic intervention implications. Examining the diversity of glia and their role in tumor biology—for example, in aggressive cancers like neuroblastoma—shows how particular glial populations might affect tumor microenvironments and the effectiveness of treatment. Research has revealed that cell populations synthesizing adhesion proteins like

CD44 are key to the examination of tumor progression and perhaps malignancy through their invasive properties, thereby demonstrating how glial cells intersect with cancer biology (Morante et al., 2019) (Figure 1.22).

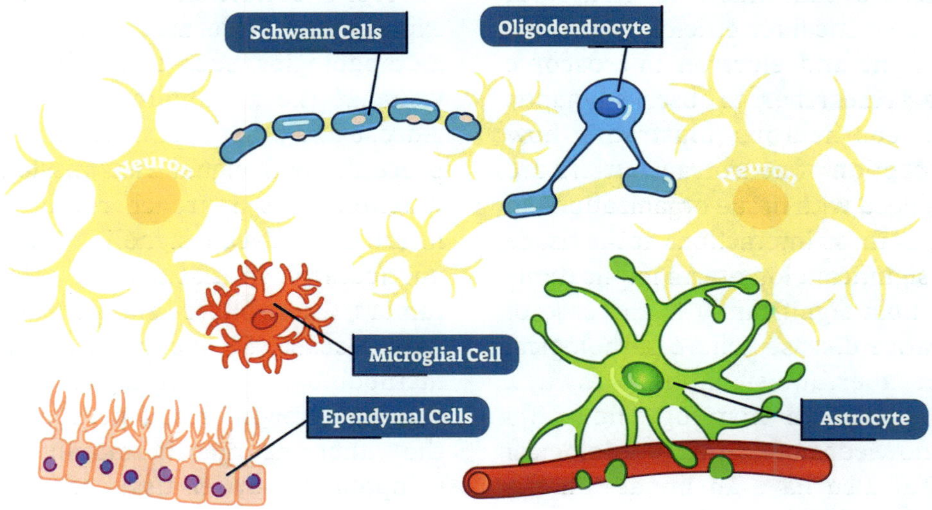

Figure 1.22. Glial cells.

Source: https://www.verywellhealth.com/what-are-glial-cells-and-what-do-they-do-4159734.

Moreover, advances in histological techniques, including intact-tissue analysis, are revealing more of the three-dimensional shape and function of glial cells in place. Traditional thin-section histology may neglect the spatial relationships that glial cells have with neuronal structures. New strategies allow volumetric tissue dynamics to be addressed, and, in doing this, a new understanding is obtained of glial cell function in complex tissue architectures (Arda et al., 2017). As research on these techniques advances, the ability to reveal novel interactions between glial cells and microenvironments rises. Not only does this enhance the knowledge of normal brain function, but also of disease mechanisms that disrupt homeostasis. A comprehensive comprehension of glial cell functions through histological examination becomes, therefore, essential to ideally treat neurological diseases and engineer targeted therapies.

1.6.3. Importance in Signal Transmission

The importance of signal transmission in human tissues is cardinal in securing physiological homeostasis. Various cell types interact through diverse pathways of signaling, such as hormonal signals, neurotransmitters, and growth factors, which each add a complex interaction network to ensure the regulation of the body's functions. Proper signal transmission guarantees that cells respond effectively to environmental stimuli and ensure internal stability. For example, interaction between immune cells and pathogens requires precise signaling to initiate proper immune responses. Without such highly coordinated interaction, tissues would be compromised, leading to disease states. The transmission of signals is a reflection not only of the necessity for cell communication but of the importance of histological studies in revealing such intricate mechanisms that underlie human health. Moreover, histological techniques have enhanced the understanding of how transmission of signals is accomplished at the microscopic level. Use of a sequence of staining processes can illustrate structural features of tissue critical for efficient signaling. For instance, light and electron microscopic techniques allow researchers to observe synaptic contact in between neurons, illustrating how release and reception of neurotransmitters are intricately packaged with tissue organization. An understanding of these interactions at the tissue level can have significant long-term implications for medicine, most significantly in the case of neurodegenerative disease, where pathological tissue involves aberrant signaling pathways. Thus, developments in histology not only improve our knowledge of normal physiological mechanisms but also have an impact on the design of therapeutic interventions to restore or mimic proper signal transmission in pathological tissues. Furthermore, recent advances in imaging science have made it possible to unmask the dynamic nature of metabolic signaling within tissues and understand the mechanisms through which cellular communication is altered under different conditions. As demonstrated in experiments performed using spectral tracing methodologies, such as STRIDE, one can now visualize the metabolic pathways utilized by glucose and other substrates and identify these processes with signal transmission and cellular function. This approach reveals the complex interplay between signaling and metabolism, particularly in tissues like the brain and tumors, where altered signaling typically occurs with disease. By inclusion of such advanced methodologies in histological studies, we can gain a better-informed perspective regarding the functions that metabolic and signaling components have in tissue health and disease, thus highlighting the crucial importance of signal transmission in the intricate mechanism of human tissues (Aagaard et al., 2018; Liu et al., 2019).

Test Your Knowledge

1. What are the main components of a neuron, and what is the function of each?
2. What are glial cells, and how do they support the nervous system?

SUMMARY

In reviewing an investigation of histology, the study of human tissues plays a critical role in both medical research and clinical practice. Histological techniques have evolved significantly, with an enhanced understanding of tissue structure and function. This evolution underscores the need for tissue engineering and regenerative medicine, emphasizing the development of artificial tissues and organs. As in the case of existing research, such as using MSCs derived from bone marrow, histological analysis can shed light on cellular and molecular features crucial to successful tissue construction. MSCs as a viable substitute source to vascular-derived cells hold promise for less invasive techniques of procurement while producing ECM as in conventional methods, underscoring potential for cutting-edge therapeutic interventions in cardiovascular medicine (Eid et al., 2017). Use to a wide variety of diagnostic and predictive environments, more specifically cardiovascular wellbeing, is demonstrated for histological concepts. Atherosclerotic plaque makeup, as explained by histological examination with the assistance of advanced imaging modalities, is a significant determinant of plaque stability and risk stratification. Both ex vivo and in vivo imaging, combined with histopathological examination, provide insightful information regarding plaque features, potentially acting as predictors of thromboembolic events. The coincidence of MRI-derived data and histological measurements emphasizes the importance of bringing together histology and contemporary imaging modalities. In addition to diagnosis, the integration may also guide targeted therapy strategy in cardiovascular medicine, towards the necessity of histological expertise in the clinic (Condon et al., 2016). Lastly, the continued emphasis on histology as a fundamental pillar in medical science guarantees ongoing advancements in understanding human disease and health. The scrupulous analysis of tissue and their intricate architecture promotes a higher level of understanding in pathological states of disease so that new forms of therapy can be designed. Since histology directs many scientific fields, from cancer to regenerative medicine, it remains a core component of biomedicine research. With increased research into tissue characteristics and their application to medical conditions, health professionals can diagnose and treat complex medical ailments more effectively, ultimately resulting in enhanced patient care and outcomes. Through this concentration of data and technological advancement, histology continues to make its invaluable contribution to medicine's future.

In histology studies, the study of human tissue gives essential information about its structure and functionality. Of prime observation is bone grafting in orthopedic procedures, particularly when graft substitutes such as recombinant human bone morphogenetic protein-2 (rhBMP-2) are used. Research indicates that rhBMP-2 can effectively enhance fusion rates in spinal reconstruction procedures compared to the use of standard autografts. In a sheep lumbar corpectomy model, studies have shown that both rhBMP-2 preparations produced a remarkable 100% fusion rate, which is significantly different from the 75% fusion in the autograft cohorts. This evidence shows the potential of rhBMP-2 to not only increase the success of grafting but also reduce the morbidity associated with autograft harvesting, making it an extremely valuable instrument for surgical use in tissue repair and regeneration (Mobasser et al., 2016). In addition to its efficacy, understanding the biological actions of rhBMP-2 on local tissue is also imperative. A critical study of the osteoclastic activity due to varied concentrations of rhBMP-2 profiles the interaction between resorption and formation of bone. The experiments revealed that an increase in the local concentration of rhBMP-2 led to temporary osteoclastic activity, initially resulting in bone resorption at the implantation site. The resorptive period, however, was followed by a healing response, with dense osteoid and new bone formation within eight weeks. Such findings point to a need to streamline rhBMP-2 application protocols to provide conducive healing environments without compromising the integrity of adjacent bones (Badura et al., 2009). Ultimately, the use of novel protein-based grafting methods, such as rhBMP-2, points to the contribution of the field of histology to the development of medical science. The innovations are not merely about making healing more accessible; they also break the conventional wisdom in tissue engineering and regeneration. The increasing evidence of the possible role of rhBMP-2 in promoting osseointegration shows a shift towards applying such biotech advances into clinical practice. This shift from grafting methodologies and the understanding of histological responses represents a new frontier in the treatment of bone disorders, thereby enhancing the outcome of patients and expanding the scope of the application of histological results (Badura et al., 2009; Mobasser et al., 2016).

KEY TERMS FROM THIS CHAPTER

- Epithelium
- Connective tissue
- Muscle tissue
- Nervous tissue
- Basement membrane
- Extracellular matrix
- Fibroblast
- Collagen fibers
- Elastic fibers
- Reticular fibers
- Stratified epithelium
- Cartilage
- Adipose tissue
- Blood
- Neuron
- Myofibril
- Sarcomere

CRITICAL THINKING QUESTIONS

1. **Which of the following is NOT a primary type of human tissue?**
   a. Epithelial
   b. Connective
   c. Muscular
   d. Skeletal
2. **What type of epithelial tissue is found lining the air sacs (alveoli) of the lungs?**
   a. Simple squamous epithelium
   b. Stratified squamous epithelium
   c. Simple columnar epithelium
   d. Transitional epithelium
3. **Which connective tissue stores energy and insulates the body?**
   a. Cartilage
   b. Bone
   c. Adipose tissue
   d. Areolar tissue
4. **Cardiac muscle tissue is characterized by:**
   a. Multinucleated fibers and voluntary movement
   b. Intercalated discs and involuntary movement
   c. Spindle-shaped cells and voluntary control
   d. Lack of striations and voluntary control
5. **Which type of tissue is responsible for transmitting electrical impulses in the body?**
   a. Epithelial
   b. Connective
   c. Muscular
   d. Nervous

Short Answer Questions

1. What are the four main types of human tissues, and what is the primary function of each?
2. What is histological analysis, and which techniques are commonly used to study human tissues?
3. How is epithelial tissue structured, and what are its main functions in the body?
4. What are the different types of connective tissue, and what roles do they play in the body?
5. Describe the three types of muscle tissue and one unique characteristic of each.
6. What are the main structural components of nervous tissue, and what is its primary function?

Answer to Critical Thinking Questions

1. (d); 2. (a); 3. (c); 4. (b); 5. (d)

REFERENCES

1. Seferovic, M., Martín, C. S., Tardif, S. D., Rutherford, J., Castro, E. C. C., Li, T., Hodara, V. L., Parodi, L. M., Giavedoni, L., Layne-Colon, D., Tamhankar, M., Yagi, S., Martyn, C., Reyes, K., Suter, M. A., Aagaard, K. M., Chiu, C. Y., & Patterson, J. L. (2018). Experimental Zika virus infection in the pregnant common marmoset induces spontaneous fetal loss and neurodevelopmental abnormalities. *Scientific Reports, 8*(1). https://doi.org/10.1038/s41598-018-25205-1
2. Aboitiz, F., Flores, O., Gil, J., Gimeno, R., et al. (2012). Anatomy of corpus callosum in prenatally malnourished rats. https://core.ac.uk/download/288912616.pdf (accessed on 14th June 2025).
3. Acosta, L., Evans, M. D., Izquierdo, F., Magnet, A., et al. (2019). Virtual libraries of tissue and clinical samples: potential role of a 3-D microscope. https://core.ac.uk/download/228195067.pdf (accessed on 14th June 2025).
4. Adamo, S. (2018). From EJTM (European Journal of Translational Myology) to EJT3M (European Journal of Translational Myology, Mobility, Medicine). https://core.ac.uk/download/158822276.pdf (accessed on 14th June 2025).
5. Adin, C. A., & Gilor, C. (2017). The diabetic dog as a translational model for human islet transplantation. https://core.ac.uk/download/323071786.pdf (accessed on 14th June 2025).
6. Aguilar Morante, D., Cabello Laureano, R., Colmenero Repiso, A., Gómez Muñoz, M., et al. (2019). CD44-high neural crest stem-like cells are associated with tumor aggressiveness and poor survival in neuroblastoma tumors. https://core.ac.uk/download/286565268.pdf (accessed on 14th June 2025).
7. Aguilera, R., Gimzewski, J. K., Rao, J., Sharma, S., et al. (2019). Piezoelectric needle sensor reveals mechanical heterogeneity in human thyroid tissue lesions. https://core.ac.uk/download/323076249.pdf (accessed on 14th June 2025).
8. Alaminos, M., Campos, A., Carriel Araya, V. S., Garzón, I., et al. (2013). Developing a practical guide for teaching histology: an evaluation of the didactic components. https://core.ac.uk/download/55734395.pdf (accessed on 14th June 2025).
9. Andre, M., Byra, M., Chang, E., Du, J., et al. (2019). Quantitative ultrasound and B-mode image texture features correlate with collagen and myelin content in human ulnar nerve fascicles. https://core.ac.uk/download/231896728.pdf (accessed on 14th June 2025).
10. Andrén, P. E., Caprioli, R. M., Castellino, S., Charkoftaki, G., et al. (2018). Yale School of Public Health Symposium on tissue imaging mass spectrometry: illuminating phenotypic heterogeneity and drug disposition at the molecular level. https://core.ac.uk/download/152438977.pdf (accessed on 14th June 2025).
11. Antal, C. E., Atkins, A. R., Becerra, C. R., Borazanci, E., et al. (2019). Targeting LIF-mediated paracrine interaction for pancreatic cancer therapy and monitoring. https://core.ac.uk/download/323062980.pdf (accessed on 14th June 2025).
12. Arda, H. E., Burns, V. M., Chakravarthy, H., Charville, G., et al. (2017). Pathways to clinical CLARITY: volumetric analysis of irregular, soft, and heterogeneous tissues in development and disease. https://core.ac.uk/download/129069108.pdf (accessed on 14th June 2025).
13. Asplund, A., Berglund, L., Björling, E., Fagerberg, L., et al. (2025). A global view of protein expression in human cells, tissues, and organs. https://core.ac.uk/download/pdf/8380022.

pdf (accessed on 14th June 2025).

14. Augustinack, J. C., Boas, D., Fischl, B., Fogarty, M., et al. (2018). Colocalization of neurons in optical coherence microscopy and Nissl-stained histology in Brodmann's area 32 and area 21. https://open.bu.edu/bitstream/2144/39279/2/nihms-1509911.pdf (accessed on 14th June 2025).

15. Badura, J., Boden, S. D., Burkus, J. K., McKay, W., et al. (2009). Short-term osteoclastic activity induced by locally high concentrations of recombinant human bone morphogenetic protein–2 in a cancellous bone environment. https://core.ac.uk/download/213087073.pdf (accessed on 14th June 2025).

16. Barbero, A., Fitzsimmons, J. S., Grogan, S. P., Mainil-Varlet, P., et al. (2006). Visual histological grading system for the evaluation of *in vitro*-generated neocartilage. https://core.ac.uk/download/18240101.pdf (accessed on 14th June 2025).

17. Basciani, S., Farcomeni, A., Franco, G., Gnessi, L., et al. (2018). Testicular histopathology, semen analysis and FSH, predictive value of sperm retrieval: supportive counseling in case of reoperation after testicular sperm extraction (TESE). https://core.ac.uk/download/188822501.pdf (accessed on 14th June 2025).

18. Baskin, L. S., Cao, M., Cunha, G. R., Ricke, W. A., et al. (2019). Reproductive tract biology: Of mice and men. https://core.ac.uk/download/323311356.pdf (accessed on 14th June 2025).

19. Bécavin, T., Keller, L., Kuchler-Bopp, S., Kökten, T., et al. (2014). Immunomodulation stimulates the innervation of engineered tooth organ. https://core.ac.uk/download/55845478.pdf (accessed on 14th June 2025).

20. Bennett, B., Dimmock, D. P., Friederich, M. W., Geurts, J., et al. (2016). Potentially diagnostic electron paramagnetic resonance spectra elucidate the underlying mechanism of mitochondrial dysfunction in the deoxyguanosine kinase deficient rat model of a genetic mitochondrial DNA depletion syndrome. https://core.ac.uk/download/213064759.pdf (accessed on 14th June 2025).

21. Bishop, J., Borowsky, A. D., Demos, S. G., Fereidouni, F., et al. (2017). Microscopy with ultraviolet surface excitation for rapid slide-free histology. https://core.ac.uk/download/323068262.pdf (accessed on 14th June 2025).

22. Bochsler, V. S., Galloway, S. B., Harley, R. A., Kramarsky-Winters, E., et al. (2007). *Coral Disease and Health Workshop: Coral Histopathology II.* https://core.ac.uk/download/11017972.pdf (accessed on 14th June 2025).

23. Boucheron, L. E., Can, A., Gurcan, M. N., Madabhushi, A., et al. (2009). Histopathological image analysis: A review. https://core.ac.uk/download/46378.pdf (accessed on 14th June 2025).

24. Bric, J. D., & Toth, J. M. (2019). An evaluation of the host response to an interspinous process device based on a series of spine explants: Device for Intervertebral Assisted Motion (DIAM®). https://core.ac.uk/download/322826130.pdf (accessed on 14th June 2025).

25. Camilleri, J., Cappello, F., Lung, C. Y. K., Rappa, F., et al. (2016). Assessment of the interaction of Portland cement-based materials with blood and tissue fluids using an animal model. https://core.ac.uk/download/323186322.pdf (accessed on 14th June 2025).

26. Carlotti, F., Chuva de Sousa Lopes, S. M., de Koning, E. J. P., de Melo Bernardo, A., et al. (2014). Lymph angiogenesis and angiogenesis during human fetal pancreas development.

https://core.ac.uk/download/55800083.pdf (accessed on 14th June 2025).

27. Chatdarong, K. (2003). *Reproductive Physiology of The Female Cat.* https://core.ac.uk/download/11694645.pdf (accessed on 14th June 2025).
28. Chen, S., Einspanier, R., & Schoen, J. (2013). Long-term culture of primary porcine oviduct epithelial cells: Validation of a comprehensive *in vitro* model for reproductive science. https://core.ac.uk/download/288114161.pdf (accessed on 14th June 2025).
29. Condon, B. C., Brierley, J. B., Santosh, C., McCabe, C., Brennan, D., Graham, D. I., Hadley, D. M., et al. (2008). Potential use of oxygen as a metabolic biosensor in combination with T2*-weighted MRI to define the ischemic penumbra. https://core.ac.uk/download/110100.pdf (accessed on 14th June 2025).
30. Condon, B., Foo, S. Y., Forbes, K. P., Holmes, M., et al. (2016). Atherosclerotic carotid plaque composition: A 3T and 7T MRI-histology correlation study. https://core.ac.uk/download/42369960.pdf (accessed on 14th June 2025).
31. Cozart, D., Hesse, D., Nichols, R., Szymik, B., et al. (2017). *UGA Anatomy and Physiology 1 Lab Manual* (3rd ed.). https://core.ac.uk/download/217306564.pdf (accessed on 14th June 2025).
32. Curry, V., Fenwick, S. A., Hackney, R., Harrall, R., et al. (2001). Expression of transforming growth factor-beta isoforms and their receptors in chronic tendinosis. https://core.ac.uk/download/2776656.pdf (accessed on 14th June 2025).
33. Darbre, P. (2019). Breast cysts and aluminum-based antiperspirant salts. https://core.ac.uk/download/286352822.pdf (accessed on 14th June 2025).
34. Eid, K., Grunenfelder, J., Hoerstrup, S. P., Kadner, A., et al. (2017). A new source for cardiovascular tissue engineering: Human bone marrow stromal cells. https://core.ac.uk/download/85215011.pdf (accessed on 14th June 2025).
35. Erturk, A., Labate, A., Seehaus, A., Silva, A. C., Khan, A. R., Jeurissen, B., Yang, B., et al. (2018). Voxel-wise comparisons of cellular microstructure and diffusion-MRI in mouse hippocampus using 3D Bridging of Optically-clear histology with Neuroimaging Data (3D-BOND). https://core.ac.uk/download/160499868.pdf (accessed on 14th June 2025).
36. Grange, S. (2011). *Current Issues and Regulations in Tendon Regeneration and Musculoskeletal Repair with Mesenchymal Stem Cells.*
37. Hedley, J., Murphy, B., Priestnall, S. L., Stapleton, D., et al. (2018). Odontoameloblastoma with extensive chondroid matrix deposition in a guinea pig. https://core.ac.uk/download/161124292.pdf (accessed on 14th June 2025).
38. Hermansson, A. (2007). Effects on the reproductive system in domestic fowl (*Gallus domestics*) after embryonic exposure to estrogenic substances. https://core.ac.uk/download/11695140.pdf (accessed on 14th June 2025).
39. Lavezzi, A., Paradiso, B., & Simonato, M. (2018). From fix to fit into the autoptic human brains. https://core.ac.uk/download/168403449.pdf (accessed on 14th June 2025).
40. Leveson-Gower, D., & Ly, D. (2025). *Bion-M2 PI 1-Pagers.* https://core.ac.uk/download/pdf/286393560.pdf (accessed on 14th June 2025).
41. Liu, Y., Miao, Y., Min, W., Qian, X., et al. (2019). Spectral tracing of deuterium for imaging glucose metabolism. https://core.ac.uk/download/323065665.pdf (accessed on 14th June 2025).

42. Matusch, A., Mencacci, A., Armitage, A. E., Brown, A. J. P., Thomson, A. M., Raab, A., Ibrahim, A. S., et al. (2013). Fungal iron availability during deep seated candidiasis is defined by a complex interplay involving systemic and local events. https://core.ac.uk/download/18601303.pdf (accessed on 14th June 2025).

43. Menzel, A., Freed, A. D., Gent, A. N., Ambrosi, D., Balzani, D., Kiousis, D. E., deBotton, G., et al. (2012). Analytical and numerical analyses of the micromechanics of soft fibrous connective tissues. http://arxiv.org/abs/1201.0421 (accessed on 14th June 2025).

44. Mobasser, J. P., Schwartz, D. G., Toth, J. M., Williams, R., et al. (2016). Instrumented lumbar corpectomy and spinal reconstruction comparing rhBMP-2/compression-resistant matrix, rhBMP-2/absorbable collagen sponge/ceramic granules mixture, and autograft in two different devices: A study in sheep. https://core.ac.uk/download/213087657.pdf (accessed on 14th June 2025).

45. Porter, A. E., Lalwani, A., Chen, C. G., Currey, J. D., Brauer, D. S., Chin, E. N., Filvaroff, E., et al. (2010). Tissue-specific calibration of extracellular matrix material properties by transforming growth factor-beta and Runx2 in bone is required for hearing. https://core.ac.uk/download/30695366.pdf (accessed on 14th June 2025).

46. Reis, C. P. da S. e S. (2011). *P2 Purinoceptors Signaling in Fibroblasts of Rat Subcutaneous Tissue*. https://core.ac.uk/download/15568458.pdf (accessed on 14th June 2025).

47. Riley, G. P. (2005). Chronic tendon pathology: Molecular basis and therapeutic implications. https://core.ac.uk/download/2776642.pdf (accessed on 14th June 2025).

THE INTEGUMENTARY SYSTEM

2

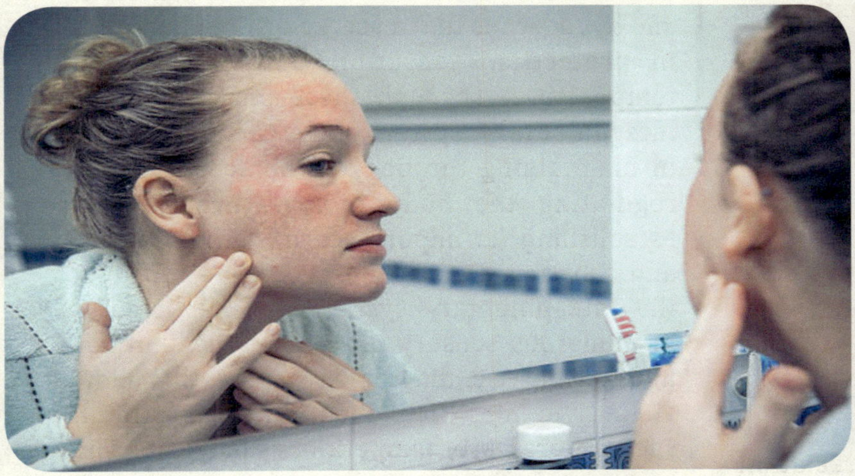

LEARNING OBJECTIVES

After studying this chapter, you will be able to:

1. Identify and explain the anatomy of the skin
2. Explain the functions of the integumentary system
3. Explain the forms of skin appendages
4. Recognize and explain common integumentary disorders
5. Explain the maintenance of homeostasis by the integumentary system

Introduction

The integumentary system, comprising the skin, hair, nails, and glands, is the body's outermost layer and thus forms the body's first line of defense against damaging environmental pressures. Protection, temperature control, and perception are among its primary functions. It is essential to understand the intricate structure and crucial functions of the integumentary system since not only does it guard underlying tissues, but it also significantly assists in body homeostasis overall. It is composed of a number of layers, the outermost of which is the epidermis, and then the dermis, which has blood vessels, nerves, and connective tissue. The complexity of the integumentary system highlights its significance in various body processes, and interference with this system leads to harmful health complications; thus, the necessity for thorough research on its characteristics and functions in medicine and health sciences (Stewart et al., 2016; Fambrough et al., 2018). For better comprehension of the integumentary system, the discussion of its development and its evolutionary significance is vital.

The system is believed to have evolved as a mechanism of defense, allowing organisms to survive in varied environmental conditions. In humans, skin has evolved to cope with climate change and UV exposure, and its lovely diversity in thickness and pigmentation. Moreover, the integumentary system's ability to heal and regenerate proves its complex cellular mechanisms. Appreciation of these adaptations not only offers a window into human biology but also creates an entry point for medical research to target conditions like skin cancer and other dermatological diseases. This evolutionary insight emphasizes the significance of the integumentary system as a crucial force in the survival and adaptation of organisms, building a critical link between environmental influences and biological development (Stewart et al., 2016; Fambrough et al., 2018).

Educational models centered around the integumentary system offer excellent learning opportunities for active learning by the students. Instruction of the system based on real-life applications ensures a deeper appreciation of the functions and importance of the integumentary system in health. Demonstrating how the integumentary system interacts with other systems within the body enhances understanding by the students and encourages teamwork, which is a vital aspect of STEM education. Adopting problem-based learning enables students to transfer theoretical concepts to real-life situations and hence consolidate their learning process. Since the integumentary system is an essential component of human health and disease, the use of such educational methods becomes imperative in the education of future healthcare providers. Engaging students in discovery learning not only imparts skills but also instills a lifetime passion for scientific inquiry and better appreciation of the issues surrounding human biology (Stewart et al., 2016; Fambrough et al., 2018).

Definition of the Integumentary System

The integumentary system is one of the most vital and ubiquitous organ systems in the human body, primarily to defend the inner parts from external injury. It consists of the skin, hair, nails, and certain glands, ultimately creating a protective layer between the inner world of the body and the external world. The biggest organ, the skin, is composed of numerous layers like the epidermis, dermis, and hypodermis that all serve distinct purposes in protection, sensation, and maintaining temperature. Through these structures, the integumentary system plays a crucial role in maintaining the body in homeostasis and regulating the body temperature, further establishing its importance in general health and function. Beyond its protective function, the integumentary system also participates in numerous sensory processes. The skin has multiple nerve endings and receptors that allow an individual to feel environmental stimuli such as pressure, temperature, and pain. The body requires sensory feedback to respond to threatening stimuli and engage appropriately with its environment (Figure 2.1).

Further, the integumentary system also facilitates such vital processes as vitamin D synthesis, which is responsible for bone growth and metabolic functions. Due to its protective and sensory features, the integumentary system indicates its significance in ensuring body integrity and its enhancement of overall health. In addition, the integumentary system is an active, not a passive, barrier; it is dynamic and subject to several physiological changes during an individual's lifetime. Age, environmental exposure, and overall health can modify the function and structure of this system. For example, as people age, their skin becomes less elastic and drier, which results in wrinkles and other telltale symptoms of aging. Furthermore, a deeper comprehension of the role and application of the integumentary systems in daily life is made possible by educational approaches that focus on the practical applications of biological principles, especially through the study of bodily systems (Stewart et al., 2016). By facilitating a collaborative learning experience that creates a discovery environment, students can optimize learning on how the integumentary system interacts with other body systems and enhance interest in the sciences (Stewart et al., 2016).

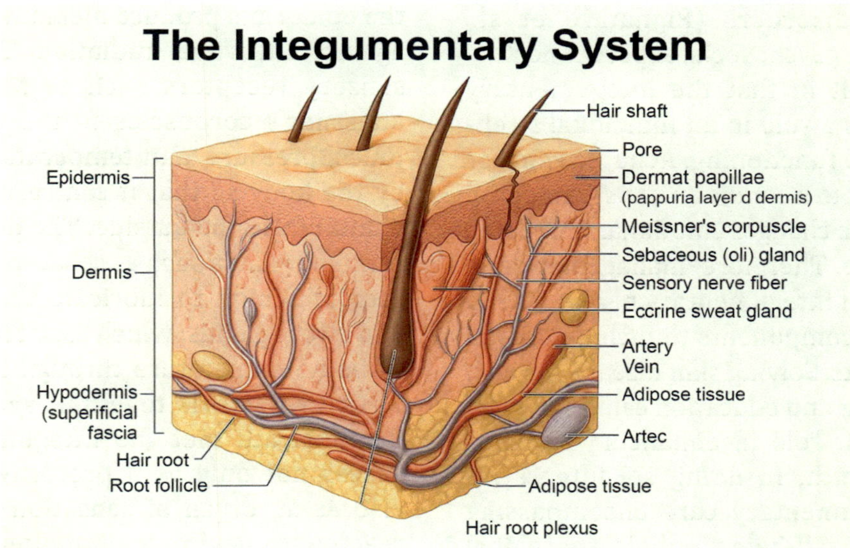

Figure 2.1. Integumentary system.

Source: https://blogger.googleusercontent.com/img/b/R29vZ2xl/AVvXsEgZorI-q9_X2uV5u3hcb7MCZ8cUJgl-BfkO2Bi7tQ7GmiQva5rvjpWga6zlC5GAreOJ8fWygaCTw4tUYUcrHc8yeZYSOIXOUVLVuTgMSRKPUYwEwavVPjBOLd6PSElLDHMjhAbG_lzKZwKKhiY3jE5tzMUznGcDXs5dUkvFbeq-DPAoIZwF5gCx-sahC2U/s16000-rw/Basics-of-the-integumentary%20system.webp.

Importance of the Integumentary System in Human Health

The integumentary system, including the skin, hair, nails, and its accompanying glands, is the body's first line of defense against the environment and thus highlights its essential function in human health. It covers internal organs to prevent them from being attacked by pathogens and physical damage, and acts as a shield to noxious substances. The structural integrity of the skin is paramount; any breakdown will result in infections and systemic problems. For instance, the lack of adequate pressure injury prevention education in healthcare settings highlights the need for solid knowledge of the integumentary system for caregivers. According to recent studies, patient care mistakes concerning integumentary assessment can lead to increased hospital-acquired pressure injury rates, illustrating that understanding this system can prove to be the difference in terms of patient outcomes and safety within healthcare settings (Pomerleau et al., 2021). Moreover, the integumentary system plays an important role in regulating body temperature and homeostasis. The skin keeps the body temperature within normal range by sweating and adjusting blood flow, thereby preventing heat accumulation when exercising or exposed to hot temperatures. Moreover, it plays a role in vitamin D production, which helps in calcium absorption and bone health. The relationship between skin health and overall physiological processes cannot be overstressed, as derangement of the integumentary system can lead to systemic complications. Evidence indicates that specific interventions that optimize integumentary health, such as maintaining skin integrity and strengthening barrier functions, are required to optimize overall health outcomes and prevent dermatological disorders (Pignataro et al., 2013). Finally, the psychosocial aspect of healthy skin is significant in that the integumentary system also plays a role in an individual's self-esteem and social functioning. Acne, eczema, or psoriasis can lead to a condition of psychological disturbance, which changes emotional well-being and quality of life. Therefore, management and comprehension of integumentary health extend beyond physical components to include mental health components. Solving skin disease through medical treatment and education campaigns can have a significant role in enhancing patients' psychosocial health. In doing so, integrative models of integumentary care encompassing body and mind well-being uphold the global importance of this system to human health and advocate for a multi-faceted approach to wellness and health promotion policy.

Overview of the Components of the Integumentary System

The integumentary system is a protective barrier composed primarily of the skin, hair, nails, and related glands. Organizationally, at a general level, the skin is arranged in three layers: the epidermis, dermis, and hypodermis. The outer, the epidermis, consists of keratinized stratified squamous epithelium that is protective of inner structures from environmental forces, as well as offers the mechanism for water loss prevention. This layer is beneath the hypodermis. Beneath this level is the dermis, a more substantial, highly connective tissue-rich layer providing structural support and flexibility. The hypodermis or subcutaneous layer holds the skin in place against deeper tissue and serves as a site of fat storage, insulating and energizing. This triad organization allows the integumentary system to function in ways significant to homeostasis and overall health, including protection, sensation, and thermoregulation. Apart from its structural components, the integumentary system also has varied special cells and structures that facilitate its function. For instance, melanocytes found in the epidermis produce melanin, which protects against ultraviolet radiation. The presence of sensory receptors such as Merkel cells and Meissner's corpuscles in the dermis enables touch, pressure, and temperature to be sensed by the body so that it can respond suitably to stimuli from the outside. The dermal layer also contains glands such as sebaceous glands, which secrete sebum to lubricate the skin and hair, and sweat glands, which assist in the regulation of body temperature through sweating. These structures work together synergistically to demonstrate that the integumentary system serves not only as a protective covering but also as an organ of sensation and regulation, reacting to environmental alterations. Further, the integumentary system is responsible for numerous basic physiological processes of the body, including wound healing and immunity. Upon injury, the skin responds with a multi-stage process of repair that includes clotting, inflammation, and regeneration of tissue. The keratinocytes also play a key role in this healing process, migrating into the injured area to re-establish the skin layer and close the wound. The integumentary system also creates a home for immune cells, such as the Langerhans cells. These antigen-presenting cells assist the immune system in recognizing and reacting to pathogens more efficiently. This immunological function further emphasizes the primary role of the integumentary system to overall body health. The varied functions controlled by this system highlight its worth as something greater than bare physical defense, preserving body integrity through a constant dynamic interrelationship of form, sensory perception, and the processes of healing.

2.1. Structure of the Skin

Learning Outcome

1. Discuss the epidermis: layers and functions
2. Explain the dermis: composition and role
3. Define hypodermis: significance and characteristics

The structure of the skin is very organized and plays a critical role in general health as an integral part of the integumentary system. Comprising three broad layers—epidermis, dermis, and subcutis—the skin performs several functions like protection, sensation, and thermoregulation. The epidermis, the outermost layer, comprises mainly keratinocytes that provide a powerful barrier against the external world. Beneath the epidermis is the dermis, a connective tissue layer abundant with collagen and elastin fibers that give the skin strength and elasticity. The subcutis or hypodermis is primarily composed of fat tissue and is responsible for insulating the body and for shock absorption. Together, these layers create a , complex structure that not only shields internal organs but also accommodates shifts in the body's surroundings, highlighting the skin's crucial role in survival. Beyond its protective structure, the skin harbors a dense microbial community known as the skin microbiome. This microbial community plays a critical role in health by modulating immune responses and protecting against pathogenic microbes. The majority of microbes exist in a mutualistic relationship with the human body; they are needed for normal body functions as well as homeostasis, particularly against external insults (Gillen et al., 2014). The skin microbiome reflects the complexity of the skin beyond the physical layers of skin and plays a vital role in the integrity of integumentary systems. It is a balance of these microbial communities that is necessary, for an imbalance will lead to infection and disease of the skin, hence emphasizing the importance of both anatomical and biological aspects of skin structure. Moreover, skin structure is not only a barrier but also an adaptive organ with evolutionary significance. Fossilized skin structures, as revealed through research, show that the integumentary modifications of contemporary species have their origins in their ancestors, which paint a picture of centuries of evolutionary changes (Benton et al., 2018). This inheritance provides insight into how different species, including birds and reptiles, have evolved advanced skin adaptations to ensure their survival. For instance, the existence of feathered epidermis in non-avian dinosaurs shows complex integumentary evolutions that were paramount for thermoregulation and protection from environmental stress. Thus, the study of the skin structure along evolutionary time lines informs us on the multifunctionality of this basic organ and how it integrates into the general scheme of the integumentary system.

2.1.1. Epidermis: Layers and Functions

The epidermal layer, the outermost layer of the skin, is a critical barrier between the external environment and the internal body. It consists primarily of keratinocytes and is crucial in protecting against physical, chemical, and microbial assaults. This layer is subdivided into several sub-layers, including the stratum corneum, stratum granulosum, stratum spinosum, and stratum Basale, each of which is specialized in its functions. The stratum corneum of flattened dead keratinocytes constitutes the primary first line of defense. In addition, the epidermis also includes melanocytes, which produce melanin, protecting against ultraviolet radiation. The diversity and complexity in the epidermis are critical to maintaining homeostasis, preventing loss of water, and modulating immune responses, impacting health and wellness overall, as evidenced by its relationship with the skin microbiome (Gillen et al., 2014) (Figure 2.2).

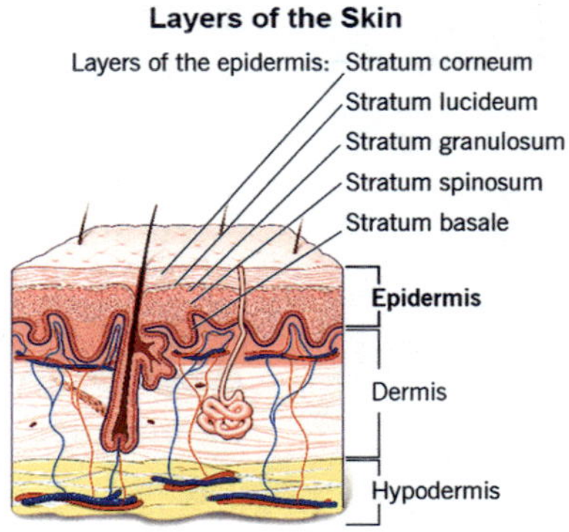

Figure 2.2. The epidermis is the top layer of your skin.

Source: https://my.clevelandclinic.org/-/scassets/images/org/health/articles/21901-epidermis.

The epidermis has a role beyond mere physical defense because it is also significant in biochemical activities crucial to skin health. In its layers, the epidermis contains cells that can sense external change and provide for sensory perception. The inclusion of Merkel cells, for instance, heightens the skin's sense of touch, pressure, and temperature. In addition, the epidermis is responsible for the production of critical vitamins, such as vitamin D, through the interaction of UV light with skin molecules.

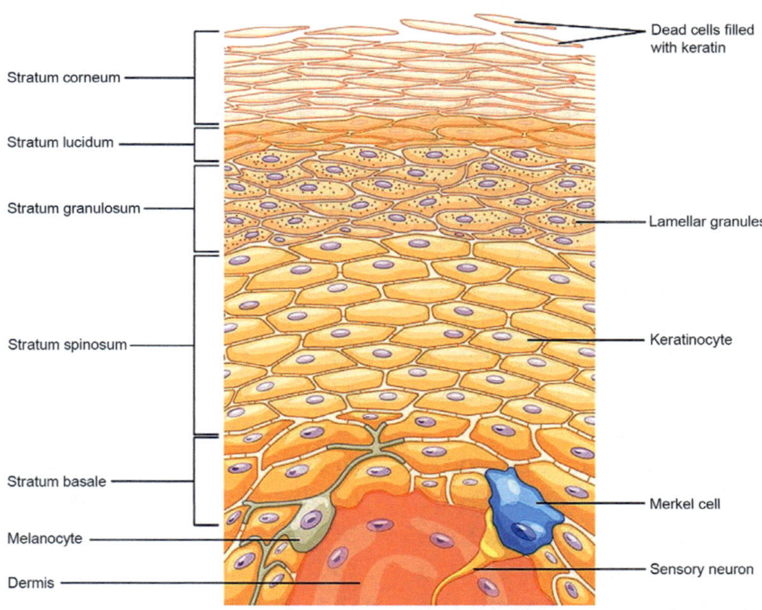

Figure 2.3. The layers of the epidermis are formed by keratinocytes at different levels of maturation.

Source: https://teachmeanatomy.info/wp-content/uploads/Layers-of-the-Epidermis-Skin-Ultrastructure.jpg.

The production of these vitamins is crucial in numerous body functions, such as calcium metabolism and immune function regulation. The interaction of the functions demonstrates the epidermis' key role in both sensory and metabolic processes and illustrates its significance beyond structure alone in the integumentary system. The connection of the epidermis with the body's microbiome further emphasizes its multifunctional role in health. The epidermal microbiome, a group of microorganisms that live on the skin surface, plays a symbiotic role in maintaining the immune response as well as defending the body against pathogenic infection. The epidermis, through this balance, not only defends against potential disease but also allows for beneficial microbial interaction to promote healthy skin. Studies indicate that this association can reveal new therapeutic modalities, such as probiotics, to leverage the skin microbiome for increased benefit to health (Gillen et al., 2014). The epidermis, therefore, is more than a defensive shield; it is an active participant in a networked web of functions essential to the maintenance of total health and resistance to environmental variation, as witnessed by its evolutionary advancements and intercommunications with other systems (Figure 2.3).

2.1.2. Dermis: Composition and Role

The dermis is a fundamental framework of the integumentary system and consists primarily of connective tissues that provide structural support and elasticity to the skin. It is found beneath the epidermis and is typically divided into two layers: the papillary dermis and the reticular dermis. The papillary layer comprises loose connective tissue that has a network of blood vessels, lymphatics, and nerve endings responsible for sensation and the uptake of nutrients. Conversely, the reticular layer, made up of dense, irregular connective tissue, contains bigger blood vessels, wider collagen fibers, and elastin that give the skin elasticity and reinforce it. The complex makeup enables the dermis to withstand mechanical stress, as the skin maintains its integrity as a barrier against environmental stresses and pathogens. The dermis does more than only provide structural support; it also carries out essential physiological tasks that preserve general health (Figure 2.4).

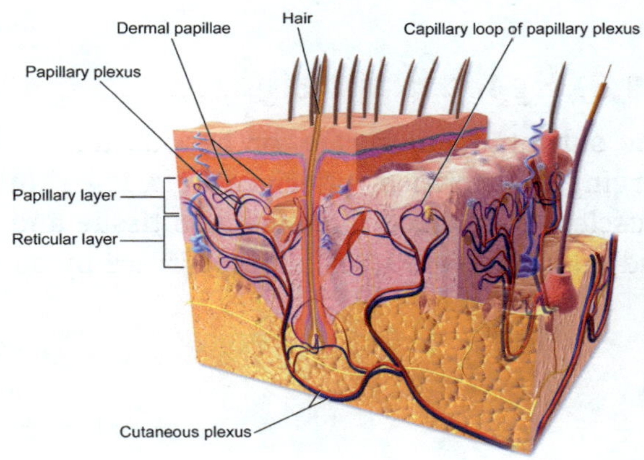

Figure 2.4. Illustration of dermal circulation and layers.

Source: https://en.wikipedia.org/wiki/Dermis#/media/File:Blausen_0802_Skin_DermalCirculation.png.

Of particular interest here is the role played by the dermis in thermoregulation, where blood vessels exhibit vasodilation or vasoconstriction to allow for temperature changes so that heat would be dispersed accordingly. In addition, the dermis contains a complex array of sensory receptors that perceive stimuli from the external environment, including touch, pain, and temperature, thus contributing to the response mechanisms of the body. The presence of a richly developed lymphatic network in the dermis also plays its role in defense through the immune system, effectively screening out pathogens and maintaining fluid balance. As a whole with the epidermis, the dermis contributes to the total hardness of the skin, demonstrating not just its structural importance but also its significant role in homeostasis and hemostasis. The focal point of dermal function and integrity is the dynamic skin microbiome, which consists of diverse microorganisms that reside on and within the skin. These resident microbes form a symbiotic relationship with the host, inhibiting pathogenic infection and regulating immune response. A well-balanced skin microbiota is essential to maintain the integrity of the skin because dysbiosis can trigger a variety of skin diseases, such as eczema and acne. The interrelation between the dermal constitution and the skin microbiome articulates the complexity of the integumentary system, as they both have a dynamic interaction in which they determine the effects of health. Understanding the structure and function of the dermis, particularly concerning microbiome and immune system, leads to new therapeutic approaches that foster healthy skin and minimize disease (Gillen et al., 2014; Kirby et al., 2020).

2.1.3. Hypodermis: Significance and Characteristics

The subcutaneous tissue, or hypodermis, is a crucial component of the integumentary system, serving as a critical interface between skin and the body's deeper tissues such as bones and muscles. Comprised of connective tissue and adipose tissue, the hypodermis serves as insulation and maintains the body's temperature by conserving heat.

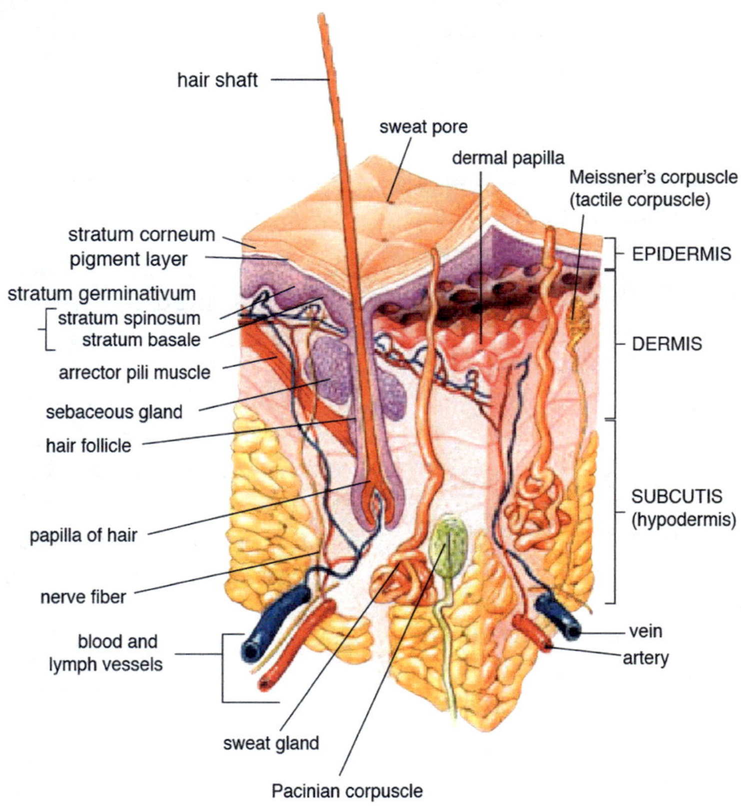

Figure 2.5. The hypodermis is the lower layer of skin.

Source: https://en.wikipedia.org/wiki/Subcutaneous_tissue#/media/File:Skin.png.

This layer also acts as a buffer, protecting the more vulnerable tissues underneath it from mechanical damage. The presence of the larger blood vessels and nerves within the hypodermis further enables communication and supply between the skin and other organ systems, highlighting its basic function in the overall health and functioning of the skin. Therefore, an understanding of the hypodermis is not only essential to comprehending the anatomy of the integumentary system but also for knowing its broader physiological importance (Pádua et al., 2019) (Figure 2.5).

Interestingly, the hypodermis facilitates energy storage that is crucial for maintaining cellular metabolism and fuel during times of energy deficiency. The hypodermal fat serves as a reservoir for lipids that may be mobilized when the body needs energy, particularly during extended fasting or vigorous exercise. Furthermore, the distribution of adipose tissue in the hypodermis is distinct in each individual and is influenced by genetic, hormonal, and environmental factors. The variation can affect the shape and structure of the body and also determine the susceptibility to diseases like obesity and metabolic syndrome. The hypodermis, therefore, performs a multi-dimensional role not only in structural support and protection but also in energy homeostasis and regulation of temperature. Appreciation of these aspects underscores the need for a healthy hypodermis as a component of overall integumentary health (Wilk-Blaszczak et al., 2018). Additionally, the hypodermis plays a role in the sensation and immune response of the skin, helping the body's first line of defense against pathogenic influences. It contains specialized nerve endings that are crucial for sensing pain, temperature, and pressure, enabling the skin to react to external stimuli. It is particularly significant because it allows for immediate reflexive reactions to harmful or threatening stimuli, which may lead to general safety. Furthermore, the hypodermis contains immune cells such as macrophages and adipocytes that are involved in the local immune system and wound healing. By providing structural support, energy storage, sensation, and immune function, the hypodermis significantly enhances the overall function and resilience of the integumentary system as a whole, demonstrating its significance in maintaining both skin health and total physiological homeostasis (Pádua et al., 2019).

Test Your Knowledge

1. What are the main layers of the epidermis, and what function does each layer serve?
2. What components make up the dermis, and how does it support the skin's structure and function?

2.2. Functions of the Integumentary System

Learning Outcome

1. Define protection against environmental hazards
2. Discuss regulation of body temperature
3. Explain the sensory perception and communication

The integumentary system, such as the skin, hair, nails, and glands associated with them, performs a variety of critical functions necessary to health and well-being. One of the basic functions of the skin is that it acts as a covering against the outside world. It keeps out pathogens, toxins, and physical abrasion, thereby safeguarding the internal tissues and organs. The skin's organization with a layered composition by the epidermis, dermis, and hypodermis facilitates protection. The skin also hosts a rich diversity of microbes constituting the skin microbiome that is crucial in maintaining the immune system as well as homeostasis within the body, so even beyond offering a covering for the human body, there is importance attached to the organ (Gillen et al., 2014). Another essential role of the integumentary system is temperature regulation, which is mostly achieved by processes like vasodilation and sweating. Skin contains an enormous network of blood vessels and sweat glands that work together to maintain thermal balance. In a rise in body temperature, skin blood vessels dilate, thereby providing greater blood flow to the surface and promoting loss of heat through radiation and evaporation. On the other hand, during low temperatures, vasoconstriction takes place, minimizing blood supply to maintain body heat. This dynamic regulatory process ensures that functions in the body are carried out optimally in varying environmental conditions. In addition, the integumentary system works in association with other systems, like the circulatory and nervous systems, to adequately react at different temperatures, indicating its pivotal contribution to homeostasis beyond mere insulation (Anglani et al., 2010). The integumentary system also performs the role of sensory perception and has a vital role to play in terms of interaction with the surroundings. The skin has a range of sensory receptors embedded within it that can sense touch, pressure, temperature, and pain. The receptors send signals to the nervous system that allow the body to respond appropriately to external conditions. This sensory feedback is essential in protective reflexes, such as removing a hand from a burn. In addition, production of vitamin D by the skin in response to sunlight emphasizes the function of metabolism, specifically in calcium and phosphate homeostasis. These varied functions of the integumentary system collectively illustrate its complexity as well as its essential contribution to human survival and health (Figure 2.6).

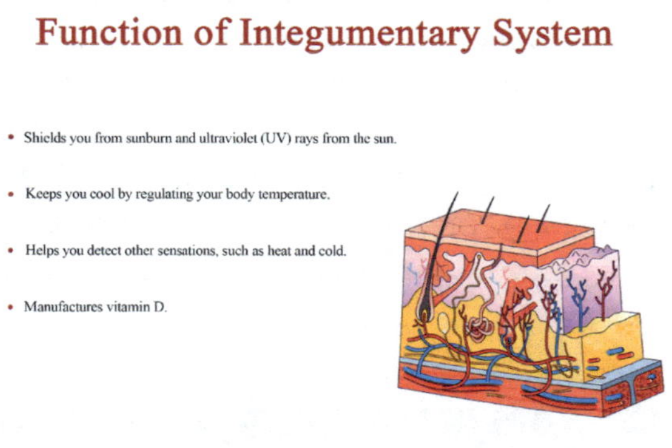

Figure 2.6. Integumentary system functions.

Source: https://www.lybrate.com/topic/integumentary-system-image.

2.2.1. Protection Against Environmental Hazards

The integumentary system is a protective defense system that maintains the body's security from a host of environmental hazards like ultraviolet rays, disease-causing agents, and physical injury. Comprising the skin, hair, nails, and accessory glands, the integumentary system is not just a physical barrier of protection but also plays a crucial role in immunity. The stratum corneum, the outer layer of the body, is the body's first line of defense and prevents harmful microorganisms from entering the body. On top of that, the skin itself also secretes essential chemicals, such as vitamin D, through exposure to sunlight, which is vital for health. This dual purpose illustrates the fundamental role played by the integumentary system in gaining homeostasis while also protecting against the environment, and its value in overall well-being. Additionally, the intricate dynamics of integumentary systems allow it to react and adapt to various types of environmental stimuli. For instance, when exposed to dangerous UV radiation, melanin creation in the skin increases, providing a darkened shield that protects against damaging radiation and minimizes cellular injury. Here, strategic responses like increased keratinization enhance the skin's resistance to mechanical abrasions and chemical irritants. Such a response is critical in workplaces where dangers are imminent. Notably, current studies reveal that understanding how previous perceptions of practices of care have been understood, for example, through models in which social and environmental settings are considered, provides us with a better understanding of how protective responses may vary (Sparozic et al., 2020). This adaptation and responsivity blend reflects the integumentary system's underlying role of delivering survivability across a broad spectrum of environments. Advances in biomedical technology also reflect the new reality of protection protocols associated with the integumentary system. Emerging designs, such as the hybrid epidermal enhancement (HEE) space suit, reflect how contemporary solutions seek to replicate the integument's protective capabilities while delivering optimum human performance under hostile conditions. The HEE suit integrates human physiology and anthropometrics to offer greater mobility and temperature management in environments that are very dangerous to the integument (Jessup et al., 2015). In imitating the natural processes of the skin, such technologies not only protect astronauts from cosmic radiation and temperature variations but also encourage further research into what the integumentary system can contribute to protective technology in general. This convergence of technology and biology represents a fundamental leap in our knowledge of defense against environmental risks.

2.2.2. Regulation of Body Temperature

Body temperature regulation is a fundamental process of the integumentary system that is crucial to homeostasis and the integrity of physiological stability in the context of external environmental changes. The skin is not only a protective covering but a significant zone for thermoregulation through a variety of physiological processes. For instance, the epidermal layer has numerous sweat glands that, in response to thermal stress, secrete sweat to cool the body through evaporative cooling. Furthermore, the blood vessels of the dermis can dilate or constrict due to temperature changes to lose or retain heat, respectively. This delicate process of thermoregulation preserves enzymatic activity and metabolic processes, allowing the body to thrive under varying environments and conditions, thereby demonstrating the importance of the integumentary system in sustaining life and maintaining the proper functioning of other body systems. The skin microbiome is essential for controlling body temperature in addition to sweating and vascular modulation. The skin's resident community of diverse microorganisms contributes to skin barrier integrity, which is vital for avoiding moisture loss and excessive heat loss. Resident skin bacteria in the complex ecosystem can also influence local immune responses and contribute to inflammation processes that can impact thermoregulation. Evidence has indicated that the healthy microbiome of the skin not only protects against pathogens but also assists in regulating skin temperature through metabolic processes, producing heat or synthesizing products that modulate thermoregulatory responses. Such a symbiotic relationship between the integumentary system and the skin microbiome thus underscores the intricacy of temperature regulation as an essential aspect of general health (Gillen et al., 2014). Moreover, integumentary system regulatory mechanisms extend beyond mere physiological processes to incorporate evolutionary adjustments that have had an impact on the regulation of temperature in vertebrates. Some of these include variations in integumentary structures such as fur in mammals, feathers in birds, and scales in reptiles. These have particular thermal functions, enhancing an organism's adaptations to its environment. The latest scientific studies suggest that the development of gene regulatory networks (GRNs) of these structures has been evolutionarily conserved and reflects an ancient common origin across the vertebrate lineage. The homology establishes the importance of integumentary structures not just for thermoregulation but also as evolutionary gadgets that have enabled vertebrates to occupy various environments and thermal regimes (Cooper et al., 2017). Each component of the integumentary system, therefore, contributes to an integrated system of body temperature regulation.

2.2.3. Sensory Perception and Communication

The integumentary system plays a significant role in sensory perception, and it is crucial in the scenario of interacting with the external world as well as in communication. Skin carries numerous sensory receptors that trigger a response to various stimuli like touch, temperature, pain, and pressure. The vast network of nerve endings enables individuals to successfully translate and react to their body sensations, thereby enhancing their awareness of the environment.

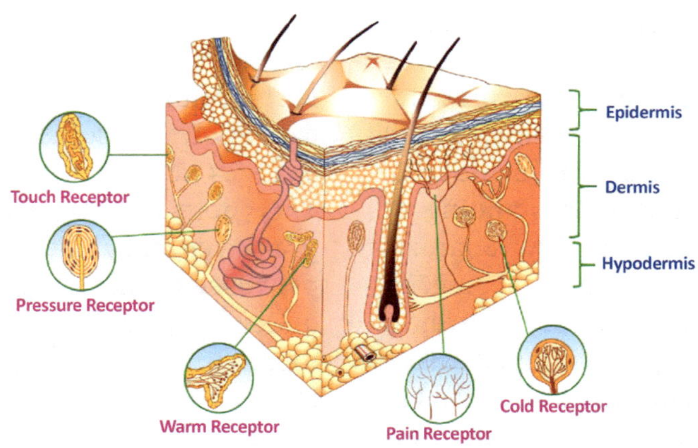

Figure 2.7. Schematic of the skin anatomy with cutaneous sensory receptors.

Source: https://www.researchgate.net/figure/Schematic-of-the-skin-anatomy-with-cutaneous-sensory-receptors_fig4_349459034.

For example, skin receptors feed back information regarding threats that might be dangerous, i.e., heat or pointy objects, leading eventually to appropriate behavior. Moreover, the ability to perceive these sensations allows for non-verbal communication since humans use tactile feedback and messages to convey feelings and intentions. Thus, the sensory roles of the integumentary system significantly contribute to both individual survival and communication between individuals. The sensory functions of the integumentary system also influence effective communication by words and deeds. The largest organ, skin, serves not just as a protective covering but as a conduit for the expression of emotions through changes in physiology. Flushing or pallor can be an indication of emotional reactions such as embarrassment or fear. In addition, the tactile properties of skin support relational dynamics when individuals touch one another because touch can convey comfort, empathy, or closeness. In this sense, sensory experience through the skin is key to understanding and reacting to social cues, particularly in establishing meaningful relationships among individuals. Furthermore, the integumental display of pigments, as in the case of some animal pigmentation, can also serve as a visual signal in mate choice and status, reflecting the multifaceted role of sensory perception in communication and behavior (Camarero et al., 2016) (Figure 2.7).

Skin integrity should be preserved not only for protective functions but also for the sensory input which is the foundation for communication. Pressure ulcers, for instance, are of concern in critical care settings because they violate the protective barrier and sensory function of the skin. Intact skin preserves rich sensory experience vital for effective communication; damage can impair these processes. As evidenced by research on critical care environments, implementing prevention will markedly reduce the occurrence of pressure ulcers and consequently preserve the physiological and communicative aspects of the integumentary system (Schindler et al., 2010). Hence, an understanding of the dependence of sensory awareness, communication, and skin integrity upon each other is an essential part of healthcare professionals' and other associated professionals ' work as it highlights the importance of maintaining skin integrity as a foundation of general health and interaction.

Test Your Knowledge

1. In what ways does the integumentary system help regulate body temperature?
2. How does the skin contribute to sensory perception and communication with the external environment?

2.3. Skin Appendages

Learning Outcome

1. Discuss hair: types and functions
2. Understand the nails: structure and purpose
3. Define glands: sweat and sebaceous glands

Skin appendages, made up of hair follicles, sebaceous glands, sweat glands, and nails, play a significant role in providing overall health and functioning. Hair follicles also serve as protective structures, but also as significant members for thermoregulatory and sensory purposes. Each hair follicle goes through growth, rest, and shedding cycles, which are influenced by hormonal and environmental considerations. The sebaceous glands of these follicles secrete sebum, an oily secretion that hydrates the skin and hair, preventing excessive dryness and inhibiting microorganism growth. This cooperation between skin appendages further enhances the barrier function of the skin, guarding against external threats while fostering overall integumentary homeostasis, which is vital to the coherence and resistance of the body (Abe et al., 2021). Sweat glands, being of an eccrine and apocrine type, contribute to the skin's protective functions. The eccrine glands are distributed throughout the body and are primarily responsible for thermoregulation through sweating. The process of cooling helps maintain the internal temperature constant during exercise or exposure to heat. On the other hand, apocrine glands are found only in specific areas, such as the armpits and groin, and secrete a thicker secretion that can function as an environment for bacterial proliferation and hence body odor. Dietary influences and hormonal changes control the activity of these glands. Dysregulation of the skin appendages can potentially lead to hyperhidrosis or bromhidrosis, which proves their importance in health and disease (Pessemier et al., 2021). Nails, usually overshadowed, are also essential skin appendages with protective as well as functional roles. Composed mainly of keratin, nails envelop the distal phalanges and enhance the sensitivity to perform precise tasks, such as grasping or manipulating objects. The structure of the nails also helps in sensory perception of the fingers and aids in generating a tactile response that is essential for everyday interaction with the world. Further, the health of the nails can reveal intrinsic health conditions; changes in color, texture, or rate can signal systemic disorders. Proper assessment of skin appendages and intricate functions, thus, warrants their significance in the integumentary system, affecting physical as well as aesthetic aspects of human health and wellness (Abe et al., 2021).

2.3.1. Hair: Types and Functions

Hair, a prototypical feature of the integumentary system, is multifunctional and crucial for physiological and social interaction in numerous vertebrates. Hair exists in many different forms—human hair, animal fur, functional structures like quills or feathers—reflecting the diverse evolutionary past of this epithelial appendage. Hair primarily comprises a protein molecule called keratin, which provides hair with its structural strength and durability. Hair may also be present to serve as an insulator, enhancing thermoregulation by serving to trap air close to the skin. Additionally, hair is a sensory organ; the follicle has nerve endings that enable the sense of touch and external stimuli to be registered, thereby allowing the animals reaction with its surroundings. Hair growth is based on genetic and molecular processes that have been formed through millions of years (Figure 2.8).

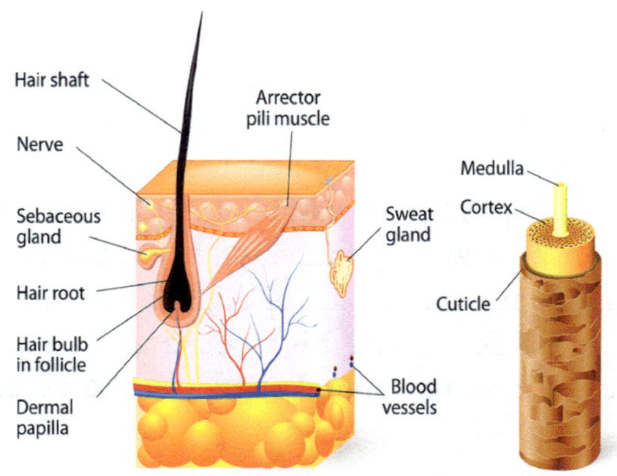

Figure 2.8. Hair anatomy.

Source: https://nurseslabs.com/wp-content/uploads/2017/06/Hair-Anatomy-Integumentary-System-Anatomy-and-Physiology-for-Nurses.png.

Present research has revealed a conserved pathway of hair follicle development across various vertebrates, with the critical significance of specific signal proteins like fibroblast growth factors (FGFs) and sonic hedgehog (shh) in triggering hair placode. These signaling mechanisms are essential as they regulate the thickness, density, and functional adaptations of the hair and are a representation of an organism's environment and lifestyle. In addition to producing heat and sensory stimulation, hair is also implicated in camouflage and communication. For instance, various species utilize color variation in their hair as danger or mate signals, demonstrating the power of structural properties of hair on the social life and reproduction of many species, including human beings. Functions and structures of hair also extend to specialized forms that attest to the diversity of the integumentary system. For example, vibrissae, or whiskers, are special hairs in most mammals with an increased sensory function, particularly in nocturnal and burrowing mammals. Similar to this, certain creatures have hair-based defense adaptations, such as the stiff quills of porcupines or the spines of some marine species that contain venom. The evolutionary significance of hair textures shows an in-depth biological legacy, as established through studies that looked into molecular mechanisms of hair development in species, bridging structural variability and functional adaptation through conserved genetic processes (Cooper et al., 2017; Adissu et al., 2019). Thus, hair not only reflects the integumentary system's sophistication but also its role within the general ecological adaptation and survival model.

2.3.2. Nails: Structure and Purpose

The nail structure is a protective and functional component of the integumentary system. The nail is predominantly composed of keratin, the fibrous protein of the skin and hair, and is made up of numerous elements. The exposed nail plate is upheld by the nail bed, which is filled with plenty of blood vessels and nerves. Beneath the nail plate lies the nail matrix, in which new nail cells are formed and which supports nail growth and regeneration. Such a unique arrangement not only safeguards the distal phalanx of fingers and toes from damage but also allows for sensory perception, which enhances tactile functions. As such, nails are functional extensions of the skin, illustrating the complexity of the integumentary system and underscoring its role in overall human well-being and health (Figure 2.9).

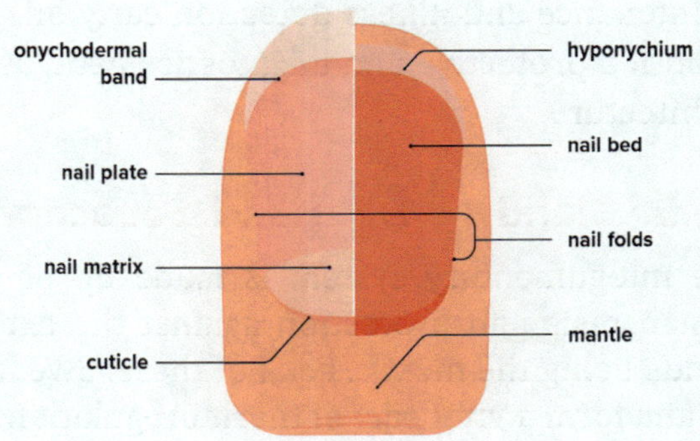

Figure 2.9. Structure of nails.

Source: https://media.post.rvohealth.io/wp-content/uploads/sites/3/2024/11/3598932-nail-anatomy-1024x736.png.

Apart from their structural role, nails play other roles that are supplementary to human functionality and well-being. Their most notable role is that of protection, whereby they protect the underlying tissue from physical injury and infection. The hardness of the nail's surface provides a protective shield from pathogens since it is an integral part of the body's defense system. Additionally, nails facilitate dexterous movements through stabilizing the fingertips, which are crucial for gripping objects and performing delicate tasks. Nails also contribute to personal hygiene and social interaction through expressing personal style and self-cleaning. Thus, nails are not merely a functional part of the integumentary system but also interactive machines with a capacity for influencing numerous aspects of a person's daily life and social being. Furthermore, nail health may also be a reflection of an individual's overall health, reflecting systemic illness not immediately apparent. Changes in coloration, texture, or growth in the nails may be indicative of many different health issues, from nutritional deficits to generalized illness. Color changes, for example, can be a sign of a lack of oxygen in the blood or liver dysfunction, while brittle nails may be a prelude to thyroid disorders or malnutrition. Therefore, monitoring nail health is a pivotal element of self-examination and health promotion. Indicators of the interface between nails and wellness can be predictors for guiding clinical and individual aspects of care, once again emphasizing the integumentary system's role in wellness maintenance and illness detection early on. Here, the multidimensional role of the nails is evident as both a protective and diagnostic agent, as part of the total human biology and control of health architecture.

2.3.3. Glands: Sweat and Sebaceous Glands

The integumentary system is made up of various structures necessary for the maintenance of homeostasis and protection against the external environment, with sweat glands and sebaceous glands being the most crucial of these. Sweat glands, which are primarily found in the dermis layer of skin, form a vital part of thermoregulation based on the process of perspiration. During increased body temperature, sweat is expelled and released onto the skin surface, allowing for evaporative cooling. In addition to thermoregulation, sweat secretion plays a vital role in metabolite excretion and skin hydration. Sweat content consists of water, salts, and organic substances that play a role not only in thermoregulation but also in the maintenance of the skin microbiome, where resident microorganisms use the nutrient burden of sweats to gain, which improves skin health as well as disease prevention (Gillen et al., 2014). Sebaceous glands are, however, intimately associated with hair follicles and secrete an oily secretion known as sebum. Sebum serves to grease the hair and skin, enhancing the barrier against water and protecting against invasion by microbes. Sebum secretion is primarily responsible for keeping the skin moist and preserving its integrity because sebum transports lipids, which are essential for building a protective barrier to resist external forces (Gillen et al., 2014) (Figure 2.10).

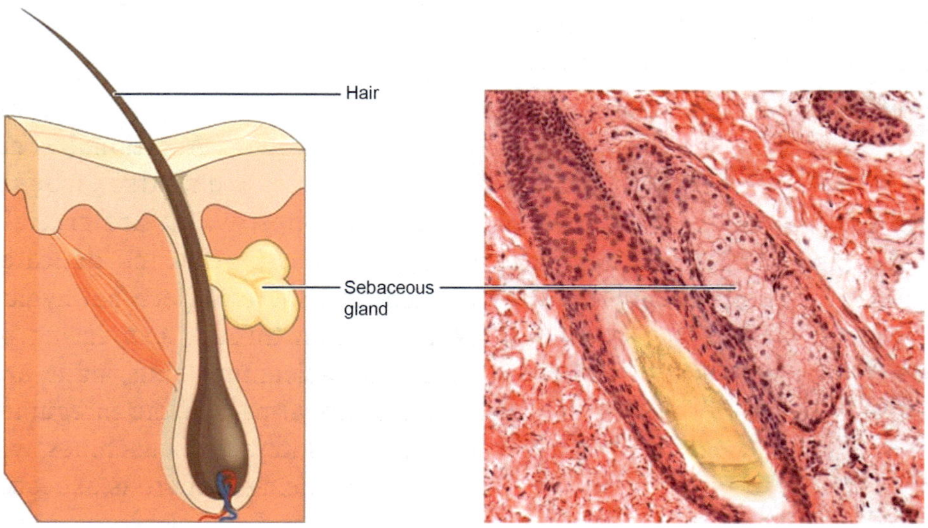

Figure 2.10. Sebaceous gland.

Source: https://biologydictionary.net/wp-content/uploads/2017/06/Sebaceous-Glands.jpg.

Moreover, the regulatory mechanisms controlling sebaceous gland functioning could also be regulated by hormonal changes, in particular more so at puberty, when the development of acne usually accompanies increased sebum secretion. Understanding the structure and functioning of these glands provides a profound appreciation of their role in supporting the integumentary system and maintaining healthy skin. The coordination of sweat and sebaceous glands also serves to demonstrate the intricacy of skin functioning. Though sweat glands are primarily involved in thermoregulation and elimination of wastes, sebaceous glands contribute to the hydration of the skin by secreting sebum. This dual mechanism not only controls water balance but also influences the skin microbiota, which can contain both beneficial and disease-causing microorganisms (Gillen et al., 2014). For example, sebum overproduction can lead to a rich medium for acnegenic bacteria, while balanced sebum promotes the growth of beneficial microbial populations that enhance skin resistance. The same phenomena are shown in rodent model studies, such as the sexual dimorphism of scent glands, where hormone influence on the physiology of the skin is reflected in morphological and secretory differentiation. Thus, their interaction emphasizes the importance of both glandular systems in controlling homeostatic as well as immune functions of the integumentary complex (Figure 2.11).

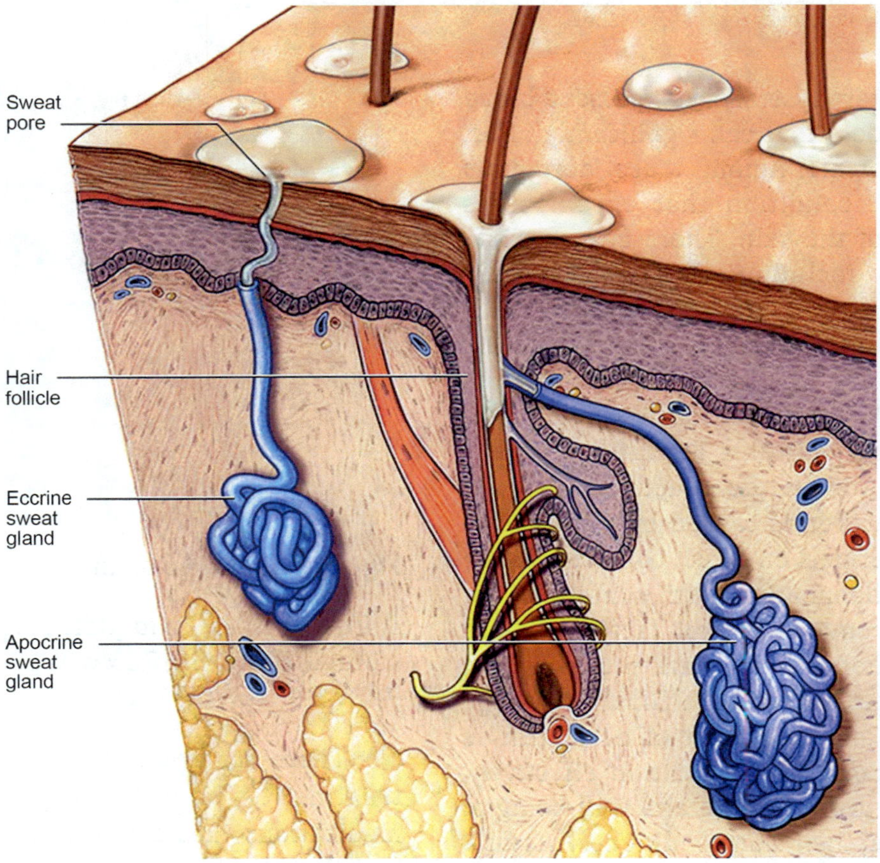

Figure 2.11. Sweat glands.

Source: https://www.mayoclinic.org/diseases-conditions/hyperhidrosis/multimedia/sweat-glands/img-20007980.

Test Your Knowledge

1. What are the different types of hair found on the human body, and what are their primary functions?
2. Describe the basic structure of a nail and explain its functional significance.

2.4. Common Integumentary Disorders

Learning Outcome

1. Explain the causes of acne and evaluate various treatment options
2. Identify the symptoms of eczema and describe effective management strategies
3. Analyze common triggers of psoriasis and discuss available therapeutic approaches

The integumentary system encompasses a broad range of disorders that can significantly affect one's quality of life. Among these, dermatitis is a prevalent condition that encompasses inflammation of the skin. There are a variety of dermatitis, including atopic dermatitis, contact dermatitis, and seborrheic dermatitis, that include redness, itchiness, and flakiness of the skin. Atopic dermatitis, which is seen in children, is a chronic condition associated with allergic rhinitis and asthma, indicating systemic susceptibility to allergic reactions. Contact dermatitis, however, is caused by exposure to irritants or allergens on direct contact, leading to localized inflammation. Both conditions are worsened by environmental factors, where patient education on skin care practices and trigger avoidance is necessary. Thus, knowledge of the causes and treatment of dermatitis is essential to manage the condition effectively, improving the overall health and well-being of the patients and their skin conditions. Psoriasis is another primary integumentary disease that poses a special challenge, mainly because of its chronic and sometimes recurrent nature. It is an autoimmune disease that results in a surfeit of skin cell growth, which produces thick, red patches with silvery scales. The pathogenesis of psoriasis is multifactorial, with an interplay of genetic predisposition, immune dysfunction, and environmental factors like stress and infections. Visibility of psoriasis also results in psychological distress due to stigma or appearance-related anxiety (Figure 2.12).

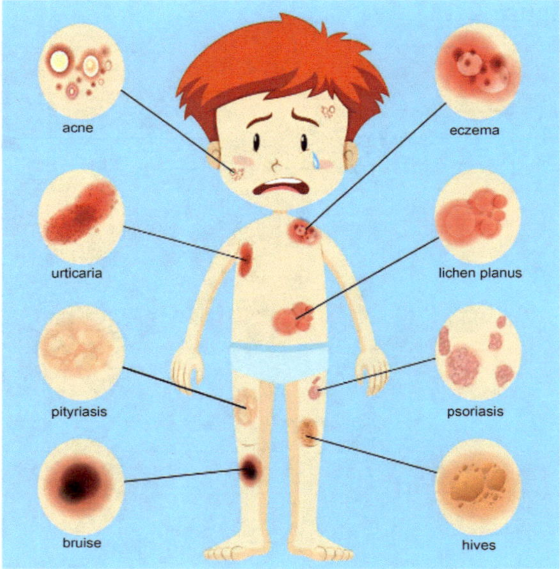

Figure 2.12. Common integumentary disorders.

Source: https://qndqdermacare.com/public/storage/Blogs/5lHRGMwAT185ZJzWj8d2R4CqRPDwFQHWWGtY3Ixd.png.

There are existing treatments like topical treatment, phototherapy, and systemic medications that act to reduce inflammation and plaque. Significantly, the progress in biologic therapies has left new hope for those who have moderate to severe psoriasis, demonstrating that reasonable disease control can really make a difference with quality of life and skin status over the long term. Burns is another critical group of integumentary disorders and have significant impact on the integrity and function of the skin. Burns can range from superficial to deep, partial, and full thickness, with clinical importance varying depending on the depth and extent of the total body surface involved.

The treatment plan for burn victims should be integrative, addressing not only physical trauma but also the psychological effects of such trauma. For instance, in severe partial-thickness and complete-thickness burns, good wound treatment is necessary to allow healing and prevent infections. Good nursing care practices are required, as evident in the case study of a client who had sustained major burns and inhalation of smoke, where careful assessment and creative wound management strategies are required (Cox et al., 2015). By considering both the psychological and physiological demands of burn injuries, medical personnel can more effectively enhance patient recovery and rehabilitation outcomes.

2.4.1. Acne: Causes and Treatments

Acne is an inflammatory skin condition caused by intricate interactions of the sebaceous glands, hormones, and the skin's resident bacteria. The underlying cause of acne is excessive sebum production by hormonal fluctuations, particularly in adolescence, which leads to clogged pores. These conditions favor the growth of Propionibacterium acnes, a bacterium that causes inflammation leading to various types of acne such as blackheads, whiteheads, and cystic acne. Genetics, nutritional factors, and stress are some of the factors that exacerbate these hormonal alterations, producing more severe outbreaks. The understanding of these etiological factors is essential in the treatment and management of acne because it accounts for the severity of this broad cutaneous disease, which occurs in individuals of all ages (Figure 2.13).

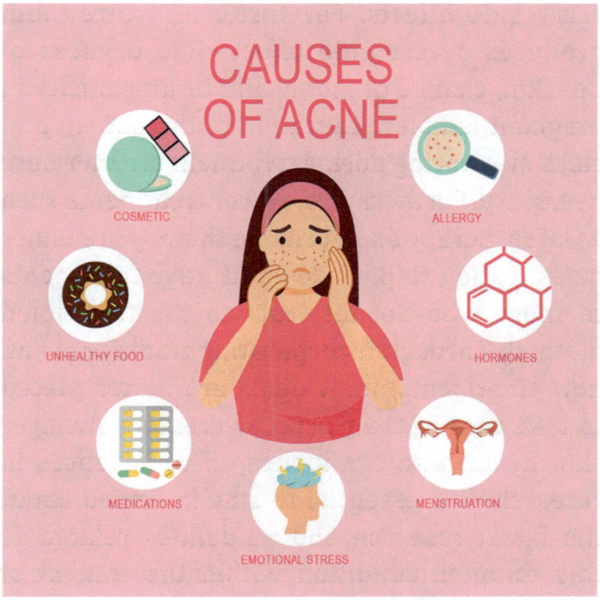

Figure 2.13. Common cause of acne.

Source: https://cdn.shopify.com/s/files/1/0591/2988/8965/files/causes-of-acne.jpg?v=1725536129.

Acne treatment is as diverse as its cause and involves topical and systemic treatment. Both retinoids and antibiotics can be applied for topical treatment, with retinoids helping to purge pores and reduce inflammation, and antibiotics targeting the bacterial component of acne. However, more severe forms like cystic acne typically need systemic treatment. According to research, isotretinoin, or Accutane, is the best medical treatment for cystic acne among doctors. Not only does the medication decrease sebum excretion, but it also addresses inflammation and bacterial elements responsible for the formation of acne.

Dietary modifications and skin care rituals, on the other hand, can be introduced as an adjunct to such medications, creating a well-rounded method of addressing not only the physical but also the emotional aspect of acne. Even though numerous treatments exist, acne control is a challenge since some drugs carry side effects. For instance, isotretinoin produces severe side effects like dryness of the skin, change of mood, and teratogenicity in pregnant females. Education of the patient and close monitoring during treatment are therefore necessary. Furthermore, newer treatments such as laser therapy and hormone therapy are under investigation to provide alternative treatments to those who do not react to the traditional method. Through incorporating traditional and new treatments, individuals are better placed to take care of their acne by creating stronger skin health and confidence. With advances in research, it is essential to stay informed about the latest research and guidelines related to this common condition within the context of the entire integumentary system.

2.4.2. Eczema: Symptoms and Management

Atopic dermatitis, also known as eczema, is a complex dermatological condition because of the multifarious symptoms and response to therapy. The condition is typically characterized by intense itching, erythema, and inflammation. It can manifest as papules, erythematous macules, and vesicles that tend to coalesce and form large plaques in some presentations. It can cause secondary lesions, which are responsible for weeping, crusting, and additional discomfort. This dynamic symptomatology not only is physically distressing but also potentially bears a significant psychological price, such as anxiety and depression, complicating further the treatment of eczema. It is crucial to understand the dynamic profile of these symptoms to develop effective management plans, which must be individualized for the patient with eczema having varying pathological features, as summarized in recent studies analyzing patient reports from internet forums (Hristidis et al., 2020) (Figure 2.14).

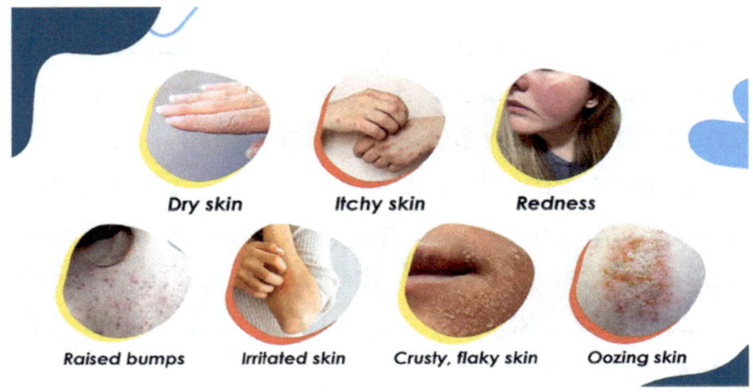

Figure 2.14. Common eczema symptoms.

Source: https://happycappyshampoo.com/wp-content/uploads/2025/04/Common-Eczema-Symptoms.jpg.

Management of eczema is a complex approach with both symptomatic relief and long-term control receiving the highest priority. Topical corticosteroids are employed most commonly to reduce inflammation and itching, and are the cornerstone upon which therapy is based. Moisturizers also play an equally significant role in the reconstitution of the skin barrier and moisturizing dry, damaged skin present in eczema patients. Second-line medications, including calcineurin inhibitors, may be applied in cases where topical corticosteroids fail to provide sufficient efficacy or are associated with side effects. Newer therapies, including biologics, target specific mechanisms within the inflammatory pathway, with a possible benefit for people with moderate to severe eczema. The integration of these treatment modalities requires an individualized regimen developed in consultation with medical practitioners, bearing the patient's specific symptom profile and psychosocial needs (Anand et al., 2023). Alternative and complementary treatments also find mention in the management of eczema, with traditional medicine providing additional treatment modalities. Interestingly, Ayurveda provides perspectives that are supplementary to contemporary dermatological trends, most notably in its integrative model for skin conditions such as eczema, known as Vicharchika in Ayurvedic literature. The ancient system focuses on a divergence from purely pharmacological management through the incorporation of lifestyle changes, dietary adaptation, and herbal medicine. Current case series have demonstrated the efficacy of Ayurvedic therapy in the relief of eczema symptoms through treatments such as bloodletting and personalized herbal formulations (Anand et al., 2023). Such evidence regarding holistic therapy suggests that holistic management of eczema is essential and, perhaps, synthesizing modern and conventional practices would enhance patient outcomes while keeping physical and mental facets of the disease in mind.

2.4.3. Psoriasis: Triggers and Therapies

The intricate relationship between psoriasis, which is an autoimmune, long-standing disease, and the integumentary system is at the core of unraveling its etiology and potential treatments. Psoriasis manifests in erythematous scaly plaques as a result of the augmented proliferation of keratinocytes, accompanied by differentiation, in effect remodeling the skin's architecture (Eckert and Ruhl, 2016). Environmental triggers such as stress, infections, and some drugs have been found to exacerbate the symptoms of psoriasis, emphasizing the dominant role of environmental triggers in interfering with the skin's capability to attain homeostasis. Not only does it affect the epidermis, but it also produces inflammatory reactions that can potentially complicate skin integrity. It is thus critical to understand these triggers in the development of focused treatments designed to restore balance in the integumentary system. There have been many therapeutic modalities that have been explored to alleviate the burden of psoriasis, especially considering its physical and psychological consequences. Traditional treatment has consisted of topical therapy, phototherapy, and systemic medication, targeting the pathophysiologic processes of the disease (Figure 2.15).

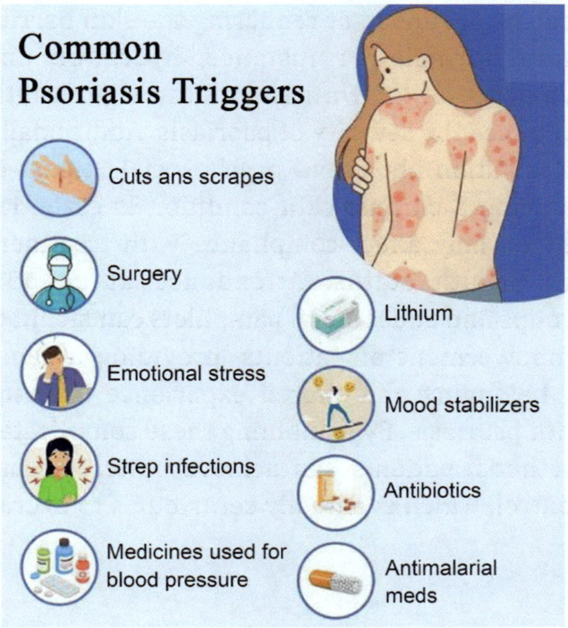

Figure 2.15. Common psoriasis triggers.

Source: https://www.mehektaguldermaclinic.com/template/mehektaguldermaclinic_com/images/Infographics/info-common-psoriasis.webp.

These treatments have some drawbacks, however, such as less-than-ideal efficacy and side effects. Recent research has identified non-psychoactive compounds, such as cannabidiol (CBD) in Cannabis sativa, as potential alternatives for treatment. Preliminary data suggest that CBD can reduce inflammation and itching and improve hydration and normalize keratinocyte function, thus addressing core aspects of psoriasis pathology directly (Andronic et al., 2024). The examination of such alternative treatments is a significant advance in the psoriasis armamentarium, to enhance quality of life in affected individuals. Lifestyle modifications, independent of the use of drugs, can play a crucial role in the treatment of psoriasis and the minimization of flare-ups.

Patients are encouraged to include a multimodal regimen consisting of dietary modification, stress reduction measures, and skin care measures specifically aimed at rendering the skin barrier more normal. For instance, hydration and avoidance of known irritants can significantly influence the severity of psoriasis. Additionally, information about the psychosocial impact of carrying a chronic skin condition is essential, as this may affect compliance with treatment and health status. Attendance at support groups and educational pamphlets can facilitate empowerment of patients, providing a sense of belonging and shared experience in living with psoriasis. By combining these complicated methods, patients can achieve better disease control, which eventually contributes to overall integumentary system health (Figure 2.16).

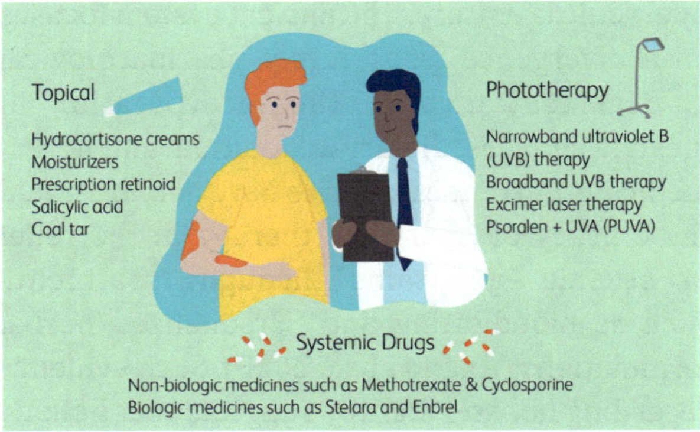

Figure 2.16. Treatment option for psoriasis.

Source: https://www.verywellhealth.com/thmb/NAWuKN7_QjtwEkj0nzoi4ddry8w=/1500x0/filters:no_upscale():max_bytes(150000):strip_icc()/psoriasis-and-inflammation-5202286_final-01-5be7bfc0a23b497a9e5ef10c7e187598.jpg.

Test Your Knowledge

1. What are the common causes of acne and the typical treatment options available?
2. What symptoms characterize eczema, and how is it generally managed?

2.5. The Role of the Integumentary System in Homeostasis

Learning Outcome

1. Define maintaining hydration and barrier function
2. Discuss the immune response and skin health
3. Explain the vitamin D synthesis and its importance

The integumentary system, comprised primarily of the skin, hair, nails, and glands, is an essential component of homeostasis in the human body. Temperature control, one of its primary functions, is critical to the normal operations of metabolic processes. By means such as vasodilation and vasoconstriction, the integument controls blood perfusion to the skin. Vasodilation permits heat release through the skin under body overheating, and vasoconstriction helps to retain heat under cold conditions. Moreover, the sweating process not only keeps the body cool but also plays a critical role in ensuring electrolyte balance, showing the complex role of the integumentary system in homeostasis. Understanding such processes shows how significant the integumentary system is in preventing thermoregulatory disease and maintaining overall internal stability. In addition to thermoregulation, the integumentary system also protects, shielding the body from external environmental trauma in the form of pathogens, chemicals, and physical injury. The skin's epidermis, particularly its outer keratinized layer, constitutes formidable resistance to microbial penetration and drying. Protection is the most critical aspect of homeostasis, as its loss would lead to infection or unregulated fluid loss, either of which would destroy internal stability. Further, specialized skin cells, such as Langerhans cells, become directly engaged in immune processes, strengthening the body's defense mechanisms. The combination of this barrier function and immune surveillance highlights the importance of skin integrity for health and wellness and demonstrates the system's dynamic role in preserving homeostasis. Additionally, the integumentary system plays a crucial role in sensory perception, which in turn helps the body respond to stimuli and maintain homeostasis. Skin contains many receptors with sensory properties that are responsive to variations in temperature, pressure, vibration, and pain. It is also essential for immediate protective reflexes like withdrawal from noxious stimuli to prevent damage and promote survival. In addition, sensory feedback enables the body to adapt to environmental change, thus allowing appropriate physiological response. This intricate relationship between the sensory input and physiological response is a perfect example of the system's function to facilitate homeostasis. Knowledge about how the sensory function of the integumentary system responds with other homeostatic processes is a testament to the interconnectedness of the body systems, an example of how all-encompassing the function of the integument in maintaining one's health and stability is.

2.5.1. Maintaining Hydration and Barrier Function

The integumentary system is a vital function in the maintenance of hydration and barrier integrity and serves as the body's first line of defense against environmental hazards. Its key structural component, the epidermis, is responsible for this protective function through several layers that effectively restrict water loss. The outermost layer, the stratum corneum, consists of dead keratinized cells that form a barrier, preventing excess transepidermal water loss (TEWL). This obstacle is crucial for maintaining adequate hydration levels within the body, which allows it to function in various physiological processes. Its interruption is known to lead to conditions like xerosis or dermatitis, and therefore, the integumentary system has an essential role to play in fluid homeostasis and skin integrity. Aquaporin water channels (AQPs) also contribute to the function of the integumentary system in maintaining hydration. These channels enhance the movement of water across cell membranes in the epidermis and primarily support the hydration level of the skin (Figure 2.17).

Importantly, AQP regulation and expression are essential in the regulation of skin cell water balance. Studies have indicated that AQP function is not only passive but also that AQPs play a regulatory role to maintain cell volume and osmotic balance, especially during external fluctuation in hydration. Besides, as we learn more about the AQP mechanism of action, we develop an additional understanding of therapeutic targets to combat skin hydration problems, highlighting the interconnectedness between biology and medical technology (Rebecca et al., 2008). Along with the hydration of skin, the barrier also plays a vital role in preventing the entry of detrimental pathogens, allergens, and pollutants. Any disruption of this barrier can lead to increased vulnerability to skin infection and systemic disease. An understanding of the support that hydrates provide to the skin barrier illuminates the interrelatedness of integumentary functions. Adequate hydration enhances the skin's elasticity and strength and reduces the likelihood of damage or compromise. Moreover, the AQPs function as facilitators of water flow to highlight the utility of research in such channels as therapeutic targets. In totality, hydration and effective barrier function are crucial for overall integumentary health, enabling protection and homeostasis functions while paving the way for future therapeutic innovation in dermatologic practice (Bill et al., 2014).

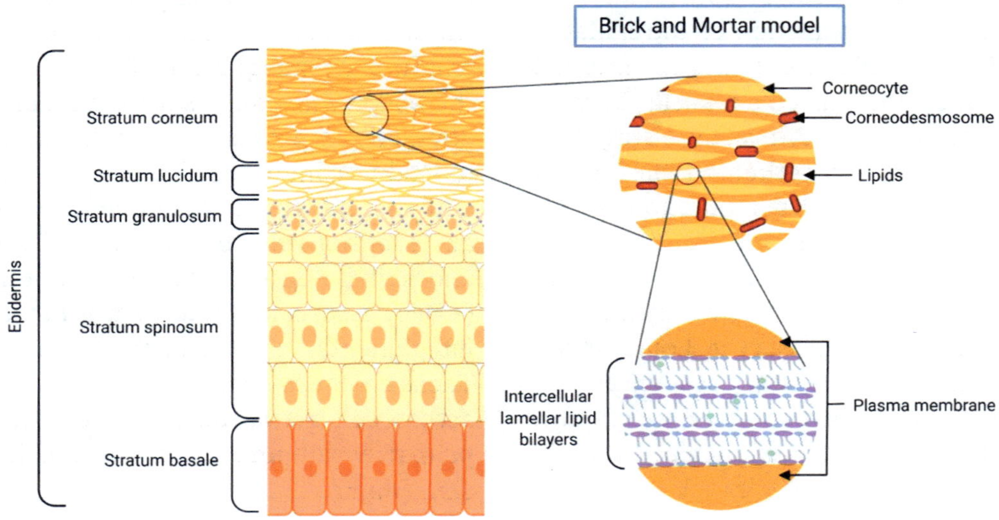

Figure 2.17. Schematic structure of the skin barrier and "brick and mortar" model.

Source: https://www.creative-bioarray.com/skin-barrier-function-and-hydration.htm.

2.5.2. Immune Response and Skin Health

The skin is the primary internal-external barrier, and it has a central role in the immune response and overall skin health. The largest organ of the integumentary system is not merely a passive barrier but is actively engaged in immune functions. The skin contains diverse immune cells, including Langerhans cells, which are dendritic resident cells that identify pathogens and activate the immune response. In addition, the skin microbiota, which is made up of millions of microorganisms that colonize the skin surface, is critical to maintaining a healthy immune response. Skin diseases and disorders are caused by abnormalities in the microbial environment, underscoring the need for a better understanding of how microbes interact with the skin. (Gillen et al., 2014). Skin health is thus crucial to a successful immune response as well as the overall health of the body. The microbiome of the skin is inherently linked with the immune system, since healthy bacteria on the skin don't just fight against and destroy harmful pathogens but also regulate immune responses. When these microbes coexist, the skin develops an impervious shield against inflammation and infection. When the normal balance of the skin is disturbed, whether by external influences or poor hygiene, it can lead to inflammation and increased susceptibility to the development of a skin disorder such as atopic dermatitis or acne. Research has established that an understanding of the skin's microbiome can inform new probiotic therapies for the restoration of microbial balance and hence enhancing skin health (Gillen et al., 2014) (Figure 2.18).

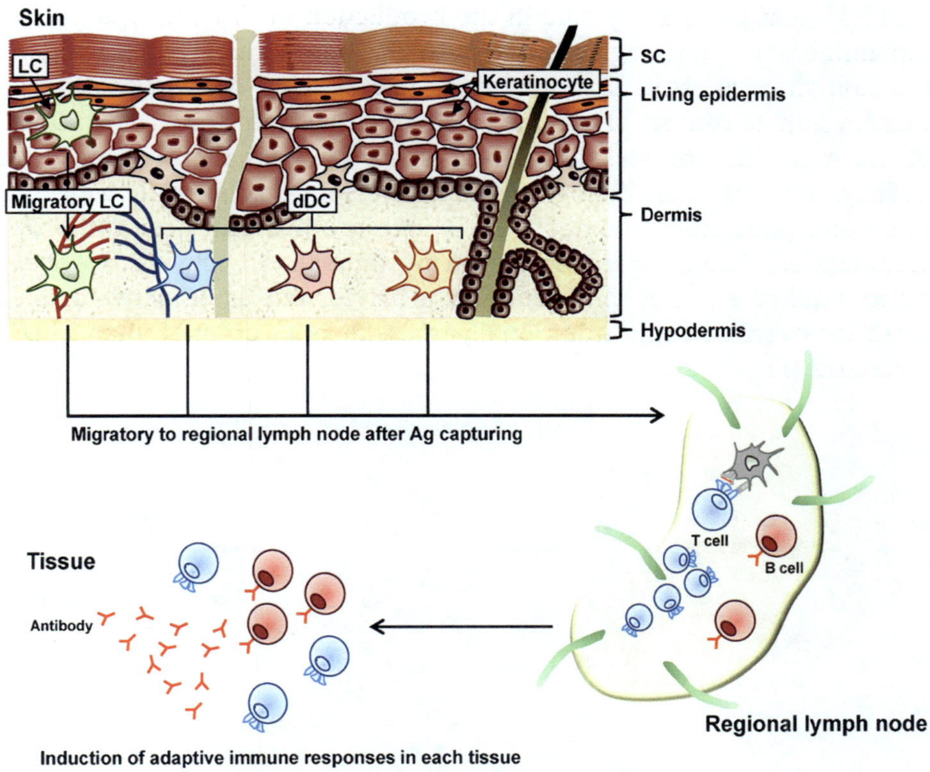

Figure 2.18. Skin immune system. The skin is enriched with various immunocompetent cells such as LCs, keratinocytes, and several dDCs. Keratinocytes are mainly involved in the induction of innate immunity.

Source: https://www.researchgate.net/figure/Skin-immune-system-The-skin-is-enriched-with-various-immunocompetent-cells-such-as-LCs_fig1_236075194.

These treatments could be helpful for chronic skin disease sufferers, emphasizing the importance of skin care, taking a holistic approach to both the health of the microbes and immune function. Additionally, more recent studies have identified the influence of lifestyle factors in the determination of immune outcomes, as well as skin health. Diet, stress, and environmental pollutants can all affect the skin microbiome and the efficacy of the immune system. For instance, an antioxidant diet may aid in promoting skin health through decreased oxidative stress and inflammation, which are critical for optimal immune competence. Similarly, immune dysregulation caused by chronic stress has been linked with adverse skin conditions reflective of internal inflammation. Therefore, a complex system encompassing nutritional, psychological, and hygiene factors must be employed to promote skin health and a healthy immune response. Identification of these connections not only aids in the prevention of skin disease but also in a fuller understanding of the multifaceted functions of the integumentary system in good health and well-being.

2.5.3. Vitamin D Synthesis and Its Importance

The integumentary system plays a key role in the production of Vitamin D, a nutrient that plays a critical role in numerous physiological processes. The mechanism begins when ultraviolet B (UVB) light from sunlight strikes the skin, which stimulates the 7-dehydrocholesterol, a naturally produced chemical in skin, to convert to previtamin D3. Heat-activated previtamin D3 is transformed into vitamin D3 through this process.. This fat-soluble vitamin is then broken down further by the liver and kidneys into its most biologically active form, calcitriol. Calcitriol is necessary for regulating calcium and phosphorus homeostasis, which are necessary for the proper growth of bones and mineralization. The special role played by the skin to convert UV rays into Vitamin D also indicates its vital role in not only acting as a barrier but as an active agent in metabolic functions required for overall health. Additionally, the effects of optimal vitamin D levels extend beyond bone structure (Figure 2.19).

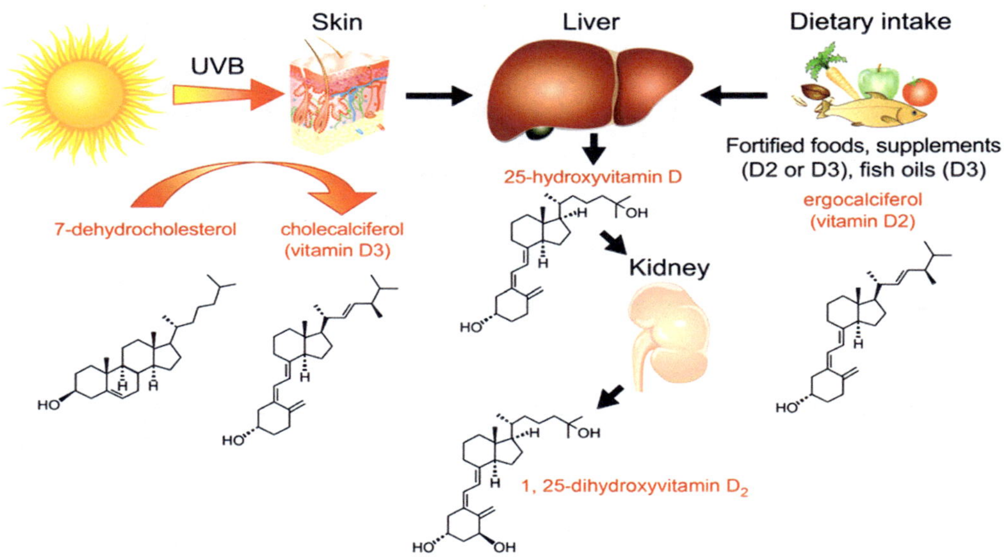

Figure 2.19. Vitamin D synthesis and metabolism. Vitamin D is photosynthesized in the skin and is also acquired by dietary intake.

Source: https://www.researchgate.net/profile/Vin-Tangpricha/publication/237096135/figure/fig2/AS:669656549433353@1536669971517/tamin-D-synthesis-and-metabolism-Vitamin-D-is-photosynthesized-in-the-skin-and-is-also.png.

Research has established that the vitamin plays a part in the avoidance of several chronic illnesses, including autoimmune diseases and certain cancers. Infection with vitamin D deficiency has been linked to increased risks of these diseases, suggesting that the part played by the skin in vitamin D synthesis is more critical to the body's general health and disease resistance. Moreover, the interactions between vitamin D and immune response have been of particular interest, particularly in light of the current public health environment. Emerging evidence suggests the therapeutic value of vitamin D to enhance immune response and inhibit inflammatory signaling, and emphasizes the need to study vitamin D status in clinical populations. Hence, vitamin D production through sunlight is essential not only for physiological health but also for protection against disease. The interaction of the integumentary system with vitamin D production is particularly relevant when public health policy concerning sun exposure is taken into consideration. As numerous variables such as geographical location, complexion, and way of life have significant effects on vitamin D synthesis, understanding of these factors becomes a prerequisite for developing appropriate health interventions. For instance, darker populations may require more exposure to sunlight to acquire adequate amounts of vitamin D due to the extra melanin that safeguards the skin better against UV radiation, also inhibiting vitamin D synthesis. Additionally, supplementation and food sources are essential to treating vitamin D deficiency, especially among populations with a greater risk due to limited sun exposure. With diet and lifestyle being an integration that must be accomplished for good health, recognizing the role the skin plays in such a multifaceted process solidifies the significance of the integumentary system beyond that of merely a barrier, but as a part of human health and well-being.

Test Your Knowledge

1. How does the skin maintain hydration and protect its barrier function?
2. What role does the skin play in the immune response to protect the body?

SUMMARY

The integumentary system is a critical barrier between the exterior world and the human body, having an enormous array of vital functions. This complex system, comprised mainly of skin, hair, nails, and accessory glands, protects deep tissues from infecting organisms and damage as well as thermoregulation and sensation. The intricate interdependence of the components of the integumentary system supports the necessity of understanding its function within the context of global body systems. Understanding how skin health impacts one's general health enables medical professionals to better treat various dermal diseases, with an emphasis on preventive over reactive treatment. Moreover, the integumentary system's connection to the other body systems supports the use of an integrative model of health. Skin interacts with the endocrine system through the secretion of hormones that regulate most body functions. Moreover, thinking of the integumentary system as an integral part of the overall human system is itself situated in the general framework of body systems, which are described as interdependent subsystems that engage in complex causal relationships (Smith et al., 2004). This holistic approach promotes interdisciplinary collaboration in medical science and clinical practice, hence enhancing patient outcomes. Current studies must continue exploring the totality of functions of the integumentary system, especially how it intersects with emerging medical technologies and interventions. Advances in dermatology science, or regenerative medicine and individualized skin care, hold the promise of improved health strategies. As institutions like Kean University place more importance on interdisciplinary studies in the science of biology, students and researchers are well-equipped to understand better the connotations of the integumentary system to human health. By integrating knowledge among systems, as discussed in initiatives like the BA Biology 2021 at Kean University (Kean University, 2021), we can develop new avenues of treatment and innovation that improve healthcare quality and enhance overall quality of life.

The integumentary system, comprised mainly of the skin, hair, nails, and associated glands, is significant to the health and homeostasis of the body overall. As the body's first line of defense, the skin protects inner structures from invaders like pathogens, environmental toxins, and physical damage. This is a necessary barrier, particularly with all the exposures our environment is currently subjected to. Also, the integumentary system helps to regulate body temperature through processes such as perspiration and vasodilation. The system, by controlling heat loss or gain, assists the body in adapting to a change in the external conditions, showing how relative it is compared to concerns over aesthetics or superficial functions. The integumentary system also facilitates sensory perception. The skin has numerous nerve endings that allow individuals to feel stimuli such as touch, pressure, pain, and temperature. This feedback through sensation is essential for a response to one's surroundings and is vital to survival because it prevents injury and facilitates responsive action to altering situations. The proprioceptive nature of skin receptors assists an individual to have a better sense of body position and movement, and enables improved coordination. Furthermore, the sensory components of the integumentary system can affect psychological and emotional well-being, further reinforcing its more general relevance in health and quality of life, but one often not noticed. Instructional techniques that incorporate experiential learning experiences can significantly enhance understanding of the integumentary system's complexity and function. For instance, through studies, it has been discovered that students who have undergone model-building experiences show increased confidence and recall about the anatomy and physiology of integumentary systems. In addition to improving student participation, active learning strategies also help ensure proper comprehension of the intricate relationships within the system. Further, including such strategies in the curriculum also helps in meeting various styles of learning, hence creating a more comprehensive learning process. As brought out in recent education reviews, supplementing anatomy classes with interactive methods can lead to enhanced academic performance and long-term retention (DeOliveira et al., 2022; Khan et al., 2023).

KEY TERMS FROM THIS CHAPTER

- Epidermis
- Hypodermis
- Melanocytes
- Merkel cells
- Stratum spinosum
- Stratum corneum
- Sebaceous gland
- Nails
- Papillary layer
- Dermis
- Keratinocytes
- Langerhans cells
- Stratum basale
- Stratum granulosum
- Hair follicle
- Sweat gland
- Sensory receptors

CRITICAL THINKING QUESTIONS

1. **Which of the following is NOT a function of the integumentary system?**
   a. Protection
   b. Temperature regulation
   c. Blood cell production
   d. Sensory reception
2. **What is the outermost layer of the skin called?**
   a. Dermis
   b. Hypodermis
   c. Epidermis
   d. Subcutaneous layer
3. **Which pigment is primarily responsible for skin color?**
   a. Hemoglobin
   b. Melanin
   c. Keratin
   d. Collagen
4. **Sweat glands that help regulate body temperature are called:**
   a. Sebaceous glands
   b. Apocrine glands
   c. Eccrine glands
   d. Ceruminous glands
5. **Hair and nails are primarily made of which protein?**
   a. Collagen
   b. Elastin
   c. Keratin
   d. Melanin

Short Answer Questions

1. What are the three main layers of the skin, and what is the primary structure of each?
2. List three major functions of the integumentary system.
3. What are skin appendages, and how do they support the skin's functions?
4. Name two common disorders of the integumentary system and describe their key symptoms.
5. How does the integumentary system contribute to maintaining homeostasis in the body?
6. What role does melanin play in protecting the skin, and which cells produce it?

Answer to Critical Thinking Questions

1. (c); 2. (c); 3. (b); 4. (c); 5. (c)

REFERENCES

1. Abe, Y., & Nishizawa, M. (2021). Electrical aspects of skin as a pathway to engineering skin devices. *APL Bioengineering*, *5*(4). https://doi.org/10.1063/5.0064529Accettola, E., Bogdan, A., Callahan, S., Chawda, P., et al. (2023). *Introduction to Health Assessment for the Nursing Professional: Part II*. https://core.ac.uk/download/622362029.pdf (accessed on 14th June 2025).
2. Achiraman, S., Akbarsha, M. A., Archunan, G., Ponmanickam, P., Rajagopal, T., Rajanarayanan, S., Saibaba, G., et al. (2020). Histomorphology perspectives of preputial and clitoral glands of soft-furred field rat *Millardia meltada*. https://core.ac.uk/download/478160414.pdf (accessed on 14th June 2025).
3. Adissu, H., Berberovic, Z., Clary, D., Eskandarian, A., et al. (2019). Genome-wide screening of mouse knockouts reveals novel genes required for normal integumentary and oculocutaneous structure and function. https://core.ac.uk/download/323068723.pdf (accessed on 14th June 2025).
4. Anand, R. J., Lawrence, D. T., Girish, K. J., & Tripaty, T. B. (2023). Ayurvedic management of Vicharchika (eczema)–A case report. https://core.ac.uk/download/617189495.pdf (accessed on 14th June 2025).
5. Andronic, O., Balta, M. D., Bejan, G. C., Busnatu, S., Stanescu, A. M. A., & Toma, C. (2024). The perspective of cannabidiol in psoriasis therapy. https://core.ac.uk/download/616639462.pdf (accessed on 14th June 2025).
6. Anglani, R., Bianco, S., Forge, D., Guimer, R., Makse, H. A., Herrick, R., Horster, M., et al. (2010). Modularity map of the network of human cell differentiation. http://arxiv.org/abs/1001.5292 (accessed on 14th June 2025).
7. Benton, M. J., Foley, T., Hone, D. W. E., Johnson, M., et al. (2018). Fossilized skin reveals coevolution with feathers and metabolism in feathered dinosaurs and early birds. https://core.ac.uk/download/158350376.pdf (accessed on 14th June 2025).
8. Bill, R. M., Bland, C., Conner, A. C., Conner, M. T., et al. (2014). Human aquaporins: Regulators of transcellular water flow. https://core.ac.uk/download/20043992.pdf (accessed on 14th June 2025).
9. Camarero, P. R., Galván, I., Mateo, R., Negro, J. J., et al. (2016). Porphyrins produce uniquely ephemeral animal coloration: A possible signal of virginity. https://core.ac.uk/download/80862957.pdf (accessed on 14th June 2025).
10. Chanson, M., Martin, P. E., O'Shaughnessy, E. M., Watanabe, M., et al. (2018). Connexin communication compartments and wound repair in epithelial tissue. https://core.ac.uk/download/293885271.pdf (accessed on 14th June 2025).
11. Cooper, R. L., Fraser, G. J., Martin, K. J., Rasch, L. J., et al. (2017). Developing an ancient epithelial appendage: FGF signaling regulates early tail denticle formation in sharks. https://core.ac.uk/download/83941916.pdf (accessed on 14th June 2025).
12. Cox, A. (2015). *Thermal Burns and Smoke Inhalation Injuries*. https://core.ac.uk/download/58826490.pdf (accessed on 14th June 2025).
13. Day, R. E., Kitchen, P., Owen, D. S., Bland, C., Marshall, L., Conner, A. C., Bill, R. M., et al. (2008). Human aquaporins: Regulators of transcellular water flow. https://core.ac.uk/download/20043992.pdf (accessed on 14th June 2025).

14. De Pessemier, B., Grine, L., Debaere, M., Maes, A., Paetzold, B., & Callewaert, C. (2021). Gut–skin axis: Current knowledge of the interrelationship between microbial dysbiosis and skin conditions. *Microorganisms, 9*, 353–353. https://doi.org/10.3390/microorganisms9020353 (accessed on 14th June 2025).

15. DeOliveira, S. (2022). Student engagement and performance assessment as associated with three types of integument system laboratory activities. https://core.ac.uk/download/525047802.pdf (accessed on 14th June 2025).

16. Elliott, C. (2019). Risk benefit analysis of treatments for cystic acne. https://core.ac.uk/download/286536282.pdf (accessed on 14th June 2025).

17. Fambrough, V., & Gibson, L. (2018). *Anatomy and Physiology I & II (UNG)*. https://core.ac.uk/download/217306203.pdf (accessed on 14th June 2025).

18. Fonteh, A. L. (2018). *Erotic Aciduria*. https://core.ac.uk/download/213462592.pdf (accessed on 14th June 2025).

19. Gillen, A. L. (2014). *The Wonderfully Made Design of The Skin and Its Microbiome*. https://core.ac.uk/download/220159123.pdf (accessed on 14th June 2025).

20. Hristidis, V., Hua, M., Sadah, S., Talbot, P., et al. (2020). Health effects associated with electronic cigarette use: Automated mining of online forums. https://core.ac.uk/download/286729292.pdf (accessed on 14th June 2025).

21. Jessup, J. M. (2015). *Hybrid Enhanced Epidermal Spacesuit Design Approaches*. https://core.ac.uk/download/235078804.pdf (accessed on 14th June 2025).

22. Kean University. (2021). *Kean Program Review–BA Biology 2019*. https://core.ac.uk/download/480706856.pdf (accessed on 14th June 2025).

23. Khan, M. (2023). *Development of Curriculum of Anatomy for BDS Students in UZ, Harare: A Survey-Based Study*. https://core.ac.uk/download/587960449.pdf (accessed on 14th June 2025).

24. Kirby, A. C. (2020). *A Characterization of The Integumentary Skeleton of Lizards (Reptilia: Squamata)*. https://core.ac.uk/download/376910272.pdf (accessed on 14th June 2025).

25. McLaughlin, J., Monteleone, G., O'Neill, C., Paus, R., et al. (2016). The gut-skin axis in health and disease: A paradigm with therapeutic implications. https://core.ac.uk/download/74196754.doc (accessed on 14th June 2025).

26. Pádua, M. S. F. P. de. (2019). *Study of The Effects of The Culture Condition in The Permeation of Reconstructed Human Skin*. https://core.ac.uk/download/243511874.pdf (accessed on 14th June 2025).

27. Pomerleau, T. A. (2021). *Strategies to Prevent Hospital Acquired Pressure Injuries in The Intensive Care Unit*. https://core.ac.uk/download/490617094.pdf (accessed on 14th June 2025).

28. Schindler, C. A. (2010). *More than S.K.I.N. Deep: Decreasing Pressure Ulcer Development in The Pediatric Intensive Care Unit*. https://core.ac.uk/download/67759746.pdf (accessed on 14th June 2025).

29. Smith, B. (2004). *Bodily Systems and The Spatial-Functional Structure of The Human Body*. https://core.ac.uk/download/226757085.pdf (accessed on 14th June 2025).

30. Sparozic, F. R. (2020). *A Snapshot of Care: Creating Models of Care for Individuals Included in the Terry Collection*. https://core.ac.uk/download/323031781.pdf (accessed on 14th June 2025).

31. Stewart, C. (2016). *Problem Based Learning and Stem Model Design in A Secondary Biology Curriculum*. https://core.ac.uk/download/638981466.pdf (accessed on 14th June 2025).

32. Twyman, H. (2018). *Evolutionary Genetics of CYP2J19 in Red Carotenoid Pigmentation*. https://core.ac.uk/download/146491409.pdf (accessed on 14th June 2025).

33. Wilk-Blaszczak, M. (2018). *Human Anatomy Lab Manual*. https://core.ac.uk/download/622362427.pdf (accessed on 14th June 2025).

THE SKELETAL SYSTEM: OVERVIEW

3

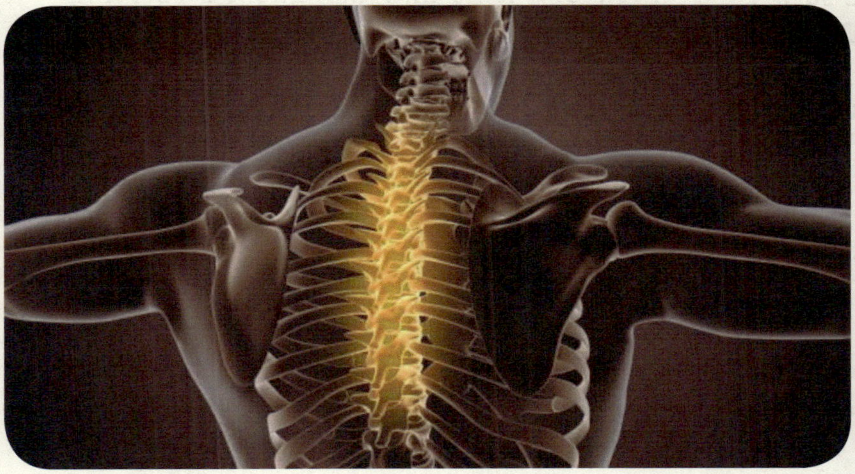

LEARNING OBJECTIVES

After studying this chapter, you will be able to:

1. Describe the anatomy of the skeletal system
2. Explain the functions of the skeletal system
3. Identify the bones' composition and structure
4. Discuss the development and growth of the bones
5. Recognize and describe the most common skeletal disorders
6. Analyze the role of the skeletal system in health and disease

Introduction

The skeletal system is a critical support foundation for the shape and purpose of the human body, serving an integral function throughout life from infancy to adulthood. Composed of bones, cartilage, ligaments, and other connective tissue, the intricate system provides support, facilitates movement, and protects internal organs. In addition to its mechanical roles, the skeletal system also serves as a mineral reservoir and site of blood cell development, highlighting its versatility in contributing to general health. Network analysis, a novel approach to examining biological systems, has been highlighted by recent studies as a potential method for elucidating the skeletal features and interactions within biological systems, thereby highlighting the additional aspect of studying morphological abnormalities such as Class III malocclusion. This new knowledge not only improves our comprehension of skeletal imbalances but also offers avenues for the successful targeting of therapies, representing the new interfaces between skeletal science and novel diagnostic methods (Angel et al., 2012). Aside from scientific purposes, the skeletal system is central to the evolution of species and the contextual significance of vertebrates in the field of biological science. Evidence has shown that detailed scanning and analysis of skeletal structures can illuminate the connections between body form and ecological adaptation. For instance, high-resolution ventures like ScanAllFish, an initiative whose goal is to register all current fish species, use state-of-the-art imaging techniques to reveal critical data concerning skeletal morphology.

The incorporation of technologies such as Unwind, which facilitates improved visualization of the skeletal structures, points towards immense technological progress in marine biology and related disciplines. Not only do such technological advances facilitate classification and understanding of fish anatomy, but they also underscore the role of skeletal features in evolutionary biology. The accurate representation of the shapes of bones with advanced methods of analysis is incredibly beneficial in comparative studies between different vertebrate groups, showing a clear association between integrity of structure and performance function (Chen et al., 2020). Complexity in the system's structure is further increased by the range of conditions that compromise its function and integrity. Disorders such as osteoporosis, arthritis, and skeletal deformities illustrate the complex nature of the orthopedic and rehabilitation medicine practice. Such illnesses are best comprehended through multidisciplinary knowledge encompassing biomechanics, anatomy, and pathology. Research in the field also continues to unveil the powerful impact of lifestyle, diet, and genetics on bone strength. By examining the interplay among these factors, health professionals can develop improved preventative and therapeutic interventions. The skeletal system is thus not only an anatomical and functional spine but also an active system subject to a diversity of internal and external factors that must constantly be researched and addressed by innovative solutions to common skeletal health issues.

Definition of the Skeletal System

The skeletal system is the body framework, and it participates in offering structure, support, as well as protection of internal organs. Made up of 206 bones in the adult human body, the skeletal system is not a static framework but an active, dynamic, and essential component of human physiology. It permits movement by serving as sites of attachment for muscles to enable locomotion and other bodily motions. The bones in themselves are made up of a complicated matrix of collagen fibers and minerals, predominantly calcium and phosphorus, which strengthen and harden them. This natural structure is characterized by its ability to respond to injury and stress through adaptation, repair, and remodeling, highlighting its dynamic nature as something more than just inert support but rather a functioning system continuously interacting with other body processes. Beyond providing the body with structure, the skeletal system is an integral part in the production of blood cells through hematopoiesis, a function performed primarily in the bone marrow. This movement indicates the multifunctional activities of the body of bones, much beyond protection and support. The skeleton also serves as a repository for essential minerals such as calcium and phosphate that can be released into the circulation to meet the metabolic needs of the body. This homeostatic regulation is crucial for bone health and metabolism, indicating the skeletal system's integration with other body systems. In addition, the relationship between the skeletal system and overall health is evident in conditions like osteoporosis, where weakened bones increase the risk of fractures and reduce mobility, ultimately impacting quality of life. Aside from its physiological functions, the skeletal system is highly significant to anthropology and evolution. It provides us with hints of human evolution, demonstrating adaptations to various environmental and physical demands through time. Such a relationship is well-proven in comparative analyses with other organisms, since resemblance and divergence in skeletal structures bring with them clues concerning adaptive methods throughout history. Moreover, the skeletal system plays a significant role in the investigation of developmental biology, illustrating how environmental and genetic factors influence bone development and shape. By studying skeletal system development, scientists can learn about broader processes of biology that tend towards similarity, thus making it significant not only to individual health but also to life sciences in general.

Importance of the Skeletal System in the Human Body

In the human body, the skeleton plays several functions that are critical to overall health and well-being. The most significant is that it is the structural support system of the body, which allows for an erect posture and the mounting of muscles and organs. The bone structure is also distinct in terms of thickness and density, capable of adjusting to the mechanical stress and function of the specific bone. This structural aid is required not only for maintaining the integrity of the body but also for movement by way of the operation of levers. The system of bones and joints permits a great range of motion (ROM) and activities to be performed, which are essential for executing everyday tasks and physical exercise. The symbiotic interaction of the skeleton and the musculature highlights the importance of the skeletal system in facilitating movement and functionality, hence a healthy lifestyle. In addition to stabilizing and facilitating movement, the skeletal system also plays a vital role in the production and storage of major substances like blood cells and minerals. Bone marrow in the cavities of certain bones is a significant hematopoietic site, wherein new blood cells develop. Hematopoiesis is the key to the oxygenation of the body, immunity, and overall health. Moreover, the bones are reservoirs of vital minerals such as calcium and phosphorus, and regulate their levels in the bloodstream. This function is particularly crucial for muscle contraction and cell signaling. The intricate equilibrium offered by the skeletal system not only enables movement but is also the foundation of numerous biochemical reactions necessary to human physiology, underscoring its multidimensional applicability. Growing research continues to emphasize the skeletal system's role in general health and regeneration. Advances in regenerative medicine and tissue engineering have put improved skeletal welfare in the limelight for effective recovery from MSK ailments. Endogenous tissue engineering, which employs the regenerative potential of the body, is gaining popularity because it can minimize the risks of transplanting foreign cells (Adam et al., 2012). Also brought out in the latest proteomic studies on the complex regulation of the metabolic pathways of skeletal muscle is the intrinsic connection between the skeletal system and metabolic well-being (Cox et al., 2015). With the expanding body of knowledge, it becomes imperative that an entire understanding of the role of the skeletal system be achieved, not only for the treatment of injury but for enabling and sustaining optimal health throughout the lifespan.

3.1. Anatomy of the Skeletal System

Learning Outcome

1. Define major components of the skeletal system
2. Explain the classification of bones
3. Understand overview of joints and their functions

The skeletal system is a sophisticated structure supporting the human body, providing for both movement and protection. Made up of 206 bones in an adult human, the sophisticated system also includes cartilage, tendons, and ligaments, all contributing to its functionality. The bones are categorized into two broad groups: the axial skeleton, which consists of the skull, vertebral column, and rib cage, and the appendicular skeleton, which includes the limbs and girdles. The classification not only assists in visualizing the body structure but also aids in understanding the varied functions various bones play in locomotion and the shielding of internal organs. In addition, the bones have twice the amount of living tissue found in other organs than the skeletal system, enabling the skeletal system to adapt to stress and influence a wide range of physiological processes, from hematopoiesis to mineral storage. Apart from its protective and supportive roles, the anatomy of the skeletal system possesses an unprecedented degree of specialization, enabling an extensive range of functions vital to health. For instance, certain bones are so formed to provide maximum leverage and control in movement, whereas others, the flat skull bones for example, give a necessary partition against body trauma. Moreover, the structure of the bones is functionally related; long bones, for example, are there for support and movement because of their cylinder shape and because they have marrow that helps in hematopoiesis. Understanding these variations in anatomy is essential for the study of sports medicine and orthopedics since they determine the course of treatment of injuries and conditions that can afflict different parts of the skeletal system. The evolution of the anatomy of the skeletal system reveals a gripping tale about the grand narrative of vertebrate evolution. Comparative studies have shown that the skeletal types across various species, even those of now-extinct archosaurs, underscore functional adaptation over time. Birds, for instance, possess unique skeletal characteristics for their complex respiratory tracts, such as pneumatic bones that reduce weight without imperiling structural support. These traits have more than anatomy merely in mind; they also reflect adaptation against evolutionary pressures. Further, the findings related to pneumaticity can help us to understand the biomechanical advantages that specific species have, as outlined in recent research that includes state-of-the-art imaging techniques (Barrett et al., 2012). This study further emphasizes the value of interdisciplinarity in the study of skeletal morphology and its implications in future developments in areas such as biomechanical engineering and prosthesis design (Rust et al., 2009).

3.1.1. Major Components of the Skeletal System

The skeletal system plays a significant role in offering structural support, defending against vital organs, and enabling movement within the human body. Consisting mainly of bones, cartilage, ligaments, and tendons, every element plays an integral part in ensuring body integrity and function overall. Bones form the framework that provides support for the body, whereas cartilage offers padding and flexibility at the surfaces of joints, enabling more effortless movement. Ligaments connect bones to bones, providing stability in joints, and tendons connect muscles to bones, enabling the force of muscle contraction to be effectively transmitted to the skeletal system. This integrated system reflects the dynamic interaction between all the components, with each one being accountable for the essential biomechanics of human movement. Moreover, the skeletal system is also divided into two broad categories: the axial skeleton and the appendicular skeleton. The axial skeleton consists of the skull, vertebral column, and rib cage and is the central axis of the body that houses the brain, spinal cord, and thoracic organs. The appendicular skeleton consists of limbs and girdles and functions in locomotion and interaction with the environment. Such a dichotomy reflects the rich diversity of functional attributes of the skeletal elements and how these come together to support a variety of movements. The axial skeleton stabilizes and supports the center of the body, while the appendicular skeleton generates mobility and flexibility. Understanding this body structure is required to comprehend how the skeletal system functions as a cohesive unit, executing its roles of elasticity and strength (Figure 3.1).

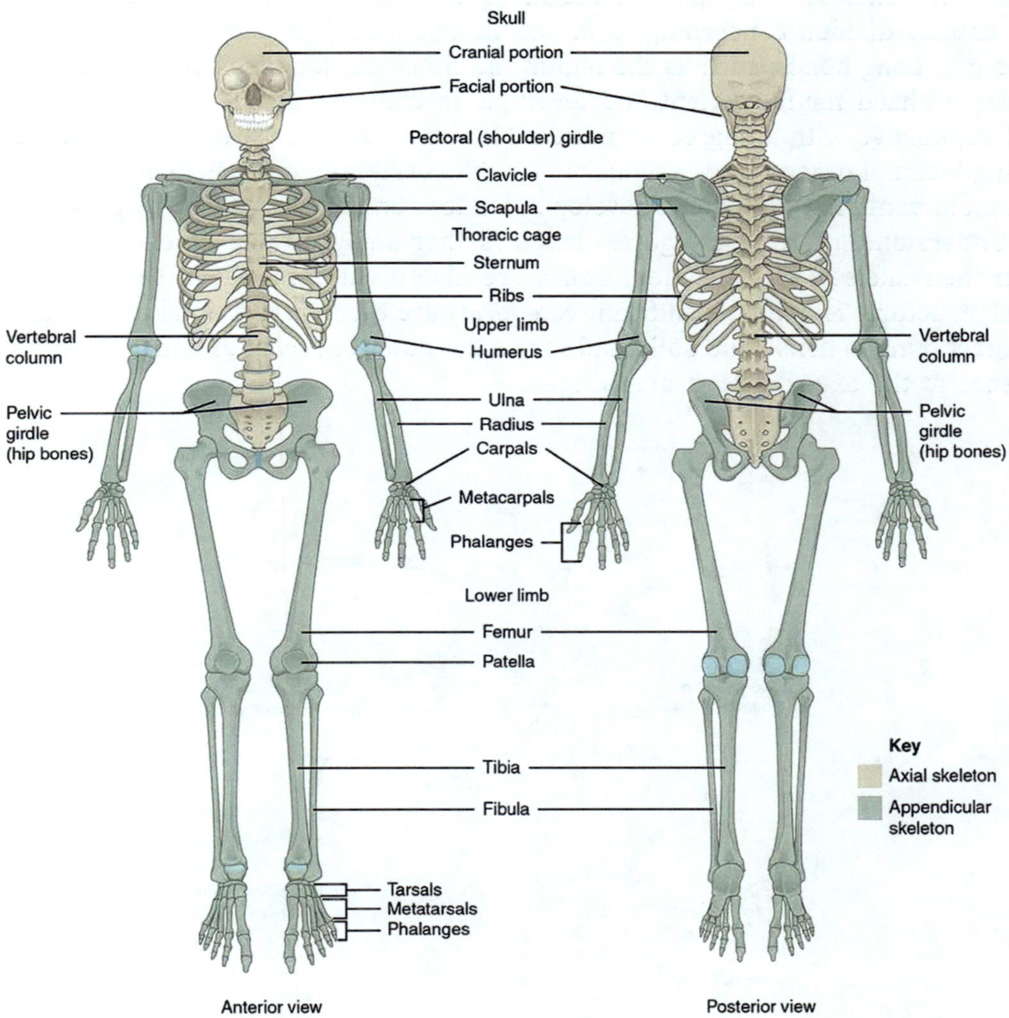

Figure 3.1. Axial skeleton and the appendicular skeleton.

Source: https://nurseslabs.com/skeletal-system/#google_vignette.

In addition, skeletal structure is not only physical; it involves biological processes essential to general well-being. Bone tissue is composed of living cells like osteocytes, osteoblasts, and osteoclasts that work to maintain, grow, and repair bones. Bones are also dynamic organs that continuously regenerate themselves based on mechanical loading and hormonal stimulation. The internal cavity of the marrow is significant for supporting hematopoiesis, or the production of blood cells, and thus directly relates the skeletal system to the circulatory system. The interdependence of the various components of the skeletal system emphasizes their mutual importance in protection, support, and enforcement of significant biological processes required in order to survive, which further speaks towards the necessity for extensive research and understanding of the skeletal system as a whole.

3.1.2. Classification of Bones

Classification of bones is a key part of acquiring the skeletal system's structure and function. Bones are usually divided concerning form and function, such as long, short, flat, irregular, and sesamoid types. Long bones, such as the femur and humerus, for instance, have a long shape and are primarily utilized for movement and leverage. In contrast, short bones like the carpals are stable and supportive with a degree of motion. Flat bones like the scapula and skull are engaged in protecting internal organs, and irregular bones like vertebrae possess many complex functions. Lastly, sesamoid bones like the patella develop in tendons and aid in reducing friction and modifying pressure. Understanding these categories helps further analyze bone functions within the body. Other than their skeletal classification, bones are also divided based on their composition and histological structure. The most significant categories are the compact and spongy (or cancellous) bone. Compact bone is dense and solid and forms the outer covering of bones, providing strength and resilience to the external pressures (Figure 3.2).

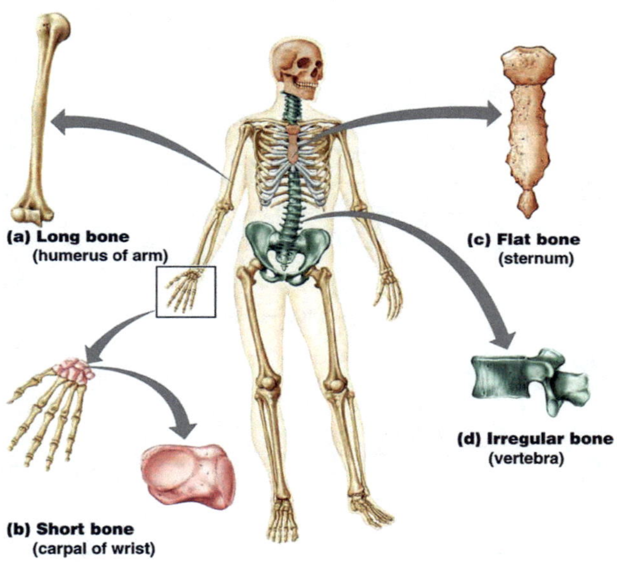

Figure 3.2. Classification of bones.

Source: https://nurseslabs.com/skeletal-system/.

It is organized into osteons, which are structural components that contain vascular canals and osteocytes. Spongy bone, on the other hand, is not as dense and is lighter and includes a network-type arrangement of framework containing bone marrow. This arrangement enhances the overall strength of bones while minimizing weight, which is essential for mobility. In addition, enhanced understanding of these compositions facilitates enhancement in medical treatments and engineering technologies for bone health and healing, as noted in bone aging research and implications for surgery and healing processes (Bagnall et al., 2014). Further, the bone classification is critical in clinical scenarios, particularly in identifying health and diagnosing disease. For instance, the distinction between the different categories of bones prescribes the procedure pursued during orthopedic treatments and surgeries. It has been established that patients with craniofacial dysmorphias exhibit unique challenges during surgery in the operating room that lead to longer stays at the hospital and complications (Allareddy et al., 2018). Practitioners can learn to modify procedures to improve outcomes for patients undergoing treatments such as orthognathic surgery by comprehending the nuances involved with each classification. Such a system of classification not only becomes a means of grasping skeletal anatomy but also a foundation of effective clinical practice and underscores the importance of bone classification in health and disease.

3.1.3. Overview of Joints and Their Functions

The human skeleton consists of an intricate system with numerous joints, each performing specific functions crucial for movement and support. Joints are functional connections between bones that facilitate flexibility and range of motion (ROM) for daily functioning. They fall into three major categories: fibrous, cartilaginous, and synovial. Fibrous joints, such as sutures on the cranium, facilitate little or no movement, thereby protecting and stabilizing cranial structures. Cartilaginous joints, such as in the vertebral column, facilitate minimal movement, to allow flexibility while maintaining structural stability. In comparison, synovial joints such as the knee and elbow are highly mobile and have a cavity in synovial fluid that serves to lubricate the joint, reduce friction, and allow tremendous versatility of movement (Shafie et al., 2016) (Figure 3.3).

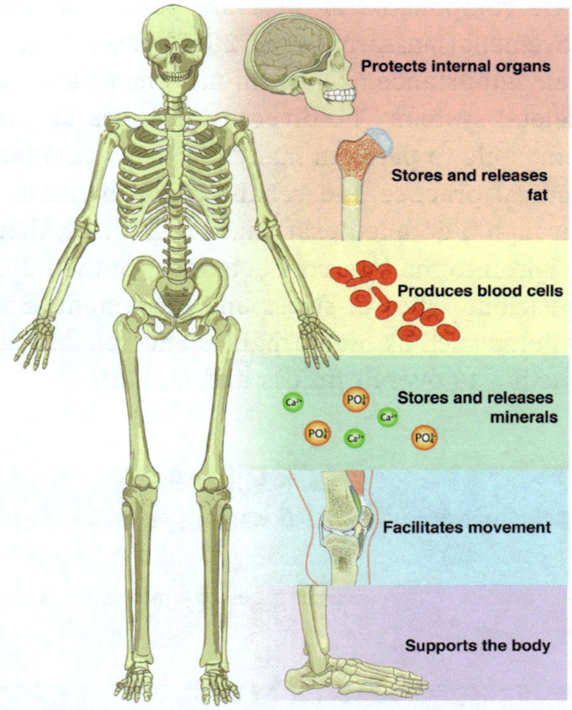

Figure 3.3. Functions of the skeletal system.

Source: https://open.oregonstate.education/app/uploads/sites/157/2019/07/mineral_storage_revised-768x938.png.

Hence, it is crucial to learn about the various types of joints in order to comprehend their functions in the skeletal system. Joints not only facilitate movement; they assist in supporting the body's weight and maintaining its posture. For example, the joint of the knee base supports the body's weight during walking, running, and jumping, which underscores its importance in locomotion and sports. In addition, some joints form the hub of load transmission between one part of the body and another, which is fundamental in successful movement. The intricacies of the joints' structure, including cartilage and ligaments, are vital for the stability and operation of the joints. Ligaments assist in connecting bones and stabilizing the joints, while cartilage lubricates the ends of the bones, a point that helps in protecting them against friction and damage. The interchangeability of these components is therefore paramount in enabling the dynamic but stable nature of human movement (Massaroni et al., 2020). Briefly put, the explanation of joints and their functions highlights their importance not just in movement but also in bearing weight and in enabling stability in the skeletal system. The diversity in types of joints is a reflection of the humanness of the body in being able to perform many physical activities. In addition, joint mechanisms are applied to teach medical practice and rehabilitation methods, particularly for injuries that affect joint function. Through a detailed examination of joints, their structure, and corresponding functions, one gains insight into the interconnectedness of the human body's systems and how they respond differently to various types of stress and movement (Shafie et al., 2016). This realization is the foundation of fields such as biomechanics and rehabilitation engineering, emphasizing the relevance of joint function to overall fitness and mobility.

Test Your Knowledge

1. How are bones classified based on their shapes?
2. What are the different types of joints, and what are their primary functions?

3.2. Functions of the Skeletal System

Learning Outcome

1. Explain the support and structure of skeletal system
2. Discuss the protection of vital organs
3. Define facilitation of movement of skeletal system

The skeleton carries out several essential functions that are fundamental to maintaining overall health and enabling body functions. Among its key is to support the structure of the body, forming the framework that gives the body its shape and enables it to move through its dynamic interaction with muscles. Bones are levers, with pivot points at the joints; this sophisticated system allows extensive movement, from simple functions like walking to intricate athletic motion. The skeletal system also aids in the protection of organs, such as the heart and lungs, which are shielded by the ribcage, and the skull that encloses and protects the brain. This role of protection emphasizes the importance of the skeletal system not only in facilitating mobility but also in sustaining the integrity of life-sustaining physiological systems. Apart from structural support and protection, the skeletal system is further tasked with the production and storage of essential substances. Bone tissue is a crucial site for hematopoiesis, where the formation of blood cells occurs in the bone marrow. This process is vital for maintaining healthy circulating blood, which is paramount in oxygen transport and immune response within the body. Furthermore, bones serve as reservoirs for minerals such as calcium and phosphorus, which are required for a variety of biochemical processes, such as maintaining the structure of cells and DNA. The regulated release of these minerals into the bloodstream provides homeostasis and facilitates essential functions like nerve impulses and muscle contractions to be carried out effectively. The dual role of the skeletal system in hematopoiesis and mineral deposition is accountable mainly for overall metabolic fitness. New evidence has also re-emphasized the role of the skeletal system in regulating vascular processes and helping with overall body homeostasis. The interlink between bone and marrow vascular niches underscores their key role in supporting stem cell function and maintaining the well-being of skeletal cell microenvironment. Bone vasculature is responsible for the delivery of nutrients and oxygen, and secretion of angiocrine factors that promote survival and self-renewal of many stem and progenitor cells. When its function becomes impaired, it may lead to serious health disorders like skeletal aging and several bone diseases. Understanding of the inter-relationship between the vascular network and the skeletal system can provide better insight into disease pathology and therapeutic potential for bone-related diseases concerning bone integrity and health, emphasizing the complexity in the function of the skeletal system as designated by recent studies in the area (Arnott et al., 2016; Chatzis et al., 2020).

3.2.1. Support and Structure

The skeletal system is the fundamental structure of the human body, and it ensures the support as well as the structural integrity required.

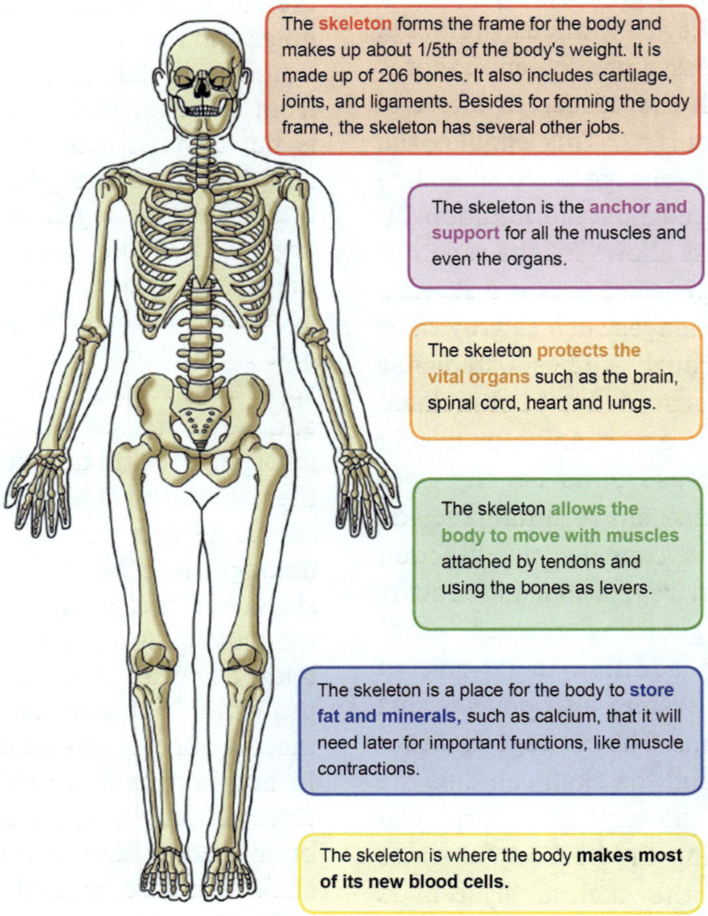

Figure 3.4. Support and structure of the skeletal system.

Source: https://www.exploringnature.org/db/view/An-Introduction-to-the-Skeletal-System.

Composed of bones, cartilage, ligaments, and tendons, the skeletal system is not only involved in posture and stability but also the facilitation of movement. Bone formation provides a stable framework that resists various forces exerted by muscles upon functioning. This integration of the muscular and skeletal systems is essential for movement, as humans are capable of performing daily functions with ease. The configuration of the skeletal system offers elasticity and dissipates the stresses of weight-bearing activities, demonstrating the delicate balance between support and mobility inherent in human biomechanics (Figure 3.4).

One of the most intriguing aspects of the skeletal system is its dynamic nature. Bones are not fixed structures; they continuously remodel under mechanical stress, a phenomenon that is accomplished through the concerted effort of osteoclasts and osteoblasts. This enables the skeletal infrastructure to change to accommodate functional demands throughout life. Additionally, the remodeling process allows for the repair of small cracks and emphasizes that the skeletal system can adapt to changes such as growth or physical training. Through studies, osteogenic activity has been demonstrated to be stimulated by mechanical loading, e.g., running or weight training, and to increase bone density over time. Moreover, in discussions regarding skeletal health, it is critical to consider the function of diet and hormonal regulation, influencing bone strength and guarding against injury and degeneration. In addition to its role of support, the skeletal system also plays a part in guarding vital organs. The rib cage encloses the heart and lungs, and the skull contains the brain, demonstrating the requisite interplay of structure and covering in the body. Besides providing covering, the skeletal system is involved in the hydraulic leverage, which facilitates more efficient movement through the joints. Ironically, the joints are composed of cartilage and ligaments, which together provide cushioning and stability along with freedom of motion. However, weakening due to age, trauma, or disease is a natural consequence, and a better understanding of how to maintain and repair skeletal function is needed. Continuous research and advances in medicine and technology aim to develop further therapeutic techniques that enhance the skeletal system's structure and operation, thereby improving overall well-being.

3.2.2. Protection of Vital Organs

The skeletal system plays a pivotal role in protecting life-critical organs throughout a series of physiological processes. Notably, the rib cage offers efficient protection to the lungs and heart, encasing them within a robust framework that minimizes potential damage from external forces. This osseous structure is not a static armor; it has an active effect and dissipates energy in the event of trauma, thereby preventing damage from reaching these organs. The intercostal muscles, found between the ribs, also contribute to the strength of this protective mechanism by allowing for expansion and contraction in the process of respiration so that the lungs can continue to function and be protected. These mechanical benefits incorporated into the skeletal system emphasize the importance of bone structure in contributing to the body's overall physical resistance to damage. Another equally significant cranial skeleton forms a covering for the brain, perhaps the most delicate and vital organ of the human body. The skull offers not merely physical shock protection but also houses several structures that are very significant to neurological function. In addition to bony shielding, the meninges, three protective layers of tissue, also shield the brain from trauma and infection. The intricate skull structure created by united bones adds strength and stability to the skull and reduces the likelihood of concussions and traumatic brain injury. Notably, abnormalities in the integrity of the skull have significant consequences, and this highlights the necessity of cautiousness regarding the preservation of bone integrity to maintain this protective apparatus. The functional interdependence of the skeletal apparatus and protection of the brain demonstrates the intricate relationship between form and function in human anatomy. The pelvis is another vital protective structure of the skeletal apparatus that safeguards the reproductive organs, bladder, and lower intestines. Its bowl-like structure provides all the necessary support and protection from external pressures and trauma, with evidence of the pelvis's evolutionary advantages. Additionally, its role in movement and balance cannot be overstated; it enables movement while ensuring the safety of these vital organs from potential damage. Its bony structure is reinforced by dense connective tissues and muscles for added protection. In this regard, the adaptability of the skeletal framework to encircling soft tissues accentuates the holistic nature of body defenses. It is thus essential that an appreciation of the skeletal system's role in safeguarding critical organs be gained to illuminate not only anatomical associations but also guide clinical practice about skeletal integrity and prevention of injury (N/A, 2025; Poudel et al., 2011).

3.2.3. Facilitation of Movement

The skeleton enables movement by creating a structure to support the body and containing muscles that will allow motion. Bones, which are held together by joints, provide rigidity that enables movement while maintaining flexibility through areas of articulation.

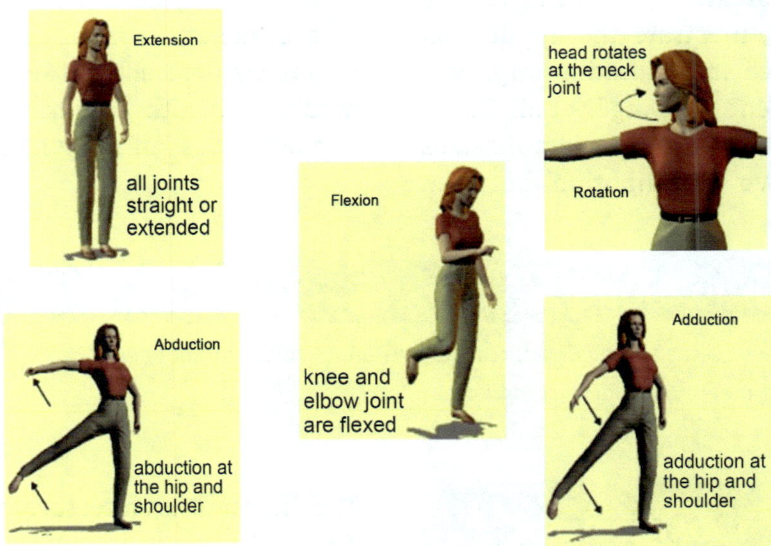

Figure 3.5. Synovial joint movement.

Source: https://present5.com/presentacii-2/20171208/9718-011_skeletal_system.ppt/9718-011_skeletal_system_38.jpg.

This movement from structure to mobility accommodates various movements ranging from delicate movements such as writing to more active movements such as running or jumping. Joints, which are differentiated based on ROM, further attest to this capability. For instance, hinge joints in the knees and elbows provide movement along one plane. In contrast, ball-and-socket joints in the hips and shoulders provide wider ROM, providing for activities that involve greater flexibility and agility. The bone and joint structural composition is thus at the forefront in the overall efficiency of the human body in facilitating movement. Muscles, which are closely linked to the skeleton, exert force on bones to produce motion. Each muscle is connected to bones with tendons, and when contracted, they tug on the skeletal system, articulating motion at a joint. This relationship between the muscular and skeletal systems is significant; it is not the presence of bones that permits movement, but the functional interaction between muscles and the skeletal system. Furthermore, advancements in movement biomechanics have highlighted the significance of functional movements that are typically applied in rehabilitation and exercise interventions. Techniques such as vibration training, potentially enhancing muscle power and balance, illustrate the application of emerging research in facilitating improved capacity for movement (Rittweger et al., 2010) (Figure 3.5). This new dialogue emphasizes the role of effective coordination between skeletal and muscular structures in order to support functional movement across various populations, particularly in rehabilitation. Interestingly, movement facilitation goes beyond mechanical interaction, involving aspects of health and well-being. A well-functioning skeletal structure supports mobility, which is essential in allowing people to maintain independence, particularly among the elderly. Evidence indicates that preventive measures and interventions regarding bone health, such as vibration exercises and resistance training, can significantly enhance bone density and muscular strength, thus reducing the risk of fractures and falls (Carnes et al., 2013). These findings highlight the relationship between movement facilitation and physical health, indicating that leading an active lifestyle is a factor that influences general health. Therefore, understanding facilitation of movement in terms of the skeletal system, as well as revealing its mechanical actions, encourages a holistic model of health comprised of diet, exercise, and awareness of body mechanics.

Test Your Knowledge

1. How does the skeletal system provide support and structure to the human body?
2. In what ways does the skeleton protect vital organs?

3.3. Bone Composition and Structure

Learning Outcome

1. Discuss the types of bone tissue
2. Explain the bone cells and their functions
3. Describe the role of minerals in bone health

The intricate architecture and composition of the bone greatly influence its function in the skeletal system. Bone tissue or osseous tissue is composed primarily of a matrix of collagen fibers, which provide tensile strength, and hydroxyapatite minerals, which provide hardness and resistance to compression. The mineral composition, being mainly calcium phosphate, is crucial to the resistance of bones to stress and to their role in the integrity of the skeleton. Cortical and trabecular bones are two principal types of bone with distinct structural characteristics. Cortical bone, dense and complex, is the outer covering of the bones, providing them with protection and stiffness. In contrast, trabecular bone, located within, is less dense with a system of struts that enhances shock absorption and flexibility. Such a dynamic structure enables bones to adapt to varying physical needs in the course of a human's life. Mechanical loading of bones also plays a vital role in shaping their structure and composition. The basis of Wolff's Law is that bone will remodel to match the loads under which it is placed; increased mechanical loading leads to bone formation, and decreased loading produces resorption. For example, individuals who engage in weight-bearing exercise have denser and stronger bones, as these exercises stimulate osteoblast activity and mineral deposition. Conversely, lack of mechanical loading, such as microgravity or prolonged periods of immobilization, can lead to pathological changes in bone structure and density. Microgravity-induced effects on spaceflight have been investigated to understand how loading conditions can redistribute bone tissue to create demineralization in certain regions while causing hypermineralization in others. The study reveals the importance of mechanical loading in maintaining the skeleton (Arnaud et al., 2025). Besides, the physiological processes of bone remodeling demonstrate the balance between bone resorption and formation as of utmost importance to the health of the skeleton. Osteoblasts that form bone and osteoclasts that resorb it simultaneously exist to maintain constant remodeling at all stages of life. Hormonal control, including parathyroid hormone and calcitonin, also controls this dynamic equilibrium, responding to the body's calcium needs. In addition, lifestyle aspects such as age, diet, and exercise can affect bone health significantly. For instance, inadequate dietary consumption of calcium or vitamin D can lead to suppression of bone growth and accelerated bone loss during aging, which in turn can lead to osteoporosis. Current studies have shown that such losses are compensable by interventions such as nutritional supplementation and exercise and can enhance bone health overall and therefore the quality of life in older persons (Fairman et al., 2018). Such intricate interrelation between composition, structure, and biological function sees the skeletal system's key function in maintaining human mobility and health.

3.3.1. Types of Bone Tissue

The skeletal system possesses the striking variability of bone tissues, each of which possesses its own structural as well as functional features. The two broad categories of bone tissue include compact bone and spongy bone. Compact bone or cortical bone is dense and acts as the outer covering of bones. It provides strength and support, contributing to resistance to compressive forces. highly organized structure, consisting of osteons or Haversian systems, is very closely packed and plays a crucial role in supplying nutrients and removing waste. Spongy bone, or cancellous bone, however, can be found in the middle regions of bones and has a porous lattice-like structure. This structure provides for efficient storage of bone marrow in which blood cell development occurs. Both of these types of bone tissue have crucial roles to play in the maintenance of the skeletal system's general integrity and functioning, allowing it to react to various stressors. Apart from their major types, bone tissues are also categorized based on composition and functions. Compact and spongy bone, for instance, both contain specialized cells responsible for the maintenance of bone and for remodeling it: osteoblasts, osteocytes, and osteoclasts. Skeletal homeostasis depends on the delicate balance between osteoblasts, which generate bone, and osteoclasts, which allow bone resorption. The dynamic nature of these cells reflects the plasticity of bone tissue to respond to physiological needs, including mechanical loading or hormonal stimulation. Not. Surprisingly, research has demonstrated that advancing our understanding of these cell mechanisms can lead to improved solutions in the treatment of MSK disorders, where diseases like degeneration or trauma harm bone structure (Adam et al., 2012) (Figure 3.6).

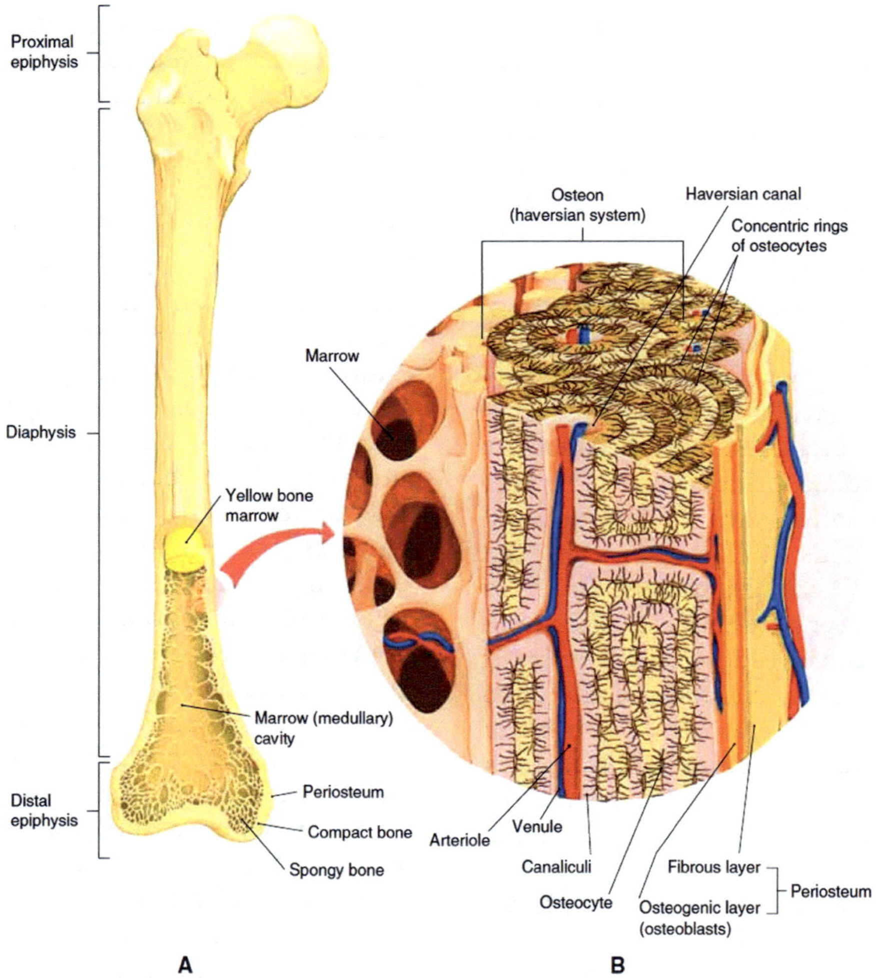

Figure 3.6. Bone tissue. (A) Femur with distal end cut in longitudinal section; and (B) Compact bone showing haversian section.

Source: https://www.brainkart.com/article/Types-of-Bone-Tissue_18679/#google_vignette.

Therefore, the relationship between the inherent nature of the different bone tissues and their cellular content underscores their significance in disease and health. The emerging breakthroughs in tissue engineering and regenerative medicine have shed new light on the areas of bone tissue types and their applications. Technologies that are based on the principles of the construction of bone tissue are being explored to identify their function in the repair and regeneration of injured skeletal tissues. These approaches usually include the construction of composite scaffolds that mimic the bone structure of the body, which is vital for smooth integration and function during clinical application. To ensure functional applications, the customized scaffolds have to incorporate heterogeneous tissue requirements, thus making them engineering challenges, such as provision of effective load-carrying function and sustaining biological compatibility (Gomez et al., 2006). With ongoing research, the confluence of material science and biology may also introduce new solutions to improve the healing potential of bone tissue, which can have promising opportunities for therapeutic interventions in the future in the context of the skeletal system.

3.3.2. Bone Cells and Their Functions

Understanding the skeletal system necessitates an in-depth exploration of the bone cells and their intricate functions. The three fundamental cell types that are accountable for bone formation and maintenance are osteoblasts, osteocytes, and osteoclasts, all playing a quintessential role in bone homeostasis. Osteoblasts contribute to bone matrix production and mineralization, enabling bones to build up and heal. These form osteoid, an organic nonmineralized matrix, which is then mineralized to hard bone tissue. The most frequent bone cells are osteocytes, which are formed by osteoblasts embedded in the mineralized matrix. As a functional ecosystem, osteocytes communicate with each other and other bone cells, making essential processes such as the regulation of calcium homeostasis and response to mechanical stress possible, for bones to be made strong and intact despite varying physical requirements. Osteoblasts and osteocytes, in addition to osteoclasts, are the major players of the remodeling process in the skeletal system. They are composed of multinucleated large cells that have a central role in bone resorption, which is the breakdown of mineralized bone matrix (Figure 3.7).

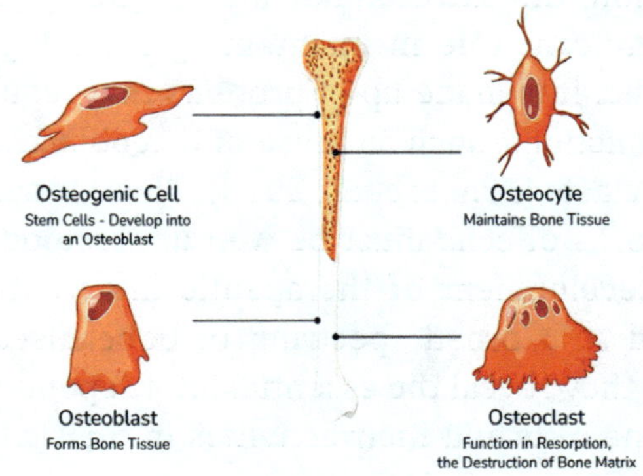

Figure 3.7. Types of bone cell.

Source: https://media.geeksforgeeks.org/wp-content/uploads/20240326131028/Types-of-Bone-Cells.webp.

Osteoclasts accomplish this by secreting bone-resorbing enzymes and acids that liberate calcium and phosphate into the circulation. This active process of bone turnover is crucial for maintaining the balance between osteoblastic bone building and osteoclastic bone resorption, a balance essential to both skeletal health and adaptation to mechanical load. This delicate balance is disrupted by a variety of bone diseases, osteoporosis among them, wherein the bones lose their density due to over-resorption. Thus it is critical to understand the function and control of bone cells for the preservation of the structure of the skeleton and overall health. In addition, the intricate interaction between the bone cells is greatly influenced by the vasculature of the bones, a critical support mechanism for bone metabolism. In addition to providing vital nutrients and oxygen, bone blood vessels also establish microenvironments that support stem and progenitor cell survival. The complex functions of bone vasculature in regulating osteogenesis and hematopoiesis have been better understood through recent research, bringing to the forefront that pathological vascular niches are the bases of skeletal aging and diseases (Chatzis et al., 2020). In addition, the extracellular matrix (ECM) plays a significant role in maintaining the integrity of bone. It is made up of proteins that regulate cell functions, such as those of osteoblasts and osteoclasts (Arnott et al., 2016). These intricate networks of cells must be well understood for the development of therapeutic interventions aimed at a broad spectrum of bone diseases since they reveal the essential interdependence of bone cells and their activities in the skeletal system.

3.3.3. The Role of Minerals in Bone Health

Minerals play a crucial role in maintaining healthy bones as structural units that serve to uphold the skeletal system's functions. Of particular mention are calcium and phosphorus because they predominantly make up hydroxyapatite, a mineral compound that gives bones hardness and stiffness.

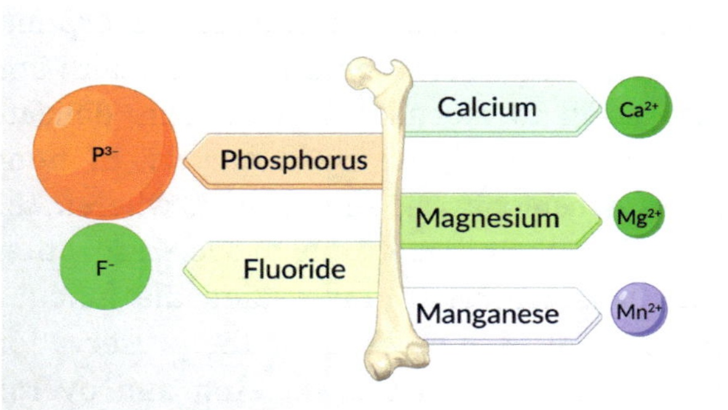

Figure 3.8. Minerals for bone health.

Source: https://www.jove.com/files/media/science-education/science-education-thumbs/14021.jpg.

Adequate consumption of these essential minerals is pivotal in the development and maintenance of bone density, particularly during growth phases in children and adolescents. Furthermore, mineral imbalances result in diseases such as osteoporosis, in which diminished bone mass increases the risk of fractures. Knowing the biochemical mechanisms involved in mineral metabolism, especially via diet and supplementation, is crucial in formulating efficient ways of encouraging superior bone health at all stages of life and preventing skeletal diseases (Figure 3.8).

In addition to calcium and phosphorus, several other minerals, such as magnesium, zinc, and fluoride, are also crucial for bone function. Magnesium, for instance, lends structural support to the bone via its role in osteoblastic activity and aids in the conversion of vitamin D to its active form so that calcium can be absorbed more easily. Zinc contributes to bone remodeling and supports collagen synthesis and other bone matrix formation. Apart from this, fluoride, introduced to dentistry, has also been suggested to strengthen bone mineralization.

The interrelationship of these minerals is complex; therefore, a deficiency in one of them can undermine the overall quality of the bone. The interplay of numerous minerals underscores the importance of adopting a holistic diet in nutrition, emphasizing the significance of proper diet in maintaining healthy bone architecture throughout life. Existing studies have centered on how environmental conditions affect mineral metabolism, such as changes under the conditions of space travel, for example. Results from research indicate that astronauts experience profound changes in bone mineral content due to the absence of gravitational stress, with greater bone loss and calcium excretion (Schneider et al., 2025).

This phenomenon highlights the significance of understanding bone loss mechanisms, emphasizing the need for adequate development of countermeasures to safeguard bone density following prolonged exposure to microgravity. Besides, anthropogenic influence studies, i.e., radionuclide exposure, have demonstrated the possible utility of bone mineral content in reconstructing ancient environmental conditions and potential health threats following death (Cook et al., 2014). These results illustrate the multifaceted function of minerals in not only sustaining bone health but also as an informative source for both current-day health assessment and previous research.

Test Your Knowledge

1. What are the different types of bone tissue, and how do they differ in structure?
2. What are the main types of bone cells, and what functions do they perform?

3.4. Development and Growth of Bones

Learning Outcome

1. Explain the bone formation processes
2. Describe factors influencing bone growth
3. Understand the changes in the skeletal system with age

Bone growth and development are dynamic and complex processes that start during fetal life and continue through early adulthood. The early fetus's skeleton is constituted primarily of cartilage, which gradually matures to become bone using a process known as endochondral ossification. This is an extremely significant alteration since it allows bones to grow in length. Mechanical stress due to fetal movements is a substantial component in this process and is known to influence the structure and alignment of bone. Limited fetal movements have been found to lead to developmental deformities, such as dysplasia of the hip and arthrogryposis, establishing the role of biomechanics in the development of the skeleton (Nowlan et al., 2015). During this period, uterine conditions, including levels and space of amniotic fluid, have significant impacts on the fetus's capacity to move freely and thus affect bone development. With maturation of the adult, bone growth takes place through modeling and remodeling. Bone modeling is a modification in the form of the bone, which is essential when growth is happening at a fast rate. In contrast, remodeling is significant for bone integrity and strength maintenance throughout life. Osteoblasts and osteoclasts are the two primary cells that are involved in such actions. Osteoblasts build new bone tissue, while osteoclasts degrade old bone, allowing a properly balanced equilibrium to ensure bone health. Nutrition and exercise also have an essential role because appropriate calcium nutrition and weight-bearing exercise are required for maximum bone density and development. Hormonal effects, particularly growth hormone and sex steroids, also cause bone formation and thus make skeletal maturity synchronous with total physical and hormonal growth throughout childhood (Stark et al., 2013). In adult life, bone density reaches its peak in the late twenties but begins to decline due to the natural aging process. This reduction can result in diseases like osteoporosis, in which bones are more porous and prone to fractures. Knowledge of the temporal dynamics of bone development and factors controlling bone development processes is critical for creating treatments to maintain sound bones and prevent bone diseases. Advances in medicine and technology over the past decade have encouraged research in pharmacological methods that could replicate hormonal effects on bone or increase the mechanical properties of available bone tissue. Secondly, a complete understanding of mechanical and biological interaction in bone development can lead to improved treatments for disorders resulting from defective bone growth or bone density issues, which is a key juncture between developmental biology and clinical practice in the field of orthopedics (Nowlan et al., 2015).

3.4.1. Bone Formation Processes

Bone formation, or ossification, is a complex physiological process that is necessary for the growth and maintenance of the skeletal system. It occurs primarily by two distinct mechanisms: intramembranous and endochondral ossification.

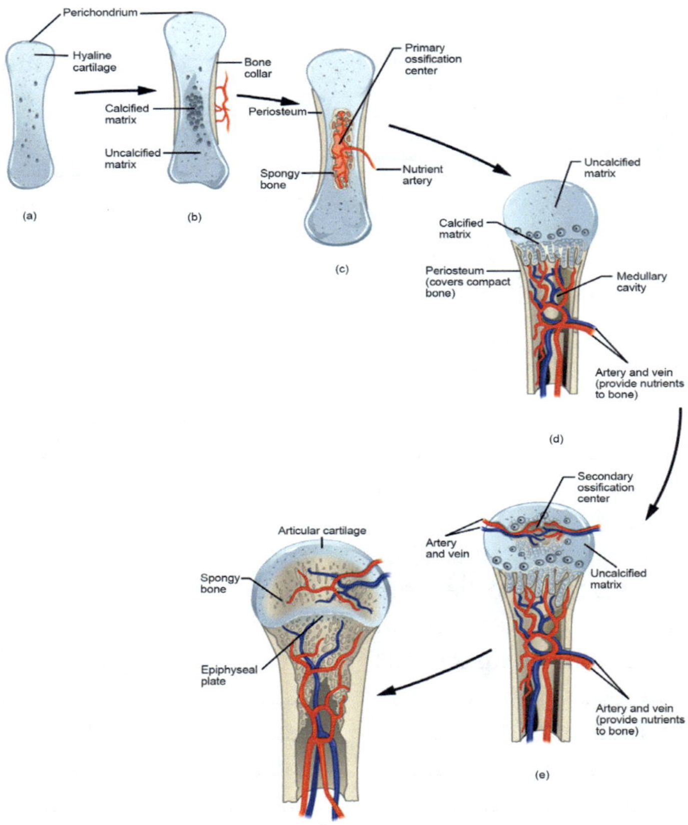

Figure 3.9. Endochondral ossification follows five steps. (a) Mesenchymal cells differentiate into chondrocytes that produce a cartilage model of the future bony skeleton; (b) Blood vessels on the edge of the cartilage model bring osteoblasts that deposit a bony collar; (c) Capillaries penetrate cartilage and deposit bone inside cartilage model, forming primary ossification center; (d) Cartilage and chondrocytes continue to grow at ends of the bone while medullary cavity expands and remodels; (e) Secondary ossification centers develop after birth; and (f) Hyaline cartilage remains at epiphyseal (growth) plate and at joint surface as articular cartilage.

Source: https://open.oregonstate.education/aandp/chapter/6-4-bone-formation-and-development/.

Intramembranous ossification gives rise to flat bones, such as those that form the skull, by direct transformation of mesenchymal tissue to bone. In contrast, endochondral ossification is the mechanism through which bone tissue substitutes hyaline cartilage, and this happens to a great degree in the formation of long bones. The two processes are intensely regulated by vascularization and the coordinated activity of various cell types, such as osteoblasts, osteoclasts, and chondrocytes, to facilitate proper mineralization and structural integrity of the skeleton. In addition to these important ossification processes, bone tissue exhibits remarkable environmental responsiveness. Mechanical loading and changes in gravity significantly influence bone formation and resorption. For instance, research has established that reduced weight-bearing conditions, such as those that occur in space, can lead to decreased bone mineral content and structural changes in the bones. These responses are not uniform across different skeletal regions; particular changes have been noted in tissues based on their metabolic activities and composition. The femur and tibia, for example, showed differences in vascular response and mineral content during hypogravity, illustrating that the response of the skeletal system is tissue-specific and intricate (Doty et al., 2025) (Figure 3.9). The development of endogenous tissue engineering methods further supports the potential for the application of the body's intrinsic regenerative capabilities in bone formation. Current techniques seek to leverage a patient's cells, thereby reducing complications of exogenous cell transplantation, such as cost, risk, and cellular compatibility (Adam et al., 2012). Through the activation of osteoblast precursor cell activity and optimization of the physiological conditions, researchers try to maximize endogenous repair processes and the efficiency of bone regeneration. This focus on endogenous repair processes is a significant breakthrough in the field that can be used to develop new therapies for MSK disorders while proving the dynamic adaptability of the skeleton in sustaining homeostasis and facilitating recuperation.

3.4.2. Factors Influencing Bone Growth

Bone growth is a polyfactorial process regulated by several intrinsic and extrinsic factors. The fundamental rudiments are genetic predisposition, where specific genes regulate functions like osteoblast activity and bone remodeling.

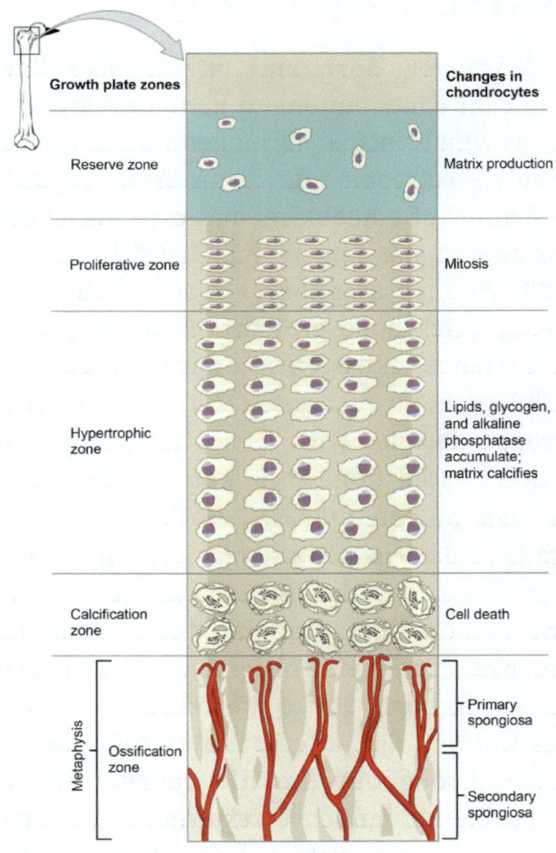

Figure 3.10. The epiphyseal plate is responsible for longitudinal bone growth.

Source: https://open.oregonstate.education/aandp/chapter/6-4-bone-formation-and-development/.

Nutrition also plays a crucial role; correct intake of calcium and vitamin D is required for sufficient mineralization of bones. Insufficient amounts of calcium might hinder bone growth, resulting in disorders like rickets in children. Besides, body exercise significantly increases bone density and strength because weight-bearing exercises stimulate an osteogenic response. This intricate interaction demonstrates the mechanism by which genetic, nutritional, and lifestyle factors synergize to define health outcomes for the bone structure. Therefore, understanding of these aspects is fundamental in developing strategies of enhancing good bones and preventing disorders of bone linked with poor bone development (Figure 3.10).

Moreover, hormonal effects also have significant contributions to bone development and growth. Principal hormones such as growth hormone, estrogen, and testosterone regulate the actions of osteoblasts and osteoclasts and thus affect bone density and skeletal integrity. Sex hormones at puberty reach their peak, driving quick bone growth and development. For instance, estrogen is bone-protective by inhibiting bone resorption. Since the level of estrogen declines with menopause, there can be accelerated bone loss, and this increases the risk of osteoporosis. Both insulin and parathyroid hormones also play a role in calcium homeostasis, and that is necessary for optimal bone health. Understanding these hormonal influences can provide insight into bone density changes throughout the life course and guide interventions that attempt to sustain skeletal health throughout the life course. Finally, environmental influences external to the body also play a strong role in bone formation. For example, physical exercise is crucial, since research has established that inactivity can lead to lower bone density. On the other hand, regular performance of resistance and weight-bearing exercises increases the density of bones and lowers the risk of fracture. Exposure to sunlight also affects vitamin D production, which is responsible for calcium absorption and, therefore, has a favorable effect on bone density. Recent research has also linked metabolic disorders such as obesity to changes in bone density. Chiesa et al. (2017) published a correlation of bone health and non-alcoholic fatty liver disease (NAFLD), suggesting that metabolic syndromes have the potential to cause a cascade effect on the skeleton. These publications indicate the need to adopt a multidisciplinary approach in studying variables that influence bone development, recognizing the multidimensional nature of bone health (Augello et al., 2010).

3.4.3. Changes in the Skeletal System with Age

The process of aging profoundly influences the skeletal system and leads to a series of morphological and functional alterations. With increasing age, bone density typically decreases as a consequence of a loss of bone mass, which makes bones susceptible to fractures. Loss is, in part, caused by hormonal changes such as decreased levels of estrogen in postmenopausal women that influence mechanisms of bone remodeling. Furthermore, the bone system also experiences a decline in collagen and other elements of the ECM, which are essential for bone strength and resilience. These age-related variations not only compromise structural integrity but also make individuals more susceptible to diseases such as osteoporosis and osteopenia. Thus, it is essential to understand such modifications to create preventative programs and interventions that will maintain skeletal health in the elderly, hence enhancing their quality of life. In addition, the interaction between muscle and bone status is more evident with advancing age. Muscle mass loss, or sarcopenia, has a profound effect on the skeletal system. This condition is characterized by a reduction in the number of motor units and atrophy of the muscle fibers, particularly the type II fibers, which are necessary for explosive strength and stability. Progressive loss of muscle mass over time causes impaired functional strength and heightened risk of falls, particularly after the sixth decade of life, with the rate of loss increasing exponentially. This interdependence highlights the importance of frequent physical activity, as regular resistance training can reverse some of the adverse effects associated with aging. Despite the existence of disrupted exercise-induced signaling due to age, physical exercise benefits remain robust and profoundly influential in preserving muscle and bone health. They are therefore a foundation for healthy aging interventions (Malone et al., 2016) (Figure 3.11).

In addition to muscle wastage, the skeletal system also suffers from biochemical and cellular changes with advancing age. Redox homeostasis disruption, for instance, results in faulty cellular signaling, which plays a critical role in the healthful development and upkeep of bone. The age-related changes resulting from oxidative stress also affect not only muscle tissue but also bone metabolism, with resultant impaired bone formation and increased bone resorption. In addition, senescent gene expression changes may alter the pathways that regulate skeletal integrity and contribute further to bone density and quality loss. It is essential to elucidate these intricate molecular pathways to create targeted interventions that can enhance the strength and function of the skeleton as individuals age. By further investigating the processes underlying such changes, scientists can better guide public health programs and clinical interventions aimed at maximizing life-long skeletal health and preventing age-related bone disease (Ptitsyn et al., 2009).

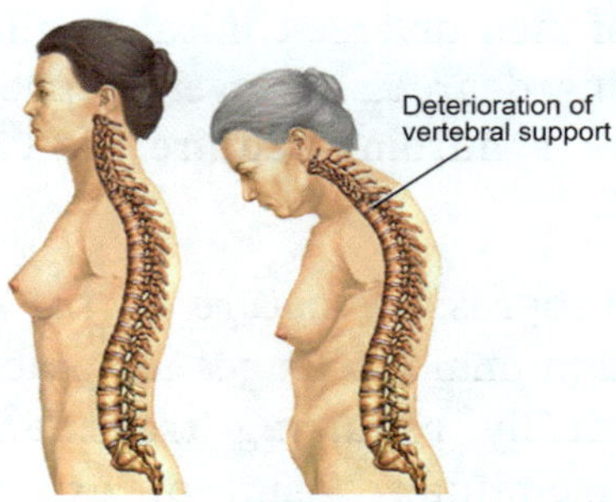

Figure 3.11. Aging changes in the bones.

Source: https://ssl.adam.com/graphics/images/en/17287.jpg.

Test Your Knowledge

1. What are the primary processes involved in bone formation?
2. How does the skeletal system change as a person ages?

3.5. Common Skeletal Disorders

Learning Outcome

1. Understand osteoporosis and its impact
2. Define arthritis and joint health
3. Explain the fractures and healing processes

The skeletal system, while primarily designed for support and movement, can suffer from a variety of disorders that disrupt its regular function. Common skeletal disorders have varied issues, impacting the general health and quality of life of the patient. Osteoarthritis (OA) is one such extremely prevalent condition, which is characterized by cartilage breakdown and the underlying bone, leading to pain, stiffness, and reduced mobility. This degenerative joint disease most commonly affects weight-bearing joints such as the knees and hips. Osteoporosis, where there is decreased bone mass and a heightened risk of fracture, is also one of the primary risks, particularly among older persons. Interaction between lifestyle factors such as diet and physical activity and hereditary predispositions leads to these disorders, which require an integrated approach to prevention as well as therapy. Morquio A syndrome is a rare lysosomal storage disorder that demonstrates how skeletal disorders may be linked with complex systemic features, too. The disease causes a variety of skeletal and joint deformities, along with significant non-skeletal complications like respiratory distress and cardiac disease. Because of their diverse clinical manifestations and varying degrees of severity, people with Morquio A syndrome require individualized treatment.

The progressive nature of the disorder creates additional challenges for practitioners, most typically requiring treatments from a multidisciplinary team of experts such as geneticists, orthopedic surgeons, and pulmonologists. Such whole-person management is critical to optimize patient outcomes and quality of life in individuals with this disorder (Berger et al., 2014). Greater understanding of fetal movement and its relationship with bone development underscores the importance of mechanical forces in skeletal development. It has been established through studies that normal fetal movement plays a crucial role in the normal formation of the skeleton because unusual or reduced movements have led to developmental disorders such as arthrogryposis and hip dysplasia. The mechanical environment for the fetus, based on amniotic fluid volume and fetal position, plays a significant role in movement ability and consequent skeletal formation. Hence, making the biomechanical aspects of fetal movements a reality opens doors to applying early interventions for compromised movement. Not only does it enhance our understanding of skeletal development, but it also informs clinical practice to reduce the occurrence of skeletal malformations (Nowlan et al., 2015).

3.5.1. Osteoporosis and Its Impact

Osteoporosis is a significant public disease, particularly among the elderly, that is characterized by increasing bone density and strength loss. It significantly increases the risk of fracture, which can cause severe morbidity and a decrease in the quality of life. When the support of the skeletal system decreases, impaired patients typically experience disabling pain and loss of independence, illustrating the extent to which osteoporosis may disable one. Osteoporosis, in America, is estimated to affect millions of Americans, primarily postmenopausal women, fundamentally altering the progression of their health. Systemic osteoporosis needs an overall understanding of both its physical and socio-economic implications, as the healthcare cost associated with fractures due to osteoporosis is high and is continually escalating as aging takes hold of society.

The pathophysiology of osteoporosis is a complex interplay of the activities of osteoblasts and osteoclasts, bone-building and bone-destructive cells, respectively. An imbalance in this equilibrium can lead to reduced bone mineral content, rendering bones porous and weak. Hormonal disturbance, for example, in the reduction in estrogen levels in women after menopause, is the key factor in the progression of this disorder. Furthermore, lifestyle factors—namely, insufficient exercise, poor diet, and excessive alcohol intake—tend to exacerbate the risk factors for osteoporosis. More recent research indicates that interventions supporting routine weight-bearing exercise and dietary enhancements can improve bone health, specifically through the preservation of a sound body composition. For instance, the regulation of osteoblast function concerning weight control may yield promising results in maintaining skeletal integrity, calling for comprehensive health approaches (Baldari et al., 2016) (Figure 3.12).

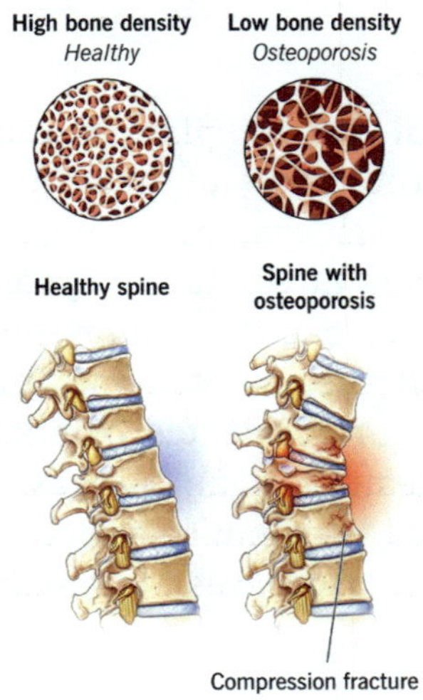

Figure 3.12. If you have osteoporosis your bones are much more fragile and weaker than they should be.

Source: https://nurseslabs.com/skeletal-system/#google_vignette.

Furthermore, osteoporosis is also complicated by overall metabolic disease states, adding to the intricacy of treatment. Of particular interest is the relationship between obesity and bone, indicating how excess body weight influences osteoblast function and bone remodeling processes. Existing evidence shows that active obese individuals are more likely to maintain their bone density compared to inactive obese individuals, hence suggesting that lifestyle changes can reverse the detrimental effect of obesity on the skeleton (Ajbage et al., 2015). This suggests a feedback mechanism where increased physical well-being not only enhances skeletal robustness but ultimately improves general well-being. Thus, treatment of osteoporosis not only encompasses attention towards pharmacological therapies but also commitment to lifestyle alteration that strengthens the bones and prevents future exacerbations, showing the multifaceted nature necessary for effective treatment of this widespread disease.

3.5.2. Arthritis and Joint Health

The complex interaction of many factors is a major contributor to arthritis and joint health, which are central to the skeletal system.

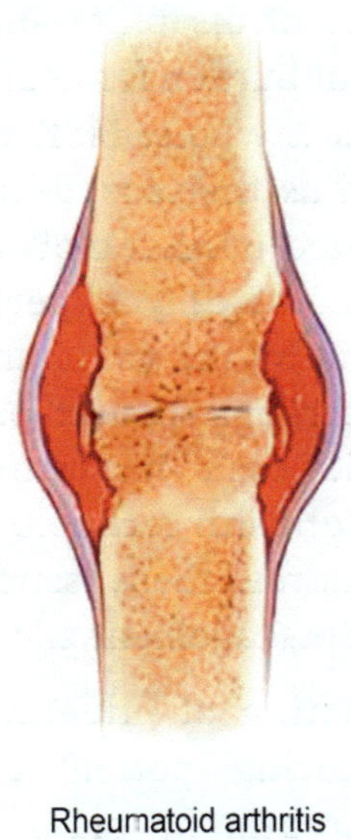

Figure 3.13. Rheumatoid arthritis.

Source: https://www.mayoclinic.org/diseases-conditions/arthritis/symptoms-causes/syc-20350772#dialogId12996992.

Arthritis is made up of over 100 distinct disorders, and the two most frequent are OA and rheumatoid arthritis (RA). OA, in which cartilage and underlying bone loss typically result from wear and tear with aging. Conversely, RA is an autoimmune disease that results in inflammation and joint deterioration due to the body's immune reaction against its tissues. Progress has identified the role of autophagy, which is a cellular process involved in the recycling of parts, in the control of immune reactions associated with RA. This autophagic process deregulation has been implicated in the pathophysiology of numerous autoimmune diseases, underlining the significance of an appreciation of such processes in ensuring that arthritis management is adequately carried out (Alessandri et al., 2018) (Figure 3.13).

Joint health is at the core of mobility and overall well-being, particularly among populations with MSK disorders. Arthritis is a leading cause of disability and chronic pain and a significant burden for healthcare systems and society as a whole. MSK disorders have been classified as the second-highest cause of morbidity-related burden globally. The impact of arthritis is not only experienced by the patient but also by the community and family of the patient through reduced productivity and increased health costs. Innovative care models incorporating eHealth technologies have been proposed to address these issues and enhance MSK condition management, including arthritis.

The utilization of eHealth can facilitate remote monitoring, patient education, and tailor-made treatment plans that improve outcomes with minimal burden on healthcare resources (Andrew et al., 2016). In managing joint health, it is essential to institute a multifaceted intervention covering prevention and management. Regular exercise as much as an individual can handle, together with an anti-inflammatory nutrient-rich diet, might decrease the risk of developing arthritis. Education about protecting one's joints and self-management also empowers individuals to take control of their health. The recent advances in therapy in the form of biologics and DMARDs are significant milestones for treating RA and preserving joint function. By integrating these therapies with lifestyle modification and eHealth technologies, healthcare providers can generate an integrated paradigm intended to enhance the quality of life of arthritis patients and support improved joint health, ultimately supporting long-term skeletal well-being.

3.5.3. Fractures and Healing Processes

The skeletal system plays a crucial role in providing the body of human beings with continuity and mechanical support, and fractures pose a serious threat to the system. Fractures tend to happen because of high-impact trauma, repetitive stress, or systemic bone disease, and create various levels of discontinuity in bones. Thereafter, healing processes take place, characterized by a multi-aspectual interaction of biological processes to re-establish bone continuity.

The first step is the inflammatory response, which offers the route for the accumulation of hematoma and signaling molecules to attract necessary cells to the fracture site. The inflammatory stage is critical because it is the foundation for the subsequent healing stages and speeds up tissue regeneration and remodeling, as it epitomizes the body's marvelous ability to regenerate after injury. As the healing process continues, there is a series of defined stages, including the hard and soft callus stages. During the soft callus stage, granulation tissue is formed, later to be replaced by a cartilage-like matrix, serving as a temporary scaffold for bone healing. This phase is an essential step for stabilizing the fracture and enabling new blood vessels to infiltrate the area, hence enhancing the supply of oxygen and nutrients needed for tissue regeneration. The transition to hard callus stage entails transformation of this cartilage into mineralized bone, which is regulated by osteoblasts that are specialized cells (Figure 3.14).

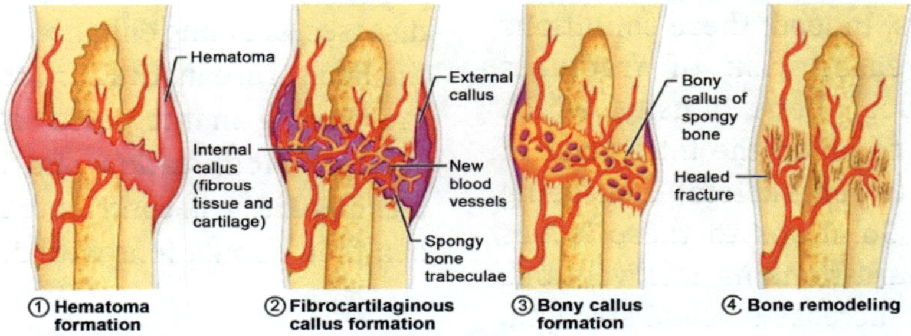

Figure 3.14. Fracture healing.

Source: https://upload.orthobullets.com/topic/9009/images/fractue%20healing.jpg.

In this multifaceted change, there is a requirement for angiogenesis, or new blood vessel formation, indicating that it plays a critical role in healing at the cellular level, as research on the role of such processes in skeletal regeneration has indicated (Lam et al., 2016). The employment of tissue engineering, however, has in recent years explored new approaches to fracture healing and regeneration. Conventional methods are generally marred by challenges in their lengthy ex vivo cultures of autologous cells and the hazards associated with transplanting foreign cells. There has thus been a move to endogenous tissue engineering techniques, which leverage the natural regenerative capacity of the body and aim to exploit the patient's cells to heal tissues. These strategies try to overcome the limitations of traditional methods by stimulating the body's repair mechanisms without employing an enormous range of exterior interventions. It is crucial for the comprehension of these new strategies to plan future therapy for enhancing the repair process and facilitating successful recovery of fractures in MSK tissues (Adam et al., 2012).

Test Your Knowledge

1. What is osteoporosis, and how does it affect bone health?
2. How does arthritis impact joint function and mobility?

3.6. The Skeletal System in Health and Disease

Learning Outcome

1. Explain the importance of nutrition for bone health
2. Understand the exercise and its effects on the skeletal system
3. Define preventative measures for skeletal disorders

The skeletal system is a vital infrastructure of the human body and is tasked with structural support, enabling movement, and protecting internal organs. It is composed of bones, cartilage, ligaments, and tendons that together achieve a myriad of body functions. In good health, the skeletal system remodels itself continuously, which keeps the rate of activity of osteoblasts and osteoclasts in equilibrium to allow for metabolic demands as well as mechanical stresses. However, many factors, such as lifestyle, dietary deficiencies, and age, will disrupt this equilibrium, leading to diseases such as osteoporosis. Indeed, these conditions present with increased risk of fractures as a result of reduced bone density, which highlights the need to grasp the intricacies of the relationship between skeletal well-being and overall health. Solutions to these issues in the form of forward-thinking interventions can reduce risk and increase skeletal strength. Although skeletal diseases usually result from changes that occur with aging, they may also be caused by numerous non-age-related processes, including genetic factors and lifestyles. For instance, sedentary living with gluttony would exacerbate the loss of bone and muscle, leading to cumulative skeletal frailties. Motor unit losses and muscle fiber atrophy, especially the type II fibers, contribute significantly to increased risk of falling as well as related fractures, mostly in older people. This loss of functional strength and power, beginning gradually but compounded leaps and bounds after the sixth decade of life, calls for caution and prudent preventive measures. Regular exercise, especially progressive resistance training, has been shown to reverse these untoward effects, maintaining muscle mass and bone density, both of which are crucial for the preservation of mobility and independence (Malone et al., 2016). In addition, the significance of an integrative approach to skeletal health cannot be stressed enough. The interaction between diet components, exercise, and medicinal therapy characterizes the optimal strategy for the prevention and management of skeletal disease. Adequate intake of nutrients such as calcium and vitamin D is mandatory, since these nutrients are essential to bone remodeling and health. Furthermore, improving medical knowledge provides insight into the multifaceted nature of disease and health, highlighting the importance of tailored healthcare practice. For instance, systems of medical knowledge can support the diagnosis of diseases of the MSK system through the association of patient symptoms with potential diseases, enabling enhanced decision-making for the healthcare institution (Minchin et al., 2006). Prioritizing an integrated solution that includes lifestyle modification and innovative medical technologies will contribute to improved skeletal health in populations with diverse backgrounds.

3.6.1. Importance of Nutrition for Bone Health

Nutrition is also accountable for maintaining optimal bones because bone structure relies on a synergy of nutrients for growth and bone density. Nutrients like vitamins and minerals, calcium, and vitamin D play a considerable role in bone mineralization and the structural skeleton. Calcium is the principal building element of bone tissue, while vitamin D facilitates the intestinal absorption of calcium and consequently its integration into bone matrix. Inadequate intake of these nutrients leads to disrupted bone mineralization, further increasing the risk of osteoporosis and fractures later on. Moreover, adequate nutrition aids the repair and remodeling needed in maintaining healthy bones throughout life. Nutritional nuances must be known to achieve lifelong skeletal health and the avoidance of age-related bone disorders (Figure 3.15).

Current research observes the role of lifestyle, including diet, on bone health, particularly in those who suffer from obesity. Research suggests that obese individuals with a sedentary lifestyle can have their osteoblast function altered, leading to diminished bone mineral density and bone strength. However, by adopting a good diet and exercise routine, these detrimental effects can potentially be reversed. For instance, a weight-bearing exercise program, accompanied by higher intakes of nutrient-rich foods that are high in calcium and vitamins, promotes better osteoblast function as well as general skeletal health. Such an intervention can promote adaptive benefits, which means that nutrition not only plays a vital role in bone structure but also in metabolic health related to obesity (Baldari et al., 2016).

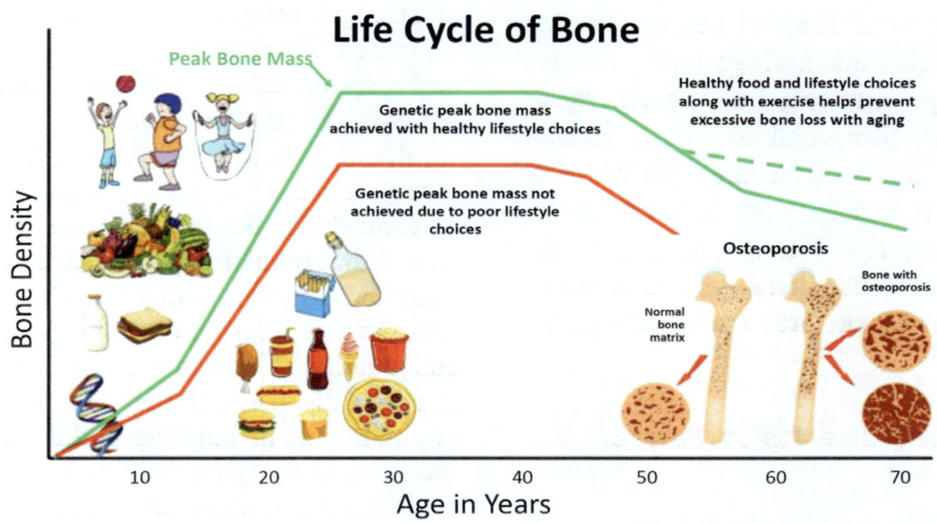

Figure 3.15. Lifelong nutrition for healthy bones.

Source: https://spinehealth.org/article/lifelong-nutrition-for-healthy-bones/.

Therefore, addressing nutrition in the context of bone health potentially offers significant therapeutic possibilities, particularly in those at great risk for osteoporosis and resultant complications. Further, the interface between diet and bone health is not simply at the level of the straightforward ingestion of isolated nutrients. Fresh evidence is that an overall dietary approach, encompassing a broad array of micronutrients and macronutrients, is paramount to optimizing bone health. Dietary regimens incorporating whole foods, such as fruits, vegetables, lean meats, and healthy fats, provide a synergistic effect contributing to bone metabolism.

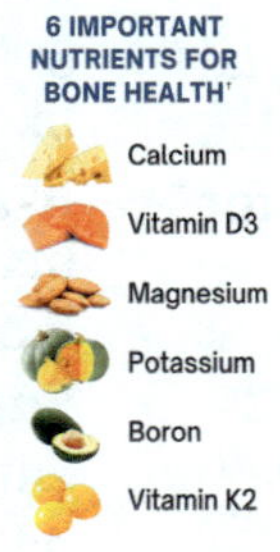

Figure 3.16. Six essential nutrients for maintaining bone health.

Source: https://external-content.duckduckgo.com/iu/?u=https%3A%2F%2Fcdn.shopify.com%2Fs%2Ffiles%2F1%2F0010%2F0250%2F4310%2Ffiles%2F6_important_nutrients_for_bone_health.png%3Fv%3D1664297577&f=1&nofb=1&ipt=fca2a1266e9514c659425f38bbd7f8397cc20392e7268d4609d8b7dd8d97f62d.

Nutrient interactions, such as the role of magnesium and zinc in calcium metabolism and the activity of antioxidants in reducing oxidative stress in bone cells, illustrate the complexity of achieving optimal skeletal health via diet. Additionally, nutrition interventions provided to the target populations, i.e., the elderly or individuals with chronic illnesses, can further enhance bone health outcomes (Fairman et al., 2018). Overall, these results reinforce the necessity of complete dietary planning in the development of robust skeletal structures and the prevention of skeletal maladies (Figure 3.16).

3.6.2. Exercise and Its Effects on the Skeletal System

Engagement in regular physical exercise is essential to the improvement of skeletal health and the insulation of the negative effects of aging on the skeleton.

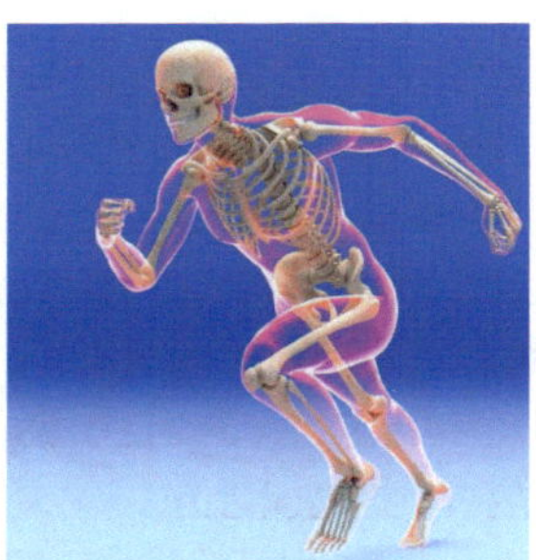

Figure 3.17. Illustration of the human skeletal system in motion, highlighting the interaction between bones and muscles essential for mobility and structural support.

Source: https://external-content.duckduckgo.com/iu/?u=https%3A%2F%2Fwww.thoughtco.com%2Fthmb%2FwJNPNSaSEF5cdBZ02rdfQ5mqwnQ%3D%2F1500x1000%2Ffilters%3Afill(auto%2C1)%2Fskeletal_sys-5bd5e9fac9e77c00267ae289.jpg&f=1&nofb=1&ipt=06fa547336f752d4f66bdf807a0826d5b4d60691c5576fa052e65e5fef518f11.

Exercise stimulates bone remodeling, a process through which old bone is replaced by new bone material, which keeps the skeleton strong and intact. Weight-bearing exercise, such as running or strength training, places mechanical stress on bones, which in turn stimulates osteocytes and osteoblasts to construct bone density and formation. The process of adaptation is significant, particularly as individuals age older, as major losses of bone density lead to conditions like osteoporosis. Studies have shown that regular physical exercise is a critical intervention to minimize age-associated bone loss and thus improve overall skeletal well-being and quality of life across the lifespan, which is especially true for the risk-exposed elderly population as highlighted in the background of the process of aging and exercise adaptations as discussed in literature (Malone et al., 2016) (Figure 3.17).

3.6.3. Preventative Measures for Skeletal Disorders

Preventive measures against skeletal disorders are essential in minimizing the risk of diseases like osteoporosis, arthritis, and scoliosis. A preventive approach begins with maintaining proper nutrition, such as the intake of calcium and vitamin D, which play essential roles in bone health. A main component of bone health is calcium, which is found in dairy products, leafy greens, and fortified foods, and vitamin D aids in calcium absorption and bone mineralization. Regular physical activity, particularly weight-bearing exercises, is also significant in the maintenance of strong bones and density. Engaging in strength training and aerobics enhances not only muscular support to bones but also balance, which plays a significant role in preventing falls and subsequent fractures. The combination of proper diet and exercise forms a sound basis for skeletal health and longevity, ultimately reducing the prevalence of skeletal disorders over time. In addition to diet and exercise, lifestyle modifications are also critical in avoiding skeletal disorders. Abstinence from smoking and limited alcohol consumption are particularly crucial as both these habits have been linked with reduced bone density and increased risk of fracture. Nicotine and heavy alcohol intake interfere with the uptake of calcium into the body and also affect hormone levels that regulate bone metabolism negatively. Secondly, maintaining a healthy body weight is crucial; being underweight can lead to osteoporosis, and overweight status can further exacerbate joint stress. Routine screening of general health that monitors bone condition is also vital, especially in those at higher risk due to family history or previous trauma. Early identification of probable issues can be made easier with early treatment according to individual needs by this preventive approach to health care. Lifestyle plays a crucial role, but multidisciplinary management and screening further maximize prevention against skeletal disorders. Coordination among healthcare professionals, such as primary care physicians, nutritionists, and physical therapists, can ensure an integrative strategy tailored to the specific patient's needs. For example, imposing consensus guidelines, like those for Mucopolysaccharidosis (MPS) VI, is a reflection of the need for collaborative decision-making in the management of bone health and related disorders. These guidelines span a spectrum of interventions, from enzyme replacement to recommendations for routine monitoring, demonstrating how evidence-based care can optimize patient outcomes. By promoting collaboration in the healthcare response, the topic of skeletal health and prevention is augmented, ultimately achieving a future with decreased rates of disabling skeletal disorders (Phillips et al., 2024; Akyol et al., 2019).

Test Your Knowledge

1. How does regular exercise benefit the skeletal system?
2. What are some common preventative measures for reducing the risk of skeletal disorders?

SUMMARY

The study of the skeletal system reveals that this complex structure is the basis for human locomotion, defense, and general physiological stability. The skeletal system is not just a storage for vital minerals but also has essential functions in hematopoiesis as well as supporting soft tissues. Understanding the organization and functions of the bones offers more insight into the significance of maintaining a healthy skeleton during the various phases of life. A healthy diet and exercise maintain the mechanical strength as well as bone density of the bones, thereby minimizing the risks of disorders such as osteoporosis, especially when individuals enter their elderly phase. As research goes on, it becomes increasingly evident that proactive care of the skeletal system positively affects overall well-being and longevity. The interrelationalities of the skeletal system with other bodily systems reinforce even more the critical nature of homeostasis and overall health. For instance, efficient calcium metabolism enabled through the skeletal framework is directly involved in muscle function, transmission through nerves, and even cardiovascular function. It is understandable in the context of these relations that the imperative of a health-conscious lifestyle, particularly for the young, is to prevent degenerative changes in old age during adulthood. Proper weight-bearing exercise enhances not only muscle strength but also bone remodeling, thereby making the skeletal structure stronger. To this end, skeletal health can be maintained through interventions that can considerably reduce fracture and fall occurrence, especially among the elderly, underscoring the necessity for awareness and preventive interventions throughout the population. Lastly, one must note the influence that technological and medical developments have had on the management and comprehension of skeletal disorders. Progress, such as in the development of skeletal-based action recognition models, shows promise in areas of overlap between skeletal science and computer science. The discovery of key motion patterns using sophisticated analysis techniques can potentially result in improved judgments regarding MSK health and rehabilitation plans, ultimately leading to improved clinical results for patients. Moreover, the understanding of physiological alterations with aging, such as alterations in muscle fiber composition and motor unit functioning, underscores the significance of exercise prescription in older individuals. Physical exercise is the fundamental countermeasure to the decline based on both the skeletal and muscular systems, culminating in enhanced quality of life and functional independence.

To grasp the complexity of the skeletal system, one needs to highlight its manifold functions essential for human survival and overall health. The skeletal system provides structural support, facilitates movement, and protects organs, in addition to being a location for mineral storage and hematopoiesis. Bones, as the body's framework, serve as points of attachment for muscles, facilitating locomotion as well as various complex movements. The understanding of these functions transcends mere anatomical knowledge, since in recent years technology has begun to exploit this intricate system for a variety of applications, ranging from robotics and computer vision to specialized fields like orthotics and physical therapy. The analysis of the skeletal system from these contexts can be utilized to comprehend its contribution to facilitating human activity as well as technological innovations in motion analysis and interactive systems. The incorporation of sophisticated technologies into the examination of the skeletal system has provided valuable insights that are usable across broad disciplines, especially in computer vision. Methods extracted from skeletal analysis play a key role in constructing effective models for human action recognition, which has gained prominence as a research area in artificial intelligence. Through methods that encode skeletal data as graph-based information, researchers can obtain high-level semantic representations, ultimately feeding these into strong action recognition models such as the A^{2}GNN mentioned in recent literature. This new approach not only emphasizes the role of the skeleton in human movement analysis but also enhances our capability towards building automated systems that can identify complex gestures, thereby bridging the gap between human interaction and technological reply, which is particularly significant in areas like human-computer interaction (HCI) and human-human communication (HHC). In addition, advances in skeletal system research emphasize the significance of deep learning methods like long short-term memory recurrent neural networks (LSTM-RNNs) to interpret body language and emotion detection. Analyzing gesture dynamics and motion patterns through two-dimensional and three-dimensional models, scientists are making new advances in behavioral analytics and emotional computing. These methods clarify the connection of body movements and emotional states, thereby enriching the understanding of non-verbal communication. Implementation of such networks points out their ability to model sequences over time, and hence, modeling dynamic body movements and activities is most appropriate. While the skeletal system continues to be a focal point of interest for anatomical as well as computational objectives, its interdisciplinary uses provide a framework for continued exploration into the realm of human behavior and technological impact on society while serving to accentuate the connection between biology and advanced computational techniques in the context of new research (Cui et al., 2017; Massaroni et al., 2020).

KEY TERMS FROM THIS CHAPTER

- Axial skeleton
- Compact bone
- Periosteum
- Osteon
- Osteoblast
- Bone marrow
- Ligaments
- Synovial fluid
- Articular cartilage
- Appendicular skeleton
- Spongy bone
- Endosteum
- Osteocyte
- Osteoclast
- Cartilage
- Joints
- Metaphysis
- Bone remodeling

CRITICAL THINKING QUESTIONS

1. **How many bones are there in the adult human skeleton?**
   a. 198
   b. 206
   c. 210
   d. 220
2. **Which of the following is part of the axial skeleton?**
   a. Femur
   b. Pelvis
   c. Skull
   d. Humerus
3. **The longest and strongest bone in the human body is the:**
   a. Tibia
   b. Femur
   c. Humerus
   d. Radius
4. **What type of joint is found in the shoulder and allows for a wide range of motion?**
   a. Hinge joint
   b. Pivot joint
   c. Ball-and-socket joint
   d. Gliding joint
5. **Which of the following bones protects the brain?**
   a. Sternum
   b. Vertebrae
   c. Ribs
   d. Cranium

Short Answer Questions

1. What are the two main divisions of the skeletal system, and what bones are included in each?
2. List three primary functions of the skeletal system.
3. What are the major components of bone tissue, and how do they contribute to bone strength and flexibility?
4. How do bones grow and develop from infancy to adulthood?
5. Name two common skeletal disorders and briefly describe their causes or symptoms.
6. How does the skeletal system interact with other body systems to maintain overall health?

Answer to Critical Thinking Questions

1. (b); 2. (c); 3. (b); 4. (c); 5. (d)

REFERENCES

1. Adam, C. (2011). Endogenous musculoskeletal tissue engineering - a focused perspective. *Cell and Tissue Research, 347*(3), 489–499. https://doi.org/10.1007/s00441-011-1234-2Ajbage, J. O., Heijsters, G., Politis, C., Salem, A., et al. (2015). Coronectomy of deeply impacted lower third molar: Incidence of outcomes and complications after one year follow-up. https://core.ac.uk/download/55765860.pdf (accessed on 14th June 2025).
2. Akyol, M. U., Alden, T. D., Amartino, H., Ashworth, J. L., et al. (2019). Recommendations for the management of MPS VI: Systematic evidence- and consensus-based guidance. https://core.ac.uk/download/323074857.pdf (accessed on 14th June 2025).
3. Alessandri, C., Barbati, C., Ceccarelli, F., Colasanti, T., et al. (2018). Autophagy and rheumatoid arthritis: Current knowledges and future perspectives. https://core.ac.uk/download/188823161.pdf (accessed on 14th June 2025).
4. Allareddy, V., Fletcher, S., Metalwala, Z., Okunseri, C., et al. (2018). Orthognathic surgical outcomes in patients with and without craniofacial anomalies. https://core.ac.uk/download/213086834.pdf (accessed on 14th June 2025).
5. Andrews, P. B., Ballance, P. F., Boreen, T. D., Buckeridge, J., Caron, V., Dunham, R. J., et al. (2004). Contrasting carbonate depositional systems for Pliocene cool-water limestones cropping out in central Hawke's Bay, New Zealand. https://core.ac.uk/download/29194757.pdf (accessed on 14th June 2025).
6. Arnaud, S. B., & Morey-Holton, E. (2025). Skeletal responses to spaceflight. https://core.ac.uk/download/pdf/42812904.pdf (accessed on 14th June 2025).
7. Arnott, J. A., Doane, K., & Planey, S. L. (2016). CCN family: Matricellular proteins in cartilage and bone development. https://core.ac.uk/download/322426577.pdf (accessed on 14th June 2025).
8. Augello, A., & De Bari, C. (2010). The regulation of differentiation in mesenchymal stem cells. https://core.ac.uk/download/177373.pdf (accessed on 14th June 2025).
9. Bagnall, A., & Davis, L. (2014). Predictive modelling of bone age through classification and regression of bone shapes. https://core.ac.uk/download/29107719.pdf (accessed on 14th June 2025).
10. Baldari, C., Bimonte, V. M., Di Luigi, L., Donini, L. M., et al. (2016). Physical activity and hypocaloric diet recover osteoblasts homeostasis in women affected by abdominal obesity. https://core.ac.uk/download/80310762.pdf (accessed on 14th June 2025).
11. Barrett, P. M., Butler, R. J., & Gower, D. J. (2012). Reassessment of the evidence for postcranial skeletal pneumaticity in Triassic archosaurs, and the early evolution of the avian respiratory system. https://core.ac.uk/download/12175752.pdf (accessed on 14th June 2025).
12. Baumann, C. W., Ferrington, D. A., Kwak, D., Thompson, L. V., et al. (2017). Downhill exercise alters immunoproteasome content in mouse skeletal muscle. https://open.bu.edu/bitstream/2144/40890/8/Downhill%20Exercise....accepted%20files.pdf (accessed on 14th June 2025).
13. Berger, K. I., Giugliani, R., Harmatz, P., Hendriksz, C., et al. (2014). International guidelines for the management and treatment of Moquino A syndrome. https://core.ac.uk/download/323073271.pdf (accessed on 14th June 2025).

14. Briggs, A. M., Australian and New Zealand College of Anesthetists, Barber, B., Bediang, G., Bender, J. L., Dear, B. F., Bossen, D., et al. (2016). Use of eHealth technologies to enable the implementation of musculoskeletal models of care: Evidence and practice. https://core.ac.uk/download/195654086.pdf (accessed on 14th June 2025).

15. Carnes, D., Homer, K., Pincus, T., Rahman, A., et al. (2013). Pain management for chronic musculoskeletal conditions: The development of an evidence-based and theory-informed pain self-management course. https://core.ac.uk/download/18327865.pdf (accessed on 14th June 2025).

16. Chatzis, A., Chen, J., Hendriks, M., Kusumbe, A. P., et al. (2020). Bone vasculature and bone marrow vascular niches in health and disease. https://core.ac.uk/download/346582880.pdf (accessed on 14th June 2025).

17. Chen, M., Chen, Z., Mason, D., Degener, P., Hong, S., Hormann, K., Jacobson, A., et al. (2020). Unwind: Interactive fish straightening. http://arxiv.org/abs/1904.04890 (accessed on 14th June 2025).

18. Chiesa, C., Donini, L. M., Lenzi, A., Pacifico, L., et al. (2017). Non-alcoholic fatty liver disease connections with fat-free tissues: A focus on bone and skeletal muscle. https://core.ac.uk/download/98335830.pdf (accessed on 14th June 2025).

19. Ciocci, M. C., Saldien, J., Vanderborght, B., Vandevelde, A., et al. (2013). Systems overview of Ono: A DIY reproducible open-source social robot. https://core.ac.uk/download/55820385.pdf (accessed on 14th June 2025).

20. Cook, G. T., & MacKenzie, A. B. (2014). Radioactive isotope analyses of skeletal materials in forensic science: A review of uses and potential uses. https://core.ac.uk/download/16462920.pdf (accessed on 14th June 2025).

21. Cox, J., Deshmukh, A., Mann, M., Murgia, M., et al. (2015). Deep proteomics of mouse skeletal muscle enables quantitation of protein isoforms, metabolic pathways, and transcription factors. https://core.ac.uk/download/53515988.pdf (accessed on 14th June 2025).

22. Cui, Z., Ji, R., Li, C., Xu, Y., et al. (2017). Action-attending graphic neural network. http://arxiv.org/abs/1711.06427 (accessed on 14th June 2025).

23. Doty, S. (2025). Effects of microgravity on rat bone, cartilage and connective tissues. https://core.ac.uk/download/pdf/42822714.pdf (accessed on 14th June 2025).

24. Fairman, C. M., Galvão, D. A., Hart, N. H., Kendall, M., et al. (2018). The potential therapeutic effects of creatine supplementation on body composition and muscle function in cancer. https://core.ac.uk/download/213607833.pdf (accessed on 14th June 2025).

25. Gomez, C., Shokoufandeh, A., Starly, B., Sun, W., et al. (2006). Transferring unit cell-based tissue scaffold design to solid freeform fabrication. https://core.ac.uk/download/287648706.pdf (accessed on 14th June 2025).

26. Lam, S. (2016). *Bone Growth Following Demineralized Bone Matrix Implantation Requires Angiogenesis*. https://open.bu.edu/bitstream/2144/14320/9/Lam_bu_0017N_10371.pdf (accessed on 14th June 2025).

27. Malone, J. K. (2016). *The Effects of Ageing and Exercise on Skeletal Muscle Structure and Function*. https://core.ac.uk/download/228176394.pdf (accessed on 14th June 2025).

28. Massaroni, C. (2020). *An Original Framework for Understanding Human Actions and Body Language by Using Deep Neural Networks.* https://core.ac.uk/download/296244558.pdf (accessed on 14th June 2025).

29. Matsakas, A., & Sfyri, P. (2017). Crossroads between peripheral atherosclerosis, western-type diet and skeletal muscle pathophysiology: Emphasis on apolipoprotein E deficiency and peripheral arterial disease. https://core.ac.uk/download/151162087.pdf (accessed on 14th June 2025).

30. Minchin, R. (2006). *Enriched Property Ontology for Knowledge Systems: A Thesis Presented in Partial Fulfilment of The Requirements for the Degree of Master of Information Systems in Information Systems, Massey University, Palmerston North, New Zealand.* https://core.ac.uk/download/148645462.pdf (accessed on 14th June 2025).

31. N/A. (2025). *Aerospace Medicine and Biology: A Continuing Bibliography with Indexes (Supplement 309).* https://core.ac.uk/download/pdf/42832898.pdf (accessed on 14th June 2025).

32. Nowlan, N. C. (2015). Biomechanics of fetal movement. https://core.ac.uk/download/76995826.pdf (accessed on 14th June 2025).

33. Phillips, M. C. L., & Picard, M. (2024). Neurodegenerative disorders, metabolic icebergs, and Mito hormesis. https://core.ac.uk/download/631285722.pdf (accessed on 14th June 2025).

34. Poudel, B. (2011). *Cell-Based Gene Therapy for Mending Infarcted Hearts.* https://core.ac.uk/download/1589844.pdf (accessed on 14th June 2025).

35. Ptitsyn, A., & Kanatous, S. (2009). Transformation of metabolism with age and lifestyle in Antarctic seals: A case study of systems biology approach to cross-species microarray experiment. https://core.ac.uk/download/pdf/1569887.pdf (accessed on 14th June 2025).

36. Reutter, D. J., & Vicary, J. (2019). A classical groupoid model for quantum networks. http://arxiv.org/abs/1707.00966 (accessed on 14th June 2025).

37. Rittweger, J. (2010). Vibration as an exercise modality: How it may work, and what its potential might be. https://core.ac.uk/download/11141396.pdf (accessed on 14th June 2025).

38. Rust, C., Whiteley, G., & Wilson, A. (2009). Experimental making in multi-disciplinary research. https://core.ac.uk/download/100323.pdf (accessed on 14th June 2025).

39. Sánchez, A., Scala, A., Caldarelli, G., McNamara, J. A., Franchi, L., Scazzocchio, M., & Auconi, P. (2012). Using networks to understand medical data: The case of class III malocclusions. https://core.ac.uk/download/12097174.pdf (accessed on 14th June 2025).

40. Schneider, V. B. (2025). *Space Medicine Considerations: Skeletal and Calcium Homeostasis.* https://core.ac.uk/download/pdf/42821460.pdf (accessed on 14th June 2025).

41. Shafie, A. A., Akhtaruzzaman, M., & Khan, M. R. (2016). *A Review on Lower Appendicular Musculoskeletal System of Human Body.* https://core.ac.uk/download/201684568.pdf (accessed on 14th June 2025).

42. Stark, J. M. (2013). *Efficacy of Probiotics for Reducing the Incidence of Lameness in Broilers Grown on Wire Flooring.* https://core.ac.uk/download/72842771.pdf (accessed on 14th June 2025).

AXIAL SKELETON

4

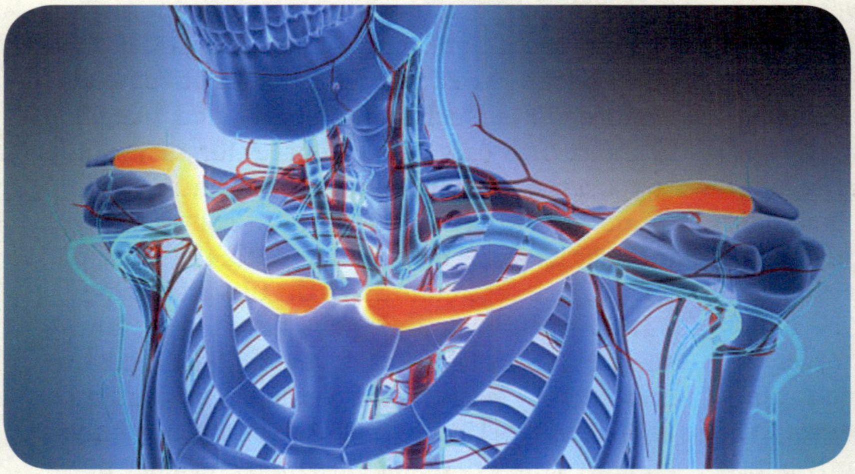

LEARNING OBJECTIVES

After studying this chapter, you will be able to:

1. Identify the structures of the axial skeleton
2. Describe the functions of the axial skeleton
3. Describe the anatomy of the skull
4. Describe the structure and function of the vertebral column
5. Describe the anatomy and function of the rib cage
6. Discuss the development and growth of the axial skeleton

Introduction

The axial skeleton refers to a central structure of the human body that consists primarily of the skull, vertebral column, and ribcage. The structural skeleton is necessary for several functional purposes, including the protection of vital organs, the support of the body posture, and facilitating movement. The brain and sensory organs are contained within the skull, while the vertebral column protects the spinal cord and provides mobility of the torso. Additionally, the ribcage shields the heart and lungs, which demonstrates the axial skeleton's central role in general health and function. Understanding the anatomy and mechanical properties of the axial skeleton is essential to the field of musculoskeletal (MSK) biomechanics and allied medical sciences such as orthopedics and rehabilitation, so the importance of this skeletal component in health as well as disease states becomes apparent. The mechanical properties of the axial skeleton have been the subject of significant research interest, namely in age-related alterations and stiffness of bone tissue. In older ages, their bones can have alterations that affect structural integrity in general, such as cortical bone stiffening. Current experimental evidence demonstrated cortical bone tissue stiffening in aged bone, which conventional multiscale elastic material models could not explain. This has resulted in new strategies in biomimetic material design through the modeling from the hierarchical structure of bone architecture (Gerisch et al., 2016). Through investigations into mineral fusion and composition's influence on mechanical properties, researchers are learning about the necessity of adaptive design in therapy intervention as well as enhancing the knowledge about skeletal health in terms of aging and injury. In addition to its mechanical characteristics, the axial skeleton's role in energy absorption and impact resistance is a research area of interest. A sample includes studies on equine hoof biomechanics and health, which have demonstrated how variations in skeletal configuration influence how the body reacts to ground contact and impact forces. It is postulated that the structural organization of hooves, particularly the contact between the radius and the ground, could significantly alter energy absorption capability. Although findings indicate that trimming of specific structures could be irrelevant to these parameters under certain conditions, alteration in biomechanical response is a critical area of research (Haazelager et al., 2025). These findings contribute to an overall appreciation of the functionality and adaptability of the axial skeleton, enriching literature on structural integrity in the context of varied biomechanical demands.

Definition of the Axial Skeleton

The axial skeleton is the central framework of the human body, composed of the skull, vertebral column, and rib cage. The axial skeleton is the central skeleton that holds up the head and trunk and contains a protective covering for essential organs such as the brain, spinal cord, and heart. The skull, comprised of multiple fused bones, includes the brain and comprises the facial structure. The backbone, composed of a series of vertebrae, is the axial skeleton that plays several different functions, including the protection of the spinal cord, functioning as a structural element, and the provision of flexibility and movement. Aside from protection, the axial skeleton is also instrumental in producing posture as well as the varied means of locomotion, which ultimately leads to body stability and integrity. There is great specialization in the vertebral column as it is specialized into zones: cervical, thoracic, lumbar, sacral, and coccygeal. Each zone has unique features adapted to specific functional requirements, such as flexibility and weight support. The cervical vertebrae, for instance, support the head and allow for maximum range of motion (ROM) in the neck. In contrast, the thoracic vertebrae articulate with the ribs to form the rib cage that guards the thoracic organs. The lumbar vertebrae provide stability and support for the significant weight of the lumbar area, thereby securing the possibility of standing and mobility. This regional diversity not only enhances the axial skeleton's total efficiency but also indicates evolutionary specializations for the support of a diversity of activities, evincing the dynamic relationship between function and structure along the skeletal system. The rib cage, yet another key member of the axial skeleton, consists of 12 pairs of ribs articulating with the thoracic vertebrae. This bony structure has several critical functions, such as protecting valuable internal organs in the thoracic cavity, i.e., the lungs and heart. The curvature of the ribs also offers the mechanism to expand and contract the respiratory apparatus, which naturally facilitates breathing. Ribs also act as attachment points for those muscles essential for respiration, thus reducing the reliance of the axial skeleton upon muscle systems. Although very much recognized for their protective and respiratory functions, ribs are also tasked with the role of delivering biomechanical stability to the thoracic region. Together, these components emphasize the axial skeleton's crucial role in maintaining the body's function, structure, and resilience against a variety of types of physical stress, thereby building a foundation necessary for human activity and survival (Figure 4.1).

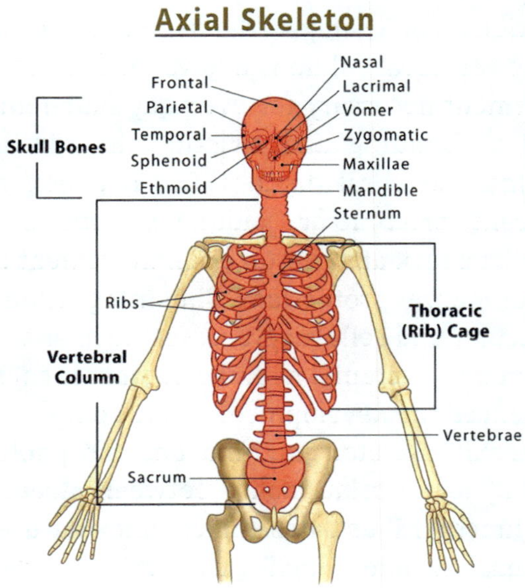

Figure 4.1. Axial skeleton.

Source: https://www.theskeletalsystem.net/wp-content/uploads/2022/11/Axial-Skeleton-Labeled.jpg.

Importance in Human Anatomy

The axial skeleton is a critical part of the human body, providing vital support and protection for the most essential organs. The skeletal framework, comprising the vertebral column, rib cage, and skull, is a requirement for posture and stability. The vertebral column is the central axis of the body, providing flexibility and strength. In its oval form, every vertebra is shock-absorbing to permit movement while shielding the spinal cord, a critical pathway for neural transmission. The rib cage provides additional protection by surrounding the thoracic cavity and thereby protecting the heart and lungs from harm. The axial skeleton, therefore, not only plays structural roles but also intersects with several physiological processes required for a state of existence. In addition, the importance of the axial skeleton also extends into the realm of pathology and disease study. For instance, studies on neurodegenerative conditions such as Alzheimer's disease (AD) show that alterations within the axial frame bear significant cognitive health consequences. White matter microstructural abnormalities and diffusion tensor imaging (DTI) changes have been reported concerning corpus callosum integrity and other tracts involving the axial skeleton. Through the study of brain volumetric parameters, researchers are now identifying correlations between axial anatomical health and neurological illnesses, thereby illustrating the skeleton's role beyond structural function only. These views underscore the importance of the axial skeleton in physical and cognitive terms, assigning anatomical integrity to greater concern in health sciences, including the evolving notion of dementia pathologies (Alves et al., 2012). The association of the axial skeleton with contemporary health issues attests to its significance in human anatomy, particularly in assessing the progression of disease over time. Anthropological investigations suggest that cancer, for example, may have been much rarer in the past than among populations today. Still, methods of identifying such disorders in human bones are far from optimal. Current techniques rely mainly on gross examination of skeletal tissues and can overlook sophisticated factors in disease initiation (Gardner et al., 2020). By refining interdisciplinary methods involving bioarchaeological and epidemiological knowledge, scholars can better interpret the meanings of skeletal health throughout human history. The shifting perspectives not only better tell us about the significance of the axial skeleton but also more clearly illuminate the intersections of shape with broader themes of human illness and health formation over the centuries.

4.1. Components of the Axial Skeleton

Learning Outcome

1. Discuss the skull component of the axial skeleton
2. Explain the vertebral column
3. Define rib cage

The axial skeleton is composed of key components that support the framework and protect vital organs. It comprises the skull, vertebral column, ribs, and sternum that make up the central body axis together. The brain and sensory organs are enclosed in the skull, which contains cranial and facial bones responsible for their intricate makeup. The vertebral column, consisting of individual vertebrae, not only contains the spinal cord but also confers mobility and flexibility without sacrificing posture in a standing position. The function of these elements underscores their need in the protection of the neurological tissue, along with serving as the points of origin for other muscle groups to move and to distribute tension throughout the body's central axis.

The sternum and the ribs form the thoracic cage, a critical protective structure of thoracic organs, particularly the lungs and the heart. The ribs, typically 12 pairs, in the back connect with the thoracic vertebrae and are categorized as true ribs, false ribs, and floating ribs, with varying physiological functions. The sternum, or breastbone, plays a vital role in providing a central point of attachment for the ribs, which guarantees stability of the ribcage while breathing occurs. An understanding of the components of the thoracic region within the axial skeleton illuminates the way the arrangement of these bones not only protects vital organs but also facilitates respiratory mechanisms. The intricateness in the makeup and arrangement of these skeletal elements highlights the processes of evolution that safeguard the thorax, yet allow basic functions of the body. Additionally, the axial skeleton is not merely used for static purposes; its components are extensively involved in dynamic functions. For example, the segmented design of the vertebral columns allows for a degree of movement necessary for everyday functioning, such as bending and twisting. In addition, the intervertebral discs (IVDs) between two adjacent vertebrae are padding structures that support shock absorption upon movement and spinal nerve protection. The integration of molecular and cellular processes, such as those referred to in cranial neural crest mesenchyme, influences the development of the components of the axial skeleton and functional morphology. This dynamic relationship between structure and function illustrates the complex nature of the axial skeleton, highlighting how it evolves under mechanical and environmental stress and then directs adaptations for enhancing survivability and functionality under a spectrum of environmental conditions.

4.1.1. Skull

The skull is extremely highly significant part of the axial skeleton and is both a protective covering for the brain and the base of the facial structure. The intricate bony framework consists of several points of interfusion between various cranial bones, and all contribute to its intricate structure. The development of the skull occurs through a series of complex embryological processes, including the migration and differentiation of cranial neural crest mesenchyme. These neural crest cells give rise to the tissue that forms the shape and the function of the skull, providing the cellular framework underpinning the different structures of the cranial cavity. Aberrations during this process of development may lead to severe defects or variations, demonstrating the intricate relation between skull shape and its resulting evolutionary adaptations, which corresponds to the specific environmental niches occupied by different species (Abzhanov et al., 2019) (Figure 4.1).

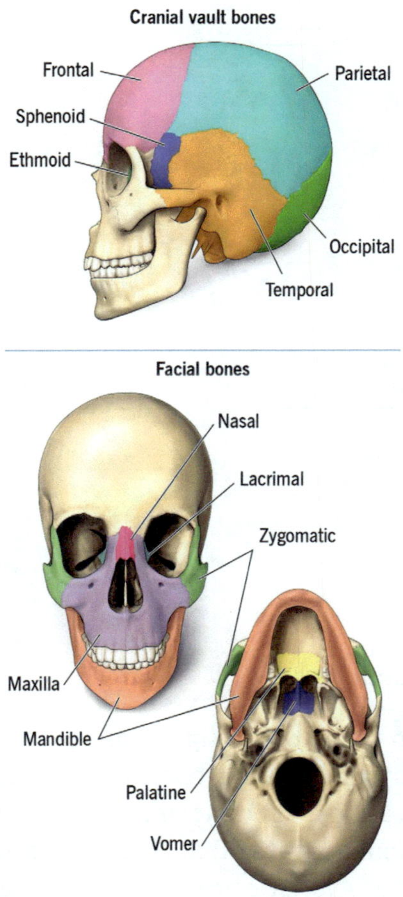

Figure 4.2. Skull anatomy.

Source: https://my.clevelandclinic.org/-/scassets/images/org/health/articles/skull-anatomy.

The diversity in skull structure between species is staggering, particularly if considered concerning evolutionary processes. Members of the order Felidae, for instance, have extremely differentiated skull morphology that correlates with their ecological niches and dietary specializations. These not only constitute superficial differences but also play vital roles, such as during sensory perception and feeding. The relationship of skull morphology to environmental pressures illuminates the role of the skull as part of the overall axial skeleton, since it is a primary interface of an organism with its surroundings. Biomechanical stress during life may also sculpt skulls, indicating the dynamic character of the bony structure in responding to behavioral and environmental forces (Alvarez et al., 2016). From the viewpoint of general function within the axial skeleton, the skull's role extends beyond simple protection of the brain. The skull harbors sensory organs and is also involved in jaw development, which is critical for the consumption of food and communication with the world at large. This three-dimensional function is indicative of the skull's advanced design, which fuses protective, sensory, and mechanical functions into a single construct. Furthermore, the axial skeleton, including the skull, exhibits allometric relations that illustrate how different parts, like the cranial and vertebral, can be susceptible to distinct evolutionary pressures, as has been shown elsewhere. The allometric relations provide insights into functional morphology in the axial skeleton, demarcating its significance not only for adaptation in a single species but also for larger evolutionary trends across taxa (Alvarez et al., 2016).

4.1.2. Vertebral Column

The vertebral column, or backbone, is a critical structure of the axial skeleton that provides structure, support, and protection to the spinal cord. This intricate sequence of vertebrae contributes significantly to various biological processes to enable flexibility, mobility, and stability in the organism. Vertebral columns are categorized into distinct sections, such as cervical, thoracic, lumbar, sacral, and caudal vertebrae. Each segment reacts to diverse mechanical stresses and support functions, based on an evolutionary response to ecological pressures and modes of locomotion (Alvarez et al., 2016) (Figure 4.3).

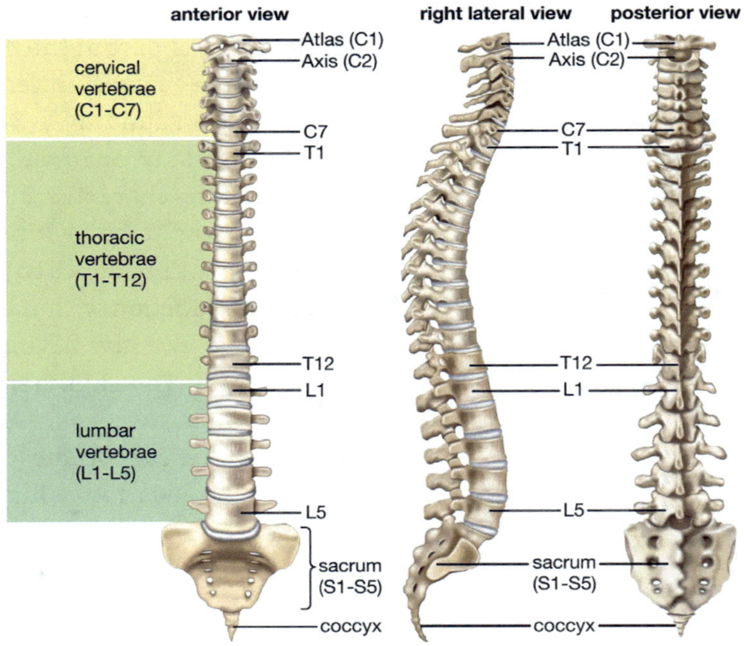

Figure 4.3. Human vertebral column.

Source: https://www.britannica.com/science/vertebral-column.

In the model of vertebrate development, resegmentation is one of the significant processes that patterns the axial skeleton in tetrapod evolution. The combination of the two neighboring somite halves to form a single vertebra is the phenomenon, thus creating a solid morphological foundation for structural support and locomotion. Recent research has demonstrated that resegmentation is not just a recently evolved character of tetrapods but an ancient characteristic present in jawed vertebrate skeletal elements such as cartilaginous fishes. In this study, tracing of cell lineages identified that, like tetrapods, certain vertebrae in skates form through a process of resegmentation, thereby illustrating the continuity of vertebral development throughout evolution across taxa (Criswell et al., 2020). The functional implications of vertebral column morphology extend beyond mechanical properties; they influence the overall health and survivability of the organism. Alterations in the shape and arrangement of the vertebrae could influence not only locomotion and agility but also elements of respiratory function and neurological health. For example, the structural acclimations within the lumbar regions of different felid species, since they directly correspond to their locomotion and habitat utilization, reflect how evolutionary pressures can condition anatomical structures. In addition, these acclimations suggest the importance of further research on the evolution and mechanics of the vertebral column as they indicate the biomechanical necessities and the ecological affiliation that characterizes various vertebrate clades (Alvarez et al., 2016).

4.1.3. Rib Cage

The rib cage is a component of the axial skeleton that plays a significant role in the mechanism of respiration and houses vital organs. Composed of 12 pairs of ribs, the sternum, and the thoracic vertebrae, the rib cage offers a protective casing for the lungs and heart while enabling the mechanism of breathing. Each of the ribs forms a posterior articulation with the thoracic vertebrae, and the rib cage is both stable and mobile in structure. On inhalation, the intercostal muscles elevate the rib and increase the thoracic cavity, thus lowering pressure and permitting air to enter the lungs. It is this dynamic association between the ribs and associated musculature that is essential to adequate respiration, emphasizing the multifunctional aspect of the rib cages in terms of support and movement in the axial skeleton. In exploring the evolutionary significance of the rib cage, one finds major adaptations among species.

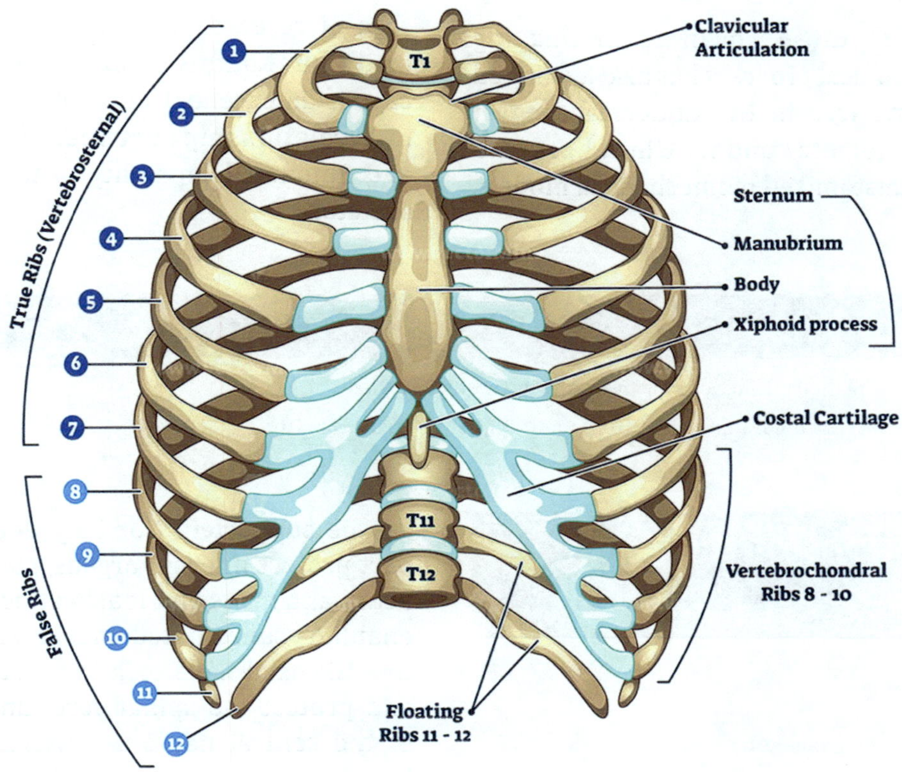

Figure 4.4. Rib cage.

Source: https://external-content.duckduckgo.com/iu/?u=https%3A%2F%2Fvectormine.b-cdn.net%2Fwp-content%2Fuploads%2FRib_Cage.jpg&f=1&nofb=1&ipt=d56a53433f1fa8e08c9a591d9f541a65c9c1824aaf623dfa76dd2859448c1dba.

The form of the rib cage is not rigid, as it has adapted to various environmental and functional demands. For instance, in mammals, the ribs have elongated and flattened to increase the thoracic cavity volume to facilitate better respiration. This is indicative of overall adaptive tendencies within the axial skeleton that harmonize locomotory schemes and metabolic costs. Current studies also indicate that the segmented nature of the rib cages is responsible for their role, providing additional flexibility yet maintaining a general protective structure around the thoracic organs. The discovery of an ossified, multipartite sternum in ancient synapsids reveals that this line of evolutionary development began earlier than previously documented, meaning the typical rib cage morphology we observe today has its beginning deep in evolutionary history (Bendel et al., 2022) (Figure 4.4).

Along with these advances in imaging techniques, technical progress has also facilitated significant advances in the understanding of rib cage morphometry and its clinical practice implications. Customized biomechanical models, derived from low-dose radiographs, present new opportunities for research and treatment of rib cage disorders, such as scoliosis. This technique enables clinicians to create patient-specific models that perfectly fit individual anatomy, optimizing treatment efficacy while minimizing radiation exposure. By separating and examining the rib cage within these models, researchers have demonstrated a powerful way of learning about how it works and creating new treatments. These applications reveal the rib cage's significance, not only as an anatomical structure but also as a significant area of research within anatomy and clinical medicine (Koutras et al., 2022). Overall, the rib cage is an excellent illustration of the complex interrelationship between structural form and functional capability in terms of the axial skeleton.

Test Your Knowledge

1. What are the primary functions of the skull in the human body?
2. How is the vertebral column structured, and what is its main function?

4.2. Functions of the Axial Skeleton

Learning Outcome

1. Discuss the axial skeleton's support for the body
2. Define the protection of vital organs
3. Explain the axial skeleton's facilitation of movement

The axial skeleton has several essential functions that are vital for supporting the body's structural integrity as well as allowing its movement. It includes the skull, vertebral column, ribs, and sternum, and it gives the bones the basic structure around which the body can be supported. Not only does this skeletal part protect internal organs, such as the brain, heart, and lungs, but it also attaches to muscles, enabling coordinated movement. Apart from this, the axial skeleton also functions to envelop and protect the spinal cord, an essential part of the central nervous system. Its protective function is of critical importance, as any injury to the vertebral column would lead to severe neurological deficiency. The axial skeleton also provides the body with shape and posture, which is critical in enabling activities ranging from mere locomotion to sophisticated athletic effort. Another crucial function of the axial skeleton is its involvement in hematopoiesis, which is the process of the formation of blood cells. Specifically, the bones of the axial skeleton are occupied by red bone marrow, which is responsible for the generation of erythrocytes, leukocytes, and thrombocytes. This position also highlights the importance of the axial skeleton beyond mere structural support, as it directly impacts the body's ability to provide oxygen, fight off infections, and clot blood. The generation of blood cells is particularly critical during growth periods and following injury that demands higher production of these elements. Thus, disruptions of the integrity or function of the axial skeleton, e.g., as with disease or trauma, can have widespread effects on overall health. Through these intricate functions, the axial skeleton is invaluable to physical stability and physiological function. Finally, the axial skeleton plays a vital role in communication and sensory function. The cranial bones of axial skeletons protect the brain and provide bases for attachment of facial muscles that allow for expression and speech. The axial skeleton further supports sensory organs of the head, such as the eyes and ears, which are crucial for vision and hearing, respectively. Such roles highlight the axial skeleton's vital role in environmental interactions that allow for enhanced behavioral responses. Under an evolutionary framework, the axial skeleton's adaptations, like its role in skull design and jaw structure, have far-reaching implications for species-specificity of behavior and dietary adaptations. By facilitating protection as well as sensory interaction, the axial skeleton is at the center of not only individual survival but also of ecological processes in complex organisms, harmonizing functionality with evolutionary biology in fascinating ways (Berkes et al., 2018; Abzhanov et al., 2019).

4.2.1. Support for the Body

The axial skeleton comprises basic components that play priceless roles of supporting and protecting the body. The structure is mainly composed of the skull, vertebral column, sternum, and ribs, and provides the function of providing the structure required for posture support and facilitating movement. The vertebral column, particularly, not only protects the spinal cord but also supports the body through its vertebral structure, which makes it flexible as well as stable. This separation is essential since it supports various ranges of motion while concurrently accommodating shocks and minimizing the risk of injury. The ribs also contribute towards protecting the thorax, which accommodates crucial organs such as the heart and the lungs, thereby acting as a protective guard from external trauma and environmental risks. Thus, the axial skeleton is a beautiful design that resists protection against structural support, reflecting its significance in the human body's overall biomechanical design (Figure 4.5).

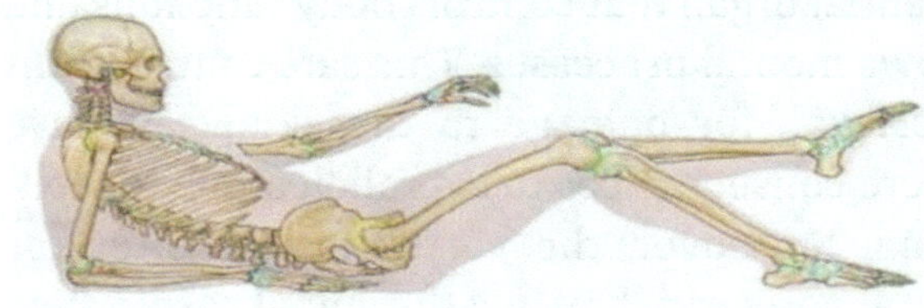

Figure 4.5. Framework that support body and cradles its soft organs.

Source: https://external-content.duckduckgo.com/iu/?u=https%3A%2F%2Fimage.slidesharecdn.com%2F4-140503111803-phpapp02%2F95%2F4-skeletal-system-2-638.jpg%3Fcb%3D1399118231&f=1&nofb=1&ipt=10325c4f6b127c72a4b34715c347c2e859fe34ec1d817b60ac93de79d7a62a4f.

In addition, the axial skeleton plays a crucial role in facilitating the movement of the human body. Vertebrae joints provide enhanced flexibility while providing strength, which is essential in various body activities from simple movement to advanced sporting movements. Coordination of the components of the skeleton, including ligaments and cartilage, enhances movement while ensuring the body's structure is strong against everyday stresses. For instance, the IVDs play a crucial role not just for shock absorption but also to permit bending and twisting of the spine. This functional relationship illustrates how the axial skeleton design not just supports the body weight but also functions with the muscles and connective tissue that enclose it to enable a wide range of movement. Thus, the axial skeleton is not simply a passive framework but is essential in allowing mobility and overall function of the body. In addition to its mechanical function, the axial skeleton is involved in supporting physiological processes crucial for life. The axial skeleton has bone marrow in which hematopoiesis—the production of blood cells—occurs and thus has a function in the body's circulatory and immune functions. The skull houses the brain, an essential organ that controls body functions and allows mental processes. This safe containment is crucial, for damage to the skull can have severe consequences to overall health and well-being. Moreover, the vertebrae are sites for neural networks, housing the spinal cord, which transfers messages from the brain to the body and back, hence regulating critical activities. The multifunctional roles of the axial skeleton provide the basic framework of mechanical, physiological, and neurological functions, which speak to its significance in providing life and health in the human body. Overall, the axial skeleton has an excellent interplay of support, protection, and functional versatility.

4.2.2. Protection of Vital Organs

The axial skeleton plays a key role in the protection of vital organs as a robust framework covering structures essential to survival. Comprising the skull, vertebral column, and thoracic cage, the axial skeleton houses the brain, spine, and thoracic organs within a protective case, respectively. The cranial bones of the skull, for instance, house the brain within a hard calvarial shell and hence protect it against extrinsic trauma. This protection is crucial because the brain is responsible for so much of the body and critical processes. The vertebral column contributes to this protection by encasing the spinal cord, a central neural pathway by which the brain can communicate with the body. The axial skeleton thus not only supports these organs structurally but also contributes crucial protective components that prevent injury from collision or falling. In addition, the thoracic cage, constructed from ribs and the sternum, is functional to provide an essential barrier against harmful forces for the heart and lungs. Rigidity and flexibility in the configuration of ribs are responsible for making the thoracic cavity able to expand during respiration and yet still maintain an enveloping cover over cardiac and respiratory processes. These intercostal muscles, found between the ribs, assist in the mechanical protection of the organs within and support their function during physical exercise (Figure 4.6).

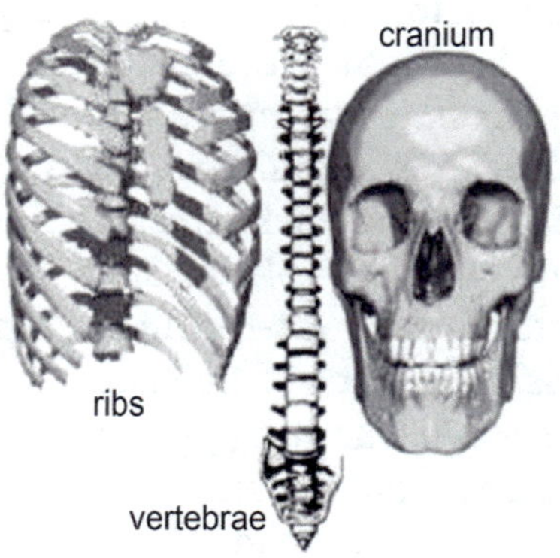

Figure 4.6. Protects internal organs and fragile body parts.

Source: https://www.slideshare.net/slideshow/4-skeletal-system/34239514.

Additionally, the joint of the ribs on the vertebrae provides contextual stability, thereby eliminating the risk of organ fracture. In this way, the thoracic cage helps to show the dynamic relationship between organ function and skeletal protection, revealing the axial skeleton's complicated aspect in offering general health. Furthermore, the shield-like function of the axial skeleton extends beyond the provision of structural support; it has a significant role in facilitating efficient physiological functions. The outward expansion of the ribcage during inspiration facilitates maximal lung capacity, which enables oxygen and carbon dioxide exchange, essential for cellular respiration. Likewise, the ribcage protective encasement of the heart shields it from any external damage. In addition, the alignment of the vertebral column is responsible for the proper alignment of nerves to allow effective transmission of impulses throughout the body. Alignment is crucial for maintaining the integrity of vital organ systems, as disruption of nerve impulses can lead to gross physiological dysfunction. Worldwide, the wide-ranging protective role of the axial skeleton underlines its central role in providing security and efficiency in human body life-supporting organ systems, emphasizing the indispensable interdependence of structure and function in the human skeleton.

4.2.3. Facilitation of Movement

The axial skeleton plays a crucial role in enabling movement by providing structural support and a framework for muscular attachment. The structure comprising the skull, vertebral column, and rib cage serves not just as a protective casing to house vital organs but also forms part of human locomotion mechanics. Each vertebra is designed to allow varying degrees of movement, making the whole spine elastic. Flexibility is essential for bending, twisting, and lifting, which form an integral part of day-to-day function. IVDs act as shock absorbers and facilitate a smooth arc of motion between vertebrae, hence making movement economical and reducing potential injury. Besides, coupled movement patterns promoted by interconnected axial skeletons are essential for complex physical activity. By stabilizing the spine during movement, muscles that originate from the axial skeleton—such as the multifidus and other core stabilizers—contribute significantly to the dynamics of movement. Myofascial tissue-caused passive tension, also referred to as human resting myofascial tone (HRMT), offers stability for posture and movement control (Evans et al., 2010) (Figure 4.7).

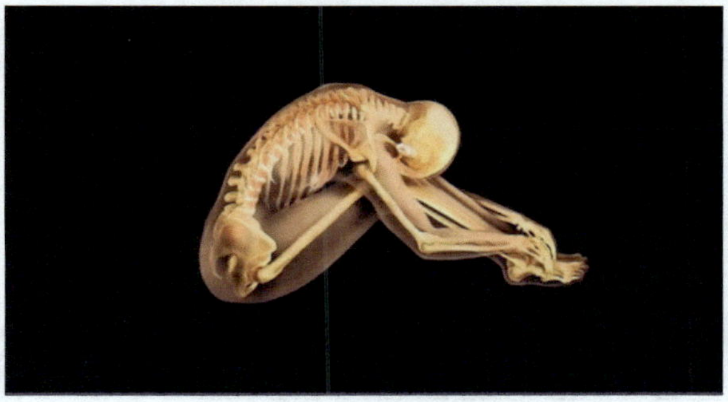

Figure 4.7. Visual representation of the human skeletal system during a seated forward bend, emphasizing spinal flexibility and joint alignment.

Source: https://cdn.storymd.com/optimized/gVAzWVuMoO/thumbnail.jpg.

This aspect of myofascial function demonstrates the way the axial skeleton is not so much a passive structure but an active participant in stabilizing the body in various states of motion. Mobilization of the axial skeleton must then be established based on a harmonious interaction between its structural components and the system of muscles so that both power and ease of movement are attained. Because modern lifestyles contribute to the sedentary nature of individuals, imbalances between forces that act on the axial skeleton can lead to dysfunction and pain. Disorders such as gluteus Medius myofascial dysfunction, which can be caused by sitting for long periods, directly impact spinal alignment and movement efficiency in general (Marsden et al., 2019). The dysfunctions reflect the strong interaction between the muscular well-being and the axial skeleton. Treatment approaches that aimed to treat these imbalances placed strong emphasis on maintaining the axial skeleton intact to enable optimal facilitation of movement. Through the treatment of myofascial triggers and mobility facilitation under specific intervention, rehabilitation can realign the axial skeleton, thus allowing it to sustain movement throughout all levels of physical action efficiently. This prolonged relationship between the axial skeleton and facilitation of movement remains a matter of significant research to optimize musculoskeletal (MSK) well-being and quality of life.

Test Your Knowledge

1. How does the skeletal system provide support for the body?
2. How does the skeletal system facilitate movement?

4.3. The Skull

Learning Outcome

1. Understand the structure and composition of the axial skeleton
2. Identify the major bones of the skull
3. Describe the role in protecting the brain

The skull is a primary element of the axial skeleton that is charged with protection as well as support to critical structures such as the brain and sensory organs. The complex bony scaffold of the skull consists of several interlocking bones that not only guard the delicate neural structures but also act as articulatory surfaces for the mandible and harbor the organs of mastication. There have been several evolutionary changes that have influenced the skull morphology, resulting in a great deal of diversity among species. For instance, jaw shape and size changes have been influenced by developmental processes that concern the cranial neural crest mesenchyme. The movement and interaction of these cells during embryonic development are essential to establishing the final form of the skull, with any irregularities potentially leading to deviations that would compromise function and health, and illustrating the intricate interplay between developmental biology and mature form (Abzhanov et al., 2019). In the study of the skull's relationship to morphology and functionality, it can be seen that various species exhibit extraordinary variations associated with adaptations to their environments. Felidae, for example, shows a wide range of body sizes and feeding behavior that is reflected in the forms and structures of their skulls. This demonstrates that the skull is not merely a static part of the axial skeleton but a dynamic structure that bears testimony to evolutionary pressures brought about by diet and environmental conditions. Morphometric study of these animals has revealed extraordinary variation in their skull characteristics, including size and shape corresponding to their hunting strategies and use of habitat. These findings demonstrate that the adaptations found in skull morphology are highly correlated with functional requirements and place emphasis on the ability of the axial skeleton to accommodate a range of ecological niches (Alvarez et al., 2016). Ultimately, the intricate design and diversity of the skull emphasize its significance as a component of the axial skeleton, as a transition between function, structure, and evolutionary history. It is imperative to understand cranial development and plasticity since this illuminates the implications for overall disease and health. For instance, any cranial deformities in development may result in jaw defects that affect feeding patterns and overall health.

4.3.1. Structure and Composition

The structure and composition of the axial skeleton are critical to understanding its function within the human body. Composed of the rib cage, vertebral column, and skull, the axial skeleton is the torso's and head's primary support system, enclosing crucial organs such as the brain and spinal cord. Bones in this region have a complex structure with compact and spongy bone; such architectural design allows for adequate strength but maintains the light weight necessary for movement. Furthermore, the integration of fibrous, cartilaginous, and synovial joints that permit movement while preserving stability facilitates the attachment between such bones. This intricate equilibrium in form and construction is crucial in preventing harm and allowing the proper physiological processes in the entire body. The mechanical characteristics of bones in the axial skeleton are similarly influenced by the loading conditions encountered by them over extended durations. Loading of the skeleton has been revealed, as per research, to play very pivotal roles in the attainment of functionally and mechanically appropriate bone formations. For instance, impact training has been proven to enhance bone density and overall strength among sports participants, particularly those engaged in sports that entail axial loading of great significance, such as running and gymnastics. Studies show that different sporting activities yield different bone geometry adaptations, where gymnasts and runners exhibit greater resistance against axial and bending forces compared to non-sport individuals. These distinctions emphasize the function of physical exercise in maintaining the structural strength and compositional resistance of the axial skeleton, thereby contributing towards enhanced bone fitness and reduced risk of fractures during one's lifespan (Cooke et al., 2011) (Figure 4.8).

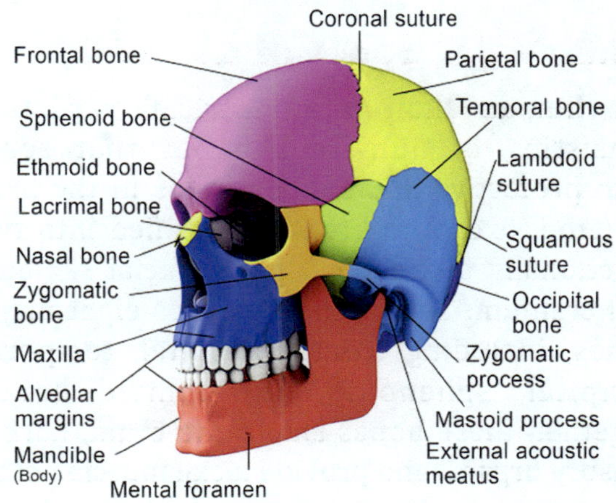

Figure 4.8. Structure and functions of the skull.

Source: https://external-content.duckduckgo.com/iu/?u=http%3A%2F%2Fwww.orthopaedics.win%2FArticle%2FUploadFiles%2F201609%2F2016092210181124.jpg&f=1&nofb=1&ipt=7eb54e9fc34697385d9243d53d41e488c8beff4737782259e7a0650d142a9698.

In addition, new evidence on the composition of axial skeletons dictates beyond mechanical strength; it dictates the prevention of disorders such as osteoporosis. The intricacy of the structure of bones, tissue composition, and external loading conditions is an articulation of the worth of an integrated health and longevity approach. Particularly, a normal lean body mass has been found to have a positive correlation with both bone mineral density and bone strength. Through the observation of the mechanical behavior of bone under varying conditions of load, ways can be designed to enhance bone health through nutritional as well as physical interventions. While the discrete particle approach to materials science can lead to a more solid understanding of material response to stress (Huerne et al., 2012), analogous ideas can also be applied to the axial skeleton. By describing the dynamics of bone response, scientists and healthcare professionals can unite to advance healthier aging and more effective prevention measures against skeletal disorders.

4.3.2. Major Bones of the Skull

The human skull is an intricate structure consisting of numerous bones that serve both protective and support roles in the axial skeleton. It can be broadly classified into two functionally distinct parts: the facial skeleton and cranium. The cranium houses eight major bones, including frontal, parietal, temporal, occipital, sphenoid, and ethmoid bones. Together, these bones shield the brain, harbor sensory organs, and provide facial muscle points of attachment. The sutures, or fibrous joints between them, are very restrictive, allowing little movement but a stability necessary to guard the brain against external damage. For this reason, the cranium is a vital component of the axial skeleton. This complex morphology is an outcome of evolutionary adaptations that create its structure, derived from neural crest cell migration during development and functional and environmental pressures on the skull and jaw (Abzhanov et al., 2019; Cozart et al., 2017). In addition to protection by the cranium, the facial bones of the skull play a key role in the overall structure and functioning of the human head. Comprising fourteen bones that are the maxillae, zygomatic bones, nasal bones, and mandible, the facial skeleton constitutes the framework of the face, housing the dental arches and supporting the delicate structures of the eyes, nose, and mouth. Noteworthy here is that the mandible itself is a movable bone of the skull that allows articulation during mastication and speech. Additionally, the intricate structure of these facial bones also contributes to individual facial characteristics and inter-population differences. An understanding of interactions between the major skull bones is necessary to understand greater complexities of the axial skeleton, e.g., how craniofacial development might be affected by gene and environmental influences, and how such differences can lead to clinical conditions that require intervention (Cozart et al., 2017; Abzhanov et al., 2019) (Figure 4.9).

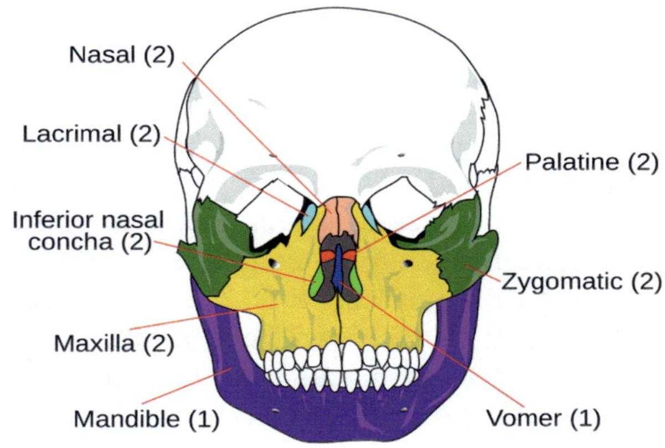

Figure 4.9. The fourteen bones that form the human facial skeleton.

Source: https://en.wikipedia.org/wiki/Facial_skeleton#/media/File:Facial_skeleton_-_en.svg.

The relationships between the prominent bones of the skull are not just structural; they also mirror the underlying biological mechanisms that drive human evolution and function. The developmental mechanisms regulating the growth of facial and cranial bones are intricate, with synchronized signaling pathways and biomechanical forces. For example, cranial neural crest mesenchyme has a crucial function in the embryonic patterning of the skull, influencing the patterning and morphology of the bones involved. From examining these complex interactions in the axial skeleton, researchers can gain insight into the evolutionary pressures that have influenced craniofacial diversity across different species. These studies also highlight how interruptions in these development processes can lead to variation and congenital abnormalities, thereby showing the importance of knowing the major bones of the skull in evolutionary biology as well as for clinical purposes (Cozart et al., 2017; Abzhanov et al., 2019).

4.3.3. Role in Protecting the Brain

The axial skeleton, made up of the skull, vertebral column, and ribcage, plays a vital role in its protective function for the brain and other vital organs. The skull itself is a sophisticated structure that is made up of interlocking bones that enclose the brain and are designed to transmit and absorb impact forces. Protection is central, as the brain is particularly vulnerable to injury. Besides, the fontanelles and cranial sutures of the infant ensure there is some elasticity, which not only facilitates the expansion of the brain but also helps the skull's capacity to withstand pressures from the outside. The intrinsic elasticity of the axial skeleton thus serves as a first-line defense, shielding the central nervous system from traumatic events that could lead to severe neurological deficits. Aside from protecting the body, the axial skeleton is tasked with keeping the brain and its health intact by its association with the central nervous system. The vertebral column protects the spinal cord, which is responsible for transmitting signals between the body and the brain. The alignment and physical condition of the vertebrae are essential for the central nervous system to function optimally, since any misalignment can cause problems such as compression of nerves. In addition, the support from the axial skeleton assists the brain in ensuring proper blood circulation, which is essential for the delivery of sufficient oxygen and nutrients. Lastly, the structural support that the axial skeleton offers is of most significance for mechanical defense as well as for general physiological support necessary for brain function. Sustaining brain function goes hand-in-hand with the axial skeleton's role in the body's structural support. With continued research revealing the complexity of signaling pathways such as WNT and retinoic acid pathways that are at the heart of developmental biology, one can discern the relevance of these mechanisms to skeletal wellbeing and, by default, brain safeguarding. For instance, disruptions in these signaling pathways lead to developmental disruptions of the skeleton as well as the nervous system, as recorded in literature. This integration of information indicates that the role of the axial skeleton as protection is more than just physical shielding; it involves a complex interaction with biological mechanisms that regulate brain development and wellness, thereby highlighting the axial skeleton's greater importance in the human body (Collette et al., 2013; Roberts et al., 2020).

Test Your Knowledge

1. What is the structure and composition of the axial skeleton?
2. Which are the major bones that make up the skull?

4.4. The Vertebral Column

Learning Outcome

1. Understand the structure and segments of the vertebral column
2. Describe the functions that IVDs serve in the vertebral column
2. Identify the common disorders affecting the vertebral column

The vertebral column is a unifying component of the axial skeleton, acting as a structural backbone and sheath of protection of the spinal cord. Comprised of 33 vertebrae in the average human body, it is classified into cervical, thoracic, lumbar, sacral, and coccygeal segments. Each segment has distinctive morphological characteristics that contribute to the functionality of the spine. The cervical vertebrae, for example, carry a significant amount of head weight and yield excellent mobility, whereas the lumbar vertebrae are responsible for stability and bearing weight. Additionally, the shape and congruity of these vertebrae create an elastic but compliant column that can be adapted to react to varying loads and movements, finally allowing optimal locomotion and posture. Therefore, the vertebral column is an advanced integration of function and form integral to the maintenance of a person's physical integrity and mobility. The vertebral column also shows marked variation in morphology between populations. Evidence indicates that there are apparent variations in the gross morphology of cervical vertebrae, particularly in relation to race and sex, emphasizing the impact of genetic and environmental factors on bone development. Studies using heterogeneous demographic samples, such as the William M. Bass Collection and the Terry Anatomical Collection, show that there exist discernible differences in these variables. This variation has some implications when it comes to the knowledge of human evolution and adaptation, as it suggests that some morphological features might have been favored on a basis of functional requirements or social organization. This evidence emphasizes the significance of the vertebral column both in individual human anatomy and on broader anthropological scales, since it indicates that it is a record of evolutionary history. Further, the dynamics of the evolution of the vertebral column inform us about mammals' locomotor adaptations. Study of vertebral morphological variation suggests that different regions of the spinal cord, especially the thoracolumbar region, bear high individual disparity patterns and are subject to evolutionary stresses. This region is also crucial for the movement functionality of mammalian life, supporting agility and adaptability. For instance, morphological difference in the lumbar and thoracic vertebrae is linked to different modes of locomotion, reflecting the evolutionary processes that have influenced these organisms. Notably, the study addresses the tension between structural variation and ecological function, illustrating that vertebral morphology is very variable, while the difference does not always define an evolutionary effect. The intricacy involved in vertebrate evolution highlights the crucial function the axial skeleton has in determining the shape of individual organisms as well as more generalized species adaptations (Haugen et al., 1994; Benson et al., 2021).

4.4.1. Structure and Segments

The axial skeleton is a fundamental component of the human skeletal system, providing the required structure and segmentation to facilitate form and function. Made up of three large segments—the skull, vertebral column, and rib cage—each segment is responsible for protecting significant organs and upholding body functions. The skull is a protective covering for the brain and houses structures that facilitate sensory perception. The vertebral column, composed of individual vertebrae, is known to create a stable yet mobile system of support for the body and allows for movement while safeguarding the spinal cord. Lastly, the rib cage also acts as a covering organ for the thoracic organs and structural support for breathing, illustrating how segmental organization in the axial skeleton is responsible for its numerous varying functions in human physiology (Figure 4.10).

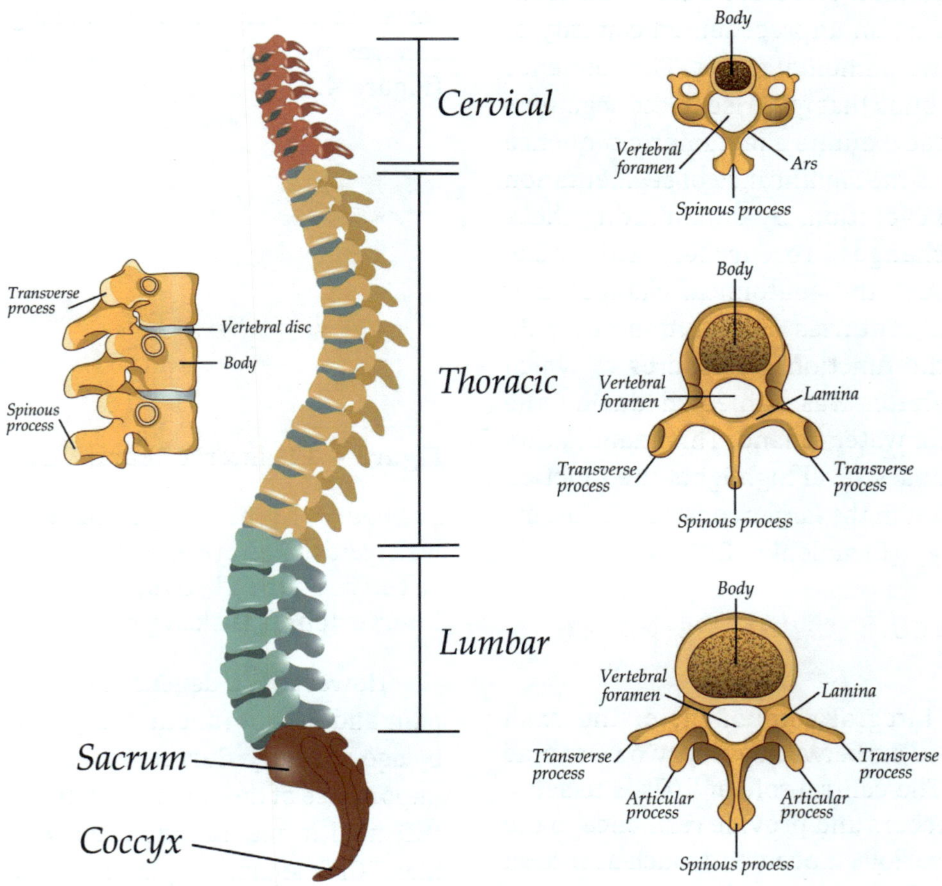

Figure 4.10. The structure of the segments of the spine.

Source: https://dspinesurgeon.com/wp-content/uploads/2022/01/structure-of-segments-spine.png.

Besides rudimentary protection, the segmented structure of the axial skeleton makes complex movements possible that are required for mundane tasks. The intricate arrangement of IVDs between the vertebrae not only makes possible flexibility and movement along various axes but also functions as a shock buffer, which lessens the load on the spinal cord. Furthermore, the articulation of the ribs with the thoracic vertebrae confers mechanical advantage for breathing and facilitates dynamic expansion and contraction of the rib cage. These characteristics are an evolutionary adaptation whereby the segmented organization of the axial skeletons not only contributes to stability but also to agility. An understanding of such structural dynamics lies at the heart of disciplines such as biomechanics and orthopedics, in which anatomical integrity needs to be maintained for the sake of injury prevention and rehabilitation. The axial skeleton also has developmental complexities in common with the tetrapod evolutionary history, indicated in its segmented form. Formation of the axial skeleton has led to significant variation in vertebral column structure among different species, showing an unprecedented capacity to respond to environmental forces. The sequence of osteogenic buds that give rise to the segments of the vertebrae exhibits a metameric sequence that underlines the significance of segmentation in vertebrate evolution. By enumerating these osteogenic changes, researchers can make inferences about the anatomical changes that occurred over centuries of evolution and gain insight into the functional pressures to which the axial skeleton was subjected during the transition from water to land. This examination at an evolutionary level highlights the function of segmentation in the larger context of anatomy and physiology (Ermolenko, 2011).

4.4.2. Functions of Intervertebral Discs

IVDs are an integral component of the axial skeleton that occur between every two vertebrae of the spine. The central role of IVDs is to serve as shock absorbers and provide resilience to the spine during various movements, such as flexion and torsion. This unique fibrocartilaginous structure possesses a gelatinous nucleus pulposus core that is enveloped by a fibrous outer annulus fibrosus. Nucleus pulposus is an internal shock absorber, redistributing compressive forces during use, with the annulus fibrosus providing tensile support to prevent excessive disc deformation. The interaction between these components allows the spine to maintain its dynamic ROM as well as to impart required stability to the vertebral column so that complete physical activity and overall mobility can be maintained. In addition to shock absorption, IVDs also play a vital role in maintaining the structural integrity of the axial skeleton. Because the spine is subjected to continuous mechanical stress throughout everyday activities, IVDs allow for the transfer of load between adjacent vertebrae and, hence, avoid potential injury and degeneration. Such fibrocartilaginous design of the discs also serves to prevent vertebral malalignment, which ensures proper posture and spinal alignment (Figure 4.11).

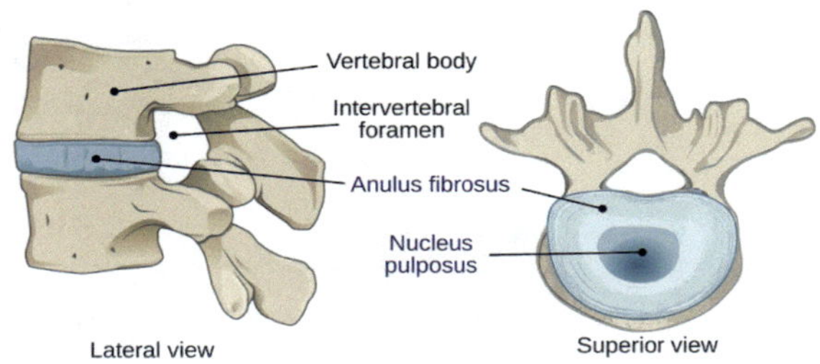

Figure 4.11. Intervertebral disc.

Source: https://upload.wikimedia.org/wikipedia/commons/thumb/3/3c/716_Intervertebral_Disk.svg/1280px-716_Intervertebral_Disk.svg.png.

However, IVD degeneration can cause chronic pain and loss of function, typically exacerbated by age or injury. Current research highlights the importance of the signaling pathways that control IVD health and function, with specific factors like TGFβ signaling playing a role in annulus fibrosus formation and maintenance (Clayton et al., 2021). Understanding these pathways has the potential to develop new regenerative therapies to prevent IVD degeneration. Furthermore, IVDs have an essential role in the biomechanics of the spine, affecting the efficiency of motion and overall health. Hydration and structure of IVDs have key functions because they offer resistance to pressure fluctuations that are intrinsic to activity. As hydration declines due to the disease process or aging, the discs lose their elasticity, which results in decreased shock absorption and increased susceptibility to trauma. This hastens the degenerative process of the spine and causes problems such as herniated discs, with significant resultant pain and disability. Investigations into genetic markers and molecular pathways that influence disc health, e.g., those that elucidate mineralization processes in IVDs, have the potential to inform us regarding spinal health better and steer multidisciplinary approaches in the management of spinal disorders (Warraich et al., 2013). The objective of the study is to identify the potential therapeutic targets, thus enhancing the quality of life of spinal degenerative disease patients.

4.4.3. Common Disorders Affecting the Vertebral Column

The vertebral column is susceptible to various disorders that may negatively impact its structural integrity and function. Among these groups of disorders are skeletal dysplasias and dysostoses, which are caused by genetic mutations during bone and cartilage development. They are characterized by varied phenotypes, which bring about complications such as vertebral malformations and growth deformities. For the majority of cases, such abnormalities are actualized by signs that involve skeletal deformities, pain, and mobility limitations, which significantly impact the quality of life of the sufferers of such conditions. The axial and vertebral columns are particularly vulnerable to genetic defects, indicating the need for advanced knowledge and new treatment modes, as the underlying molecular deficiencies remain largely unidentified despite improvements in research technologies (Doherty et al., 2016). Scoliosis, a disorder associated with the vertebral column, is characterized by an abnormal lateral curvature of the spine. It can occur idiopathically or as a complication of neuromuscular disorders, congenital abnormalities, or degenerative disease. The pathophysiology of scoliosis is a complex interaction of genetic and environmental influences leading to distorted biomechanics of vertebral growth. The effects of untreated scoliosis are chronic pain, compromised lung function, and postural abnormalities that can preclude regular daily activity and overall well-being. In recent years, extensive advances in surgical techniques, such as spinal fusion and posterior spinal instrumentation, have made it possible to treat extreme cases. Proper screening and early intervention remain paramount in the prevention of long-term complications from this prevalent disorder (Keith et al., 2007) (Figure 4.12).

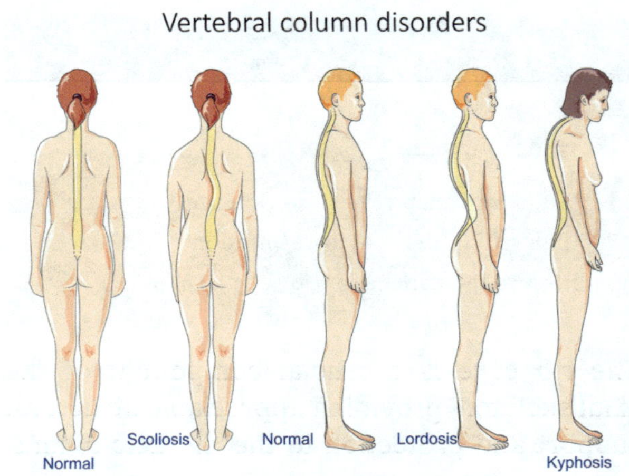

Figure 4.12. Vertebral column disorders.

Source: https://upload.wikimedia.org/wikipedia/commons/3/3b/Vertebral_column_disorders_-_Normal_Scoliosis_Lordosis_Kyphosis_--_Smart-Servier.jpg.

IVD degeneration is another common condition of the vertebral column, particularly with age. It is a degenerative disease in which the vertebral discs degenerate, and they act as cushions between the vertebrae. Its symptoms may be lower backache, reduced motility, and, in severe cases, compression of nerves leading to radiculopathy. Disc degeneration's pathogenesis is a complex process of biochemical alteration with alterations in the ECM and dehydration that progressively undermine disc structure over the long term. Preventive measures, such as maintaining a healthy weight, engaging in regular exercise, and adopting correct ergonomic practices, are essential to minimize the risk of disc degeneration. Secondly, ongoing research on regenerative therapies like growth factors and stem cell therapy provides a promising avenue for future treatment that will reverse damage associated with the discs, thereby improving overall spinal health (Doherty et al., 2016).

Test Your Knowledge

1. What is the basic structure and main segments of the vertebral column?
2. What functions do IVDs serve in the vertebral column?

4.5. The Rib Cage

Learning Outcome

1. Define the anatomy of the rib cage
2. Understand the role in respiration
3. Discuss the connection to the sternum

The rib cage is a crucial component of the axial skeleton, providing appreciable structural support and protection to the thoracic organs, including the heart and lungs. The rib cage is made up of 12 pairs of ribs, thoracic vertebrae, and the sternum, and is a semi-rigid system that facilitates respiratory mechanics. These rib bones each articulate posteriorly with the thoracic vertebrae and then curve forward to meet the sternum anteriorly, creating a flexible container that can be expanded and contracted as a human exhales and inhales. This structural organization not only defends against the organs but also serves as an anchor point for several muscles that shift during respiration, posturing, and upper limb movement, suggesting the rib cage's integral function in general cardiovascular and respiratory functions. The evolutionary nature of the rib cage suggests its flexibility between species. In recent mammals, the sternum is a distinct element of the rib cage, comprising several ossified units, the origin of which has puzzled scientists. Ancientsynapsids, for instance, possessed a unitary sternal element. At the same time, recent discoveries placed the origin of a multipartite sternum at the base of Theriodontia, showing an elaborate evolutionary past that reflects the functional diversification of the rib cage. This evolutionary explanation emphasizes the rib cage's role not merely in protection and respiration but in adapting to a range of environmental stresses and activities throughout evolution, testifying to its significance beyond mere anatomy. Advances in the methodology of medical imaging have also shed additional light on the structural complexity of the rib cage, in particular as it pertains to its biomechanical character. Patient-specific biomechanical models are now a significant tool in the treatment of such conditions as adolescent idiopathic scoliosis, where rib cage alignment and shape can have a substantial effect on breathing. From low-dose biplanar radiographs, researchers have been able to develop protocols for building patient-tailored models that accurately depict a patient's rib cage anatomy. Such an approach not only minimizes exposure to harmful radiation but also enhances the insensitivity of the models to artifacts like rib interpenetration. Such developments signify the rib cage's continued utility not only in explaining human anatomy but also in improving clinical outcomes and treatment strategies, demonstrating the connection of structure to function within the axial skeleton (Bendel et al., 2022; Koutras et al., 2022).

4.5.1. Anatomy of the Rib Cage

The rib cage, a key feature of the axial skeleton, is a crucial component that ensures thoracic cavity protection and respiratory processes. Composed of 12 pairs of ribs, the rib cage falls into three types: true ribs, false ribs, and floating ribs. The first seven pairs are true ribs and hence have costal cartilages to attach to the sternum, providing a secure as well as stable anterior anchor. In comparison, the next three sets, referred to as false ribs, do not directly connect to the sternum but are indirectly supported by the costal cartilage of the rib above. The last two sets, the floating ribs, possess no anterior connection, thus being more unrestricted but less a part of the protective group of the thorax. This body plan allows for the flexibility needed for respiration while maintaining the structure in place. Evolutionarily, the rib cage has undergone significant evolution between species in terms of respiratory biomechanics as well as locomotion. The sternum, which is part of the rib cage, has been of considerable interest to paleontologists trying to come up with its evolution in synapsids, more particularly the pectoral girdle. Evidence shows that early synapsids had a single sternal element, which evolved into the complex, segmental pattern of the sternum in modern mammals. Fresh findings of ossified sternal elements in fossilized gorgonopsians indicate that such multi-part anatomy traces to the Permian period, extending the timeline for the evolution of complex respiratory mechanisms in mammals (Bendel et al., 2022) (Figure 4.13).

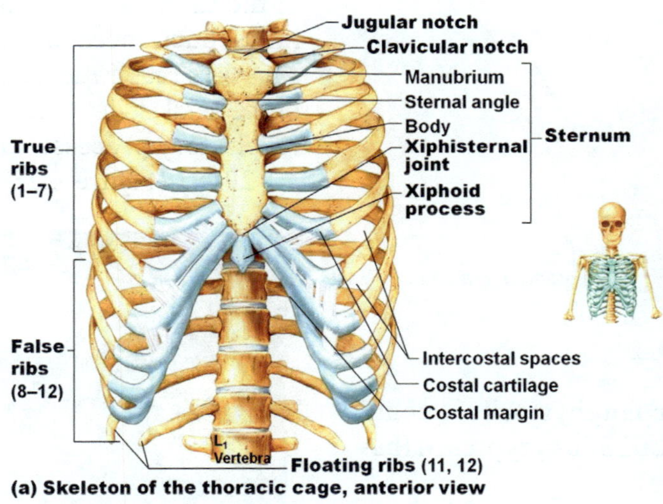

Figure 4.13. Structure of ribs.

Source: https://samarpanphysioclinic.com/rib-cage/.

These adjustments have clear implications for respiratory effectiveness and overall biomechanical function in movement. Furthermore, novel modeling techniques have added to our understanding of rib cage anatomy and its use in clinical situations, such as therapeutic intervention for adolescent idiopathic scoliosis. With the combination of low-dose radiographs and patient-specific biomechanical models, one can analyze rib cage morphology in high levels of detail while limiting radiation dose. This technique enables clinicians to build precise models of the rib cage, allowing tailored treatment plans, including the development of personalized braces. By perfectly molding the template model into the specific anatomy, this strategy presents a firm solution to the detection and treatment of deformities in the rib cage that impair lung function and posture (Koutras et al., 2022). Overall, understanding the anatomical structure and formation of the rib cage gives us a more precise comprehension of both biological and clinical settings within the field of anatomy (Figure 4.14).

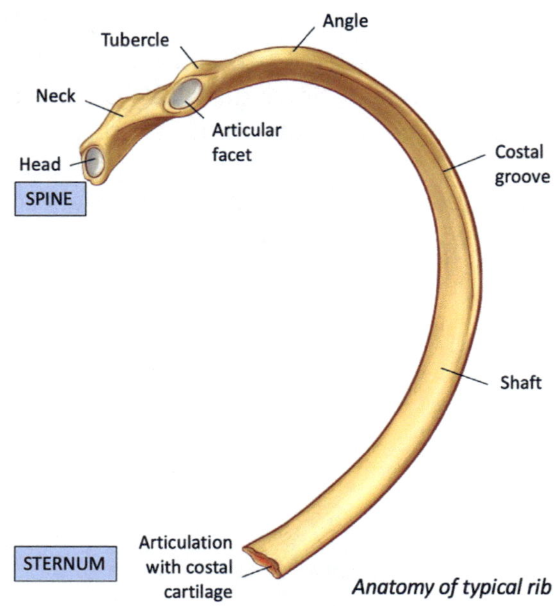

Figure 4.14. Typical ribs.

Source: https://samarpanphysioclinic.com/wp-content/uploads/2023/04/typical-ribs-768x791.webp.

4.5.2. Role in Respiration

The axial skeleton supports respiration, particularly through offering support to respiratory breathing structures. The vertebral column, which is part of the axial skeleton, provides sites of attachment for respiratory function muscles and ribs. Through protecting the spinal cord and spinal column support structure, the vertebral column ensures the effective operation of the respiratory muscles. The ribcage, composed of the thoracic vertebrae and the ribs, encloses vital organs such as the lungs and heart, while simultaneously establishing a dynamic respiratory apparatus. Its rhythmic expansion and recoil during inhalation and exhalation allow for necessary airflow, demonstrating the interconnection between bone support and respiratory mechanics (Bekish et al., 2017). Furthermore, the sternum, which is a crucial component of the axial skeleton, also demonstrates how respiratory structures are related to the skeletal system. It serves as the front attachment of ribs to create a protective shield for the thoracic cavity. The rib-sternum movement during breathing demonstrates that it is an effectively coordinated system whereby the axial skeleton facilitates lung expansion. When the muscles contract, the sternum elevates and the ribs twist outwards, increasing the volume of the thoracic cavity, thus pushing air into the lungs. Such mechanical advantage is crucial to adequate respiration, pointing to the significance of the axial skeleton towards facilitating efficient respiratory processes in the body (Chinsamy et al., 2008) (Figure 4.15).

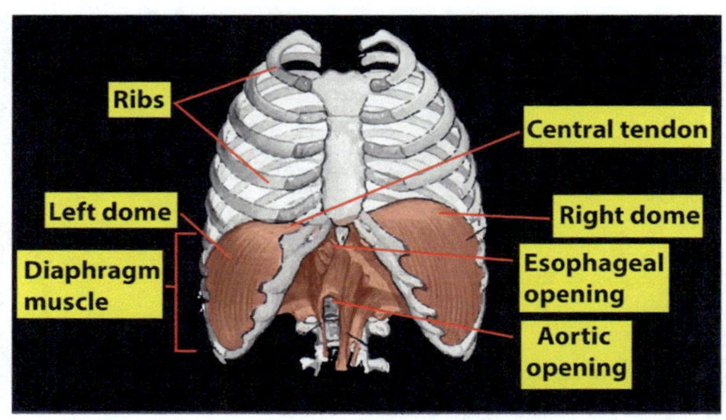

Figure 4.15. The functions of ribs and diaphragm in breathing.

Source: https://www.vedantu.com/question-sets/4503be11-2439-4f00-a641-f8d9d679f930133773128988463253.png.

Furthermore, the evolution of the axial skeleton has had cascading effects on respiratory mechanisms in all animal life. In birds, for example, pneumatic bones, which carry flight adaptations, also demonstrate evidence of a well-adapted respiratory system. The thoracic vertebrae demonstrate structural characteristics that guarantee ventilation of air sacs, optimizing gas exchange. Evidence shows that such specialized elements as the furcula and ilium are closely linked to this respiratory adaptation and act as sites of pneumatic hollowing, enabling air passage through the lungs (Chinsamy et al., 2008). This evolutionary perspective highlights the ongoing relationship between respiratory efficiency and the morphology of the axial skeleton, highlighting the axial skeleton as not only a support framework but an intrinsic component of respiratory physiology.

4.5.3. Connection to the Sternum

The sternum is a stabilizing element in the axial skeleton, particularly for mammals, whose action is embedded with the pectoral girdle of the appendicular skeleton. Its evolution is not only a morphological anomaly but a reflection of essential functional adaptations that have taken place over millions of years. The sternum in mammals comprises multiple ossified portions, which endow it with greater stability and biomechanical action. This segmental structure allows for greater mobility and flexibility of the thoracic cage, which is most important during forelimb locomotion and breathing. The evolutionary history of the sternum highlights a shift towards a single sternal element in early synapsids to a more complex structure as in present-day mammalian forms, hence constituting a milestone event in vertebrate morphology (Bendel et al., 2022).

This comprehension of this evolutionary trajectory further illuminates the overall evolution of the axial skeleton and how it is incorporated with appendicular elements. The importance of sternum research in understanding the evolution of mammalian posture and movement may be among its most fascinating features. The sternum's progressive modifications have been linked with the posteriorization of respiratory musculature, which in turn impacts secondarily the biomechanics of locomotion. As the sternum evolved, it allowed for a more vertical, upright stance, facilitating bipedal locomotion in some species and maximizing the efficiency of respiratory function.

This connection is particularly significant in vertebrate evolution, where the evolution of skeletal form can reflect broader changes in locomotion and interaction with the environment. Its multi-segmented anatomy has been proposed to have been important in mammalian dynamic breathing patterns today, designating the complex relationship between the appendicular and axial skeleton in evolutionary biology research (Bendel et al., 2022). Aside from its anatomical importance, the significance of the sternum stems from its influence on respiratory morphology among species. In bird taxa, for example, the sternum is in close relation with respiratory efficiency, as seen from the presence of pneumatic foramina through which air sacs come into contact with the postcranial skeleton. The varying morphology of the sternum relative to such respiratory structures poses interesting queries concerning the evolutionary pressures operating on diverse taxa. Understanding the nuances of sternal morphology and its role in various animals can provide valuable information regarding the evolution of respiratory adaptation, demonstrating how alterations of the axial skeleton are capable of making significant differences in overall respiratory efficiency. Hence, studies on the sternum not only explain its role within the axial skeleton but also give a better understanding of the evolutionary processes that dictate vertebrate anatomy.

Test Your Knowledge

1. What are the main anatomical components of the rib cage?
2. How does the rib cage contribute to the process of respiration?

4.6. Development and Growth of the Axial Skeleton

Learning Outcome

1. Define embryonic development of the axial skeleton
2. Explain the changes during childhood and adolescence
3. Identify the aging effects on the axial skeleton

Development and formation of the axial skeleton are critical aspects of vertebrate embryogenesis with a complex interplay of cellular and molecular mechanisms. Initially, the axial skeleton, which comprises the vertebral column, ribs, and cranial elements, initiates development during early phases of embryogenesis. In mammals, this is done through the complex migration of those mesenchymal cells that will differentiate into various skeletal components. Most significantly, the cranial neural crest mesenchyme plays a crucial role in axial skeleton formation, enabling bones and cartilages that serve as structural support and function. Dysregulation of such developmental processes not only leads to skeletal malformations but may also have an impact on the organism's general development and health, as exemplified by the need for an intimate understanding of such developmental processes to grasp implications in evolutionary biology as well as clinical implications (Abzhanov et al., 2019). In addition to cellular differentiation, the development of the axial skeleton is also significantly influenced by mechanical stresses evolving during development and functional loading. With the growth and performance of various movements, mechanical loading of the elements of the skeleton leads to dynamic remodeling of these elements. This biomechanical feedback system optimizes the shape and density of skeletal components, allowing them to withstand the applied physical stresses. Furthermore, the regulation of these biomechanical forces is closely linked to molecular signaling pathways, which coordinate the formation and adaptation of the axial skeleton. Understanding these interactions is essential because any interference could impact the development of the skeleton and lead to pathologies, which explains why it is essential to study biomechanical principles as part of learning the development of the skeleton (Bochsler et al., 2007).

Axial skeleton development also calls to mind the adaptability and diversity that exist among vertebrate animals. Environmental pressures and lifestyle modifications have led to significant disparity in the axial skeleton architecture among taxa. In the modulation of vertebral numbers and morphologies within species, for example, one can witness how evolution drives the changes of skeletal architecture towards enhancing locomotion or preservation of other physiological processes. These discrepancies provide an insight into the driving forces of evolution that shape not only the axial skeleton but also the general vertebrate body plan. The elucidation of these patterns in the development of bones and their relevance to evolution explains the strong relationship between anatomy, function, and ecological adaptation. It promotes better understanding of vertebrate biology and evolutionary past (Abzhanov et al., 2019).

4.6.1. Embryonic Development of the Axial Skeleton

The embryonic formation of the axial skeleton is a gentle and highly coordinated process that begins early in gestation. Axial skeleton formation consists of the development of the vertebral column, ribs, and their corresponding structures from mesodermal precursors. The paraxial mesoderm and notochord develop into the axial skeleton, which guides the differentiation of somites into sclerotomes to form vertebrae. Somite segments individually develop into specific vertebral elements, which set the earliest pattern of the spinal column.

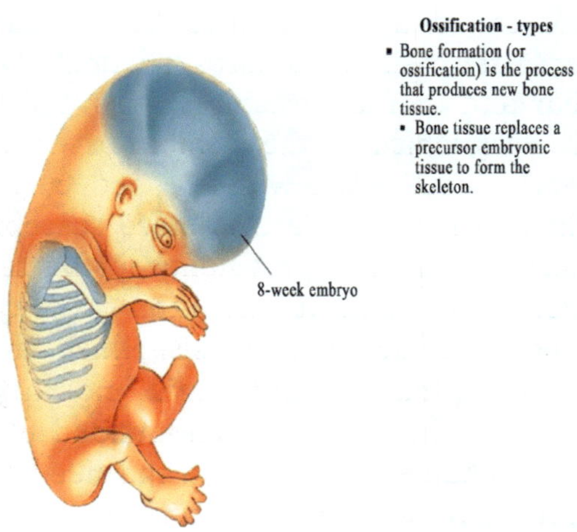

Figure 4.16. Embryonic development of the axial skeleton.

Source: https://i.ytimg.com/vi/p-3PuLXp9Wg/maxresdefault.jpg.

Furthermore, pathways for signaling, such as those involving the use of Sonic Hedgehog (Shh) and Wnt, play important roles in mediating cell fate determination and coordinating patterning of such skeletal elements so that each element gets its proper place within the developing anteroposterior axis of the embryo. With the formation of the axial skeleton, embryonic tissue interactions play significant roles in specifying vertebral elements and associated structures. The process involves not only mesodermal tissues but also neural crest cells, which contribute to the formation of structures such as IVDs and ligaments. The interactions are facilitated by molecular cues that guide the development of chondrogenic and osteogenic lineages. Particularly, developmental abnormalities can be caused by disruption of the signaling pathways, highlighting the importance of maintaining a rigid regulation during embryonic development (Figure 4.16).

For example, interference during notochord formation has been found to lead to serious defects in skeletogenesis, showing how the development of the axial skeleton is closely interlinked with other embryological events. Also, the embryonic development of the axial skeleton is a valuable model for investigating congenital malformations of scoliosis and other vertebral malformations. Investigation into the genetic component in axial development is crucial, as exemplified by the role of transcription factors in craniofacial and vertebral morphology determination. Gene knockouts, for example, can produce a variety of phenotypes that provide insight into the genetic mechanism underlying axial malformation. These findings suggest that mutations in genes that contribute to axial skeleton development may affect cell proliferation and differentiation, culminating in modified bone structure and integrity. Therefore, the intricate interaction of genes, molecular mechanisms, and embryonic cell dynamics not only shapes the axial skeleton but also instructs us about their related congenital diseases with immediate clinical significance.

4.6.2. Changes During Childhood and Adolescence

The development process during childhood and adolescence is characterized by considerable physical transformations, especially in the axial skeleton. During growth, the vertebral column goes through an ossification process that results in a change in both the size and shape of the vertebrae. The growth process is determined by hormonal changes, especially at the puberty stage, which not only affect height but also the general alignment and curvature of the spine. It is essential to understand these changing dynamics since they have a direct impact on postural development and lead to potential MSK challenges later in life. Additionally, physical activity levels and dietary intake during this critical period of growth play a vital role, highlighting the need for a balanced lifestyle to nourish healthy skeletal development. The axial skeleton, including the skull, vertebral column, and rib cage, is the body's central support system, crucial in both supporting and defending the body's organs. Development of the axial skeleton in childhood and adolescence, in addition to growth in length, involves changes in the bones' density and morphology. Recent investigations involving the use of DTI methods have emphasized the importance of changes in microstructure happening within the skeleton as the body grows up. Research findings indicate a significant age-effect on DTI parameters during vertebral formation, suggesting that bone structure and density growth can impact global body function and mechanics (Amaro et al., 2015). This knowledge may be necessary in determining risks for scoliosis or osteoporosis later in adulthood. During the period that children enter adolescence, the skeletal system undergoes a higher rate of change, influenced by genetic and environmental factors. The interaction between growth and psychosocial development is strongest at this time, as new studies indicate that psychosocial stressors can affect bone health and growth patterns. For instance, patients with 22q11.2 Microdeletion Syndrome have disturbances in both neurodevelopmental and skeletal pathways, demonstrating an intricate interaction of genetic and environmental conditions (Bearden et al., 2014). This highlights the need for active management of health during childhood and adolescence to compensate for possible skeletal deficits due to genetic susceptibility or extrinsic stressors. Understanding these complex relationships promotes a more holistic strategy to encourage healthy development in the axial skeleton during these developmental years.

4.6.3. Aging Effects on the Axial Skeleton

Aging is highly influential on the structural stability of the axial skeleton, which includes the skull, vertebral column, and rib cage. In the course of aging, vertebrae become vulnerable to the degenerative process that is characterized by a reduction in bone density and bone microarchitecture deformities. These changes increase the risk of fractures, particularly the lumbar and thoracic fractures. Also, the IVDs themselves, which are the cushions between the vertebrae, degenerate with age, reducing disc height and making the disc more susceptible to herniation. This prevalence of vertebral weakening and disc degeneration is the cause of conditions such as kyphosis, which further weakens spinal stability and mobility in elderly individuals. The compounded effects of these changes underscore the need for a deeper understanding of aging mechanisms to develop effective strategies for preventing bone loss and preserving axial skeleton function. Furthermore, the interaction between aging and axial skeleton mechanical load responses unveils key physiological adaptations. With increased age, the skeleton's capacity to respond to mechanical stimuli diminishes, and a condition of mechanoadaptation insufficiency exists. Research has indicated that disuse conditions are capable of reversibly restoring load responses in older mice, suggesting long-term mechanical unloading can impair the axial skeleton's capacity to adapt. Loading conditions are capable of having a great potential to induce new bone formation in young individuals, but with little effect in aging individuals, particularly in cortical bone. In comparison to younger people, the age-specific decline in the mechanosensitivity of the axial structures complicates restoration of bone mass and density, risking skeletal fragility and associated disorders in later life (Chenu et al., 2017). Overcoming such challenges with exercise-induced proactive loading has the potential to facilitate easier structural resilience among the elderly. Furthermore, the neural and vascular connections that are required for bone strength also deteriorate with age and affect the strength of the axial skeletons. There is also evidence that hippocampal disconnection, specifically affecting limbic tract integrity, is responsible for cognitive function's impact on bone health and density. Research has shown that pattern separation, essential for correct memory and spatial navigation, is compromised by aging and has been associated with changes in the neural networks involved in bone adaptation (Bennett et al., 2014). As declining cognition reduces an individual's tendency to be active, they are less likely to participate in physical activities beneficial to bone health, thus further exacerbating the detrimental effects of aging upon the axial skeleton. It is essential to grasp this interaction between neurological health and bone strength for developing holistic strategies for maintaining maximum aging and minimizing the adverse effects on the axial skeleton.

Test Your Knowledge

1. What are the key stages in the embryonic development of the axial skeleton?
2. How does the axial skeleton change during childhood and adolescence?

SUMMARY

When investigating the axial skeleton, it is imperative to take into consideration its intricate composition and beyond-a-doubt importance in the overall functioning of the vertebrate body. The axial skeleton, basically composed of the vertebrae, skull, and ribcage, forms the basic framework upon which the body's other systems depend. This structure protects crucial organs such as the brain and heart, while also accommodating movement and serving as a point of attachment for muscle. The evolutionary adaptations of the axial skeletons, particularly in the jaw complex of amniotes, are a couple of instances in which molecular and cellular events generate form and function over time and allow species to persist in environments that change. It has been noted in jaw evolution research that perturbation during development may lead to defects as well as remarkable adaptation, illustrating the inherent relationship between structure and success in evolution (Abzhanov et al., 2019). Furthermore, the axial skeleton itself is not a static structure; it is dynamic and sensitive to internal and external forces. This responsiveness is evident in the extensive variety of biomechanical stresses exerted on the axial skeleton, which facilitates movement and absorbs stresses placed upon it. The role of cranial neural crest mesenchyme, for example, has been quoted to be instrumental in the species-specific organization of cranial elements and therefore provides the basis for vertebrate groups' diversity. By studying these developmental processes, researchers can link evolutionary processes to the differences in anatomy among existing vertebrates, including human beings. Not only do such studies enable us to comprehend anatomy better, but they also guide the potential medical applications, particularly the treatment of developmental diseases and injuries in the axial skeleton (Abzhanov et al., 2019). Finally, the work on the axial skeleton has uses beyond anatomy and evolutionary biology, but it is also informed by the science of paleopathology, which enhances our knowledge of the health conditions of the past and their implications. The Museum of Florence's hydrocephalus case is a poignant reminder of how skeletal remains can illuminate the lived experiences of individuals in the past. This confluence of modern scientific technique with ancient inquiry permits greater penetration into pathologies that would have acted upon evolutionary lines. Intersecting these disparate fields of inquiry, the research identifies the axial skeleton's focal status not just in structural integrity but also in its capacity to reflect biological hardship borne by organisms through their evolutionary history. Last, the axial skeleton is a testament to the complexity of vertebrate anatomy and the complex means of adaptation and survival in the wild.

The axial skeleton, including the skull, vertebral column, and rib cage, plays vital functions in the anatomy of humans. To begin with, it provides structural support, safeguarding vital organs such as the brain, spinal cord, and heart. The skull, made up of cranial and facial bones, is an anatomical stronghold that provides protection as well as facilitates processes like respiration, mastication, and sensation. The vertebral column, which is constituted by a column of vertebrae, supports the upright posture as well as enables the flexibility and twisting motion of the torso. The rib cage is also involved in the dual function of housing thoracic organs and aiding respiration. Knowledge of the components and functions of the axial skeleton is essential to understand its significant contribution towards overall human welfare and movement. In addition to its stabilizing role, the structural components of the axial skeletons play an essential role in ligament and muscle attachment. Most groups of muscles that are involved in movement rely on these skeletal structures for attachment and origin. For example, rib-attached muscles are crucial in breathing movements, while muscles attached to vertebrae assist in posture regulation and dynamic movement. Equally important is how the axial skeleton works with the rest of the body's systems, namely the appendicular skeleton, meaning the limbs. The union of the axial and appendicular skeletons makes straightforward how complex the process of human locomotion is and how necessary it is for a strong, stable central skeleton to serve as the anchor from which physical mobility and activity are feasible. Finally, the axial skeleton itself is not exempt from pathology, which will critically affect overall health and function. Scoliosis, fractures, and degenerative conditions are some of the processes that weaken the integrity of the axial skeleton and propagate a downward spiral of illnesses. These deficiencies may manifest as pain, loss of mobility, or compromised protection of organs. Study of such conditions calls for high-level expertise and abilities in areas like biomechanics and pathology, and this reinforces the demand for academic study and medical research. As there is a shift in knowledge regarding the complexity of axial skeletons, it is required to encourage interdisciplinary approaches that conjoin the input of anatomy and medicine so as to develop effective interventions for its conditions. Realizing these aspects underscores the need for ongoing research and education on the axial skeleton and its related disorders.

KEY TERMS FROM THIS CHAPTER

Skull
Facial bones
Maxilla
Zygomatic bones
Cervical vertebrae
Lumbar vertebrae
Sternum
Cranium
Mandible
Nasal bones
Vertebral column
Thoracic vertebrae
Intervertebral discs
Ribs

CRITICAL THINKING QUESTIONS

1. **Which of the following bones is NOT part of the axial skeleton?**
   a. Skull
   b. Sternum
   c. Pelvis
   d. Vertebral column
2. **How many cervical vertebrae are found in the human body?**
   a. 5
   b. 7
   c. 12
   d. 14
3. **The bone that forms the lower part of the nasal septum is called the:**
   a. Vomer
   b. Maxilla
   c. Mandible
   d. Zygomatic
4. **What is the function of the intervertebral discs?**
   a. Protect the spinal cord
   b. Connect ribs to the sternum
   c. Allow movement of the limbs
   d. Absorb shock between vertebrae
5. **The thoracic cage is composed of:**
   a. Clavicle, scapula, and sternum
   b. Ribs, sternum, and thoracic vertebrae
   c. Pelvis, ribs, and femur
   d. Ribs, humerus, and scapula

Short Answer Questions

1. What are the main components of the axial skeleton?
2. What are the primary functions of the axial skeleton?
3. Describe the structure and key functions of the skull.
4. How is the vertebral column organized, and what roles does it play in the body?
5. What bones make up the rib cage, and what is its main function?
6. How does the axial skeleton develop and grow from infancy to adulthood?
7. Why is the axial skeleton important for protecting vital organs?

Answer to Critical Thinking Questions

1. (c); 2. (b); 3. (a); 4. (d); 5. (b)

REFERENCES

1. Woronowicz, K. C., & Schneider, R. A. (2019). Molecular and cellular mechanisms underlying the evolution of form and function in the amniote jaw. *EvoDevo, 10*(1). https://doi.org/10.1186/s13227-019-0131-8Allard, J., Debeir, O., Decaestecker, C., Hermand, D., et al. (2019). Characterization of *Posidonia oceanica* seagrass aerenchyma through whole slide imaging: A pilot study. http://arxiv.org/abs/1903.03044 (accessed on 14th June 2025).
2. Alvarez, A. R., Cuff, A., Goswami, A., Antón, M., Argot, C., Bertram, J. E. A., Biewener, A. A., et al. (2016). Cryptic complexity in felid vertebral evolution: Shape differentiation and allometry of the axial skeleton. https://core.ac.uk/download/36779280.pdf (accessed on 14th June 2025).
3. Alves, C. E., Alves, G. S., Engelhardt, E., Fußer, F., et al. (2012). Different patterns of white matter degeneration using multiple diffusion indices and volumetric data in mild cognitive impairment and Alzheimer patients. https://core.ac.uk/download/14528092.pdf (accessed on 14th June 2025).
4. Amaro, E., Anés, M., Barker, G., Bressan, R. A., et al. (2015). Age-effects in white matter using associated diffusion tensor imaging and magnetization transfer ratio during late childhood and early adolescence. https://core.ac.uk/download/45312686.pdf (accessed on 14th June 2025).
5. Barrett, P. M., Butler, R. J., & Gower, D. J. (2012). Reassessment of the evidence for postcranial skeletal pneumaticity in Triassic archosaurs, and the early evolution of the avian respiratory system. https://core.ac.uk/download/12175752.pdf (accessed on 14th June 2025).
6. Bearden, C. E., Chow, C., Jalbrzikowski, M., Karlsgodt, K. H., et al. (2014). Altered white matter microstructure is associated with social cognition and psychotic symptoms in 22q11.2 microdeletion syndrome. https://core.ac.uk/download/323077572.pdf (accessed on 14th June 2025).
7. Bekish, V. J., & Zorina, V. V. (2017). *Biology*. https://core.ac.uk/download/80152204.pdf (accessed on 14th June 2025).
8. Bekish, V. J., Logishinets, I. A., & Zorina, V. V. (2017). *Practical Book on Biology*. https://core.ac.uk/download/80152210.pdf (accessed on 14th June 2025).
9. Bendel, E. M., Fröbisch, J., Kammerer, C. F., Luo, Z. X., et al. (2022). The earliest segmental sternum in a Permian synapsid and its implications for the evolution of mammalian locomotion and ventilation. https://core.ac.uk/download/611857947.pdf (accessed on 14th June 2025).
10. Bennett, I. J., Huffman, D. J., & Stark, C. E. L. (2014). Limbic tract integrity contributes to pattern separation performance across the lifespan. https://core.ac.uk/download/305124377.pdf (accessed on 14th June 2025).
11. Benson, R. J., Figueirido-Castillo, F. B., Martín-Serra, A., Pastor, J. F., et al. (2021). Serial disparity in the carnivoran backbone unveil a complex adaptive role in metameric evolution. https://core.ac.uk/download/621566417.pdf (accessed on 14th June 2025).
12. Berkes, S., Blaschke, K., Brendolan, A., Britanova, O., Buck, A., Bush, J. O., Capellini, T. D., et al. (2018). Pbx loss in cranial neural crest, unlike in epithelium, results in cleft palate only and a broader midface. https://core.ac.uk/download/323072849.pdf (accessed on 14th June 2025).
13. Bochsler, V. S., Galloway, S. B., Harley, R. A., Kramarsky-Winters, E., et al. (2007). *Coral Disease and Health Workshop: Coral Histopathology II*. https://core.ac.uk/download/11017972.pdf (accessed on 14th June 2025).

14. Buchanan, G., Ma, M., & Rea, P. M. (2014). A multimedia package for patient understanding and rehabilitation of non-contact anterior cruciate ligament injuries. https://core.ac.uk/download/16461708.pdf (accessed on 14th June 2025).

15. Chenu, C., Collinson, R. S., De Souza, R., Javaheri, B., et al. (2017). Prolonging disuse in aged mice amplifies cortical but not trabecular bones' response to mechanical loading. https://core.ac.uk/download/132194058.pdf (accessed on 14th June 2025).

16. Chinsamy, A., Bezuidenhout, A. J., King, A. S., Müller, B., Britt, B. B., et al. (2008). Evidence for avian intrathoracic air sacs in a new predatory dinosaur from Argentina. https://core.ac.uk/download/pdf/8193605.pdf (accessed on 14th June 2025).

17. Clayton, S. W. (2021). *TGFβ Provides the Backbone of Embryogenesis: Elucidating the Role of TGFβ Signaling and Its Downstream Effectors on Spinal Column Development*. https://core.ac.uk/download/640972654.pdf (accessed on 14th June 2025).

18. Collette, N., Economides, A., Gale, N., Harland, R., et al. (2013). Sost and its paralog Sostdc1 coordinate digit number in a Gli3-dependent manner. https://core.ac.uk/download/323081486.pdf (accessed on 14th June 2025).

19. Cooke, C. B., Gannon, L., Hind, K., Truscott, J. G., et al. (2011). Bone cross-sectional geometry in male runners, gymnasts, swimmers and non-athletic controls: A hip-structural analysis study. https://core.ac.uk/download/29019048.pdf (accessed on 14th June 2025).

20. Cozart, D., Hesse, D., Nichols, R., Szymik, B., et al. (2017). *UGA Anatomy and Physiology 1 Lab Manual* (3rd ed.). https://core.ac.uk/download/217306564.pdf (accessed on 14th June 2025).

21. Criswell, K. E., & Gillis, J. A. (2020). Resegmentation is an ancestral feature of the gnathostome vertebral skeleton. https://core.ac.uk/download/305121129.pdf (accessed on 14th June 2025).

22. Doherty, T. B. (2016). *Investigation of Uncharacterized Spondylocostal Dysostosis Using Whole Exome Sequencing*. https://open.bu.edu/bitstream/2144/14656/7/Doherty_bu_0017N_10488_web.pdf (accessed on 14th June 2025).

23. Echols, M. S., Hedrick, B. P., Lawson, A. B., Martinez, M. A., et al. (2024). Variation in air sac morphology and postcranial skeletal pneumatization patterns in the African grey parrot. https://core.ac.uk/download/640946457.pdf (accessed on 14th June 2025).

24. Ermolenko, A. (2011). *Development of Human Limbs*. https://core.ac.uk/download/pdf/289771.pdf (accessed on 14th June 2025).

25. Evans, T., Ghandour, Y., Masi, A. T., Nair, K., et al. (2010). Clinical, biomechanical, and physiological translational interpretations of human resting myofascial tone or tension. https://core.ac.uk/download/pdf/8560636.pdf (accessed on 14th June 2025).

26. Galassi, F. M., Nesi, G., Ottini, L., Pietragalla, G., et al. (2018). The antiquity of hydrocephalus: The first full paleo-neuropathological description. https://core.ac.uk/download/188829525.pdf (accessed on 14th June 2025).

27. Gardner, E. (2020). *Cancer in Ancient Human Populations: Methods and Practice in Bioarcheology and Paleopathology*. https://core.ac.uk/download/323062037.pdf (accessed on 14th June 2025).

28. Gerisch, A., Grimal, Q., Penta, R., Raum, K., et al. (2016). Can a continuous mineral foam explain the stiffening of aged bone tissue? A micromechanical approach to mineral fusion in musculoskeletal tissues. https://core.ac.uk/download/132211488.pdf (accessed on 14th June 2025).

29. Haazelager, M. B., Leeuwen, J. L. van, Muller, M., et al. (2025). The effect of trimming of the frog on the impact accelerations of the equine hoof during walk and trot. https://core.ac.uk/download/pdf/29253136.pdf (accessed on 14th June 2025).

30. Haugen, G. M. (1994). *The Cervical Spine: Race and Sex Differences.* https://core.ac.uk/download/268809086.pdf (accessed on 14th June 2025).

31. Huerne, H. L. ter, Luding, S., & Magnanimo, V. (2012). Modeling of asphalt durability and self-healing with discrete particles method. https://core.ac.uk/download/pdf/11483421.pdf (accessed on 14th June 2025).

32. Keith, A., Minelli, A., Rokas, A., Stollewerk, A., Stoltzfus, A., et al. (2007). Homeotic evolution in the Mammalia: Diversification of therian axial seriation and the morphogenetic basis of human origins. https://core.ac.uk/download/pdf/7715930.pdf (accessed on 14th June 2025).

33. Koutras, C., Nesme, M., Otaduy, M. A., Péres, P., et al. (2022). Biomechanical morphing for personalized fitting of scoliotic torso skeleton models. https://core.ac uk/download/534430093.pdf (accessed on 14th June 2025).

34. Marsden, R. S. (2019). *The Effects of Sacroiliac Manipulation and Pelvic Blocking on Active Gluteus Medius Trigger Points: A Randomized Clinical Trial.* https://core.ac.uk/download/323341134.pdf (accessed on 14th June 2025).

35. Roberts, C. (2020). Regulating retinoic acid availability during development and regeneration: The role of the CYP26 enzymes. https://core.ac.uk/download/pdf/322832230.pdf (accessed on 14th June 2025).

36. Warraich, S. (2013). *Ectopic Mineralization of Spinal Tissues in Mice Lacking Equilibrative Nucleoside Transporter 1.* https://core.ac.uk/download/61637591.pdf (accessed on 14th June 2025).

APPENDICULAR SKELETON

5

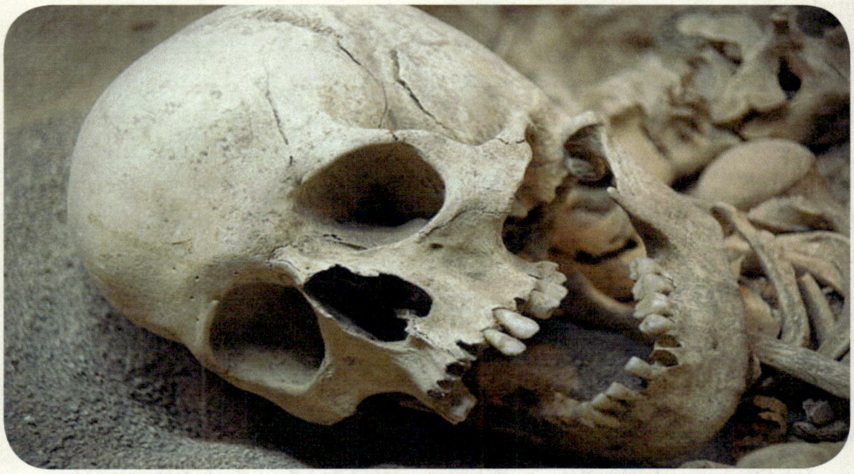

LEARNING OBJECTIVES

After studying this chapter, you will be able to:

1. Enumerate the structures of the appendicular skeleton
2. Outline the functions of the appendicular skeleton
3. Compare and contrast the appendicular skeleton with the axial skeleton
4. Summarize the development of the appendicular skeleton
5. Enumerate common injuries and disorders of the appendicular skeleton.
6. Summarize diagnostic procedures used to assess appendicular skeletal disorders

Introduction

The appendicular skeleton has a significant role in vertebrate body structure, facilitating movement and contact with the environment. It is established by limbs, girdles, and appurtenant structures and is distinct from the axial skeleton, which creates the body's central framework. The upper appendicular elements facilitate delicate manipulations and locomotion, while the lower appendicular structures are adapted for weight-bearing and terrestrial locomotion. It is necessary to understand the nuances of the appendicular skeleton as it has a direct bearing on several disciplines like biomechanics, veterinary science, and evolutionary science, as it plays a crucial role in determining an organism's ability to perform irreplaceable functions like running, jumping, and grasping. A detailed analysis of the appendicular skeleton not only showcases its adaptations for function but also the repercussions of its evolution on diverse species. Evolution and history of the appendicular skeleton have been shaped by a variety of factors, including environmental demands and specialized life habits of organisms. The of limb structures seen among mammals and birds, for instance, points to the adaptive radiations that allow such organisms to occupy various ecological niches. Research indicates that the appendicular skeleton is not a static structure but is always subject to external pressures that cause diversification and specialization in the long term. The study of skeletal transformation provides us with the knowledge of the evolutionary path of the vertebrates, in particular, how different species develop to fit into their environments. Furthermore, the appendicular skeleton warrants teaching and learning with innovative methods, as seen in research aimed at creating interactive learning materials for veterinary students to comprehend complex details of joint movement and muscle function (Buck et al., 2022). Besides, the appendicular skeleton is also essential in comprehending locomotion, which is fundamental for survival and adaptation in diverse surroundings. Its shape not only allows for movement but also maximizes biomechanical efficiency, one of the determinants for the evolutionary success of most species. For instance, birds, which have evolved specialized body shapes, possess complex respiratory systems that enable optimal activities during flight (Barrett et al., 2012). Continual research on the appendicular skeleton enables advancements in imaging technologies and techniques to elaborate on subtle anatomical relationships and functional dynamics. These findings not only add to our understanding of locomotion and locomotory patterns but also have significant implications for fields ranging from evolutionary biology to applied veterinary practice. A precise beginning to the appendicular skeleton thus serves as a basis for an appreciation of its various functions in biology and medicine.

Definition of the Appendicular Skeleton

The appendicular skeleton is a vital component of the vertebrate skeleton, and it comprises the limbs and their corresponding girdles. The framework of the skeleton involves the pectoral girdle, which is utilized to connect the upper limbs with the trunk, and the pelvic girdle, which is employed to support the lower limbs. These elements together enable a range of movement and function needed for manipulation and locomotion within the environment. Gross bones of the appendicular skeleton are characterized by possessing complex articulations and varied morphologies, due to their adapted functions in support and motion. The humerus of the arm, for instance, allows for broader range of movement, while the femur in the leg supports the body weight when walking on two legs. This skeletal diversity exemplifies the evolutionary accommodations of the appendicular skeleton across species, illustrating how some bone forms and some joint orientations facilitate survival and mobility. The developmental biology of the appendicular skeleton is a fundamental component of this system, which is regulated by genetic, environmental, and evolutionary factors. Investigation of the appendicular skeleton typically involves applying new methods, such as three-dimensional imaging and machine learning, to analyze morphological differences. For example, studies have noted that there is significant variation among appendicular elements, including that found in fossil records for the titanosaur sauropods. Variation in morphology among the bones of these specimens has been linked to functional adaptation, hence shedding light on the locomotion and diet of the early animals. The variation of the appendicular skeletons aids in reconstructing not only the biological purpose of such species but also their ecological function within habitats, forming a robust perception of anatomy and evolution (Buck et al., 2022; Páramo et al., 2021). The appendicular skeleton also forms an essential base for investigating various biomechanical characteristics involving movement. The distinctive patterns of bones and joints in this space of bone are what allow for these advanced motions, such as running, jumping, and grasping. Each of the positions of the limbs is designed for its function, and because of this fact, the appendicular skeleton is so vital to biomechanical study. This extends beyond anatomy into the field of physiology, because the attached musculature for these bones is necessary to their movements. Research has established that understanding the appendicular skeleton's composition aids in evaluating locomotor methods and habitat forms in current and past organisms. Therefore, the appendicular skeleton is not merely an assemblage of bones but a portal to comprehending mobility's evolutionary role and life's overall patterns (Buck et al., 2022; Páramo et al., 2021) (Figure 5.1).

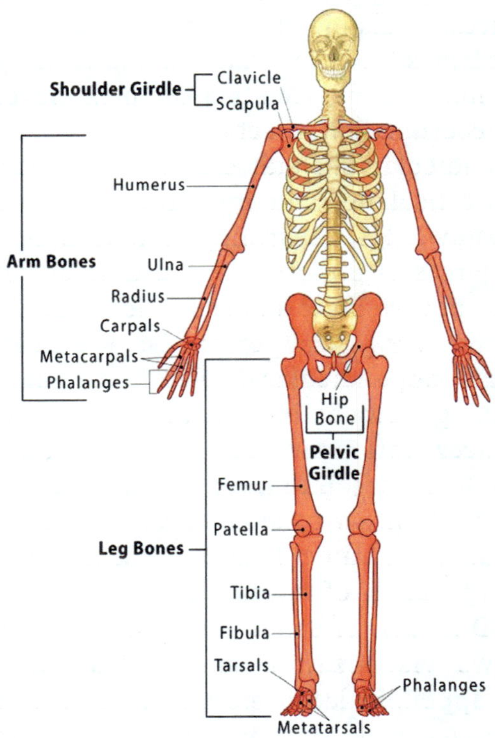

Figure 5.1. Appendicular skeleton.

Source: https://www.theskeletalsystem.net/wp-content/uploads/2022/10/Appendicular-Skeleton.jpg.

Importance in Human Anatomy

The appendicular skeleton contributes a significant amount to the overall movement and functioning of the human body, serving not only as a support for the attachment of muscles but also as an integral component of most biomechanical movements. The skeletal system consists of the limbs and girdles, facilitating an incredible range of movements crucial to activities such as walking, running, and the manipulation of objects. The plasticity of the appendicular system renders humans versatile in performing diverse activities, illustrating the role of evolution. This is exhibited when contrasting other animals' limbs, say felids, where variations in skeletal morphology are attributed to ecological and behaviorally driven adaptations, upholding the concept of integrated morphology in evolutionary biology (Goswami et al., 2018). The effect of environmental demands on skeletal form underscores the significance of the highly evolved appendicular skeleton in serving diverse functions across species. Furthermore, the evolution of appendicular skeletons has implications for human anatomy and physiology universally, illustrating interdependence between skeletal systems and functional adaptability. The arm, made up of the humerus, the radius and ulna, and the intricate set of carpals and phalanges, manifests this versatility through its ability to create sophisticated movements necessary in tools and expressions of communication. The shoulder girdle's architecture, in particular, allows for an impressive amount of range of motion (ROM), essential in many different pursuits, from sports excellence to simple daily tasks. Most importantly, the morphological variation that occurs in appendicular skeletons of other animals enlightens further on how anatomical form is shaped by functional pressures, as part of an overall biological principle whereby evolutionary lineages sculpt anatomical shapes (Paretsis et al., 2020). This interplay between anatomy and function speaks to the significance of the appendicular skeleton in human evolution and in our normal lives. In addition, knowledge of anatomy of the appendicular systems is imperative in clinical and rehabilitation environments. Anatomy knowledge of appendicular structures aids medical professionals in diagnosing and treating musculoskeletal (MSK) diseases, fractures, and injuries. Anatomy knowledge of the precise position and functional capability of upper and lower limbs, for instance, is instrumental for successful rehabilitation procedures. Furthermore, anatomical differences between the skeletal anatomy of populations underscore the importance of a critical understanding of human anatomy, particularly in adapting treatment protocols to specific needs according to variation in anatomy (Goswami et al., 2018). In conclusion, the appendicular skeleton's function is not only for support; it serves a vital role in improving human function against the environment, and its inclusion in anatomy studies and practical clinical practice is justified.

5.1. Components of the Appendicular Skeleton

Learning Outcome

1. Discuss the upper limb bones and lower limb bones
2. Define pelvic girdle and pectoral girdle

The appendicular skeleton consists of the limb bones and girdles that connect them to the axial skeleton. This skeletal division is significant in allowing movement and walking, a capacity based on evolution. An important turning point in vertebrate evolution was reached approximately 370 million years ago when limbs from lobe-finned fishes evolved, demonstrating a complex reorganization of skeletal and musculoskeletal (MSK) structure. The appendicular skeleton of the living lobe-finned fishes and early tetrapods shares very similar anatomical features, namely pectoral and pelvic limb organization. This evolution into more fragmented, module-like limbs reflects muscle diversification in functionality with a wide range of movements and flexibility in terrestrial settings, which would be necessary to thrive in changing habitats (Abbasi et al., 2018). The study of the appendicular skeleton also highlights the role of the individual components in mobility and function. The pectoral girdle, constituted by the scapula and clavicle, stabilizes the forelimbs and facilitates most significant movement needed for functions like climbing, flying, and hunting. Similarly, the pelvic girdle maintains the hindlimbs while providing the support and strength required for running and jumping. Additionally, these anatomical structures enable the precise articulation of limb bones. The joints, like ball-and-socket joints and hinge joints, facilitate complex movement and coordination of actions. The evaluation of appendicular skeletal elements, particularly their articulation and organization, contributes to knowledge regarding biomechanics and the forces of evolution in the development of limbs in vertebrate animals (Buck et al., 2022). From a pedagogical perspective, the education of the appendicular skeleton can enhance teaching methods in veterinary and biological sciences. Interactive tutorials explaining the complexity of joint movement, muscle tension, and recognition of anatomical structures, for instance, reframe learning paradigms. The incorporation of advanced visual tools, such as 3D models of bones and animated overlays, allows visualization and interaction with the appendicular skeleton structures in an improved way. This method not only assists in the identification of normal vs. abnormal form but also adds to one's knowledge about locomotion. By correlating theory to practice, such innovative instructional material promotes overall study of appendicular anatomy and helps build a richer learning experience for students (Buck et al., 2022).

5.1.1. Upper Limb Bones

The bones of the upper limb play an essential role within the appendicular skeleton's functional anatomy to provide for a lot of movement and fine motor function. Comprised of the humerus, radius, and ulna, as well as a whole series of smaller bones in the wrist and hand, these items enable gross and fine motor capabilities. As a vital link between the axial and appendicular skeletons, the humerus, a single bone in the upper arm, articulates with the scapula at the shoulder joint. It continues proximally to form the elbow joint, where it articulates with the radius and the ulna, showing the intricate relationships of the bones of the upper limb. An understanding of these components reveals not just the individual functions of each entity, but also how they contribute individually to overall mobility and manipulation, a reflection of evolutionary specializations designed to perform multiple locomotor and manipulative tasks found in human activities. The history of tetrapods from lobe-finned fishes influenced the evolution of limb bones of the upper limbs, a milestone in vertebrate morphology (Figure 5.2).

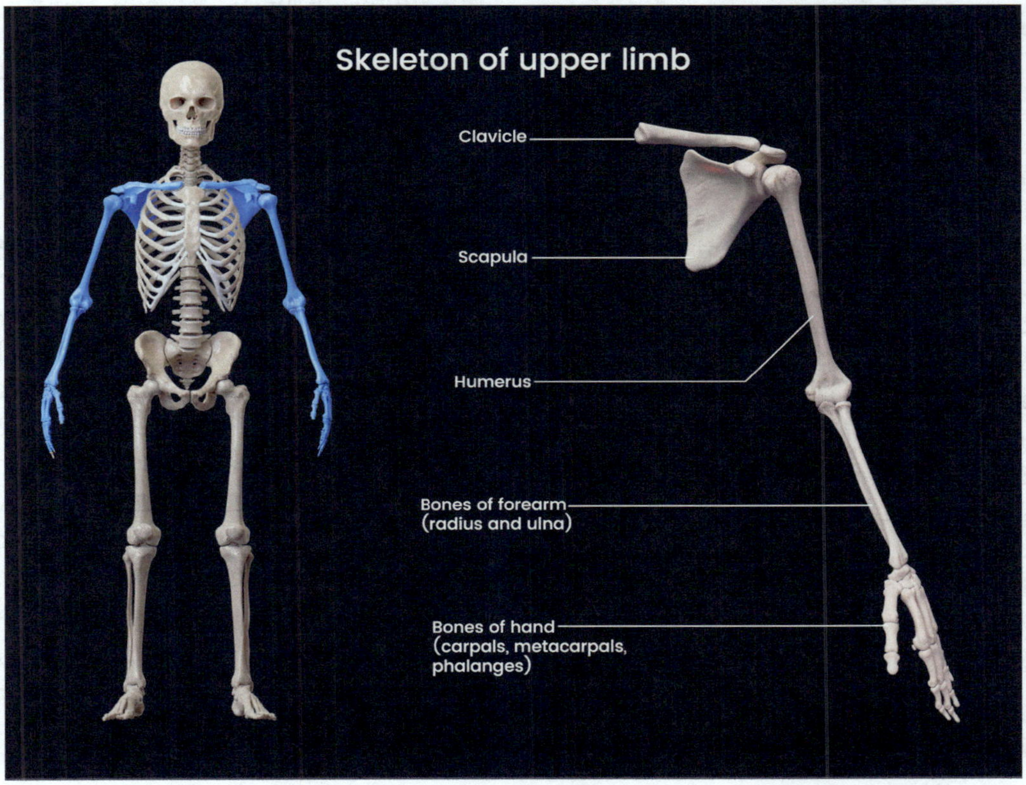

Figure 5.2. Skeleton of upper limb.

Source: https://admin.anatomy.app/Media/images/ac1538bb-1873-45cd-819e-376d6750f399_large.jpg.

As tetrapods developed onto land, their skeleton was overhauled drastically, allowing for the development of more general-purpose limbs than in their aquatic ancestors. This process can be traced to the anatomical changes that formed differentiated hindlimb and forelimb characteristics, both enhancing stability and locomotor efficiency. Specifically, analysis of contemporary species demonstrates an extraordinary modularization of limb morphology with characteristic configurations of bones in the forelimb supporting specialized capabilities, such as object manipulation and grasping. Such evolutionary patterns identify upper limb bones as adaptive devices that have arisen to meet environmental challenge and opportunity, emphasizing their role in survival and success in terrestrial vertebrates (Abbasi et al., 2018). History of extinct creatures, such as the giant short-faced bear, also gives meaning to the functional diversity of upper limb bones throughout evolution. Studies of the craniodental anatomy of *Arctodus simus* have provided insight into its paleobiology and have demonstrated not only how these bones enabled locomotion but how they adapted to various ecological niches. Applying craniodental measurements to distinguish relationships in the Ursidae family, researchers discovered evidence that while *A. simus* had robust limb structures, it did not conform to those of advanced predators. The scaling and morphology of limb bones suggest a robust omnivore capable of surviving in various environments, utilizing its upper limb bones for foraging and locomotion rather than solely for predation. These findings summarize the evolutionary narrative as represented by the upper limb bones, which signify their complexity and adaptational significance in various taxa (Figueirido-Castillo et al., 2010).

5.1.2. Lower Limb Bones

These bones of the lower limb are essential in the overall structure and function of the appendicular skeleton and serve critical biomechanical functions for locomotion and support. Comprising the femur, patella, tibia, fibula, tarsals, metatarsals, and phalanges, they all contribute to assist in performing complex motions, ranging from ambulation to jogging. The femur, the longest human bone, connects the hip joint to the knee, and the patella, or kneecap, reinforces the leverage of the quadriceps muscle during knee extension, helping in the practical mechanics of movement. This structure demonstrates how selective pressures have shaped the bone anatomy of the lower limb for terrestrial locomotor needs, and how there exist intricate interrelations and functions with the appendicular skeleton. Exploring the history of lower limb bones offers informative data on how they evolved from lobe-finned relatives of present-day tetrapods. As indicated in scholarly research, terrestrial-to-aquatic locomotory transitions needed radical remapping of muscular and skeletal systems to arrive at greater modularity and reduced anatomical integration of limb bones (Abbasi et al., 2018) (Figure 5.3).

This transition illustrates the complex interaction of environmental stress and biomechanical adaptation as early tetrapods evolved the morphology for terrestrial existence. By studying current species and their anatomical features, researchers can reverse-engineer the evolutionary trajectories that led to the formation of lower limb bones, providing rich context for considering diversity in locomotor strategy among species in the appendicular skeleton. The patella seems to be an exceptionally fascinating component of the lower limb bones, offering multiple functional advantages that increase the overall efficiency of movement. Its existence is especially notable in the sense that it increases joint leverage and provides assistance for adjacent tendons, optimizing the biomechanics of knee function (Benjamin et al., 2016). Moreover, recent research has also presented evidence for the patella's evolutionary significance by citing its presence in many different amniote groups and explaining its morphological variation. It has been proposed that this sesamoid bone might have evolved independently and therefore serve as a significant indicator of functional adaptation in mammals and reptiles. The dynamic role of the patella within lower limb anatomy serves to illustrate the broader significance of evolutionary processes in the construction of the appendicular skeleton, better informing us of both structural and functional relations between the various elements of limb anatomy.

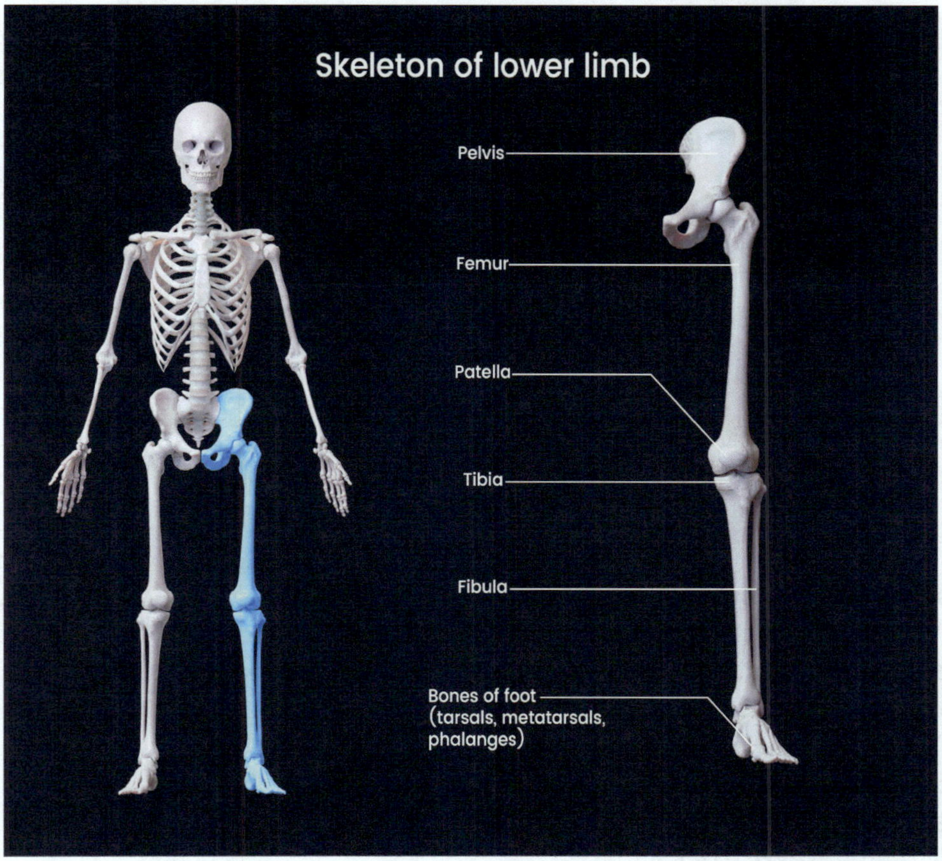

Figure 5.3. Skeleton of lower limb.

Source: https://anatomy.app/Media/images/lower-extremity-skeleton-pelvis-free-lower-limb-bones-anterior-view_20240828055159_medium.jpg.

5.1.3. Pelvic Girdle and Pectoral Girdle

Appendicular skeleton, comprising pelvic as well as pectoral girdles, is the most crucial component of vertebrate movement and functional adaptation. The pectoral girdle that supports the front limbs is far more complex, considering its evolutionary function. It not only serves as a structural support for movement but also provides for a sequence of movements that are obligatory for the execution of a whole range of actions, such as swimming, flying, and grasping. Through the process of evolution, the morphology of the pectoral girdle has undergone wide variations. It indicates a high level of adaptability and flexibility in responding to different habitats. This evolutionary dynamism emphasizes the complex interplay between form and function in the pectoral girdle as a prime consideration in the evolutionary history of vertebrates, most notably during the shift from water to land, where limb development offered greater mobility in varied ecological niches (Figure 5.4).

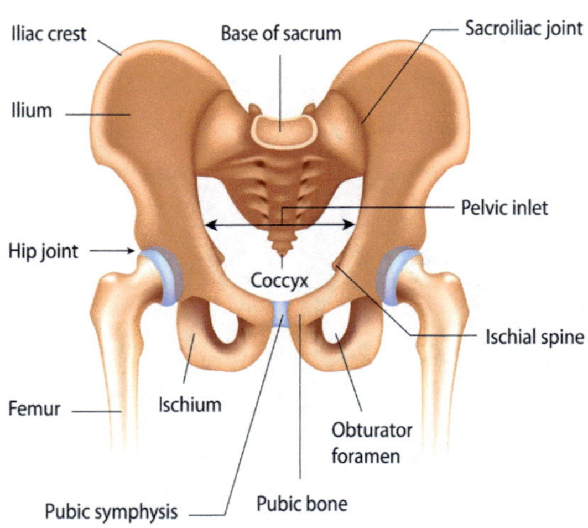

Figure 5.4. Pelvic girdle.

Source: https://womenshealthdublin.ie/wp-content/uploads/2020/09/pelvic-girdle-diagram-ireland-dublin-help.jpg.

Conversely, the pelvic girdle also experienced significant evolutionary changes but lagged behind the pectoral girdle in the transition from fin-like materials to limb-like morphology. This dichotomy can be observed in the skeletal part of the pelvic appendage, which is generally smaller or less complex compared to its pectoral counterparts. Developmentally, however, there is a high degree of anatomical congruence between early tetrapod pelvic and pectoral girdle muscles, according to comparative studies. This point of congestion during the fins-to-limbs transition implies that while the musculature was originally analogous, the terrestrial locomotion-directed evolution of the pelvic girdle was more evolutionary.

The nuanced analysis of such evolutionary events illuminates how the pelvic girdle has evolved to facilitate bipedalism and other locomotory behaviors within terrestrial environments compared to its more leisurely evolutionary history with the pectoral girdle (et al., 2018). The interaction between the pelvic and pectoral girdles is a classic illustration of the excellent evolutionary adaptation to emergent environmental challenges presented by early tetrapods.

Evidence suggests that the two girdles share a common ancestry that explains a certain degree of anatomical congruence, particularly in terms of muscle composition and functional integration. Studies have established that with tetrapod evolution, there was augmented diversification in muscle functions, which facilitated greater adaptability and flexibility in various environments. Such appendages' original modularity points to an evolutionary tactical advantage by enabling more specialized movements for particular hobbies and lifestyles. In addition, understanding the evolutionary history of these girdles, particularly through network analysis, enables researchers to reconstruct anatomical changes that occurred during the fins-to-limbs transition and subsequently improve our knowledge of vertebrate evolution (Abbasi et al., 2018) (Figure 5.5).

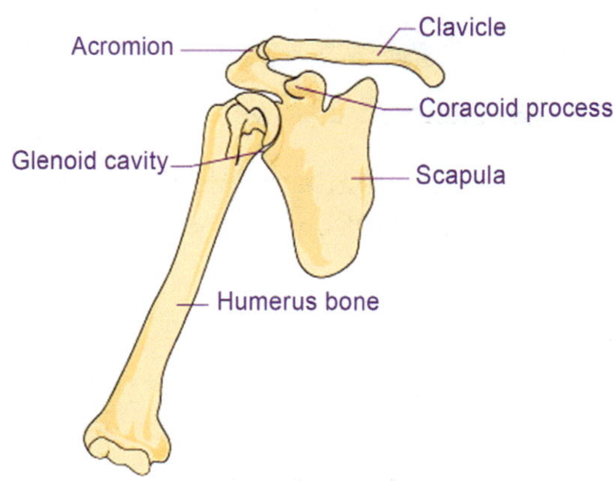

Figure 5.5. Pectoral girdle.

Source: https://cdn1.byjus.com/wp-content/uploads/2022/03/Pectoral-Girdle.png.

Test Your Knowledge

1. What are the main bones that make up the upper limb and lower limb?
2. What is the structure and function of the pelvic girdle?

5.2. Function of the Appendicular Skeleton

Learning Outcome

1. The appendicular skeleton plays a pivotal role in supporting the body
2. Explain the role in locomotion
3. Discuss the contribution to overall body stability

The appendicular skeleton has a highly significant role in the production of movement and structural support to varied aspects of bodily function. Composed of the limbs and the supportive girdles, the appendicular skeleton permits a range of movements that are necessary for locomotion as well as for manipulation of the environment. In tetrapods whose evolutionary lineage traces back to lobe-finned fishes, fin-to-limb evolution is a paradigm of a significant biomechanical innovation. This evolution required the remodeling of the skeletal and muscular anatomy to enable better mobility and the development of diverse locomotion methods in different environments. The appendicular skeleton design also helps to the capacity for complex movements while in balance and stability, particularly in terrestrial environments, and substantiates the hypothesis that its functional features are a key factor in the survival and adaptability of these animals (Abbasi et al., 2018). Central to appendicular skeletal function is the intricate relationship between bones and muscles that allows for motion. In mammals, the interaction of several groups of muscles with the skeleton allows for motion as well as specific joint function. Analysis of this function is crucial for a discipline such as veterinary medicine, where the identification of joint functional change and muscle activity can be a life-altering difference in diagnosis and treatment. Interactive learning devices that provide a three-dimensional tour of the skeleton and the dynamic vision of muscle action with locomotion facilitate comprehension of these complex interactions. By providing examples of normal and abnormal structure and function, these devices enable appreciation for the appendicular skeleton's role in injury and health and thereby emphasize its significance both in anatomical teaching and clinical practice (Buck et al., 2022). Moreover, its functional diversity is a result of the appendicular skeleton's modularity. The modularity is capable of specialized adaptations that vary depending on the type of movement required by various species. For instance, the pectoral and pelvic appendages possess different degrees of morphological adaptation to environmental requirements, such as swimming or running. This specialization is further brought out by evolutionary studies, which have demonstrated a trend towards less integrated and more modular anatomical structures. Such adaptations not only improve movement but also perform complex tasks, thereby once again substantiating the appendicular skeleton's multidimensional function in an organism's locomotion and interfacing with the environment. Lastly, the appendicular skeleton is essential not only for locomotion but also for the adaptive processes that have evolved as a consequence of numerous ecological stresses (Abbasi et al., 2018).

5.2.1. Support and Movement

The appendicular skeleton supports the body and allows movement, so it is critical for several physical activities. Its primary components are the bones of the upper limbs, pelvic girdle, lower limbs, and shoulder girdle. The skeletal components are designed to allow stability along with a high degree of mobility. For instance, the shoulder girdle permits a wide range of arm movement required for such work as basic functional movements and complicated athletics.

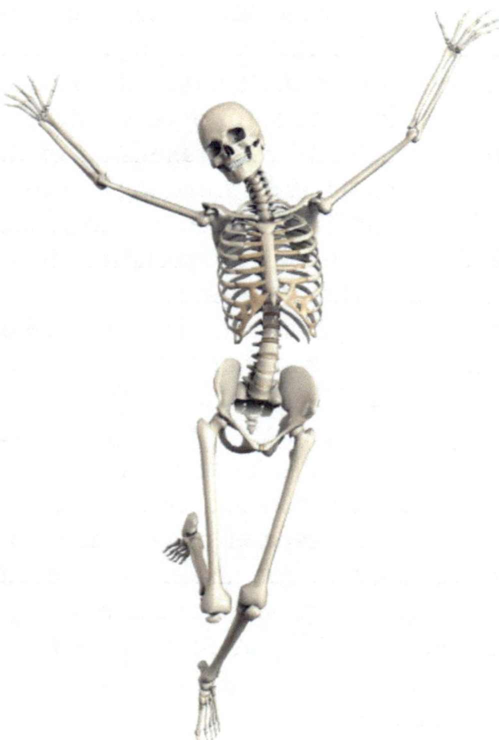

Figure 5.6. One of the most important functions of the appendicular skeleton is movement. Bones of the limbs work together with the muscular system to initiate motion.

Source: https://external-content.duckduckgo.com/iu/?u=https%3A%2F%2Fwww.albert.io%2Fblog%2Fwp-content%2Fuploads%2F2023%2F12%2Fskeleton-2504341_1280-690x1024.png&f=1&nofb=1&ipt=7c6de6d54cce7a0c1e13a1115911935ad88a1359e1048d18f6169c96b7751ba2.

The appendicular skeleton, therefore, is not only a framework upon which muscles attach but also a system of levers that amplify the force of muscular contractions to improve the body's overall capacity to move. Another interesting aspect of the appendicular skeleton is its relationship with postural stability, that is, the manner in which variations among individuals influence performance and support. Research on the appendicular skeleton components, such as the arms, has disclosed striking differences between the dominant and non-dominant sides. It was established that postural stability, as measured by procedures like inertial measurement units (IMU), exhibits remarkable differences in movement patterns and stability between individuals. The difference of acceleration and movement factors between limbs suggests the importance of such organization in precision- and balance-requiring activities (Figure 5.6).

This argument stresses the function of the appendicular skeleton's complexity to not only enable the generation of movements but also stability, especially when the visual feedback is removed, thus emphasizing its internal function in both static and dynamic types of movement (Cerny et al., 2019). The significance of the appendicular skeleton extends beyond simple capability for ordinary movement; it encompasses complicated interaction between bone development and evolutionary modification in a large number of species. Consider ceratophryid frogs, which show remarkable changes in bone production that ultimately impact their systems of eating and movement. Their evolutionary adaptations, which include new morphological features related to the appendicular skeleton, emphasize the connection between functional anatomy and ecological niches. These specializations allow the frogs to efficiently feed on large prey, showing a complex relationship between skeletal evolution and locomotory strategy concerning environmental needs. Appendicular diversification within species not only explains the capacity to carry out functions but also the forces behind movement capabilities in varying environments (Pereyra et al., 2016).

5.2.2. Role in Locomotion

The appendicular skeleton is the locomotory key to enabling a wide array of movements and functions required for adaptation and survival. It comprises the limb bones and supporting girdles. The appendicular skeleton enables stability and flexibility, and it aids in various modes of locomotion, such as walking, running, flying, and swimming. In terrestrial animals, the limbs have joints and musculature that work in combination to create coordinated movement.

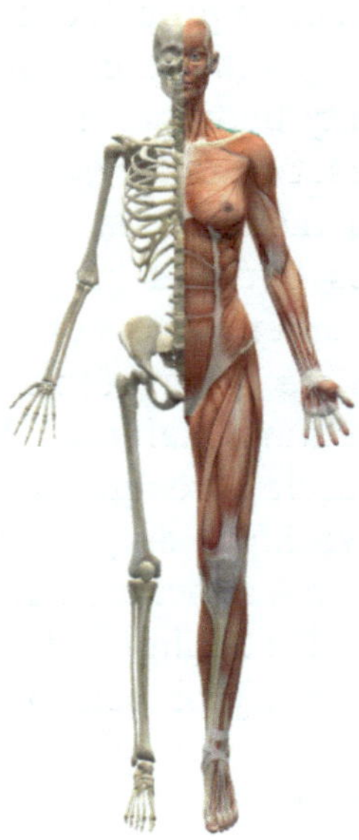

Figure 5.7. The bones in the appendicular skeleton serve as the base for the muscles to attach to to create movement.

Source: https://www.albert.io/blog/an-overview-of-the-appendicular-skeleton/.

The relationship of bones, muscles, and tendons creates leverage, significant in force production as well as in propelling the body forward. Alignment and structural support of the appendicular skeleton, therefore, directly affect an organism's capacity to move about its environment in the best possible manner. The appendicular skeleton's evolution is an account of significant adjustments to fluctuating locomotor lifestyles. With the origin of tetrapods from lobe-finned fishes, the fins-to-limbs evolution occurred through fundamental changes in form and function of skeletal and muscular components. Evolutionary progress allowed for increased mobility on land, providing the foundation for the institution of specialized running and walking routines. Abbasi et al. (2018) elucidate how anatomical innovations led to increasingly segregated but more modular limbs with increased diversification of muscle functions (Figure 5.7).

These specializations not only improved locomotion but also enabled more complex movements, like climbing or burrowing, necessary to the ecological niches occupied by various species. Notably, support for the appendicular skeleton's involvement in locomotion is also provided through pathological examination in animals. Some illustrations depict deformities or trauma that weaken limb structures, leading to severe impairments in locomotion. These results emphasize the necessity of a functional appendicular skeleton to achieve locomotion. Where bones' integrity is breached, as with experiments conducted with bovine models, the effect can have far-reaching implications for the general well-being and productivity of the subject. Bortolami et al. (2017) demonstrate these effects, where excessive lesions limit normal gait and necessitate intervention. Understanding these dynamics not only confirms the importance of limb integrity to mobility but also offers potential for investigation of healing interventions to maximize mobility and quality of life in affected species.

5.2.3. Contribution to Overall Body Stability

Appendicular skeleton contribution to body stability is most significant when biomechanical functions are considered. The appendicular skeleton, which includes limbs and their accompanying girdles, is tasked with enabling movements that facilitate a variety of postural adjustments. The mechanical rigidity of the femur and humerus bones offers weight-bearing activity that is essential for stability throughout dynamic movement. Moreover, paired arrangements, particularly in the shoulders and hips, enable smooth coordination and efficient transmission of force between the upper and lower body. As Goswami et al. (2018) note, the use of bone elements is vital for the appendicular skeleton's efficient functioning, suggesting that morphological diversity could heavily impact stability and functional capacity. Therefore, an understanding of these interconnectivities informs not just anatomical studies but also the construction of rehabilitation programs for enhancing overall body balance. The role of muscular attachments concerning the appendicular skeleton cannot be overemphasized, considering their immense contribution towards stabilizing the body. Muscles functioning around joints, such as the rotator cuff of the shoulder and gluteal muscles at the hip, provide indispensable support and control during motion. This musculature stabilizes articulations and provides proper alignment of the skeletal structures to withstand loads and conditions. These connections also have a dense network of ligaments and tendons that support them so that limbs may withstand external forces. The research from observing these musculoskeletal connections illustrates how specific exercise improves stability in individuals, particularly those already suffering from conditions or injuries. Studies have shown that particular resistance training not only adds to muscle strength but also reorganizes the appendicular skeleton's response, and the result is enhanced mechanical function and posture, as highlighted in Chee et al. (2018). Last but not least, the neuroskeletal system is linked to the overall contribution of the appendicular skeleton to the body's stability. Proprioception, which is made possible by sensory receptors in muscles and joints, is significant in matters of balance and coordination. Proprioception enables an individual to make instant readjustments to stabilize the body in physical activities. Incorporating proprioceptive training into rehabilitation protocols can be influential in affecting stability by improving the capacity of the body to react to unforeseen alterations in movement. For instance, balance challenge-evoking exercises such as single-leg stance or dynamic movement over uneven terrain uniquely activate the proprioceptive pathways of the appendicular skeleton. Hence, the integration of muscle strength, joint stability, and proprioceptive input emphasizes the role of the multifunctional appendicular skeleton in the provision of body stability and thus physical performance and injury prevention.

Test Your Knowledge

1. How does the appendicular skeleton support the body structurally?
2. What role does the appendicular skeleton play in human locomotion?

5.3. Comparison with Axial Skeleton

Learning Outcome

1. Describe the structural differences of the appendicular skeleton
2. Explain the functional differences between the axial and appendicular skeletons
3. Analyze the interrelationship between the axial and appendicular skeletons in human movement

The appendicular skeleton, whose primary role is to facilitate movement and provide support for locomotion, is relatively disparate from the axial skeleton, whose primary role is to enclose the organs of life and provide structural support. While the skull, vertebral column, and ribcage are components of the axial skeleton, the appendicular skeleton includes the limbs and girdles. This distinction highlights the special function of each skeletal system; for instance, the axial skeleton forms the body's mid-axis, and the appendicular skeleton supports a wide range of movements by joints and muscles. Awareness of such distinctions is not only crucial to vertebrate anatomy but also serves to investigate adaptive evolution responsible for the development of such skeletal structures. In tracing the evolutionary histories of these skeletal systems, one can see the beauty with which the limbs of tetrapods have evolved from the skeletons of ancestral lobe-finned fishes' pectoral and pelvic appendages. This conversion, which is pivotal in the fins-to-limbs transformation, reveals a level of anatomical organization and functional diversification that is matched by the adaptations in the axial skeleton. As suggested by research, the anatomical organization in both appendages exhibits a modularity trend consistent with an accommodation of muscle functions as tetrapods evolved to live on land. Comparative studies' use of network models shows how both systems have evolved and suggests that, although axial parts provide stability in protection and support, appendicular components have demonstrated more adaptability to a range of locomotor demands. (Abbasi et al., 2018). Increased investigation shows that appendicular skeletal muscle and skeletal structure, particularly in the pelvic limbs, exhibit distinctive patterns relative to the axial skeleton. Surprisingly, early tetrapods possessed more anatomical similarities between pectoral and pelvic regions than their ancestor lobe-finned relatives. This would mean that the evolution of the pelvic appendage from fin-like to limb-like structure lagged behind pectoral appendage evolution, essentially due to an early similarity bottleneck. Research indicates that this bottleneck is manifested in the smaller number of muscles found in the pelvic appendages as opposed to the pectoral appendages, highlighting an asymmetry in function between the two systems. Last but not least, the study of such anatomical variations not only serves to counterbalance the functional activities of the appendicular skeleton with those of the axial skeleton but also enlightens on the intricate history of vertebrate evolution (et al., 2018).

5.3.1. Structural Differences

The appendicular skeleton, consisting of the limbs and girdles that bear the limbs to the axial skeleton, exhibits typical structural dissimilarities that reflect functional adjustments in various forms. These dissimilarities are self-evident when looking at the morphology of pelvic and pectoral fins in aquatic organisms, say Raja asterias and Torpedo marmorata. It has been demonstrated by studies that the structural organization of such fins is vastly different; for instance, *T. marmoratas* pectoral fin has a unique organization because of its electric organs, subsequently reducing its surface area and altering hydrodynamic efficiency (Lanteri et al., 2023). As for *R. asterias*, it has a more traditional fin organization to generate greater lift and maneuverability in its environment. The importance of these structural variations emphasizes the evolutionary pressures that shape the form and function of the appendicular skeleton to facilitate species survival in their environments. Other structural variations exist in the organization and form of radials and fin rays that are essential to the propulsive mechanisms of these aquatic animals. In *Torpedo marmorata* and *Raja asterias*, the internal fin anatomy demonstrates a regular organization; however, there is a diversification of calcification patterns and specializations of function in these radials. For instance, in T. marmorata, the calcified tiles are organized to obtain the significant oscillatory motion, which contributes to propulsion, while *R. asterias* has more stiff structural components in dorsal tail fins, indicative of a compromise between flexibility and stiffness (Lanteri et al., 2023) (Figure 5.8).

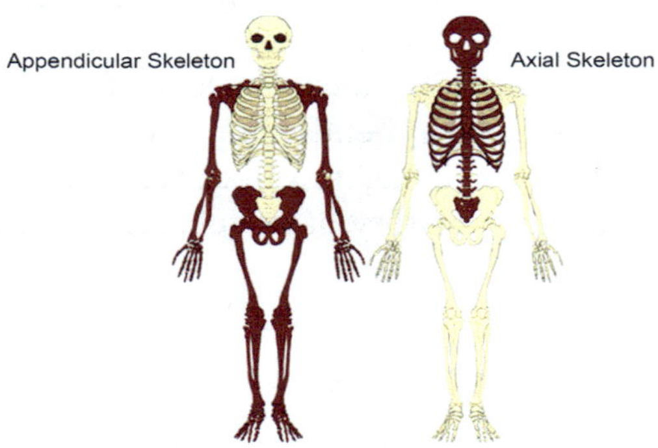

Figure 5.8. The axial and appendicular skeleton.

Source: https://www.teachpe.com/wp-content/uploads/2019/06/axial800-jpg.jpg.

These fin shape variations are not mere anatomical curiosities but are inextricably bound up with the swimming patterns and ecological roles of each species, an interesting conjunction of morphology and functional biomechanics. The periosteal features also play an essential role in the general shape and robustness of bones in the appendicular skeleton, working to emphasize even further the importance of structural differences. The periosteum is a thick layer of connective tissue that contains osteogenic cells, which are involved in the production of bone. The cells control bone growth and adaptation to changing mechanical loading, thereby influencing bone shape and density of limbs like those in limb girdles and long limb bones. Significantly, studies reveal that periosteal growth is capable of lowering fracture risk by enhancing the strength and structure of bones, particularly in weight-bearing regions such as the femoral neck and lumbar spine. Periosteal function and associated endosteal activity are a testament to a further aspect of complexity in appendicular skeletal structural dynamics, illustrating how different elements work together to offer mobility and survivability in various contexts.

5.3.2. Functional Differences

The appendicular skeleton, comprising the limbs and their associated girdles, mirrors significant functional divergences that have emerged in diverse species. Major innovations have appeared as an adaptation to the varying locomotory challenges posed by distinct taxa. The evolution of limbs from fins during tetrapod evolution involved extreme modifications of skeletal and muscular morphology. This reorganization extends not only to the intrinsic morphology of the limbs but also to the diversification of muscle function. Through the evolution of limbs from their lobe-finned origins, appendages became less integrated and more modular. They thus permitted a larger degree of movement and functional diversity in early tetrapods. This evolutionary pattern is characterized by perceiving how some anatomical features evolved to support the specialized behavior and environmental niches of various terrestrial organisms, leading to modern limb function (Abbasi et al., 2018). Secondly, functional divergence in the appendicular skeleton is also depicted through the study of some taxa, e.g., the felids. Even though overall cat morphology is not incredibly diverse, more detailed examination verifies significant dissimilarity in the limb and skull structures. These are paralleled closely by ecological niches and behavioral adaptations, which reinforce the idea that even slight morphological variations can have a pronounced effect on functionality. Regionalization of the vertebral column in carnivorans also indicates this, as the different segments respond differently to ecological stress. The integration observed between skeletal elements, especially for the vertebral column and limbs, is a reflection of evolutionary adaptations maximizing movement and specialized behavioral efficiency. Most notably, such autonomy of skeletal integration emphasizes the significance of evolutionary pressures that determine form and function in the appendicular skeleton (Goswami et al., 2018). Moreover, the functional differences of the appendicular skeleton extend beyond mere morphology into biomechanics. Structural differences in the limbs can lead to differing locomotor efficiencies, impact on agility, and accommodation to specific environmental demands. For instance, jumping animals, such as frogs, have significantly different limb proportions from more terrestrial mammals that can be specialized for endurance or speed of running. These adaptations refer to the selective forces that guide the functional arrangement of appendages concerning ecological pressures imposed on species. Such functional differentiation knowledge is not only informative for our understanding of evolutionary biology but also enhances our grasp of the fine-grained adaptability of different animal groups. This merging of form and function in the appendicular skeleton ultimately mirrors the diversity of evolutionary pressures that underpin biodiversity (Abbasi et al., 2018).

5.3.3. Interrelationship Between the Two Skeletons

The appendicular skeleton comprises the limbs and their associated girdles and is basically involved in human locomotion and agility. Its interaction with the axial skeleton is accountable for holistic skeletal functioning. Axial skeleton, comprising the skull, vertebral column, and rib cage, is primarily engaged in supporting as well as protecting the central nervous structures. This cooperation in movement is made possible by the pelvic and pectoral girdles acting to immobilize the limbs onto the body so that ease of transfer of the muscle forces from limb-initiated movements is obtained. A good example is the shoulder girdle attached to the axial skeleton, which confers a broad range of mobility in the upper limb for tasks requiring precision and strength. Such correspondence and interaction between the two skeletal components thus play a pivotal role in both anatomical stability and functional flexibility within human biomechanics. Studying the appendicular skeleton in conjunction with the axial skeleton yields knowledge of both evolutionary biology and anthropological practice. Traditionally, skeletal analyses, as in the case of Mississippian societies, highlight how social status and structure were articulated in the form of burial practice, which indicated the cultural interdependence of skeletal elements. Scientists have noted that variations in activity and social stratification are associated with skeletal development and pathology distinctive of specific groups. For example, the presence of degenerative joint diseases in the appendicular skeleton might be seen as evidence of a high degree of activity utilized in the attainment of social status, demonstrating the blending of physicality and social identity in the arena of skeletal analysis. This is one manifestation of broader inclinations in anthropology toward attention to the importance of both cultural practice and biological characteristics in the formation of human experience. The process of skeletal maturation provides an added complexity to the dynamic interaction between appendicular and axial skeletons. Epiphyseal fusion studies illuminate variation between periods as well as among social classes, which associate biological development with cultural transformation. For instance, studies reveal that skeletal maturation rates differed according to environmental and sociopolitical stresses, as one would expect to encounter in growth retardation during times of unrest. Studying epiphyseal development in skeletons from various archaeological sites, researchers found a shared pattern of fusion and revealed information on the biological age and maturational processes underlying human growth. Appreciating these differences within the appendicular skeleton sheds light on the broader picture of human resilience and adaptation, demonstrating the complex interplay between environmental factors, cultural norms, and physical structure in determining patterns in societies throughout history (Robinson et al., 1976; Dolding-Smith et al., 2023).

Test Your Knowledge

1. What are the key structural differences between the appendicular and axial skeletons?
2. How do the functions of the appendicular skeleton differ from those of the axial skeleton?

5.4. Development of the Appendicular Skeleton

Learning Outcome

1. Explain the embryonic development of the appendicular skeleton
2. Describe the processes of growth and maturation of the appendicular skeleton
3. Identify common developmental disorders affecting the appendicular skeleton

Evolution of the appendicular skeleton is a remarkable evolutionary record that speaks volumes of immense adaptation and transformation in the vertebrates. The appendicular skeleton, made up of limbs and girdles, evolved for the first time from the lobe-finned fishes some 370 million years ago. This was characterized by the evolution of limbs that were structurally distinct from their fish-like precursors. A shift from fin-based morphology to a more complex limb structure that supports terrestrial mobility was indicated by the redistribution of tetrapod muscle and skeletal morphology, which improved the efficiency of terrestrial movement. The most valuable point is the emergence of some similarity between the pelvic and pectoral appendages, indicating an evolutionary blueprint shared by both that caused diversified locomotion among these early land vertebrates (Abbasi et al., 2018). The appendicular skeletal changes at the level of evolution also encompassed changes at the level of bone structure, but included significant anatomical integration between adjacent muscles and bones. Network analysis studies have identified a trend toward more modular appendages in tetrapods, which is very different from the more dissociated structures in living lobe-finned fishes.

This modularity is a reflection of an evolutionary innovation allowing diversification of muscle function, necessary for survival in varied environments. By comparing the anatomy of present-day amphibians and amniotes with their ancient lobe-finned ancestors, scientists can reconstruct the step-by-step process of this transformation. These models of analysis tell us more about the dynamic interplay of anatomical features and functional demands that are associated with fin-to-limb evolution

(Abbasi et al., 2018). Further, appendicular skeleton evolution is linked with the emergence of specialized respiratory systems, particularly in regards to the transition from aquatic to terrestrial habitats. In birds, the development of sophisticated respiratory systems is accompanied by postcranial skeletal pneumaticity that is evocative of adaptations favorable for a highly active lifestyle. Since it is not entirely developed in all groups of vertebrates, the evolutionary history of respiratory adaptations in archosaurs, both the birds and crocodilians, reiterates a broader motif of functional optimization. These special appendicular adaptations of the bird could also be signaling evolutionary changes based on the increased metabolic cost of flight. Discussion of the interrelation of these facts both illuminates the development of the appendicular skeleton and provides a broader context in which to consider the general evolution of the vertebrates.

5.4.1. Embryonic Development

The intricate processes of embryonic growth are crucial for the formation of the appendicular skeleton, including limbs and attached structures. Limb buds emerge initially in early embryogenesis, which develop from precursor mesodermal cells. It is a crucial step toward the definition of the general shape of the limb, with signal pathways such as Sonic Hedgehog (Shh) and FGFs playing an essential role in patterning and extension. With ongoing development of the limb buds, these signaling molecules' interaction with various cell types orchestrates the process of proliferation, differentiation, and thereafter ossification to achieve complete development of the limbs. Regulation of these factors must be extremely accurate and sensitive, as disturbances can lead to congenital abnormalities in the structure and function of the limbs. In the appendicular skeleton, the equilibrium of signaling pathways is also brought out by investigations into single genetic mutations (Figure 5.9).

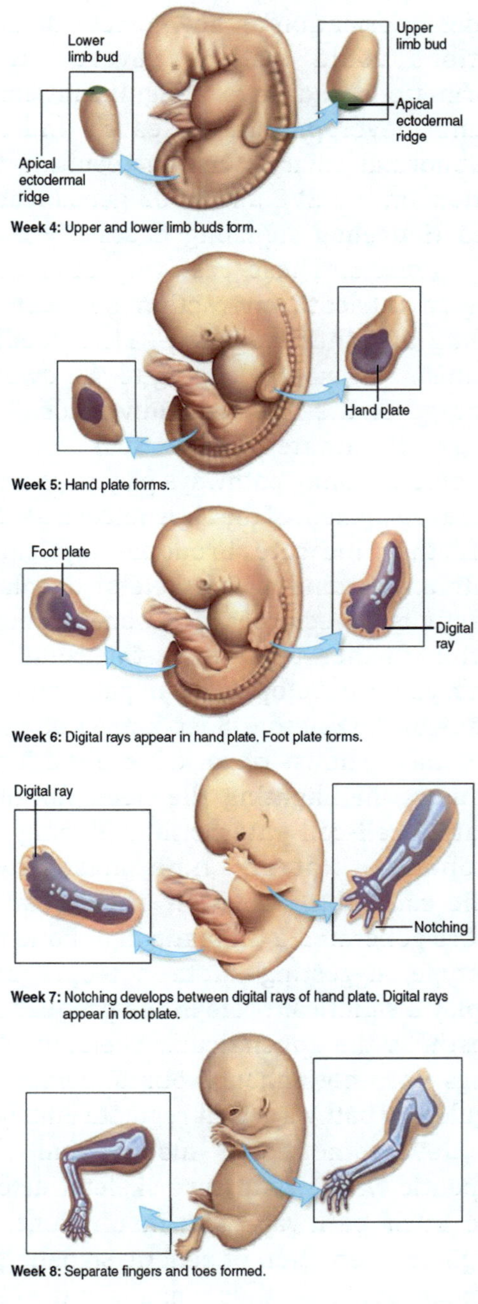

Figure 5.9. Development of the appendicular skeleton. The upper and lower limbs develop between weeks 4 and 8. Upper limb development precedes corresponding lower limb development by 2 to 4 days.

Source: https://www.pinterest.com/pin/836-development-of-the-appendicular-skeleton--788904059718998095/.

For instance, Ellis-van Creveld (EvC) syndrome provides information on how genetic signaling mutations could lead to severe skeletal malformations and have a significant impact on limb development. Research indicates that abnormal ciliary function resulting from mutations in the EVC and EVC2 genes leads to altered Hedgehog signaling necessary during embryogenesis. These resulting aberrations reveal an intricate interaction between FGF signaling and the Hedgehog-PTHrP feedback mechanism, ultimately leading to the dwarfing phenotype of the affected individuals. These findings illuminate the critical role that embryonic signaling pathways play in providing proper development of the appendicular skeleton and further indicate broader implications for our understanding of skeletal dysplasias. The activity of sclerostin, a bone formation inhibitor, further testifies to the complexity of embryonic development in patterning the appendicular skeleton. Sost knockout mouse studies have shown remarkable elevations in bone mass, highlighting the need for highly regulated cell-cell interactions during limb development. Notably, limb mesenchyme-specific conditional ablation of sclerostin by Prx1-Cre generated a dramatic high bone mass phenotype, suggesting that the osteoprogenitor cells play a significant role in the production of sclerostin in the appendicular skeleton. These findings not only enhance our understanding of regulatory pathways that regulate embryonic bone development but also reveal novel therapeutic windows to cure skeletal diseases where such pathways are insufficient. The synergistic interaction of genetic signaling and molecular regulation thus remains at the center of elucidating the complexities of appendicular skeletal development in embryonic life.

5.4.2. Growth and Maturation

The growth and maturation of the appendicular skeleton are complex processes that involve multiple cellular and molecular activities. During early development, the appendicular skeleton is formed from differentiating mesenchymal cells that become osteoblasts and chondrocytes, which establish the precursors of bones and joints. As one ages, epiphyseal plates or growth plates are essential for the elongation of long bones, like the arms and legs.

These plates are still active during childhood and adolescence and are regulated by numerous factors, including load and hormones. Knowing how such growth plates function and how they close during the end of puberty is crucial, as premature closure of growth plates can lead to abnormal and disproportionate growth and skeletal deformities. Increased knowledge of how the mechanisms regulating growth plate activity function can give hints on which therapeutic directions can be pursued to correct growth disorders in children. Sclerostin control has been a major area of focus when studying the biology of bone development, especially in relation to bone formation modulations. Sclerostin is an osteocyte-secreted protein that inhibits the Wnt signaling pathway required for osteoblast differentiation and activation and serves as a negative regulator of bone formation. Sost knockout mouse experiments have shown that the deletion of sclerostin leads to unprecedented bone acquisition, accentuating its central role in skeleton maturation and maintenance. This regulatory mechanism is also seen in the appendicular skeleton since conditional deletion of Sost in specific lineages resulted in augmented bone mass within the femur and lumbar spine. These findings suggest that sclerostin pathways may have new therapeutic approaches to enhancing bone density and preventing age-related bone loss, illustrating the delicate balance between growth regulation and skeletal maturation of the appendicular skeleton (Bajwa et al., 2018) (Figure 5.10).

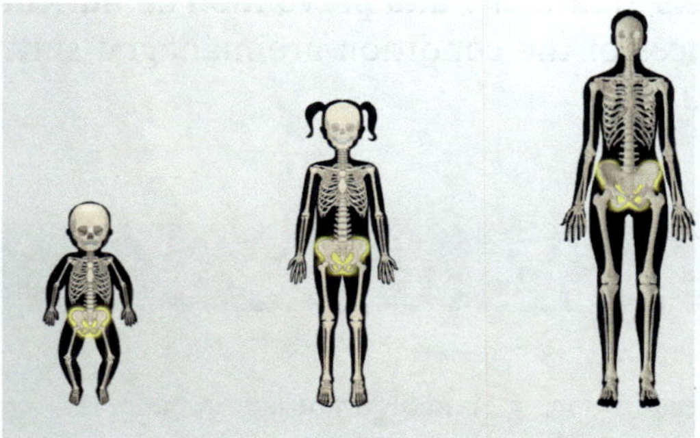

Figure 5.10. Changes in the appendicular skeleton with age.

Source: https://www.jove.com/files/media/science-education/science-education-thumbs/14057.jpg.

In addition, the role of transcription factors such as HOXA10 plays a vital role in directing osteogenic lineage commitment and bone formation. HOXA10 has been identified as an essential factor in the induction of mesenchymal cell differentiation into osteoblasts by triggering key regulators like Runx2 that orchestrate bone development. Temporal expression of HOXA10 synchronizes with key stages of osteoblast differentiation, resulting in widespread transcriptional activation of osteogenic genes. Notably, the ability of HOXA10s to induce osteoblast maturation in the absence of RUNX2 illustrates its specialist role in the development of the appendicular skeleton. This research demonstrates the importance of genetics in the establishment and maintenance of the structural integrity of the appendicular skeleton in growth and maturation. As scientists continue to unravel these molecular mechanisms, revelations that are made can provide new therapy in skeletal disease as well as a better understanding of human growth patterns (Hassan et al., 2007).

5.4.3. Common Developmental Disorders

The appendicular skeleton is essential in the comprehension of common developmental disorders, as the latter always manifest themselves through the derangement of its structure and functioning. Among the vast number of disorders related to limb development, congenital limb deformities are of the greatest importance due to their prevalence and variety. They may range from comparatively minor malformations to severe limb deficiencies and may impair the mobility and quality of life of a person. For instance, syndactyly and brachydactyly present severe challenges since anomalies in the structure and number of digits define them. They not only hinder movement but also require varied intervention strategies, such as surgical procedures or prosthetics, considering the patient's needs. The significance of skeletal fractures within developmental disorders is considerable, particularly in terms of how they can complicate involved conditions or occur as a direct consequence of them. As per research, patients who present with appendicular skeletal fractures are often also affected by variations in serum ionized calcium levels, which then can signify either metabolic or developmental issues in their skeletal status. In a study of types of fractures, comminuted and simple fractures in participants had higher levels of ionized calcium compared to control samples. This correlation emphasizes the significance of clinicians being careful with biochemical markers in patients of developmental disorders because they can signify the general bone integrity of the patient and appropriate treatment strategies for recovery and rehabilitation (Azevedo et al., 2017). Additionally, the study of congenital limb deformities still reveals rare and significant conditions warranting investigation. Reporting cases of bilateral aphalangia, brachydactyly, and unilateral ectrodactyly not only elucidates understanding of these malformations but also promotes the absolute need for thorough clinical and radiographic investigations. As these malformations remain underreported, particularly in veterinary literature, awareness and reporting are required for advancement in this field. The study of developmental disorders of the appendicular skeleton gives a way to better diagnosis, treatment, and prevention in individuals suffering from these problems, such that various instances of the condition are managed suitably in both human and veterinary medicine (Valle et al., 2016).

Test Your Knowledge

1. What are the main stages of embryonic development of the appendicular skeleton?
2. How does growth and maturation affect the appendicular skeleton during childhood and adolescence?

5.5. Common Injuries and Disorders

Learning Outcome

1. Explain the fractures of the appendicular bones
2. Discuss the joint dislocations
3. Describe the degenerative diseases affecting the appendicular skeleton

The appendicular skeleton, comprising the limbs and their associated girdles, is most susceptible to a variety of injuries and diseases due to its functional complexity and ease of movement. Fractures are the most common form of injury incurred by this part of the skeletal system, which most commonly occurs in the arms and legs during high-impact or violent activities. These are fractures that can be small, which usually mend without much medical attention, to compound fractures, which may penetrate the skin and require a great deal of medical attention. Furthermore, stress fractures, which result from repeated stress or overuse, are increasingly prevalent among athletes and other active individuals. Early detection and early intervention of such fractures are necessary because delays may lead to inappropriate healing and permanent mobility deficits in the traumatized limb. Besides fractures, the appendicular skeleton is also prone to disorders that have a profound effect on individuals' quality of life. Heterotopic ossification (HO) is one such disorder, where the development of abnormal bone in soft tissues may occur after surgeries, traumatic injuries, or burns. This condition not only leads to painful calcifications but also causes complications such as joint immobility and loss of range of motion (ROM). HO needs to be treated, and treatments usually consist of non-steroidal anti-inflammatory drugs and, in some cases, radiation therapy to manage symptoms and prevent further complications (Wolfe et al., 2012). The new developments in the molecular mechanisms of HO have opened new avenues for new forms of treatment, emphasizing the importance of ongoing research in this area to offset its effects on patient health and mobility. The other significant aspect of typical injuries and disorders of the appendicular skeleton is the prevalence of tendon and ligament ruptures, particularly in the regions around the shoulder and knee. These soft tissue injuries most frequently occur due to acute trauma or cumulative overuse and are biomechanical loads applied to these tissues under the demands of physical activities. Tears of the rotator cuff are prevalent in overhead athletes, whereas anterior cruciate ligament (ACL) injuries are frequently encountered in sports involving pivoting or brusque changes of direction. Their actions go beyond treating acute pain; they also play a role in chronic joint instability and arthritic alteration when inadequately treated. Timely diagnosis and rehabilitative management, whether through physical therapy or surgery when required, is key to restoring function and averting future injury recurrence, emphasizing the importance of multidisciplinary treatment protocols in the management of these disorders.

5.5.1. Fractures of Appendicular Bones

Appendicular bone fractures are a serious clinical problem due to their prevalence and the potential for serious complications. Appendicular bone fractures are most frequently caused by trauma, e.g., following falls, sports injuries, or motor vehicle collisions, and affect long limb bones such as the femur, tibia, humerus, and radius.

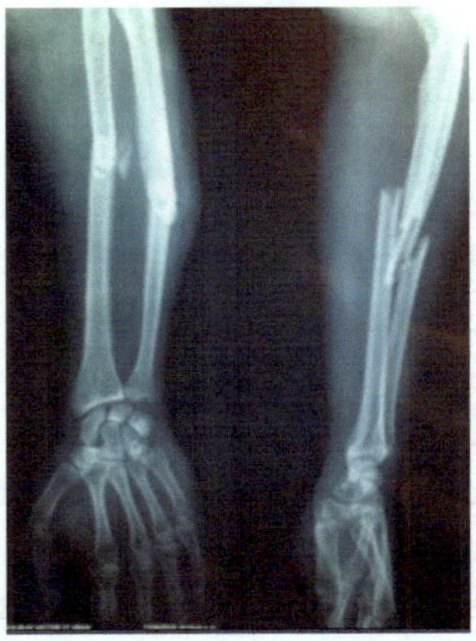

Figure 5.11. The biggest risk to the appendicular skeleton is fracture. This image depicts an X-ray taken of a forearm in which both the radius and ulna are fractured.

Source: https://www.albert.io/blog/wp-content/uploads/2023/12/fracture-bone-2333164_1280-225x300.png.

Identification of the fracture types—e.g., simple, comminuted, and compound—is essential for effective diagnosis and therapy. Clean breaks in simple fractures are breaks that do not enter the skin, while comminuted fractures consist of numerous pieces and are more challenging to treat. Each fracture type demands a unique kind of therapy, and this reflects the necessity of having proper imaging techniques as well as early intervention to ensure optimal healing and recovery. Appendicular bone fracture treatment may require a mix of conservative and surgical approaches, depending on the nature and location of the fractures (Figure 5.11).\

The majority of treatments are non-operative and consist of immobilization, stabilization, and natural healing of the fracture by cast or splints. The surgical approach is reserved for complex fractures, particularly those that are displaced or incredibly fragmented. Internal fixation with rods or plates and external fixation are frequently used methods. Also, familiarity with the mechanical and biological aspects of the healing of bone is crucial for clinicians to implement measures that allow recovery to take place. Effective management also includes close follow-up for potential complications such as infection, malunion, or nonunion, as testifies to the significance of a multidisciplinary strategy to the treatment of fractures of the appendicular bones. Fractures of the appendicular bones have implications that extend beyond the immediate physical trauma, influencing patients' quality of life and function. It has been observed through research that fractures of the appendicular skeleton act as a precursor to severe long-term consequences, including chronic pain, loss of function, and psychological disturbance. As observed in several clinical trials, especially those that were founded on the analysis of serum ionized calcium values in fracture patients (Azevedo et al., 2017), the physiological consequence of fractures also threatens metabolic disturbances, most especially in comminuted fractures that may have more severe symptoms compared to those with simple fractures. It is thus crucial that doctors concentrate on both psychological and physical recuperation in their intervention. The vast understanding of the implications involved with the fractures of appendicular bones can consequently be used to enhance the patient's care outcomes and the recovery rate.

5.5.2. Joint Dislocations

The appendicular skeleton refers to the limbs and attachments to the body trunk and is essential in mobility and stability. Among the various types of injuries that may be experienced within this framework, joint dislocations are particularly notable because they are sudden in development and often have long-term consequences. A joint dislocation happens when the bones that make up a joint are pushed out of their natural alignment, frequently as a result of degenerative processes, trauma, or excessive stress.

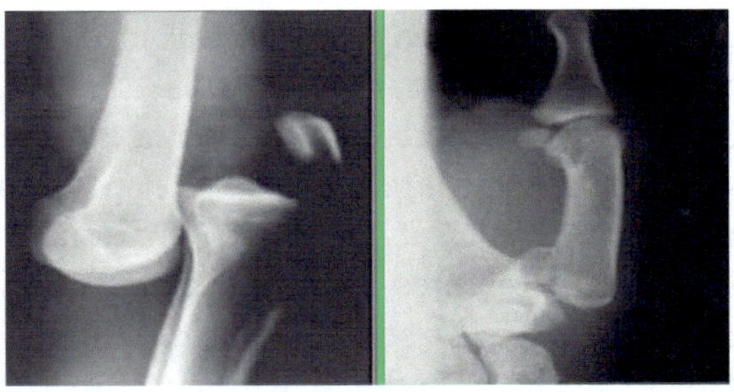

Figure 5.12. Joint dislocations.

Source: https://external-content.duckduckgo.com/iu/?u=https%3A%2F%2Fimage5.slideserve.com%2F9432434%2Fdislocation-l.jpg&f=1&nofb=1&ipt=563e44fc24f036cdafcaa397fb647213fd6f98592badad7dc1b4ae90b8e332e3.

Dislocation commonly occurs in the shoulder, elbow, and knee joints, which have anatomical configurations that allow for greater mobility but with an increased likelihood of dislocation. As a result, correct diagnosis and early treatment are necessary to return the joint to normal function and prevent complications such as nerve damage, muscle weakness, or long-term joint instability, which will occur if the dislocation is not treated early. For the appendicular skeleton, dislocated joint management can vary widely based on the specific joint involved as well as the degree of injury. For instance, acute dislocations of the shoulder often need reduction, in which bones are placed back into their normal positions, followed by immobilization to allow healing. Surgery may be needed in recurrent dislocations, often secondary to intrinsic ligamentous laxity (Figure 5.12).

Nonoperative treatments, such as physical therapy, also play a critical role in restoring the function and strength after the joint has been stabilized. Knowledge of the anatomical relationships and biomechanical forces involved with joint injuries maximizes clinicians' ability to create appropriate management protocols. For instance, a comprehensive evaluation of the whole shoulder complex, including the acromioclavicular (AC) joint, is required since injuries to this area can worsen issues of shoulder dislocation, and therefore a treatment plan for the whole body should be taken into account (Menzer et al., 2016). Moreover, dislocation of the joints extends far past temporary physical symptoms and affects people's long-term quality of life and functional ability. After initial management, recurrence potential could increase from residual joint laxity or suboptimal healing. Rehabilitation is pivotal in resolving such conditions, with provisions for strengthening of the surrounding musculature, improving joint proprioception, and restoration of the motion arc. These channels are essential for both sports persons and the general public, as well as for older individuals, who may experience dislocations not only due to sports but also from falls or other age-related causes. An appreciation of these principles of rehabilitation and the long-term care of ensuring joint health is imperative to successful recovery and prevention of injury. Continuing research into joint dislocations and treatment approaches is required to optimize outcomes and advise future practice (Bernthal et al., 2023).

5.5.3. Degenerative Diseases Affecting the Appendicular Skeleton

Degenerative disease has a significant impact on the appendicular skeleton, and typical results include chronic pain, decreased mobility, and significant alterations in the functioning of joints. Conditions such as osteoarthritis (OA), characterized by the progressive loss of cartilage and changes in supporting bone, are good examples of how these diseases impact joint structural function.

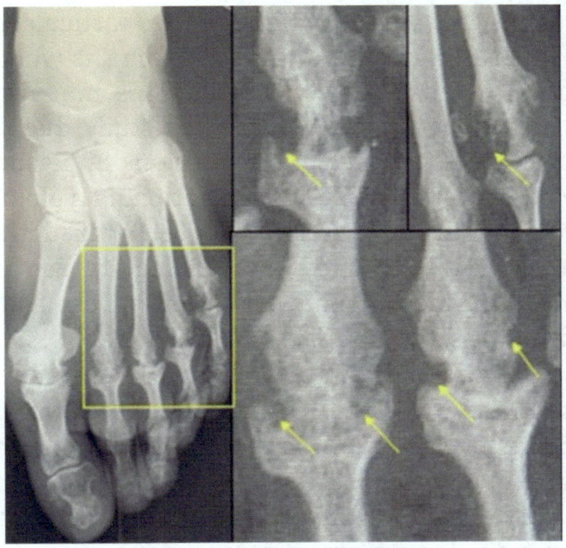

Figure 5.13. Rheumatoid arthritis.

Source: https://pub.mdpi-res.com/biomolecules/biomolecules-11-00048/article_deploy/html/images/biomolecules-11-00048-g001.png?1609578077.

This condition is prevalent in the elderly, but recent findings attribute the onset of this condition at younger ages to lifestyle conditions like obesity and heavy physical exertion. With the loss of cartilage, the bones may rub against each other, causing inflammation and further loss of the joint. Since the appendicular skeleton is so central to allowing movement, the effects of such degenerative processes are far more significant than bodily pain and tend to result in a diminished quality of life and increased reliance on medical intervention. Furthermore, long-term conditions such as rheumatoid arthritis further significantly contribute to their effect upon the appendicular skeleton. Unlike OA, which is a wear-and-tear disease, rheumatoid arthritis is an autoimmune disease leading to systemic inflammation. Such an inflammatory process may involve joints of the appendicular skeleton and be a cause for joint deformity and functional impairment (Figure 5.13).

Chronic inflammation is not only capable of destroying cartilage, but can penetrate bone tissue, creating erosive changes that radically deform joint architecture. Work in various populations indicates that congenital factors can predispose to the disease. Thus early diagnosis and ongoing surveillance are essential if symptoms are to be controlled, functional impairment prevented, and an acceptable level of activity established. In doing so, it is critical to be aware of the underlying mechanisms of such degenerative illnesses to establish therapeutic procedures. Delving further into the physical consequences of degenerative diseases, the connection between chronic systemic inflammation and joint degeneration cannot be escaped. The interaction between variables such as genetics, environmental factors, and lifestyle factors exacerbates the severity of joint diseases in the appendicular skeleton. For instance, paleopathological skeletal analysis of such archaeological sites as *Chucalissa* reveals patterns of degenerative joint disease that are common due to the mechanical stresses placed on the appendicular skeleton from engaging in various occupational activities. Individuals who did labor-intensive work were found to have increased frequencies of joint degeneration, thereby highlighting the significance of occupational and social determinants in the expression of degenerative disease in prehistoric populations, demonstrated by the frequency of nonspecific inflammation and healed fractures of the appendicular skeleton (Robinson et al., 1976). These discoveries provide a framework for appreciating how modern lifestyle decisions affect bone health in the same way, again confirming the need for preventive strategies in dealing with degenerative diseases.

Test Your Knowledge

1. How are joint dislocations in the appendicular skeleton typically diagnosed and managed?
2. What are some degenerative diseases that affect the appendicular skeleton and their main symptoms?

5.6. Diagnostic Techniques

Learning Outcome

1. Analyze the use of X-rays and imaging techniques for evaluating the appendicular skeleton
2. Explain the role of MRI and CT scans in diagnosing appendicular skeletal conditions
3. Apply physical examination methods to assess the appendicular skeleton

The study of the appendicular skeleton, i.e., the limbs and girdles that support them, requires rigorous diagnostic technique using either simple approaches or more sophisticated imaging methods to detect disorders or disease effectively. Among the most significant advances in such work is the use of computed tomography (CT) scans. The inclusion of CT has revolutionized veterinary medicine and anatomy studies by giving detailed cross-sectional images that significantly enhance diagnostic accuracy. With the use of CT, experts can dissect complex bone structure, examine the soft tissue conditions, and identify vascular irregularities with unparalleled clarity, which is most critical in the diagnosis of appendicular skeleton problems. Furthermore, the rapid development and availability of CT technology have been responsible for its broader application in clinical trials and research centers to gain valuable information about a variety of conditions that impair bone and soft tissue integrity, as highlighted by Keane et al. (2017). Another equally applicable diagnostic modality for assessing bone health, particularly in illnesses such as multiple myeloma, is whole body low-dose CT (WBLDCT). This modality is critical as a first-line imaging study due to its sensitivity to detect bone lesions of plasma cell disorders. The 2014 International Myeloma Working Group criteria also recognized the value of WBLDCT by referencing its use in evaluating the appendicular skeleton. Despite its advantages, the lack of established guidelines on the utilization of WBLDCT hinders its broader use in the clinic and research. Best acquisition and reporting practices recommendations are needed to optimize its performance and the quality of care for those patients suffering from appendicular skeletal diseases, which justifies its essential place in modern diagnostic practice as emphasized in Aquerreta et al. (2018). Other imaging modalities, such as X-rays and magnetic resonance imaging (MRI), apart from CT and WBLDCT, play a vital role in diagnosing the appendicular skeleton. Because X-rays are easily accessible, reasonably priced, and offer early information about bone fractures and abnormalities, they are typically the first technique utilized for evaluation. But MRI adds one step further in diagnosis by giving improved soft tissue evaluation, which is significant in diseases involving ligaments, cartilage, and muscle structures of the overlying regions.

Summing up these imaging techniques gives a total diagnostic process, allowing for complete examination of the appendicular skeleton. With continued developments in imaging techniques, the intersection of such methods will progressively advance diagnostic accuracy and patient care in the practice of orthopedics and sports medicine. Understanding the strengths and limitations of each technique is crucial to the development of effective therapeutic regimens.

5.6.1. X-Rays and Imaging

Imaging and X-rays are at the heart of the study and exploration of the appendicular skeleton, particularly in the way that they enable inspection of bone structure and disease. X-ray imaging enables physicians to visualize the various components of the appendicular skeleton, including the long bones of the extremities and intricate joints between them. For fracture or structural abnormalities, X-rays help in assessing the severity of the injury as well as suggesting treatment. The clarity of images captured through X-ray technology is crucial for detecting diseases such as arthritis and developmental disorders that affect limb morphology. Also, advances in imaging made it possible to offer a better resolution and visualize the soft tissues around bones to provide an image of the appendicular skeleton's functional dynamics, thereby enhancing medical results with precise diagnostic abilities (Figure 5.14).

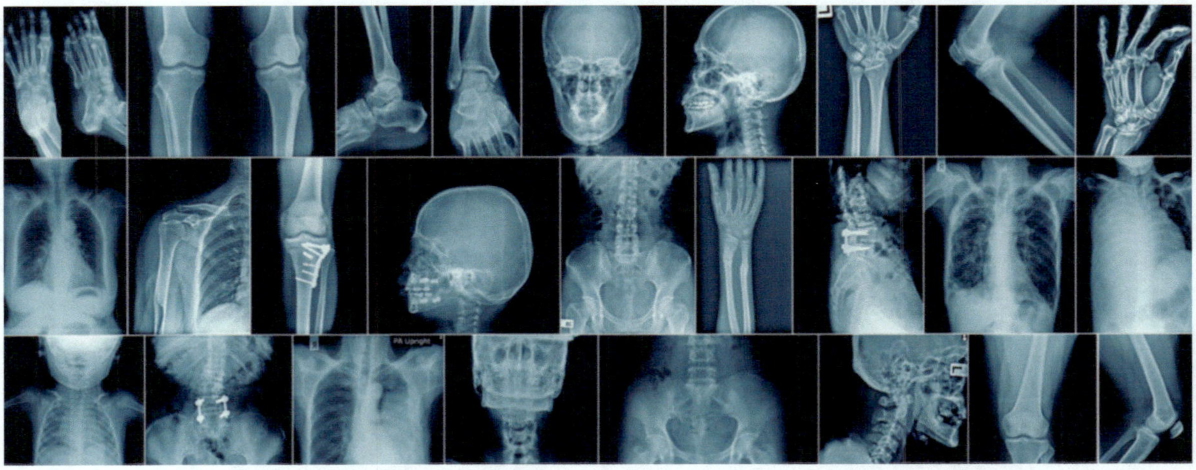

Figure 5.14. A compilation of X-ray images showing various parts of the human skeletal system, used for diagnostic assessment of bones and joints.

Source: https://external-content.duckduckgo.com/iu/?u=https%3A%2F%2Fwww.ucsfhealth.org%2F-%2Fmedia%2Fproject%2Fucsf%2Fucsf-health%2Fmedical-tests%2Fhero%2Fx-ray-skeleton-2x.jpg%3Fh%3D1112%26w%3D2880%26ha sh%3DCFA177B5092DFF1B3AC225908DF7C476&f=1&nofb =1&ipt=033d9e3443fb7ceaa3c6ca1d8d664eaa5e646dcf09a9579b09517a2c21460e50.

The use of sophisticated imaging procedures, particularly CT, has dramatically improved the knowledge of the appendicular skeleton in human and veterinary medicine. CT imaging, with its high resolution and capability to create 3D reconstructions of bone structures, has revolutionized the way clinicians examine intricate anatomical features. The incorporation of CT in veterinary medicine signifies its applicability not only for diagnosis but also in planning surgery and intervention tactics, especially among species with distinctive skeletal anatomy. In addition, it enables the investigation of bone, vasculature, and soft tissue interaction, ultimately shaping clinical practice in ways previously unknown. The integration of this state-of-the-art imaging with conventional X-rays provides a complete arsenal to health care practitioners, allowing for a more precise evaluation of skeletal well-being and the possibility of enhanced therapeutic results in appendicular injury and disease management (Keane et al., 2017). Besides conventional X-ray and CT imaging, micro-CT (μCT) has also proved to be a robust research tool for investigating the microarchitecture of the appendicular skeleton. This method provides unparalleled resolution at the microscopic level, enabling scientists to examine the delicate structural patterns of bones in different species. These analyses, as demonstrated by examinations of species such as Raja asterias and Torpedo marmorata, uncover important information concerning the differences in morphological skeletal structures, especially locomotion and functional performance. For example, the pattern and calcification of fin ray alignment in these groups highlight the evolutionary specializations of their appendicular structures, equipping us with deeper insight into biomechanics. Such minute detail not only serves to inform our understanding of comparative anatomy but also refines our knowledge of the evolutionary pressures that have confronted various species, highlighting the importance of imaging technology in skeletal research (Lanteri et al., 2023).

5.6.2. MRI and CT Scans

MRI and CT scans have proved to be indispensable diagnostic and assessment tools for the conditions of the appendicular skeleton. MRI, with increased soft tissue contrast, is superior in imaging structures such as muscles, cartilage, and ligaments that enclose bone.

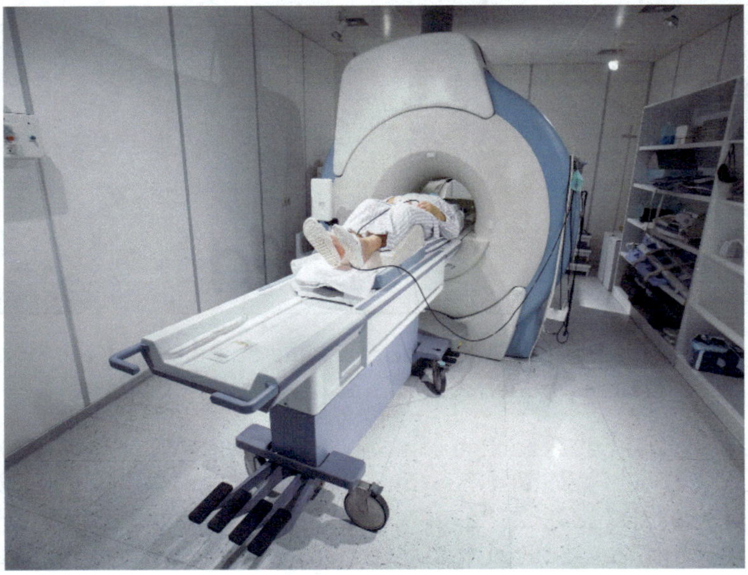

Figure 5.15. MRI scan procedure showing a patient positioned for internal imaging of bones and soft tissues.

Source: https://medanta.s3.ap-south-1.amazonaws.com/blogs/July2024/7SenHvoV2dbwfnunh3a6MBDMVJJqD1-metaTXVzY3Vsb3NrZWxldGFsIEltYWdpbmcgVGVjaG5pcXVlcyBGcm9tIFgtUmF5cyB0byBNUkkuanBn-.jpg.

This feature, which produces high-resolution pictures that can detect subtle changes not seen with traditional X-rays, is useful in evaluating sports injuries or degenerative disorders of the appendicular skeleton. CT scans, by contrast, can provide high-resolution images of bone structure, thus helping in identifying fractures, alterations in bone density, and complex joint pathologies. The union of these imaging modalities enables clinicians to formulate comprehensive treatment plans tailored to each patient's unique conditions, thus improving patient outcomes. The effectiveness of MRI and CT scans in measuring chronic conditions is also supplemented by their ability to detect complications arising from infections such as osteomyelitis. For instance, in a recent study, it was shown that 18F-FDG PET/CT scans were highly sensitive with a sensitivity of 100% for the region in the detection of appendicular skeleton chronic osteomyelitis (Dora et al., 2018) (Figure 5.15).

This tremendous sensitivity underscores the crucial role of advanced imaging techniques in diagnosing chronic infection presenting in the bone, which otherwise would be hard to assess using clinical presentation alone. Therefore, the application of MRI and CT scans not only facilitates the detection of the degree of infection but also offers valuable information about adjacent anatomical structures, so that the course of treatment is appropriately managed based on the condition of the patients. Where suspected infection is present or inflammation, the application of more than one imaging modality significantly enhances diagnostic sensitivity. A review examining the effectiveness of combined bone scanning and immunoscintigraphy found that even if there was moderate specificity, the method was very sensitive for the diagnosis of appendicular skeleton chronic osteomyelitis (Jundt et al., 2018). This finding underscores the significance of a multi-modal strategy in the utilization of imaging technology for the diagnosis of complicated diseases in the appendicular skeleton. By integrating the strengths of MRI, CT, and supporting imaging modalities, clinicians will be better equipped to understand the pathophysiology of conditions in the appendicular skeleton, leading to improved management and treatment options.

5.6.3. Physical Examination Methods

Physical examination of the appendicular skeleton involves several methods that assess the integrity of the bones, function of the joints, and strength of the muscles. ROM examination and palpation are fundamental elements of the procedure. Palpation allows the practitioner to identify abnormalities or tenderness in the bones and soft tissue structures that may indicate underlying pathology. During ROM testing, health professionals quantify active and passive movement to determine the amount of joint restrictions, pain levels, or stiffness that can be symptomatic of MSK conditions. Visual examination also plays a significant role in uncovering asymmetry, swelling, or deformity that may require diagnostic imaging. Such evaluations are not only necessary for the detection of acute conditions but also for chronic problem monitoring throughout time, thus ensuring timely intervention and informed treatment planning. A critical element in the evaluation of the appendicular skeleton is the evaluation of joint alignment and stability, primarily focusing on the shoulders, elbows, hips, and knees. Narrow examinations, such as the Lachman test of the knee, are extremely demanding tests of the integrity of the ligaments, and the apprehension test can ascertain shoulder joint stability. Special tests provide hints regarding potential injuries such as dislocation or rupture of the ligaments, which both athletic and non-athletic individuals share. For instance, joint laxity may lead to secondary wear of associated structures, again raising the risk for entities like OA or patellofemoral pain syndrome. The information gained by these sophisticated testing modalities is also critical to developing effective rehabilitation programs. Therefore, careful physical examination methods are not only invaluable to accurate diagnosis but also to enhancing general care of the appendicular skeleton. Other research on skeletal and systemic conditions explains the importance of holistic evaluation in physical exams. One example comes from research that has established that bone health is affected by metabolic illnesses such as non-alcoholic fatty liver disease (NAFLD), which can gradually lead to decreased bone mineral density (Chiesa et al., 2017). This connection points to the necessity of integrating measures that are more than purely MSK evaluation, as predictors of systemic health can quite profoundly influence the appendicular skeleton's integrity. Additionally, current research on the role of sclerostin in bone metabolism emphasizes the dynamic interplay between various tissues responsible for skeletal health (Bajwa et al., 2018). Comprehensive physical examinations, thus, have to keep in mind the broader physiological context so that clinicians can better manage both local and systemic issues that could compromise the appendicular skeleton's health and functionality.

Test Your Knowledge

1. How do MRI and CT scans complement each other in diagnosing appendicular skeleton disorders?
2. What physical examination techniques are commonly used to assess injuries or abnormalities in the appendicular skeleton?

SUMMARY

The appendicular skeleton is crucial to the generic versatility and overall efficiency of vertebrates, connecting limb development evolution to their present-day anatomical structure. The evolution from lobe-finned fishes to tetrapods was a critical moment in evolutionary history, when skeletal and muscular anatomy went through enormous reorganization towards the aim of terrestrial locomotion. As in comparative studies of modern species, this evolution led to particular modifications of appendicular anatomy, contributing to a complex and modular pattern of bones and muscles. Thus, learning these evolutionary processes not only explains vertebrate morphology but also provides an insight into which the structural adaptations facilitate different locomotor capabilities in various species, validating the appendicular skeleton's crucial role in vertebrate biology (Abbasi et al., 2018). Additionally, engagement with modern learning resources can effectively enhance the comprehension of the appendicular skeleton's complexities. The use of interactive tutorials, as proposed in the recent curriculum attempts, allows students to explore concepts that otherwise would appear either abstract or confusing. By observing features such as joint function and muscle action through an intact 3D skeleton and animated overlays, students can observe the complex interactions and anatomical relationships inherent within the appendicular skeleton. This novel method of studying fosters more learning, enabling students to distinguish between normal and abnormal forms and track locomotion dynamics more tangibly. Including such materials in classes improves the appreciation of the appendicular skeletons function and form and enhances veterinary and biological education in the long run (Buck et al., 2022). Finally, the appendicular skeleton is highly applicable to academic and medical domains. Knowledge of the evolutionary origins and functional adaptations of limbs can inform practice in fields such as veterinary medicine and physical therapy, where understanding the biomechanics of movement is relevant. Advances in imaging technology and models of education can bridge knowledge gaps so that future practitioners can leverage this knowledge for practical application. Furthermore, sustained research on the anatomical changes from aquatic to terrestrial habitats continues to provide insights into the complexity of vertebrate adaptation and evolution. Therefore, a broad comprehension of the appendicular skeleton not only proves to be practically applicable but also serves to emphasize its significance in the wider context of evolutionary biology and applied sciences (Abbasi et al., 2018; Buck et al., 2022).

The appendicular skeleton is a critical component in the aquatic-terrestrial evolutionary transition, best exemplified by the morphological patterns that define the fish-tetrapod transition. The key points of this discussion reveal that body parts of the appendicular skeleton, e.g., limbs and fins, exhibit significant morphological disparity, a reflection of the evolutionary pressures on these animals. Experiments revealed that anterior appendicular information still retains phylogenetic resolution. In contrast, posterior appendicular information typically results in loss of resolution for evolutionary relations, illustrating the complexity of determining lineage through morphological characters. These findings emphasize the necessity of examining specific parts of the appendicular skeleton in an attempt to grasp processes of evolution, thus putting the appendicular skeleton in the spotlight of phylogenetic analysis and stressing the importance of grasping limb evolution as part of vertebrate history (Adamowicz et al., 2016). In addition to its evolutionary significance, the appendicular skeleton further has significant implications to developmental biology, particularly in understanding how bone formation is influenced by gene expression. One such interesting participant is HOXA10, which was revealed to be essential in skeletal element patterning and also for subsequent bone formation processes. Experiments show that HOXA10 brings about key transcription factors, such as Runx2, that play a fundamental role in osteogenic lineage determination and bone phenotypic gene regulation. Specifically, HOXA10s induction of essential osteogenic genes evinces its central function in chromatin remodeling during osteoblast differentiation, hence establishing a link between gene regulation and physical structure in the appendicular skeleton. This gene interaction illustrates how intramolecular development processes cascade into intricate appendicular structures (Hassan et al., 2007). Furthermore, the interrelation between appendicular skeleton adaptive evolution and genetic control illustrates its complex function within organismal and phylogenetic biology. This morphological diversity observed between appendicular structures of fish and tetrapods reflects an extent of anatomical as well as functional evolution under environmental pressures and adaptive responses. Notably, the unequivocal occupation of morphospace by diverse taxa reflects the adaptive significance of appendicular structures to survive in diverse habitats. The importance of both external morphological and internal genetic control implications makes the appendicular skeleton a central dimension for study for comprehending life's evolution. Even as research continues to reveal further the intricate interactions among morphology, gene expression, and the evolutionary narrative, the appendicular skeleton is a critical component of university discussion in the fields of evolutionary biology and developmental genetics, inviting ongoing interdisciplinarity (Adamowicz et al., 2016).

KEY TERMS FROM THIS CHAPTER

- Pectoral girdle
- Clavicle
- Scapula
- Humerus
- Radius
- Ulna
- Carpals
- Metacarpals
- Phalanges
- Pelvic girdle
- Ilium
- Ischium
- Pubis
- Femur
- Patella
- Tibia

CRITICAL THINKING QUESTIONS

1. **The appendicular skeleton includes which of the following?**
   a. Skull and vertebrae
   b. Ribs and sternum
   c. Limbs and girdles
   d. Sacrum and coccyx
2. **Which bone is part of the pectoral (shoulder) girdle?**
   a. Femur
   b. Scapula
   c. Pelvis
   d. Tibia
3. **The bone commonly known as the collarbone is called the:**
   a. Clavicle
   b. Humerus
   c. Radius
   d. Ulna
4. **Which of the following bones is found in the lower limb?**
   a. Humerus
   b. Radius
   c. Femur
   d. Scapula
5. **The pelvic girdle is composed primarily of:**
   a. Ilium, ischium, and pubis
   b. Clavicle and scapula
   c. Femur and tibia
   d. Sacrum and coccyx

Short Answer Questions

1. What are the main components of the appendicular skeleton?
2. What are the primary functions of the appendicular skeleton?
3. How does the appendicular skeleton differ from the axial skeleton in terms of structure and function?
4. Describe the general process of development of the appendicular skeleton.
5. Name two common injuries or disorders that affect the appendicular skeleton.
6. What diagnostic techniques are commonly used to assess injuries or conditions of the appendicular skeleton?
7. Why is understanding the appendicular skeleton important in clinical diagnosis and treatment?

Answer to Critical Thinking Questions

1. (c); 2. (b); 3. (a); 4. (c); 5. (a)

REFERENCES

1. Esteve-Altava, B., Molnar, J. L., Johnston, P., Hutchinson, J. R., & Diogo, R. (2018). Anatomical network analysis of the musculoskeletal system reveals integration loss and parcellation boost during the fins-to-limbs transition. *Evolution, 72*(3), 601–618. https://doi.org/10.1111/evo.13430Adamowicz, L., Ahlberg, P. E., Anderson, J. S., Ausich, W. I., Baddeley, C., Bapst, D. W., et al. (2016). Comparable disparity in the appendicular skeleton across the fish-tetrapod transition, and the morphological gap between fish and tetrapod postcranial. https://core.ac.uk/download/42584850.pdf (accessed on 14th June 2025).
2. Ahlberg, P. E., Braus, H., Byerly, T. C., Clack, J. A., Coates, M. I., Diogo, R., et al. (2018). Evolution of hindlimb muscle anatomy across the tetrapod water-to-land transition, including comparisons with forelimb anatomy. https://core.ac.uk/download/161772648.pdf (accessed on 14th June 2025).
3. Allen, B., Hung, I. H., Kamiya, N., Kunieda, T., et al. (2016). Elevated fibroblast growth factor signaling is critical for the pathogenesis of the dwarfism in *Evc2/Limbin* mutant mice. https://core.ac.uk/download/74358375.pdf (accessed on 14th June 2025).
4. Allen, M. R., Burr, D. B., & Hock, J. M. (2004). Periosteum: Biology, regulation, and response to osteoporosis therapies. https://core.ac.uk/download/46959707.pdf (accessed on 14th June 2025).
5. Aquerreta, J. D., Cavo, M., Delorme, S., Dimopoulos, M. A., et al. (2018). Recommendations for acquisition, interpretation and reporting of whole-body low dose CT in patients with multiple myeloma and other plasma cell disorders: A report of the IMWG Bone Working Group. https://core.ac.uk/download/547491548.pdf (accessed on 14th June 2025).
6. Azevedo, P., Carreira, L. M., Lavrador, C., Neto, R., et al. (2017). Serum ionized calcium variations in simple and comminuted fractures in the dog's appendicular skeleton and consequent risks of a hypercalcemic condition. https://core.ac.uk/download/147568931.pdf (accessed on 14th June 2025).
7. Bajwa, J., Chang, J. C., Economides, A. E., Horan, G. S., et al. (2018). Conditional deletion of *Sost* in MSC-derived lineages identifies specific cell type contributions to bone mass and B cell development. https://core.ac.uk/download/158967696.pdf (accessed on 14th June 2025).
8. Barrett, P. M., Butler, R. J., & Gower, D. J. (2012). Reassessment of the evidence for postcranial skeletal pneumaticity in Triassic archosaurs, and the early evolution of the avian respiratory system. https://core.ac.uk/download/12175752.pdf (accessed on 14th June 2025).
9. Bashir, H., Mehmood, S., Rashid, N., Riaz, M., et al. (2018). Hybrid bone scintigraphy in gastrointestinal malignancies–Institutional experience. https://core.ac.uk/download/227107241.pdf (accessed on 14th June 2025).
10. Benjamin, M., Camp, C. L., Castanet, J., Cope, E. D., Gauthier, J. A., Haines, R. W., et al. (2016). Anatomy, morphology and evolution of the patella in squamate lizards and tuatara (*Sphenodon punctatus*). https://core.ac.uk/download/36779107.pdf (accessed on 14th June 2025).
11. Bernthal, N., Eckardt, J., Geiger, E., Greig, D., et al. (2023). Proximal femur replacements for an oncologic indication offer a durable endoprosthesis reconstruction option: A 40-year experience. https://core.ac.uk/download/622530208.pdf (accessed on 14th June 2025).
12. Bortolami, A., Crosby-Durrani, H., Gillespie, A., Verin, R., et al. (2017). An unusual presentation

of actinomycosis in a dairy cow. https://core.ac.uk/download/82984794.pdf (accessed on 14th June 2025).

13. Buck, A. (2022). *Canine Gait Analysis: Interactive Online Tutorials for Veterinary Students*. https://core.ac.uk/download/547498878.pdf (accessed on 14th June 2025).
14. Cerny, R., Hana, K., Hejda, J., Kutilek, P., et al. (2019). Methods evaluating upper arm and forearm movement during a quiet stance. https://core.ac.uk/download/288281766.pdf (accessed on 14th June 2025).
15. Chee, R., Clay, T., Feeney, K. T., Galvão, D. A., et al. (2018). Mechanical suppression of osteolytic bone metastases in advanced breast cancer patients: A randomized controlled study protocol evaluating safety, feasibility and preliminary efficacy of exercise as a targeted medicine. https://core.ac.uk/download/213607862.pdf (accessed on 14th June 2025).
16. Chiesa, C., Donini, L. M., Lenzi, A., Pacifico, L., et al. (2017). Non-alcoholic fatty liver disease connections with fat-free tissues: A focus on bone and skeletal muscle. https://core.ac.uk/download/98335830.pdf (accessed on 14th June 2025).
17. Chuliver Pereyra, M., Cruz, J. C., Fabrezi, M., Goldberg, J., et al. (2016). Developmental changes and novelties in ceratophryid frogs. https://core.ac.uk/download/159296627.pdf (accessed on 14th June 2025).
18. Della Valle, G., Di Dona, F., Fatone, G., Lamagna, F., Meomartino, L., et al. (2016). Congenital deformity of the distal extremities in three dogs. https://core.ac.uk/download/pdf/84247038.pdf (accessed on 14th June 2025).
19. Dolding-Smith, J. (2023). *Maturation of the Modern Human Skeleton*. https://core.ac.uk/download/560371254.pdf (accessed on 14th June 2025).
20. Dora, C., Eid, K., Hartmann, A., Stumpe, K. D., et al. (2018). Diagnostic value of 18F-FDG PET/CT in trauma patients with suspected chronic osteomyelitis. https://core.ac.uk/download/159156630.pdf (accessed on 14th June 2025).
21. Figueirido-Castillo, F. B., Martín-Serra, A., Palmqvist-Barrena, C. P., Pérez-Claros, J. A., et al. (2010). Demythologizing *Arctodus simus*, the 'short-faced' long-legged and predaceous bear that never was. https://core.ac.uk/download/621567857.pdf (accessed on 14th June 2025).
22. Goswami, A., & Randau, M. (2018). Shape covariation (or the lack thereof) between vertebrae and other skeletal traits in felids: The whole is not always greater than the sum of parts. https://core.ac.uk/download/154748431.pdf (accessed on 14th June 2025).
23. Hassan, M. Q., Lee, S. H., Lian, J. B., Mandeville, T. H., et al. (2007). *HOXA10* controls osteoblast genesis by directly activating bone regulatory and phenotypic genes. https://core.ac.uk/download/56518752.pdf (accessed on 14th June 2025).
24. Jundt, G., Kaim, A., Kirsch, E., Maurer, C., et al. (2018). Chronic complicated osteomyelitis of the appendicular skeleton: Diagnosis with technetium-99m labelled monoclonal antigranulocyte antibody-immunoscintigraphic. https://core.ac.uk/download/159157300.pdf (accessed on 14th June 2025).
25. Keane, M., Paul, E., Rauch, C., Rutland, C. S., et al. (2017). Computed tomography in veterinary medicine: Currently published and tomorrow's vision. https://core.ac.uk/download/80784172.pdf (accessed on 14th June 2025).

26. Lanteri, L., Manconi, R., Pazzaglia, U. E., Raspanti, M., et al. (2023). Fin systems comparative anatomy in model Batoidea *Raja asterias* and *Torpedo marmorata*: Insights and relationships between Musculo-skeletal layout, locomotion and morphology. https://core.ac.uk/download/566479463.pdf (accessed on 14th June 2025).

27. Menzer, H. M. (2016). *Treatment of Injuries and Conditions of The Distal Clavicle: A Review.* https://core.ac.uk/download/270100114.pdf (accessed on 14th June 2025).

28. Páramo Blázquez, A. (2021). *The Appendicular Skeleton Variability of the Sauropoda Titanosauria from the Upper Cretaceous of Lo Hueco (Cuenca, Spain).* https://repositorio.uam.es/bitstream/10486/692487/1/paramo_blazquez_adrian.pdf (accessed on 14th June 2025).

29. Paretsis, N. F., Pizzutto, C. S., Rosenfield, D. A., Yanai, T., et al. (2020). Osteologia bruta e radiografia digital da capivara comum (*Hydrochoerus hydrochaeris*), Carl Linnaeus, 1766 para aplicação científica e clínica. https://core.ac.uk/download/386148848.pdf (accessed on 14th June 2025).

30. Robbins, G., Gray, K., Schug, M., Mohanty, R. K., Tripathy, V., Misra, V. N., & Shinde, V. S. (2009). Skeletal evidence for leprosy in India by the second millennium B.C. https://core.ac.uk/download/pdf/288249.pdf (accessed on 14th June 2025).

31. Robinson, R. K. (1976). *Social Status, Stature, and Pathology at Chucalissa (40SY1), Shelby County, Tennessee.* https://core.ac.uk/download/268802901.pdf (accessed on 14th June 2025).

32. Wolfe, B. (2012). *Heterotopic Ossification: Cellular Basis, Symptoms, and Treatment.* https://core.ac.uk/download/58824502.pdf (accessed on 14th June 2025).

JOINTS AND LIGAMENTS

6

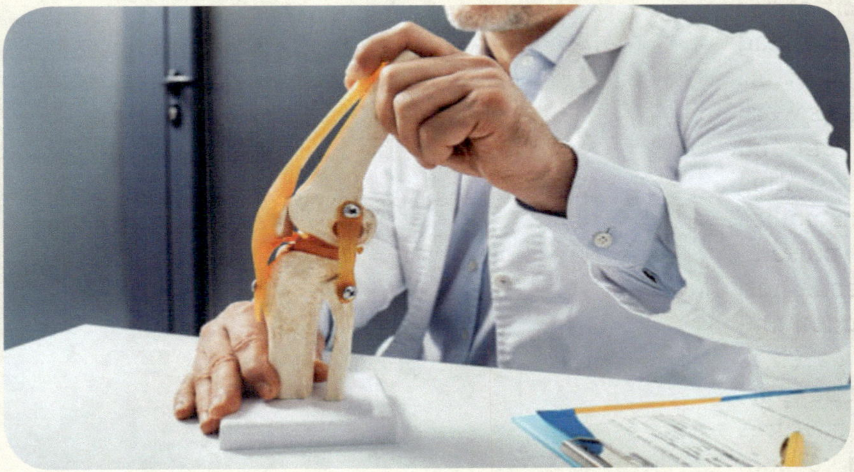

LEARNING OBJECTIVES

After studying this chapter, you will be able to:

1. Describe and classify the different types of joints
2. Define the joint composition
3. Identify the types of ligaments
4. Define the functions of the joints and ligaments
5. Describe common joint and ligament injuries

Introduction

The ligaments and complex joints play a central function in the musculoskeletal (MSK) system, providing stability, support, and mobility. Joints, the sites of apposition between two or more bones, are the functional units that provide movement from simple flexion and extension to complex rotating activities. Ligaments consist of thick bands of connective tissue and vary in their significance in binding bones together at joints to keep them stable and intact during movement. Generally, ligaments, through their individual anatomical arrangements and biomechanical characteristics, ensure joints are not injured, which can occur while engaging in physical activity. This fundamental understanding of the structure and function of the joints and ligaments shows how crucial it is to understand their anatomy and physiology, specifically in terms of overall injury and illness that can also severely impact quality of life. Further specifics of studying an individual ligament, such as the iliolumbar ligament, demonstrate their essential role in joint function and movement. The iliolumbar ligament has been described as the most stabilizing ligament in the lumbosacral interface and plays a critical role in restricting motion in sacroiliac joints. Its anatomical orientation, in that it possesses a sacroiliac component that commingles with the interosseous sacroiliac ligaments, suggests a complex interplay of the pelvic girdle to produce stability with dynamic movement. Experiments using advanced imaging techniques have elucidated the direction and orientation of this ligament, supporting the hypothesis that it helps in limiting excessive movement of the sacroiliac joints, which might otherwise lead to dysfunction or chronic pain (Entius et al., 2001). Understanding how these ligaments work is essential to design beneficial treatment and rehabilitation regimes for individuals presenting with pain or limitation caused by joint instability. The relationship between joints and muscles is more complex than simple mechanics, influencing overall patterns of dysfunction and pain in the body. Low back pain is often seen as a consequence of muscle and ligament support imbalances, such that dysfunction of structures such as the gluteus Medius can lead to pain across the low back and over the sacroiliac joint. Past research has aimed to examine treatment methods to control such issues, such as sacroiliac manipulation and biomechanical pelvic blocking, with a focus on returning normal function to both joints as well as the involved soft tissues. The findings of these studies illustrate that, as varied treatment methods yield positive clinical outcomes, MSK pain's complex nature calls for extensive knowledge of joints and ligaments and their role in health and rehabilitation (Marsden et al., 2019). With increased understanding of the structural and functional dynamics of these structures, we can further advance our practice in addressing concomitant conditions with enhanced efficiency.

Definition of Joints and Ligaments

Anatomical structures known as ligaments and joints are a vital part of the MSK system of the human body. Joints, being the junctions of two or more bones, provide for movement while also giving varying levels of stability. Joint classification often considers structure and function and divides them into synovial, hinge, ball-and-socket, and fibrous joints based on characteristics and means of movement.

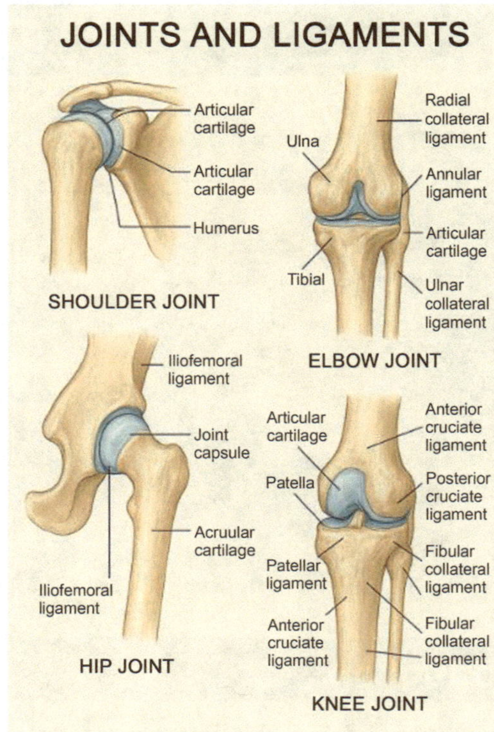

Figure 6.1. Major human joints showing ligaments and cartilage that support stability and movement.

Source: https://sdmntprwestus3.oaiusercontent.com/files/00000000-7f54-61fd-b0d0-35e85c6ac99a/raw?se=2025-05-27T13%3A34%3A55Z&sp=r&sv=2024-08-04&sr=b&scid=67cc2423-facb-56b9-84a4-2f5e90e93360&skoid=9ccea605-1409-4478-82eb-9c83b25dc1b0&sktid=a48cca56-e6da-484e-a814-9c849652bcb3&skt=2025-05-26T23%3A31%3A22Z&ske=2025-05-27T23%3A31%3A22Z&sks=b&skv=2024-08-04&sig=OR7hu9bn6HK3mpfv3lrKAhFz3rF1kTpGp8tJJjnUEAI%3D.

Although some joints allow the most significant amount of motion, such as in the shoulders, others will be relatively immovable, including the skull's sutures. It is possible to understand the diversity in joint types as a means of comprehending how they contribute toward creating the function, mobility, and overall health of the body, a complex system working together for movement and weight-bearing functions. Ligaments, on the other hand, are tough connective tissues that join bones to one another at joints, giving stability and mobility. Composed mainly of collagen fibers, ligaments vary in strength and elasticity, adapted to the specific biomechanical demands of different joints. They contribute not only to structure but also play an essential part in proprioception, the ability of the body to feel position and movement in space. A good example of the significance of ligaments is the anterior cruciate ligament (ACL) of the knee joint. Damage to the ACL frequently requires surgery and an intense rehabilitation regimen to bring about strength and function. As highlighted by recent innovations in instructional aids, a greater understanding of the function and injury of ligaments can lead to improved rehabilitation adherence, ultimately resulting in enhanced recovery outcomes (Buchanan et al., 2014) (Figure 6.1).

Integrating joint and ligament information into practice and training ensures healthier outcomes for patients. Functional anatomical knowledge generates heightened sensitivity to mechanisms of injury and rehabilitation techniques required for return to function. For example, the semantic structure of anatomical terminology, presented in studies on resources like *Terminologia Anatomica*, highlights the importance of clear communication in the healthcare setting. The connectivity of ligaments and joints is of greater importance when correctly depicted within medical educational frameworks. The structured anatomical vocabulary not only assists healthcare professionals in diagnosing and treating patients but also helps patients better comprehend the nature of their illness and the rationale behind their treatment protocol. This improved understanding is of key importance in supporting adherence to rehabilitation programs and enhancing long-term health outcomes (Rosse et al., 2000).

Importance of Joints and Ligaments in the Human Body

The intricate function and structure of joints and ligaments are crucial in maintaining the human body nicely mobilized and stable. Joints, where bones meet, allow for different forms of movement, ranging from the easy flexing of a finger to the complex movements of sports. These connections enable the skeletal system to perform functions such as supporting weight and absorbing shock when exercising, thus preventing injury. To this end, ligaments, the fibrous connective tissue between bones, serve to stabilize and limit unnecessary movement that could lead to dislocations or other forms of injury. Their role is not limited to mere support; ligaments are involved in proprioception, providing feedback to the brain on the position and movement of limbs, which is necessary for movement coordination and posture and balance maintenance. Joint protection is essential in the maintenance of joint functionality, and that is where ligaments become crucial. Ligaments support the joints by forming a strengthening web that stabilizes their structure and lowers the risk of injury. For example, the ACL in the knee assists in maintaining the proper positioning of the femur and tibia during dynamic movements such as running and jumping. When ligaments are damaged or ruptured, as happens in sports injuries, stability of the affected joint is lost, leading to pain, inflammation, and reduced mobility. In addition to preventing ligamentous injury, knowledge of joint and ligament biomechanics helps guide rehabilitation techniques so that wounded individuals can heal and resume their pre-injury activity levels. Examinations of the anatomical and functional specifics of ligaments and joints underscore their significance in human health. Research emphasizes the intimate relationship among multiple elements in the structure of joints and their respective ligaments, as shown in various models of anatomy. For instance, results from anatomical studies on ostrich knees reveal information on joint structure and how the latter can be utilized to enhance knowledge in mechanobiology, shedding light on sesamoid bone formation and its significance for joint function (Abourachid et al., 2014). Furthermore, meticulous examination of anatomical terminology reveals how precise definitions of such organs contribute to the greater body of knowledge within biomechanics, thus facilitating progress within medical informatics and patient management (Rosse et al., 2000). Since the criteria for determining the importance of ligaments and joints continue to shift, it becomes increasingly important to emphasize their roles during motion as well as overall physical health.

6.1. Types of Joints

Learning Outcome

1. Define fibrous joints and cartilaginous joints
2. Discuss about synovial joints

The human skeletal system also has various types of joints, grouped based on structure and function. The primary types are fibrous, cartilaginous, and synovial joints. Fibrous joints, such as sutures in the skull, are fixed together by dense connective tissue, allowing for minimal motion. Cartilaginous joints, such as those between vertebrae, provide minimal motion, stability, and cartilaginous cushioning. Synovial joints, being the most common and adaptive of all the joints, encompass a wide range of movements due to the lubrication of their cavities. This broad categorization supports the important connection between joint classification and functional capability in human physiology by stabilizing the skeletal support and allowing the body to carry out complex tasks. Of the three, synovial joints are particularly remarkable due to their sophistication and the variety of movements they allow. Synovial joints, with a synovial cavity, synovial fluid, and joint capsule, also consist of several types of joints: hinge, ball-and-socket, pivot, saddle, plane, and condyloid joints (Figure 6.2).

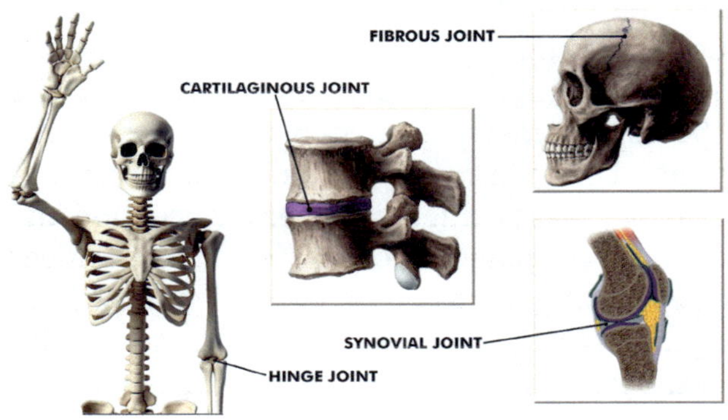

Figure 6.2. Types of joints in our body.

Source: https://i.ytimg.com/vi/XwhM_1qR4oI/maxresdefault.jpg.

Hinge joints of the elbow are responsible for flexion and extension, while ball-and-socket joints in the hip allow rotation. All the subtypes are essential for undertaking specific movements in everyday activities and sports performance. Understanding the unique features of each subtype of synovial joint provides vital information regarding their functional significance, reinforcing the relevance of detailed knowledge in the disciplines of sports medicine and rehabilitation. The importance of understanding the mechanics of different types of joints extends beyond basic anatomy and has implications for clinical practice and rehabilitation methods. As an illustration, non-contact injuries, particularly to ligaments such as the ACL, are now a prevalent aspect of sports medicine. Failure to follow rehabilitation protocols is a frequent consequence of insufficient knowledge of the structure and function of the knee joint and its associated ligaments. New technologies, for example, multimedia instructional packages with high-definition images and animation, aim to enhance patient education and compliance with rehabilitation protocols (Buchanan et al., 2014). Moreover, advancements in computational techniques, like the finite element method, provide researchers and practitioners with further understanding of joint mechanics and injury prevention, especially for challenging joints like the wrist and ankle (Gislason et al., 2010). These developments underscore the critical intersection between joint biology, biomechanics, and outcomes for the patient.

6.1.1. Fibrous Joints

It is critical to understand fibrous joints well in the study of joints and ligaments because the function of such joints is to stabilize while allowing for limited motion. Fibrous joints are characterized by the tough connective tissue that binds bones together, which forms a firm but immovable union. This type of joint is usually found in places where rigidity is more critical than movement; the sutures of the skull are a case in point, since they do indeed protect the brain by firmly anchoring cranial bones. In contrast to the very freely movable synovial joints, which possess a synovial cavity, fibrous joints depict a biomechanical system demonstrating the adaptation of the body to protection and structural support. There are three general types of fibrous joints, and these include sutures, syndesmoses, and gomphoses. Sutures are found only in the skull, where they join irregular bones together, and have little movement to accommodate growth in children. Syndesmoses are with longer connective fibers, allowing a small amount of mobility; one example is the distal tibiofibular joint, where the fibula and tibia are connected (Figure 6.3).

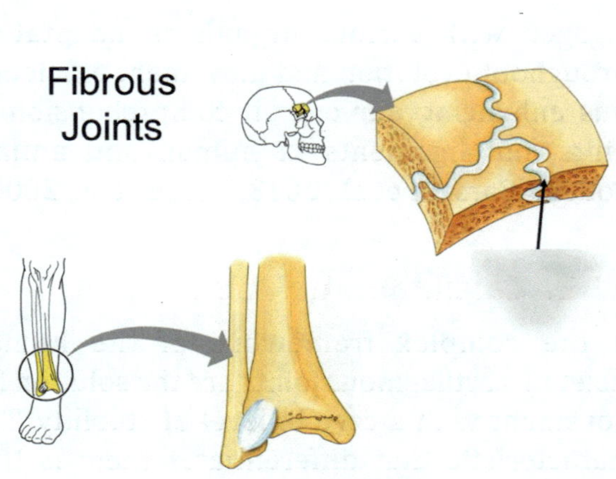

Figure 6.3. Fibrous joints.

Source: https://external-content.duckduckgo.com/iu/?u=https%3A%2F%2Fo.quizlet.com%2F6KS1sl0qnX6o5aW1i3o2cQ_b.png&f=1&nofb=1&ipt=b0d3f084a1ee9c130af63f7486a9ab817abd35d24eba10d2bcb4d59982b2b467.

Gomphoses are a specialized type whereby a pegging structure is housed within a matching socket and teeth are supported by periodontal ligaments. The combined features of these fibrous joints prove the evolutionary advantage of rigidity in regions, some areas of anatomy, and stimulate protection and stability within the skeleton. The study of fibrous joints also lends itself to an investigation of their clinical significance. Abnormalities or trauma to such joints can cause conditions such as craniosynostosis, where premature synostosis of skull sutures generates developmental abnormalities. Likewise, syndesmosis injury, which often occurs following traumatic accidents such as high-impact sport injuries, can give rise to a symptomatic yet frequently underdiagnosed syndrome known as syndesmotic ankle sprain. An understanding of the structure and role of fibrous joints is therefore relevant to health practitioners to be able to make correct diagnoses and formulate treatment protocols. Since research still widens, particularly in comparative anatomy throughout the species, the discovery to be obtained may also better inform us regarding how fibrous joints are engaged with various organisms' adaptation throughout evolution and movement efficiency, thus enhancing our overall comprehension of joints and ligaments in human and animal models (Barszcz et al., 2013; Rosse et al., 2000).

6.1.2. Cartilaginous Joints

In the complex framework of the human skeleton, cartilaginous joints are the solution for movement with a certain level of stability. The characteristic that differentiates them is that there is cartilage, a flexible connective tissue that cushions and reduces friction between the bones that make up the joint. Unlike synovial joints, which are capable of movement and lubricated by synovial fluid, cartilaginous joints do not have a high range of movement.

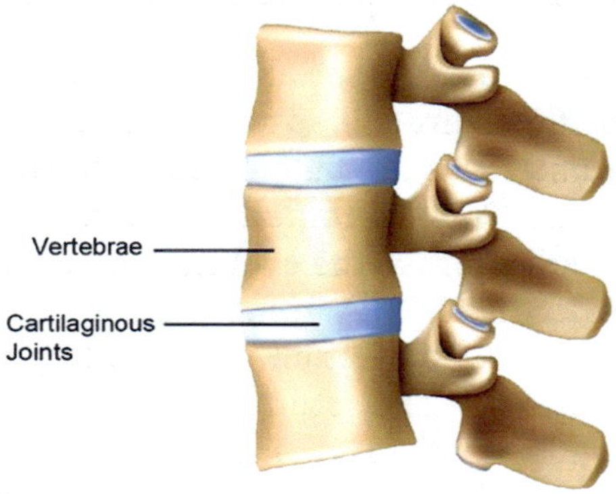

Figure 6.4. Cartilaginous joints.

Source: https://www.sawanonlinebookstore.com/cartilaginous-joints/.

They are again classified into two main groups: synchondroses, by which bones are joined by hyaline cartilage, and symphyses, which are joined by fibrocartilage. A synchondrosis is the epiphyseal plate of growing bones, while a symphysis is the pubic symphysis, joining the left and right pubic bones. This structural variation emphasizes the primary role and compatibility of cartilaginous joints in the human system's biomechanics. Cartilaginous joints are not only involved in plain mobility but, among other things, are responsible for basic functions in weight transference as well as shock absorption that is involved with ambulation and running. Cartilaginous joints, by their construction, also play the role of resilience and elasticity, allowing minute movement that becomes unavoidable with activity (Figure 6.4). For instance, the intervertebral discs (IVDs), which are symphyses, provide minimal movement between vertebrae and serve as shock absorbers during movement. This characteristic mechanical property serves not only to preserve the spinal column's integrity but also that of the vertebral joints in general. Appreciation of such mechanical advantages emphasizes the significance of cartilaginous joints in the grand scheme of joint function and health, illustrating how they satisfy the requirements of an active and sometimes physically stressful lifestyle. Beyond their biomechanical roles, there is a growing interest in understanding the pathologies of cartilaginous joints, particularly of degenerative diseases. Such diseases as osteoarthritis (OA) can severely affect cartilage, resulting in pain and reduced mobility. Alves et al. (2017) note that treatment for such disorders typically involves symptomatic relief, which is aimed at reducing pain and improving function. Advances in diagnostic methods, particularly in imaging examinations, have greatly assisted in identifying diseases that affect cartilaginous joints. These non-invasive imaging modalities allow the clinician to visualize the joint structure, facilitating evidence-based treatment programs that encompass both symptomatic management and underlying pathological change. The investigation of cartilaginous joints, therefore, not only informs greater awareness of joint mechanics but also highlights the importance of joint health in clinical practice.

6.1.3. Synovial Joints

Synovial joints are characterized by their unique anatomical features and are required to perform a wide variety of motions within the body. Synovial joints are characterized by the presence of a synovial cavity filled with synovial fluid that has numerous functions, such as lubrication and the supply of nutrients to cartilage. The bones that articulate in synovial joints are covered with hyaline cartilage, which lowers friction during motion and cushions shockFurthermore, the joint is held in place by the fibrous connective tissue capsule that surrounds it. Such a sophisticated framework allows synovial joints to be adapted to support varying degrees of motion, ranging from the significant range in the shoulder joint to the more restricted motions in the elbow. Understanding synovial joint structure and function is vital for appreciating how the body facilitates complex processes such as walking, jumping, and grasping (Figure 6.5).

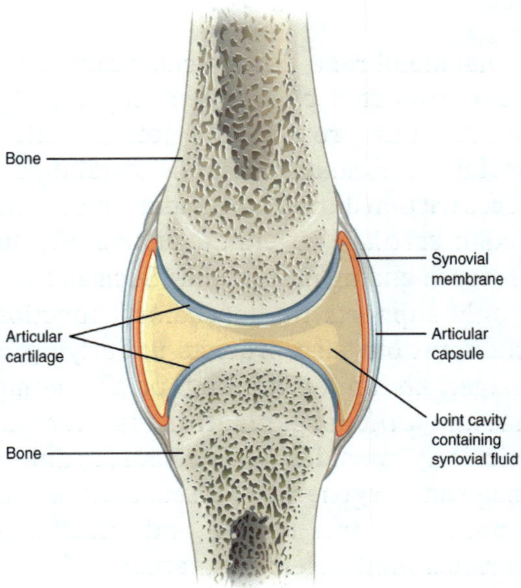

Figure 6.5. Structure of synovial joint.

Source: https://en.wikipedia.org/wiki/Synovial_joint#/media/File:907_Synovial_Joints.jpg.

The classification of synovial joints further emphasizes their diverse functions, which are primarily classified based on the type of motion they facilitate. The six major types include hinge, ball-and-socket, pivot, saddle, plane, and condyloid joints. They facilitate specific movements; for instance, flexion and extension movements are facilitated by hinge joints (e.g., elbows and knees), while rotational and multidirectional motion is facilitated by ball-and-socket joints (e.g., shoulders and hips). Synovial joint flexibility is essentialcrucial for performing various physical movements, enabling them to withstand considerable stress. Furthermore, the anatomy of each synovial joint also determines whether or not it is prone to injuries and degenerative disorders, hence becoming a focal point of study in anatomy as well as in clinical processes.

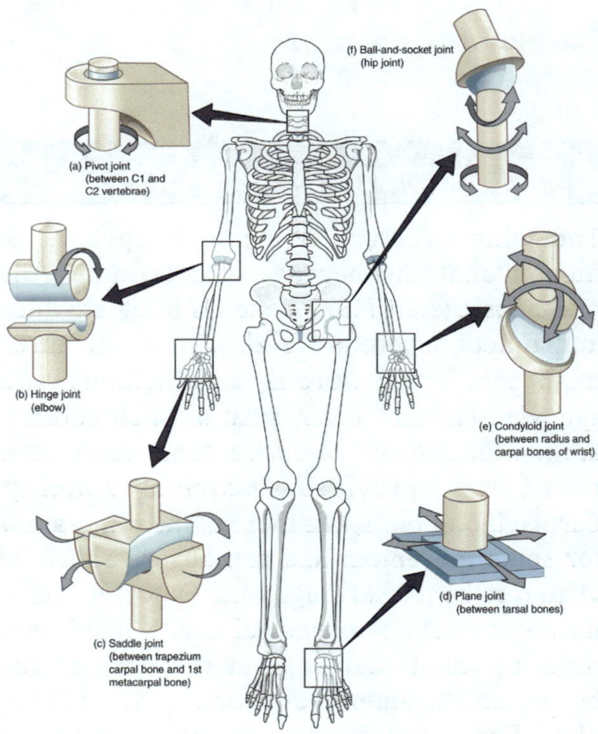

Figure 6.6. Types of synovial joints.

Source: https://en.wikipedia.org/wiki/Synovial_joint#/media/File:909_Types_of_Synovial_Joints.jpg.

This information becomes vital in setting up efficient modes of treatment and rehabilitation for joint injuries. Beyond their functional and structural significance, synovial joints are also key to the subject of anatomical nomenclature. The complexity of their attributes demands precise nomenclature, which might be explored through systems such as the *Terminologia Anatomica*. Relationships between anatomical terms concerning synovial joints, such as spatial orientation and joint fluid dynamics, may be critical to health professionals and researchers alike. Enhancing the accuracy of these term relationships can facilitate more precise communication in clinical settings and support the creation of anatomical knowledge in biomedical informatics. With the ongoing development of medical terminology, standard representations of anatomical relations need to be developed not only to advance educational performance but also to facilitate interdisciplinary cooperation in research and patient management (Rosse et al., 2000; Gielen et al., 2012). Realizing the importance of synovial joints is to present their significance not only in body health but also in the overall perspective of anatomical sciences (Figure 6.6).

Test Your Knowledge

1. Explain the articular cartilage and joint capsule
2. Discuss the synovial fluid

6.2. Structure of Joints

The joint structure is a key component of human anatomy because it determines the musculoskeletal (MSK) system's ROM, stability, and function. Joints are classified into three main categories: fibrous, cartilaginous, and synovial. Fibrous joints, such as skull sutures, are immovable and comprise dense connective tissue that provides maximum stability. Cartilaginous joints, like those of the spine, allow for some movement and can absorb shock by virtue of being cartilaginous. Synovial joints, however, possess a synovial cavity filled with fluid, articulate cartilage at the ends of the bones, and ligaments supporting the joint in place. Such intricate architecture is essential in allowing for movement while still maintaining the integrity of joints, a balance essential for the dynamic functions of the body. The synovial joint that possesses intricate architecture has a quintessential role in facilitating a wide range of movements such as flexion, extension, and rotation. Significantly, these joints are marked by their unique features, such as the joint capsule, synovial membrane, and articular cartilage. The joint is protected by the joint capsule, which supports and protects the joint, while the synovial membrane secretes synovial fluid that reduces friction during movement. Smooth tissue articular cartilage covers the ends of the bones for smooth gliding movements. Such a structure not only supports the mechanical functioning of the joint but also protects underlying bone damage. An understanding of the complex synovial joint organization is necessary, particularly considering their susceptibility to damage and degenerative disease, emphasizing the necessity for a refined and effective joint apparatus. Finite element methods of analysis have been employed in modeling joint behavior, providing insight into the structural dynamics of the joints. This numerical technique has proved to be successful in the simulation of joints like the hip and knee, but difficulty is encountered in more complex joints, e.g., the wrist and ankle. Investigation tends to be hampered, the requirement for the imposition of unphysical boundary conditions being required for numerical convergence. These difficulties emanate from the intricate interaction of soft tissue stabilizing mechanisms that control these joints, which tend to be cumbersome to model both anatomically and at a material level fully. Investigating these constraints may result in improved understanding of the stabilizing mechanisms, ultimately gaining traction in clinical practice as pertains to joint health and rehabilitation paradigms. As previously mentioned, joint structural function and integrity are crucial to overall mobility and quality of life, emphasizing the need for ongoing research in this crucialss area of study (Rosse et al., 2000; Gislason et al., 2010).

6.2.1. Articular Cartilage

Articular cartilage is significant to joint health and function as a smooth, elastic tissue that cushions movement and shock. The unique cartilage is composed primarily of water, collagen fibers, and a complex network of proteoglycans, which give the tissue its distinctive mechanical properties. Articular cartilage design supports load redistribution and minimizes friction on joint movement, offering smooth freedom of movement for all activities. However, articular cartilage is avascular with no possibility of significant repair, which makes it highly susceptible to degenerative disease such as OA. Understanding the biomechanical function of articular cartilage is crucial for comprehending joint health and developing effective treatment protocols for joint diseases. The integrity of articular cartilage is often compromised by processes such as aging, increased mechanical load, or trauma, and this can lead to OA. OA is a type of degenerative joint disease that involves cartilage breakdown and is usually characterized by inflammatory cytokines that enhance tissue loss. Specifically, pro-inflammatory cytokines like interleukin-1 and tumor necrosis factor-α have been reported to cause catabolic activity in the cartilage matrix that leads to the depletion of vital extracellular components such as glycosaminoglycans (GAGs) (Figure 6.7).

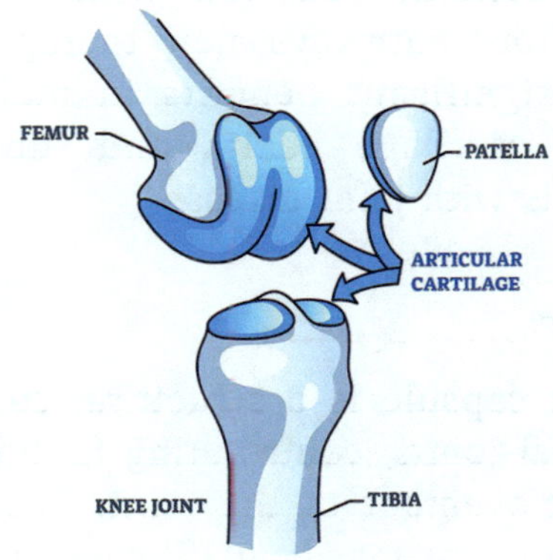

Figure 6.7. Articular cartilage structure.

Source: https://external-content.duckduckgo.com/iu/?u=https%3A%2F%2Fvectormine.b-cdn.net%2Fwp-content%2Fuploads%2Farticular_cartilage_outline_diagram-1.jpg&f=1&nofb=1&ipt=20253a9c76ad7dce2e39863c6af5be85b0eb7f9e10509d98302290f626f5f9ec.

GAG degradation not only compromises the shock-absorbing function of the cartilage but also adversely affects cell viability, leading to a vicious cycle of damage. To counteract these inflammation-driven processes is, therefore, crucial in the prevention or delay of OA and preservation of joint function. Emerging advances in therapeutic approaches have focused on reversing the disruptive effect of inflammation on articular cartilage. One of the most encouraging strategies is the inhibition of cartilage destruction initiated by inflammatory cytokines using glucocorticoids such as dexamethasone (Gislason et al., 2010). The data indicate that dexamethasone can promote cellular survival and augment GAG production, thereby countering the destructive impact induced by pro-inflammatory mediators. However, its capacity for preventing tumor necrosis factor-α-induced GAG loss still needs to be investigated. This also identifies the need for tailored therapeutic approaches that target the complex interactions in the joint microenvironment (Gislason et al., 2010).

Sparing cellular function while targeting inflammatory pathways, new therapies could provide significant benefits in maintaining articular cartilage health and function in individuals with joint disease.

6.2.2. Joint Capsule

The joint capsule is a structural component of synovial joints, contributing to stability as well as movement of the joint. The capsule is composed primarily of fibrous connective tissue, which surrounds the joint and acts as a cushion to absorb forces external to the joint as well as inhibiting excessive movement that could lead to injury. The capsule is typically bilayered, with an outer fibrous layer providing strength and an inner synovial membrane that secretes synovial fluid. This fluid plays multiple functions, including lubrication of the surfaces of the joints, delivery of nutrients, and elimination of waste, thus maintaining joint health and longevity. Structural integrity of the joint capsules is critical in maintaining normal joint function because any degradation can result in conditions like joint laxity or instability, which compromises mobility as well as overall quality of life. In addition to its protective roles, the joint capsule contributes to proprioception so that the body can sense where it is located in space. Such information is crucial to facilitate movement and balance, particularly in complex activities. With mechanoreceptors within the joint capsule, it can provide feedback on the tension and stretch at the joint, which is utilized by the central nervous system in effective motor control. In addition, the joint capsule plays its role in healing from injury. The synovial membrane can become inflamed following injury or disease, such as arthritis, leading to increased synovial fluid production or synovitis. Inflammation has a significant impact on joint function and requires proper management strategies to restore normalcy. New approaches to enjoying and managing joint injury have emerged, highlighting the role of the joint capsule in this area.

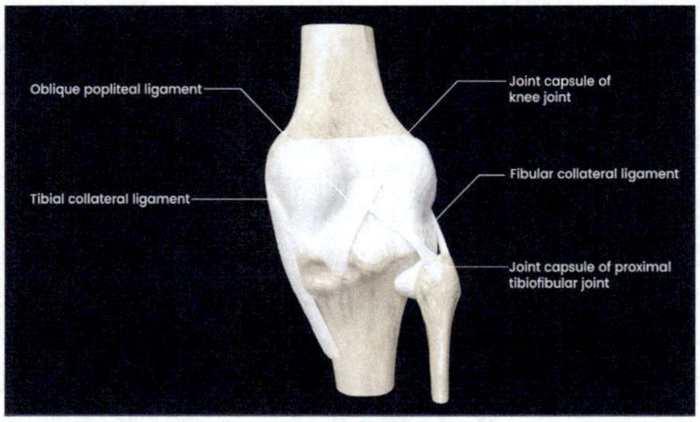

Figure 6.8. Joint capsule of knee joint.

Source: https://external-content.duckduckgo.com/iu/?u=https%3A%2F%2Fanatomy.net%2Fuploads%2Fb4e06d9e-75c7-4033-be26-dc943032bf5c.jpg%3Fwidth%3D1200&f=1&nofb=1&ipt=4c7920c9d36a06b1329599e6c87ae93fc7c48edceb4b9f1219e408ae8e9dfdfa.

Non-contact sprains of ligaments occur often among a high percentage of sporting competitors, for instance, those to the ACL, where involvement of the joint capsule also occurs. Patient information treatment programshave been implemented to educate patients on anatomy, healing, and rehabilitation techniques, aiming to optimize compliance and recovery rates. Medical professionals can also utilize advanced tools, such as 3D models and multimedia packages, to enhance patient education on joint dynamics and the healing process, particularly concerning the joint capsule. These activities not only help in improving patient adherence to rehabilitation programs but also long-term outcomes, enabling patients to return to previous levels of function with stability and confidence (Buchanan et al., 2014) (Figure 6.8).

6.2.3. Synovial Fluid

The role of synovial fluid is critical in the case of synovial joints, acting as a lubricant as well as a vehicle for the nourishment of the cartilage that surrounds the bone surfaces. The synovial membrane, an intercellular lining of the joint capsule with fibroblasts and macrophages, secretes the viscous synovial fluid. Synovial fluid not only reduces friction between the articular cartilages during movement but also absorbs shocks, thereby cushioning the joints against damage. It also has a critical role of providing nutrients and oxygen to avascular cartilage to ensure metabolic health. Synovial fluid changes in volume or composition can significantly impact joint function, leading to conditions such as OA, for which cartilage degradation could be compounded by cytokines like interleukin-1 and tumor necrosis factor α (Wallace et al., 2018) (Figure 6.9).

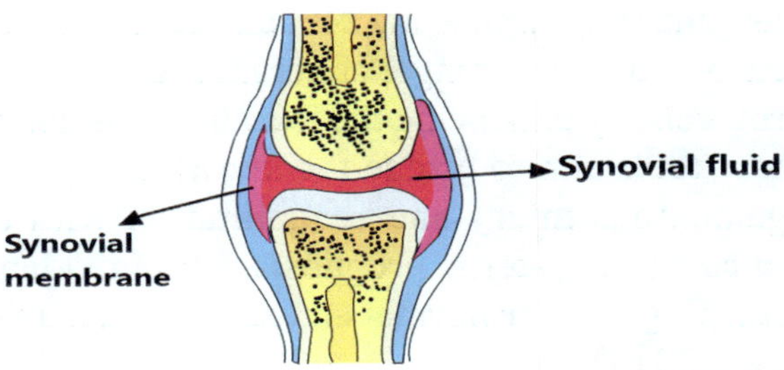

Figure 6.9. Synovial fluid.

Source: https://www.vedantu.com/question-answer/synovial-fluid-is-secreted-by-a-blood-b-class-11-biology-cbse-5f96b3a418cb6e2c518f9454.

Knowledge of such dynamics is critical to the formulation of effective treatments for joint diseases. Biochemical composition of synovial fluid is critical, since it includes hyaluronic acid, lubricin, and several proteins that give it such typical rheological properties. The concentration of hyaluronic acid is particularly crucial to the maintenance of the fluid's viscosity, which serves to protect the articulating surfaces. Under inflammatory disorders such as rheumatoid arthritis (RA), the synovial fluid composition is severely affected, with its content becoming packed with inflammatory cytokines and immune cells. The leukocyte recruitment during active RA, which is predominantly made up of monocytes differentiated into proinflammatory macrophages, is indicative of a change in the synovial environment (Alivernini et al., 2017). This alteration not only disables the lubricating capacity of the fluid but also tends to enhance degradation of the cartilage, demonstrating how synovial fluid is both a health promoter and a potential mediator of disease. In therapeutic applications, the regulation of synovial fluid properties offers options for intervention in joint disease. Glucocorticoid intra-articular injections, such as dexamethasone, are a standard treatment to decrease inflammation and pain caused by OA and allied conditions. The treatment is designed to down-regulate the inflammation process and preserve synovial fluid quality, which improves overall joint function. Dexamethasone has been reported to increase chondrocyte viability while suppressing the detrimental effect of pro-inflammatory cytokines on cartilage and synovial fluid content (Wallace et al., 2018). With increasing knowledge on synovial fluid and its relationship with cartilage, it is clear that preserving the integrity of synovial fluid is crucial for the preservation and maintenance of joints. There is a need for future research to work towards maximizing therapeutic interventions to regain the synovial fluid's protective function, thereby maximizing patient benefit in joint disease.

Test Your Knowledge

1. How does the joint capsule contribute to joint stability?
2. What role does synovial fluid play in joint health and movement?

6.3. Types of Ligaments

Learning Outcome

1. Define intrinsic ligaments and extrinsic ligaments
2. Explain the accessory ligaments

Ligaments, being part of the MSK system, are of various types depending on their structure, composition, and functions in the body. Primarily, ligaments are classified under two broad types: dense regular and dense irregular connective tissues. Dense regular ligaments are characterized by the parallel arrangement of collagen fibers, which provides them with extreme tensile strength in a single direction. These ligaments, such as the ACL, play significant roles in stabilizing joints by connecting bones to bones. Dense irregular ligaments consist of collagen fibers that are enmeshed and can absorb resistance forces from different directions. They are most commonly found in joint capsules and the periosteum, where structural support and toughness are crucial for the normal functioning of various forms of joints, including synovial and fibrous joints. Because of their contributions to proprioception and mobility, ligaments play a crucial role in joint function in addition to providing basic structural support. For instance, ligaments possess sensory receptors that are sensitive to tension and position, and report accordingly to the central nervous system. Such sensory input helps maintain balance and coordination of movement. The knee joint, for instance, exemplifies the role played by ligaments, where the ACL and posterior cruciate ligament (PCL) work together to limit excessive movement and prevent injuries such as tears or ruptures. The ACL is most vulnerable to non-contact injury, necessitating surgery for repair in many patients. Rehabilitation post-surgery is critical for a return to function; however, compliance is challenging for most patients during their recovery. Therefore, there is a need for better teaching aids explaining the ligament's role and recovery (Buchanan et al., 2014). Innovative ways of repairing the ligament and educating are continuous, especially improving patient outcomes in the event of injury. The above-listed surgeries, e.g., ACL reconstruction, tend to involve a lot of rehabilitation, which tends to be difficult as a result of issues such as patient non-compliance or lack of proper understanding of the mechanics of injury. To counter these problems, medical professionals are increasingly using sophisticated multimedia learning tools that integrate cadaveric dissection with high-quality images and 3D reconstructions. Such materials enhance patient knowledge regarding their anatomy, injury, and rehabilitation process, hence leading to stronger adherence to treatment protocols. By enhancing the learning experience, these tools aim to bridge the knowledge gap in ligamentous injury and rehabilitation with an improved long-term prognosis for individuals returning to their normal endeavors (Buchanan et al., 2014).

6.3.1. Intrinsic Ligaments

Intrinsic ligaments, an intrinsic feature of joint stability, play a vital role in the integrity of synovial joints. Intrinsic ligaments possess the feature of being attached directly to the joint capsule and providing support in the form of passive resistance with movement. In contrast to extrinsic ligaments, which link bones between joints to adjacent structures, intrinsic ligaments are located within the joint capsule to allow them to react dynamically to the mechanical stresses encountered during locomotion, such as walking or running. Their intrinsic placement permits them to have increased proprioception, allowing the body to sense and adjust to joint positioning and movement. This intrinsic organization not only provides stability to joints but also prevents the possibility of dislocation or other trauma that might be caused by severe stress or trauma to the joint. Intrinsic ligaments provide more than just mechanical stability; they also play a crucial role in important biological processes. The biochemical composition of these ligaments has specialized cells and extracellular matrix (ECM) components, which are responsible for their viscoelasticity. This is needed in the reaction of the joints to varying loads and stressors, particularly within sporting groups where forces on joints may be drastic. Furthermore, the intrinsic ligaments regulate movement in the joint by allowing controlled movement across a range of positions without excessive translation, thereby maintaining joint stability. As evident from the latest biomechanical studies, understanding the extremely intricate interaction between intrinsic ligaments' structural and functional features is paramount to the development of effective rehabilitation protocols for joint recovery following injury, since they demonstrate which regions of strengthening can enhance joint resistance as a whole (Harris et al., 2012) (Figure 6.10).

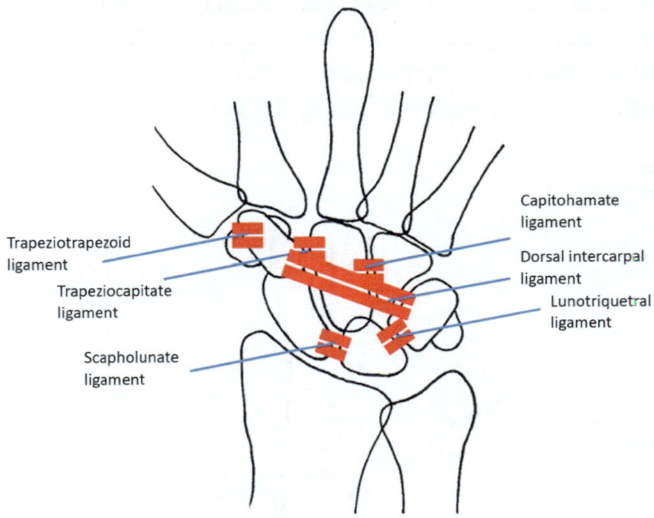

Figure 6.10. A schematic representation of the intrinsic ligaments on the dorsal side of the wrist with labels naming the ligaments.

Source: https://www.researchgate.net/figure/A-schematic-representation-of-the-intrinsic-ligaments-on-the-dorsal-side-of-the-wrist_fig2_320765538.

New developments in biomechanical modeling techniques, such as finite element analysis (FEA), have allowed researchers to analyze the dynamics of intrinsic ligaments under changing loads more precisely. New techniques hold the potential for simulation of the complex interactions among intrinsic ligaments and the joint environment, and this provides us with a deeper insight into the processes involved in stabilization. For example, finite element models have been successful in replicating the joint dynamics of joints like the wrist and ankle, pointing out the sophistication posed by their complex architectures (Gislason et al., 2010). These kinds of models demonstrate how the additional constraints affect the behavior of the ligaments, ultimately leading us to understand joint function and integrity. These findings hold not only basic significance but also critical importance for clinical practice, particularly in the development of orthopedic therapy and healing variables, underscoring the need for ongoing interdisciplinary research into the biomechanics of intrinsic ligaments.

6.3.2. Extrinsic Ligaments

Extrinsic ligaments play a crucial role in joint stability and function, as they connect bones to surrounding tissues. Extrinsic ligaments, which are located outside the joint capsule, provide the support necessary to maintain correct alignment during movement. They are primarily responsible for resisting excess motion, which can lead to injury. For instance, in the knee joint, extrinsic ligaments such as the collateral ligaments not only stabilize the joint itself but also contribute to the overall biomechanics of the leg, influencing the ROM as well as the leg's bearing load capacity. The placement of the ligaments as a strategic defense system indicates their function as the initial line of mechanical defense against stress, carrying out an intrinsic role within joint stability during complex movements and sports exercises. The dynamic interaction between extrinsic ligaments and joint function can be exemplified by their role in the stability of the ACL. Extrinsic determinants like biomechanical forces and anatomical differences have been identified to significantly affect the incidence of ACL injuries, particularly in women. According to the American College of Sports Medicine, women patients are overrepresented in the incidence of ACL injuries based on a combination of extrinsic and intrinsic factors of risk that include differences in structure and hormonal components (Gillie et al., 2011) (Figure 6.11).

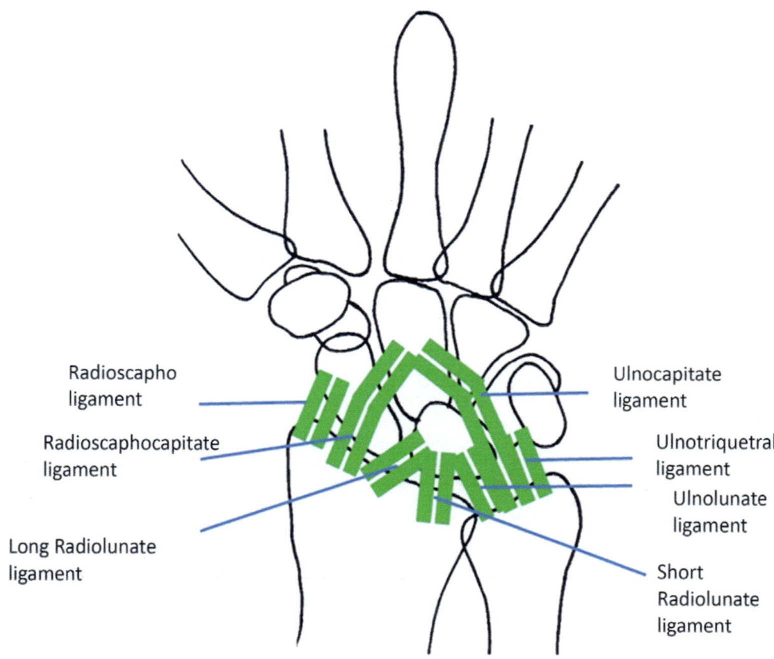

Figure 6.11. A schematic representation of the extrinsic ligaments on the palmar side of the wrist with labels naming the ligaments.

Source: https://www.researchgate.net/figure/A-schematic-representation-of-the-extrinsic-ligaments-on-the-palmar-side-of-the-wrist_fig4_320765538.

Understanding these factors can be pivotal in developing prevention strategies that address the specific vulnerabilities of female athletes. Analysis of how outside factors interact with extrinsic ligaments can help scientists create a better understanding of preventive strategies that increase knee joint stability and reduce injury rates. Additionally, advances over recent years in simulation technology, such as the finite element method, have made it possible to study extrinsic ligament mechanics at unprecedented levels of detail. These simulations have the potential to make detailed investigations of how different constraints imposed on the joints, particularly complex ones like the wrist and ankle, affect stability and overall functionality. The previous finite element study encountered difficulties in precisely simulating the complex soft tissue mechanisms due to the extrinsic ligaments' complicated nature (Gislason et al., 2010). By refining these models, researchers can gain more detailed data regarding extrinsic ligament stabilizing functions and joint health contributions. In this way, such data not only informs clinical practice but also enhances athletic training programs, ultimately enhancing the resilience and performance of joints in various populations.

6.3.3. Accessory Ligaments

Accessory ligaments have a significant role in joint stability and function since they are accessory structures that hold the primary ligaments in place. Not only are accessory ligaments a critical component of joint system stability, but they also facilitate freedom of movement by providing additional support during dynamic movement. For instance, in the knee joint, the presence of accessory ligaments such as the ligament of Wrisberg and the ligament of Humphry illustrates their function of complementing the stability of the principal cruciate and collateral ligaments. Their mechanical and anatomical positions are crucial in limiting excessive motion and the resulting harm. Thus, it is crucial to understand the role of accessory ligaments for those practitioners who want to prevent or rehabilitate joint-associated injuries that can be caused to athletes or active individuals. Besides their stabilizing functions, accessory ligaments exhibit a broad diversity of anatomical differences between species, which supports their evolutionary changes to biomechanical requirements. For example, in ungulates, the new arrangement of accessory ligaments increases their shock absorption and the ability to withstand forces involved in locomotion. Comparison of accessory ligaments in various species of ungulates, such as reindeer and caribou, brings insights to their joint mechanics and overall health.

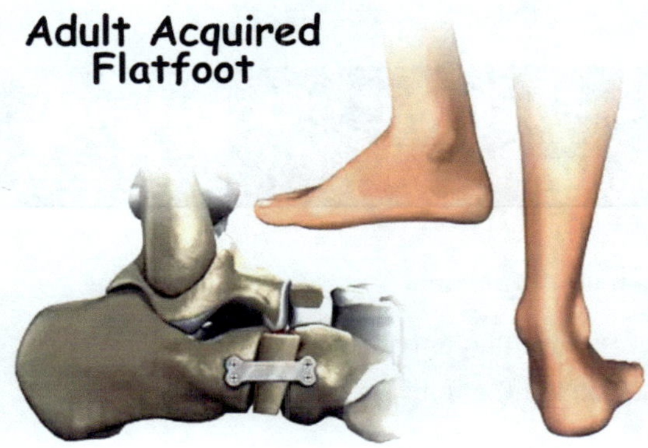

Figure 6.12. Adult acquired flatfoot deformity (AAFD).

Source: https://www.advantagephysiotherapy.com/media/img/347237/foot_acquired_flatfoot_intro01.jpg.

The information on this topic is derived from research that examines the distinct structural features of these ligaments, including their points of fixation and contact with surrounding tendons and muscles. Increased information in this regard not only encourages zoological information but also promotes veterinary practice towards improving animal welfare and functional outcomes for such animals (Hull et al., 2021). The functional importance of accessory ligaments is also relevant to the diagnosis and management of the pathology of instability in the foot, like in adult acquired flatfoot deformity (AAFD). In AAFD, the consequences of accessory ligament dysfunction can be observed, particularly the consequences on plantigrade stance and gait mechanics. When the posterior tibialis tendon and stabilizers fail, secondary effects occur in the form of disruption of accessory ligaments such as the spring ligament. Malalignments due to this failure can severely limit motion and generate crippling foot pain. Intervention to restore function must consider not only the major ligaments but also the essential accessory structures, with special reference to their role in both surgical and conservative management planning. Thus, accessory ligaments form part of the broader understanding of joint health and functional movement (Davis et al., 2019) (Figure 6.12).

Test Your Knowledge

1. What is the difference between intrinsic and extrinsic ligaments?
2. How do accessory ligaments support joint stability?

6.4. Functions of Joints and Ligaments

Learning Outcome

1. Discuss the functions of joints
2. Explain the functions of ligaments

Joints enable movement and provide flexibility by connecting bones. Ligaments stabilize joints by connecting bones and preventing excessive movement.

6.4.1. Functions of Joints

Joints are critical parts of the MSK system in human bodies and serve to connect bones and allow movement in multiple directions. The classification of joints into synovial, fibrous, and cartilaginous is typical of the myriad functions that they perform. Synovial joints, for instance, allow extensive movements like flexion, extension, rotation, and gliding movements. These features of motion are essential to daily activities, from ambulating to elite athletic function. This inherent flexibility is a result of the structural features of synovial joints, including joint capsules and synovial fluid, which lubricate the articular surfaces and decrease friction and enhance mobility. In contrast, cartilaginous and fibrous joints are less movable and more stable and serve essential roles in areas such as the ribcage and the skull, where they need to be rigid to support and to protect. The mechanical operations of joints are significantly influenced by the integrity and presence of ligaments and surrounding soft tissues, which stabilize and guide joint movement. Ligaments are tough, fibrous connective tissues that are important in keeping bones in correct alignment and offering resistance to excessive stress. Ligament tension helps to distribute forces more evenly when a joint is loaded, reducing the risk of damage The subtlety of such stabilization becomes particularly evident in joints such as the knee, which rely on sophisticated ligamentous restraints for stability during movements such as running and jumping. Appreciation of how ligaments influence joint function highlights the importance of general rehabilitation protocols following joint trauma. This is essential to restoring not only mobility, but also the ability to withstand the physical stresses placed upon these joints, so athletic function and functional capacity are preserved. Furthermore, new methods of biomechanical modeling, such as the finite element method, have advanced our understanding of how joints work and how forces applied to them influence them. This computational approach allows researchers to simulate joint behavior under various circumstances, hence providing insight into the complexity of joint mechanics. For example, experiments on the wrist joint have demonstrated that the complex stabilizing mechanisms provided by soft tissues are usually not attained in biomechanical models. These constraints highlight the difficulty scientists face in accurately modeling the anatomical and functional relationships of joints. Nonetheless, understanding that is derived through such research can lead to better treatment practices and prevention protocols for joint injury because it highlights the importance of stabilizing roles contributed by ligaments and surrounding structures to preventing joint disease and dysfunction (Gislason et al., 2010). Thus, continued examination of joint biomechanics is vital for enhancing clinical protocols and understanding the relevance of joint health in varying populations.

6.4.1.1. Movement

The intricate interaction among joints, ligaments, and motion is central to learning about human biomechanics. The joints are the focal points of union between bones that allow a series of motions from the simple bending of the elbows to the combination of motions of the knee and shoulder. Ligaments, by contrast, provide stabilization by bone-to-bone attachment and stabilize the joint during motion. This structural strengthening is essential because it maintains the integrity of the joint without compromising enough flexibility to perform complex movements. Biomechanical inquiry provides substance to this study by applying the principles of physics to the world of living tissue to reveal the underlying mechanisms that govern how ligaments and joints work with each other during dynamic motion such as running and jumping. It is worth understanding these interactions to not only enhance sport performance but to prevent injury that comes from inefficient patterns of movement (Figure 6.13).

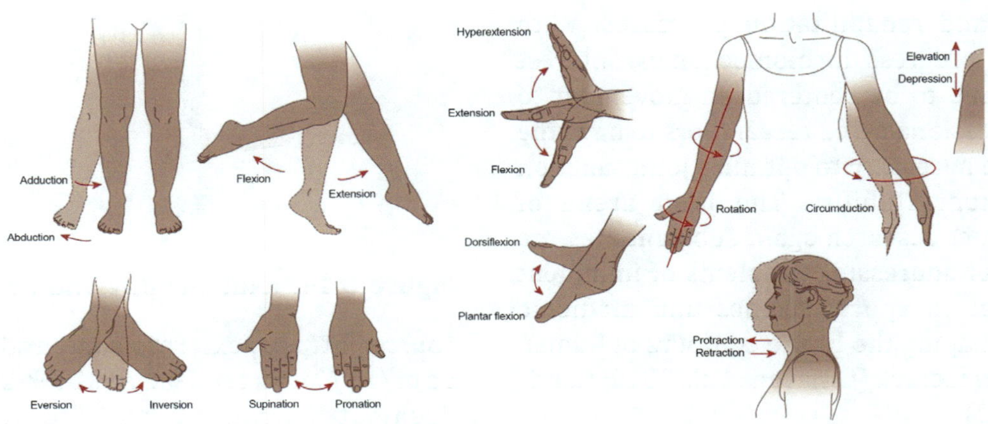

Figure 6.13. Types of joint movements.

Source: https://www.pharmacy180.com/media/article/article-Types-of-Joint-Movem-9Pn.jpg

Movement is also made more complicated by the role of stabilizing soft tissues, particularly in more evolved joints like the wrist and ankle. Experiments that have applied FEA have provided some understanding of the special character of these joints, which are prone to being modeled by more advanced mechanical models. Such a study illustrates that more rudimentary models cannot properly describe the stabilizing mechanism of such joints due to their intricate anatomical structure. Therefore, researchers have imposed constraints to further improve their simulation and achieve numerical convergence. For instance, during wrist motion, interaction between multiple bones and soft tissues provides a variety of possible motions, which necessitate extensive modeling approaches. Based on understanding such stabilizing mechanisms, researchers are able to assess joint function better and heal injuries caused by instability or overloading of tendons and ligaments. Besides, advances in biomechanical modeling techniques are revolutionizing human movement and injury prevention approaches. The integration of diverse fields like engineering, biology, and medicine has yielded new methods involving the application of inverse dynamics and MSK modeling to predict movement patterns better. These multidisciplinary studies contribute to our knowledge about how the body adapts to a range of forces during physical motion, providing clinical expertise about mechanisms of injury and rehabilitation processes. With continued progress in biomechanics, interest will continue to be centered on movement to allow professionals and researchers to have the knowledge necessary to optimize joint function and ligament stability. The joint arena of biomechanics research again substantiates the necessity of addressing problems of imminent significance in sports science and medicine and thus shaping the future contours of human movement research (Gislason et al., 2010; Harris et al., 2012).

6.4.1.2. Stability

The concept of joint stability plays a pivotal role in the maintenance of overall MSK integrity. Joints, being bony connecting structures of the bones, are entirely dependent on their anatomical configuration and the corresponding ligaments for stability. The relationship between bony articulations and the overlying soft tissue structures will be responsible for a joint's ability to withstand forces during motion. In diarthrodial joints such as the knee and shoulder, stability relies on conditions such as joint congruence and ligament placement concerning functional tasks. Alignment and strength of these ligaments should be adequate to prevent unnecessary motion that can lead to injury.

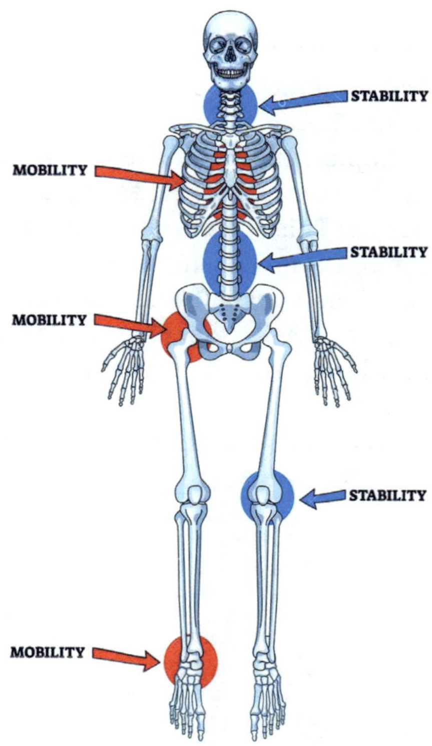

Figure 6.14. Joint stability and body mobility.

Source: https://external-content.duckduckgo.com/iu/?u=https%3A%2F%2Fthumbs.dreamstime.com%2Fz%2Fjoint-stability-body-mobility-skeletal-bone-division-outline-diagram-272771627.jpg&f=1&nofb=1&ipt=d933bcf09139acd5470361168fe0181aaeca56d2cd0bf4c0886a09cf82d32105.

Hence, it is of paramount importance to understand the nuances in joint stability so that efficient prevention techniques and rehabilitation techniques can be developed that target specific joint dysfunctions. Analysis of joint stability must consider the advanced techniques employed to simulate and investigate the behavior of a joint under dynamic loading. The finite element model has emerged as an essential simulation tool for modeling joint mechanics, particularly when examining intricate structures like the wrist and ankle. They are unique joints to stabilize due to their intricate anatomical shape and dependency on soft tissue for stability. As demonstrated in studies, e.g., those on wrist modeling, it is apparent that the specific interaction among bones, ligaments, and exerted forces plays a central role in elucidating the stability mechanisms. The context of the use of sophisticated modeling techniques offers the potential for a greater appreciation of how different constraints change may affect stability, and how, from this, arise improved therapeutic interventions for joint-related disorders. Mainly when found among athletes or individuals with repetitive stress injuries (Gislason et al., 2010) (Figure 6.14). Investigating load distribution and transfer in joints also offers additional fundamental information about stability. The wrist example illustrates how significantly load shifts between each finger during, for example, gripping actions. The research demonstrates that the principal load—to an incredibly high extent—lies on the radius and only a minimal amount from the ulna, illustrating how anatomical design governs functional load management. Understanding these complexities enables a more thorough identification of any weak points that can cause instability or harm. Furthermore, through the application of discipline-specific models, it is possible to account for individual anatomical variations and offer personal insight into joint stability (Bransby-Zachary et al., 2009). This individualized approach not only improves the accuracy of simulations but also allows for the development of more effective interventions, thereby enhancing the quality of life among vulnerable subjects to joint instability.

6.4.1.2. Load Distribution

In joints and ligaments, load distribution is a critical element that is forecast to determine the MSK system's mechanical stability and functionality. Under the forces encountered during a range of activities by the joints, how loads are distributed among the bones, ligaments, and the respective tissues significantly influences their integrity as well as susceptibility to damage. For instance, load distribution over the wrist must consider the complex interaction between several bones and soft tissues. Inefficient distribution of load can lead to high stress on individual structures, thereby enhancing the likelihood of degeneration or damage over time. Understanding the biomechanics of load distribution enhances the assessment of joint functionality, guiding therapeutic and rehabilitative interventions aimed at optimizing joint health. Development in imaging and modeling technology over the past few decades has allowed for greater insight into load distribution within various joints. FEA is currently a significant aid to the exploration and comprehension of joint behavior under specific loads and conditions. These models can now study complicated joints like the wrist, which is highly challenging due to its intricacy and the stabilizing effects of ligaments. Through subject-specific loading data, researchers can develop more accurate models of the actual biological conditions. Examples of this include load distribution studies that have shown how, during maximal grip function, there is an exceptionally high percentage of load transmission through the radius and not the ulna, highlighting the importance of accurate anatomical considerations within load-bearing analyses of the wrist (Bransby-Zachary et al., 2009). In addition, load distribution implications extend beyond understanding mechanical function to be employed in guiding practice in preventing and treating injury. By the method of FEA, researchers have delineated the relationship between ligamentous support and load distribution and identified sites of possible failure in a joint. Such studies stress the importance of including all material anatomical structures, such as ligaments and tendons, in biomechanical models if accuracy is desired. By close inspection of the loads transmission and distribution over a sequence of movements, clinicians can more effectively design rehabilitation protocols by maximal restoration of joint function and avoidance of future injury. Thus, knowledge obtained through the analysis of load distribution provides an underlying platform for optimization of preventive measures and therapeutic exercises for joint injuries (Gislason et al., 2010).

6.4.2. Functions of Ligaments

Ligaments play an essential function in providing stability and functionality to various joints in the human body. Composed mainly of dense connective tissue, they connect bones to bones and therefore play a role in the general structural support of the skeletal system. The tensile strength of ligaments enables them to stretch significantly while facilitating movement. For instance, in the knee, ligaments such as the ACL and PCL are essential for offering proper alignment and ROM. Not only do these ligaments prevent excessive movement that may cause injuries, but they also facilitate dynamic movements such as running and jumping, indicating their multipurpose function in joint health and mobility. In addition to providing stability, ligaments have a fundamental function in proprioception, or the sense of body position in space. Through proprioceptive nerve endings, ligaments are directly involved in the feedback loop that informs the central nervous system about joint movement and position. This information is vital to coordinating muscle function and proper body mechanics in a wide range of activities. For instance, during sudden changes of direction, such as during sports, the proprioceptive feedback through ligaments allows for timely compensations and thereby limits injury. Moreover, understanding the proprioceptive functions of ligaments is not only crucial to athletes but also to rehabilitation therapy since optimal use of this feedback system can be utilized to aid in recovery as well as improve function following injury. Lastly, ligaments are vital tissues in injury repair, with inherent strength and flexibility. While their limited blood supply can facilitate dysfunctional healing, enhanced therapeutic measures aim to encourage healing in ligamentous tissue. Knowledge of the biologic and biomechanical nature of ligaments is essential in the determination of effective treatment protocols, particularly in sports medicine. For example, three-dimensional anatomical investigations of ligaments, such as the studies of the ostrich knee joint, yield important information about their structural complexity and functional significance (Abourachid et al., 2014). Understanding these aspects of anatomy can inform the design of rehabilitation programs aimed at not only repairing but also enhancing ligament function, which is valuable for both prevention of injury and optimization of movement through a variety of activities (Rosse et al., 2000).

6.4.2.1. Joint Stabilization

Effective joint stabilization is crucial for maintaining functional mobility and preventing injury. Joints, being components of the MSK system, are reliant on coordination among ligaments, tendons, muscles, and neuromuscular control to maintain their stability during motion. Ligaments, which connect bones, are a significant source of stability by restricting excessive motion. The various categories of joints, including synovial and fibrous joints, exhibit contrasting mechanisms of stabilization according to the structural composition as well as their functional necessity. For instance, the stability of the knee joint, relying heavily on the ACL and PCL, is critical to running and jumping activities. Thus, understanding these stabilizing mechanisms can be helpful in the development of effective rehabilitation strategies for individuals who have joint instability or injury (Figure 6.15).

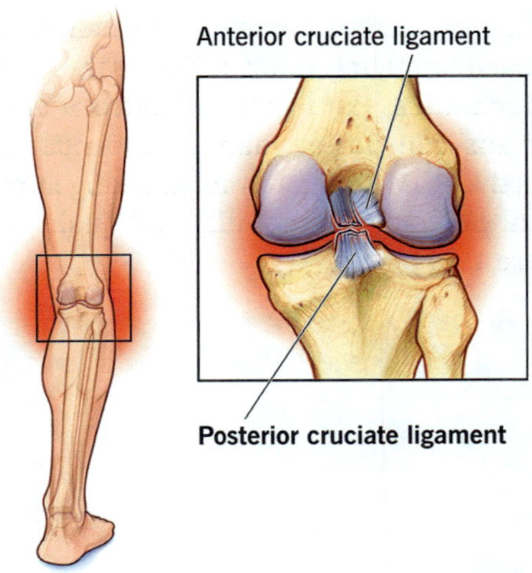

Figure 6.15. A tear of the posterior cruciate ligament (PCL), a ligament in the knee.

Source: https://my.clevelandclinic.org/-/scassets/images/org/health/articles/21793-posterior-cruciate-ligament-tear.

In clinical use, measurement and enhancement of joint stabilization are essential, particularly in the event of injury or surgery. Therapy strategies typically involve a combination of physical therapy, strengthening, and, in some cases, surgical repair to achieve appropriate joint function. A case in point is the closing wedge ostectomy operation (CWO) to treat cranial cruciate ligament rupture in dogs, and the complexities involved in attaining dynamic stabilization of the joints. By surgical adjustment of the tibial plateau angle, the demand for the injured ligament is eliminated, and cranial tibial thrust under weight-bearing loads is thus reduced (Borges et al., 2016). Similarly, targeted rehabilitation protocols can reinforce the stabilizing musculature, offering greater stability and re-injury protection. These multimodal approaches showcase the application of joint stabilization in veterinary and orthopedic medicine alike. Also, as the understanding of joint stabilization evolves, it has broader implications extending beyond clinical care into sports science and the prevention of injury. Sporting individuals are particularly vulnerable to joint injuries due to the bodily toll imposed on their bodies through sporting competition. By focusing on proprioception and neuromuscular training, therapists can significantly enhance joint stability, leading to improved sporting performance and decreased rates of injury. In addition, biomechanical studies of joint movement only continue to uncover the exact forces necessary in action, which allows for the development of particular strengthening regimens. As highlighted in the literature detailing pelvic injuries and rehabilitation, stabilization to the best possible amount is paramount for rehabilitation and recovery (Shyshchuk et al., 2014). Briefly, the intricate relationship between joints, ligaments, and stabilization systems is significant to both performance and health across diverse populations.

6.4.2.2. Limiting Range of Motion

Joint limiting ROM is a fundamental term that is both an anatomical aspect and a critical clinical consideration. ROM describes the amount of motion which can be produced by a joint around a specific axis, and is defined by the structural organization of the bones, muscles, and ligaments about the joint. When assessing joints and ligaments, it is essential to identify the factors that may be causing the restriction of ROM. Restrictions can be due to anatomical limitations, such as joint capsules and ligaments that provide stability but restrict motion. Hypermobility, on the other hand, leads to increased vulnerability to injury, demonstrating the delicate balance of flexibility and stability in joint movement. These factors reveal a multifaceted interrelation between biomechanics and anatomy in the delivery of peak performance at minimal risk of trauma.

Another crucial element of restriction in ROM is its relationship with injury mechanisms. Joint injuries usually occur from overlarge or uncoordinated movement past the physiological limits of the joint (Figure 6.16).

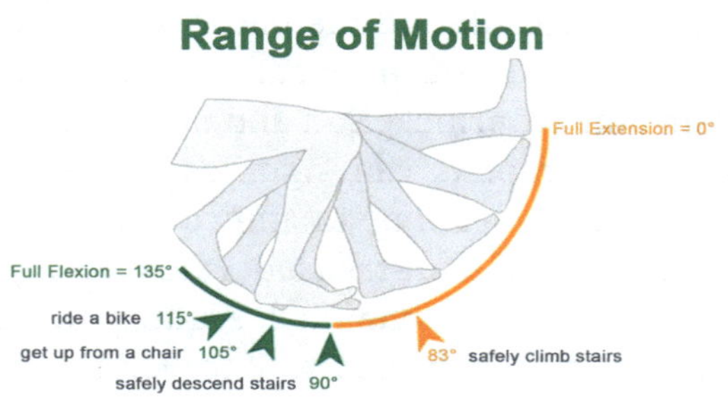

Figure 6.16. Range of motion (ROM).

Source: https://x10therapy.com/wp-content/uploads/2017/09/ROM-1024x576.png.

For example, the shoulder joint is in so much danger due to the enormous amount of motion it enjoys, yet at what cost is flexibility paid? It takes mindful exploration of muscle and ligament mechanics to figure out how particular movements, such as abduction and adduction, affect stress on these tissues. Current investigations employing newer model techniques, including FEA, have clarified the stresses that the shoulder joint undergoes while undertaking routine movements, thereby shedding light on how anatomical constraints influence ROM as well as susceptibility to injury (Krishna et al., 2014). The analysis highlights the importance of accounting for joint function not only within the mobility domain but also in the prevention of injuries. Finally, the use of ROM restrictions carries on into clinical settings where an understanding of joint mechanics is utilized in aiding rehabilitation regimens. Inter-ossicular dysfunction, for instance, can lead to extreme movement and functionality limitations through related pathologies. Critical examination of these dynamics informs effective intervention practices, such as the development of prosthetic devices that account for the adaptability required in joints (Baird et al., 2013). Ergonomic interventions, coupled with directed therapy, can maximize recovery by addressing both the structural and functional potential of the involved joints. By embracing a multidisciplinary approach, applying information from anatomy, biomechanics, and rehabilitation science, clinicians can better manage the nuances of restrictive ROM, ultimately maximizing improved patient outcomes in mobility and quality of life (Figure 6.17).

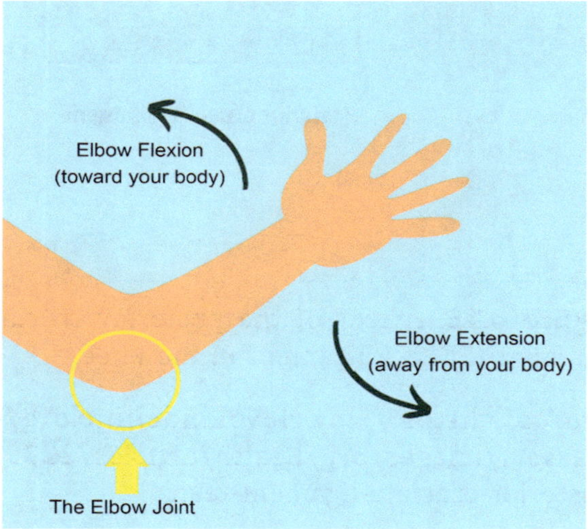

Figure 6.17. Demonstrating elbow flexion and extension.

Source: https://www.onestep.co/resources-blog/the-importance-of-range-of-motion.

6.4.2.3. Supporting Joint Structure

The support of the joint structures is essential to their stability and function. Joints, where two or more bones are apposed, rely heavily on a system of supporting musculature, tendons, and ligaments to maintain their integrity during movement. Ligaments, which consist of dense connective tissue, bind bones to one another and contribute to the stability of joints by limiting excessive movements that can lead to injury. The intricate structure of these connective tissues forms an intricate biomechanical system that responds to varying forces, thus yielding mobility and protection. Such an association is important in emphasizing the role of the understanding of ligament form and function, as it has a direct bearing on the health of the joint. Full appreciation of these supportive tissues is the solution to clinical practice progress, particularly in developing preventive maneuvers as well as rehabilitation procedures for trauma related to joints. In addition to the anatomical details of joint support, information about the behavior of the structures under various conditions is given by biomechanical studies. The finite element technique, a computer-intensive method, has found extensive application to simulate joint mechanics, particularly for complex joints like the shoulder and elbow. Later studies that incorporated this technique have demonstrated that simple joints could be relatively well modeled, but that more complex articulations, such as the wrist, are not quite so simple due to their geometric complexity and related soft tissue support systems. This often involves accepting non-physiological boundary conditions to allow numerical convergence in the models being employed. Such problems direct us towards the need to further improve our anatomical description and understanding of these support elements in an attempt to make relevant simulations that can give way to clinical knowledge and practice (Gislason et al., 2010). Furthermore, establishing a standardized and integrated presentation of anatomical connections has immense potential to enhance our understanding of joint function and stability. The Terminologia Anatomica, while being a valuable tool for anatomical nomenclature, also lags in explicit modeling of part-whole relations that might support dynamic coupling between joints and supporting tissues. By overcoming such deficits, researchers can offer the coupling of anatomical information to medical informatics, which is essential to the formation of controlled medical terminology (CMT) initiatives. These projects aim to create machine-readable representations of the biomedical concepts, including the specific anatomy of joints and ligaments. Enhancing the mapping of anatomical terms to their context-dependent meanings will not only improve educational performance but also enable enhancements in clinical technologies aimed at improving the health of joints and optimizing the effects of treatments (Rosse et al., 2000).

Test Your Knowledge

1. What are the primary functions of joints in the human body?
2. How do ligaments contribute to joint stability and movement?

6.5. Common Joint and Ligament Injuries

Learning Outcome

1. Discuss the sprains and strains
2. Understand the dislocations

Injuries to the ligaments and joints are common across numerous sporting and everyday activities and have a vast impact on physical function and quality of life. Among all injuries, the ACL tear is one of the most common, specifically in athletes who engage in high-impact activities like soccer and basketball. Non-contact ACL tears are likely to occur due to either changes in direction or sudden stops, and they are very possible to impede an individual's participation in sports. The process of cure typically involves surgeries and rehabilitation regimens. However, the patients find it challenging to adhere to the patterns of rehabilitation, most commonly with premature return to activity, which will undermine the integrity of the graft and lead to re-injury. This underscores the necessity for improved patient education during the healing process and realistic timelines of return to sport-related activities, as highlighted in current clinical guidelines (Buchanan et al., 2014). Another category of severe joint injuries is those that occur to the shoulder and ankle, with sprains and dislocations among them. Ankle sprains, for example, occur when the ligaments responsible for keeping the ankle stretched and in place are stretched or torn, usually due to misstepping or uneven landings. This is especially true in sports because most games entail abrupt movements that might put undue strain on the ankle joint. Shoulder dislocations, similarly, are more likely to occur due to trauma or falls, and these injuries can lead to considerable joint instability if not properly treated. Both the mechanisms and consequences of these types of injuries need to be comprehended to prevent and rehabilitate them. By utilizing prevention techniques such as appropriate warm-up and strength training, athletes can decrease the likelihood of such common injuries. Furthermore, appropriate rehabilitation education is essential in guiding athletes through their return-to-play options (Fabbri et al., 2016). In considering the significance of these injuries, it is clear that both short-term and long-term management plans are essential for successful recovery and prevention. According to current literature, the cooperative effect of surgical repair combined with other supporting operations, like lateral extra-articular tenodesis, can improve stability in the presence of ACL injuries along with other instabilities in the knee. For instance, elite female soccer players have shown positive outcomes following this two-faceted approach, with greater subjective and objective measures of stability and function. These outcomes highlight the importance of individual athlete profile utilization in the form of patient-specific treatment planning, particularly among high-risk groups. With advancements in technology, it will be essential to develop cutting-edge teaching materials and rehabilitation protocols to maximize patient compliance and long-term outcomes of recovery for patients with typical joint and ligament injury (Buchanan et al., 2014).

6.5.1. Sprains

Sprains are a form of injury that occurs when ligaments, which are supportive tissues in joints, get stretched or even torn. This can occur as a result of sudden motion or sports accidents, leading to pain, swelling, and limited mobility in the affected area.

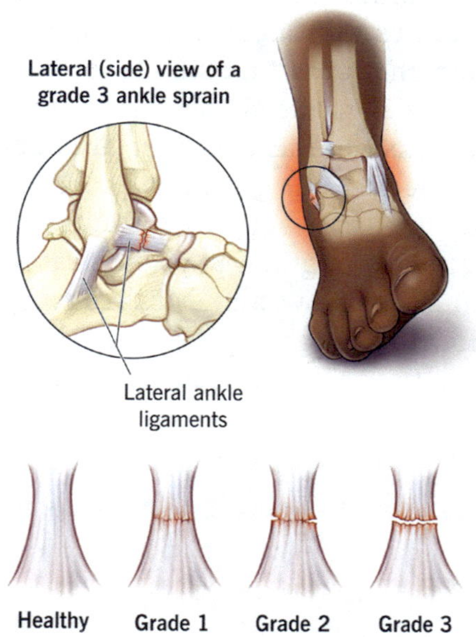

Figure 6.18. Ankles are one of the most commonly sprained joints.

Source: https://my.clevelandclinic.org/health/diseases/sprains.

Ankle sprains, for instance, are among the most frequent sports injuries, accounting for approximately 14% of all such injuries. They most frequently occur due to inversion or supination mechanisms, wherein the foot is inverted in a manner that it twists inwardly, resulting in stress to the lateral ligaments. It is essential to understand the mechanisms of sprains as it can guide measures of prevention and treatment protocols suitably, emphasizing protection of the joint in engagement in sports (Millas et al., 2018) (Figure 6.18). The effects of sprains extend beyond immediate physical discomfort; they can significantly impact an athlete's performance and might lead to long-term issues if inadequately addressed. A literature review indicates that not only does spraining cause abrupt cessation of sports activity, but it can also place individuals at risk for subsequent injury or chronic instability in the event of poor rehabilitation. This highlights the importance of comprehensive injury management practices, encompassing education on proper warm-up techniques, strengthening exercises, and the use of appropriate equipment, including supportive footwear. The inclusion of these elements can reduce the likelihood of recurrence, which is crucial as a previous history of sprain could double the risk, as supported in recent research (Millas et al., 2018). Furthermore, the management of sprains typically involves conservative treatment with a focus on rest, ice, compression, and elevation (the rice protocol). While immobilization has been a routine recommendation in the past, present-day practices are shifting towards active rehabilitation to prevent joint stiffness and promote recovery. Established treatments, such as acupuncture and herbs, have shown promise in pain and inflammation relief, particularly when used within cultures that adopt these practices as part of sports medicine. Prevention and management are ultimately integral to the maintenance of athletic function and joint integrity, a significant area of study within the broader topic of joints and ligaments (Anandacoomarasamy et al., 2009).

6.5.2. Strains

Strains, or the overextension or rupture of tendons or muscles, are a common injury that can hurt joint function and overall mobility. Frequently, the product of acute trauma or repetitive stress, strains range in their levels of severity from mild soreness to crippling injuries that require lengthy rehabilitative care. Understanding the anatomy at work, such as how muscles and tendons function together with ligaments within the joints, is key to effective treatment and prevention.

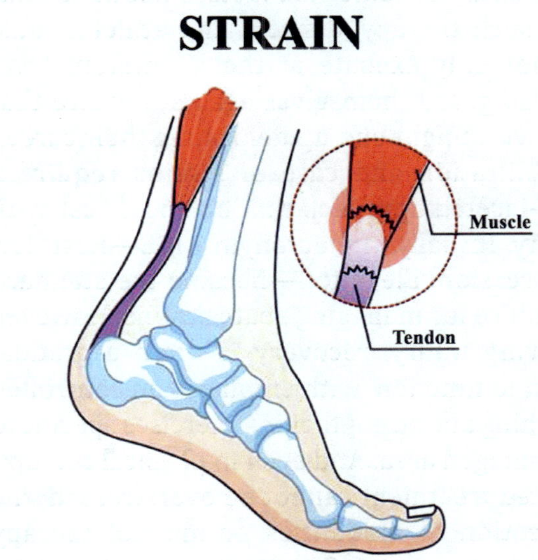

Figure 6.19. Strain (injury).

Source: https://therapia.com.au/wp-content/uploads/2019/04/sprains-vs-strains-840x546.jpg.

When the human body performs exercise that involves flexibility and strength, strains become increasingly likely, particularly in vigorous dance or sporting activity, in which dynamic movement places considerable tension on such structures. MSK biomechanics analysis is crucial in demonstrating how strains occur and can be avoided through proper conditioning and technique (Harris et al., 2012). Strains commonly happen in sports and recreation environments as a result of inadequate warm-up or conditioning that results in strength and flexibility imbalances. Interestingly, dancers frequently struggle with strains due to the strenuous nature of their dance style, highlighting the need for affordable education on injury prevention (Batenhorst et al., 2020) (Figure 6.19). Individualized strength exercise and stretching regimens can effectively increase the resistance of the muscles and tendons supporting weak joints and thereby prevent strains. The incorporation of biomechanical analysis can also enable a comprehensive analysis of body movements and identify specific risk factors about strains. With such therapy, dancers and athletes alike can not only execute at their optimum level but also guard themselves against injuries that otherwise might end up deforming their career. Rehabilitation and care of strains require a multi-faceted approach that balances rest with activity. Initially, the acronym RICE—Rest, Ice, Compression, Elevation—became the standard procedure for managing acute strains. However, following injury, recovery is often a gradual return to function, with emphasis on controlled stretching and strengthening exercises specific to the damaged area. And even in physical therapy, targeted treatment cannot be overstressed; the application of modalities or manual therapy techniques can significantly accelerate healing. With further advancements in biomechanical studies, they continue to uncover better methods of injury prevention and recovery, thus making it an easier path for victims of strain to heal and return to their maximum working capacity, which then enables them to continue with their activities based on the stability of joint and ligament strength (Harris et al., 2012).

6.5.3. Dislocations

Dislocations are a serious problem when it comes to joints and ligaments because they entail the complete displacement of a bone from its standard articulation with a second bone. It can result from a variety of reasons, including trauma, sports injuries, and falls.

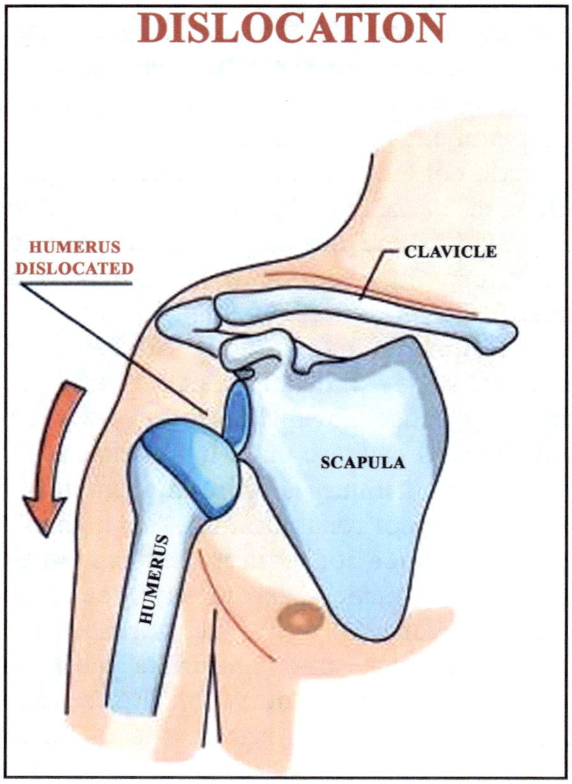

Figure 6.20. Dislocation.

Source: https://www.carehospitals.com/ckfinder/userfiles/images/dislocation_a.webp.

The consequences of a dislocation can even extend beyond pain and discomfort; they may result in severe aftermaths like ligament tear, nerve injury, or instability of the joint if left untreated. The anatomical predisposition of some joints, like the shoulder and the knee, makes them particularly vulnerable to dislocations. For instance, repetitive motion and impact force in the shoulder may result in dislocations, emphasizing the need for preventive measures such as strength training and proper technique in sports. Dislocations must be treated early, as if left late, they may result in chronic pain or permanent disability. In the treatment of dislocations, emergent medical care is necessary. Diagnosis is typically made by examination and then imaging modalities such as X-rays to look for associated fractures (Figure 6.20). The primary objective of treatment is the reduction of the dislocated joint, followed by immobilization to facilitate the healing of surrounding tissues and ligaments. Depending on the severity and frequency of dislocations, surgical treatment may be considered to provide joint stability and function. For instance, recurrent dislocations of the shoulder can be treated surgically to avoid their recurrence. Proper rehabilitation following reduction is essential, consisting of return of ROM and strength and progressive reintroduction of loading activity of the affected joint. The clinician's cognizance of the subtleties of dislocation management will enable the prevention of possible complications and return to full activity. Emerging technologies in orthopedic implant technology, particularly biodegradable magnesium-based implants, are revolutionizing the treatment of joint dislocation and related injuries. These implants are gaining more and more popularity due to their favorable mechanical properties and potential to stimulate osteogenesis, which enhances the healing process in dislocated joints. Comparative studies have determined that magnesium-based materials may surpass traditional orthopedic implants in biocompatibility and degradation behavior and facilitate a quicker recovery process. Research indicates that the implants can effectively stabilize and heal progressively as they are absorbed and eliminated by the body, thus eliminating the need for additional removal surgery. With the continued developments in joint stabilization and repair, the integration of new and innovative solutions like biodegradable materials will be crucial in optimizing patient outcomes after dislocation, vindicating the merit in adopting technological advancement in orthopedics (Wang et al., 2020).

Test Your Knowledge

1. What is the difference between a sprain and a strain?
2. What are the common causes of joint dislocations?

SUMMARY

The intricate relationship between ligaments and joints is at the heart of maintaining the structural and functional capacity of the MSK system. The importance of comprehending the sophistication inherent in these components has been highlighted, with illustrations given of how they are implicated in not only movement but also overall well-being and health. The assessment also underscores that disparities in ligamentous arrangement and joint anatomy could have far-reaching clinical implications, ranging from OA to scoliosis. Integrated comprehension of such associations fosters enhanced diagnostic and therapeutic management, thus maximizing patient care outcomes in healthcare settings. Lastly, the recognition of the important role of joints and ligaments directs attention to the absolute necessity for continued research in this field to unravel the complexity of MSK disease. Additionally, the value of improved imaging modalities in the diagnosis of joint and ligament disease has become increasingly apparent. The improvements in modalities such as MRI are significant, as they provide valuable information that allows accurate diagnoses and treatment plans specifically, as in the instance of such conditions as carpal boss, imaging outcome in correspondence with clinical presentation supports the need to utilize comprehensive diagnostic tests (Mespreuve et al., 2017). In addition to conventional practice, the incorporation of innovative techniques—such as the application of FEA during surgical design—enhances understanding of mechanical interaction within the spine and related structures, as evidenced by studies into scoliosis treatment (Polanco et al., 2022). All these interdisciplines emphasize the importance of a multiparty strategy to support treatment models and increase surgical success linked with joints and ligaments. Ultimately, cultivating knowledge of the anatomy, function, and pathologies of joints and ligaments is vital in clinical practice and research evolution. The controversy surrounding advanced imaging modalities and biomechanical investigations highlights the growing appreciation for the complexities present within these MSK components. When researchers and clinicians come together to elucidate these critical constituents further, the potential for developing targeted interventions and preventive treatments grows exponentially. Continued study of the interactions among joints, ligaments, and associated anatomical structures is critical if MSK disease states are to be successfully treated. With continuing advances in medical technology and research methods, the future of joint and ligament treatment holds promise for the quality of life for millions of individuals.

In the process of deconstructing the complexity of joints and ligaments, elementary human strength modeling becomes an essential aspect in exploring the complexities. of factors come into play in describing strength, such as body joint orientations and positions, and isometric and dynamic strength differences. Such factors are not only , but also crucial for theoretical models, but also for coping with practical applications, especially biomechanics and rehabilitation. The intricacies of strength measurement encompass an enormous range of factors, including muscle size, group membership, and training practice or fatigue effects. These factors indicate that even though the strength modeling capacity can provide information regarding the possibility for tasks and demands of strength, the intricate dynamics of an individual's strength pose a formidable challenge to describe, and thus, the need for more sophisticated models in research as well as clinical interventions (Badler et al., 2025). Further studies in joint modeling specifically highlight the paramount relevance of MSK dynamics in describing human movement. In contrast to most existing modeling that is focused on gross motion, recent advances have developed algorithms for the analysis of the fine-scale interactions of body anatomical joints. Body local flexibility has a significant impact on movement analysis, giving vital information about joint loading and tissue behavior. This dynamic technique is essential for orthopedic use, where a precise understanding can inform surgical techniques as well as rehab strategies. Joint modeling improvements, including linear and non-linear dynamic analyses, refine the capacity to simulate typical joint behaviors under conditions. These developments provide further insight into joint laxity and the nature of soft tissue interactions, ultimately to lead to improved clinical outcomes and a better understanding of joint mechanics (Esat et al., 2009). Due to the challenges in joint modeling, scientists have come up with methodologies that encompass complicated tissue deformations and contact geometries. The creation of joint analysis collision detection algorithms demonstrates these developments by allowing accurate simulation of joint interaction about motion dynamics. Through the determination of how body tissues react to force—either linear or non-linear models—scientists are in a better position to predict joint behavior for different loads. The inclusion of short path algorithms accelerates the analysis of soft tissue movement and the resultant forces on joints. These developments thus facilitate an improved understanding of the biomechanical functions of joints and ligaments, justifying the necessity of accurate modeling in study and clinical practice. Therefore, biomechanical modeling continues to evolve and set the pace for further comprehension and treatment strategies in ligament and joint wellness (Esat et al., 2009).

KEY TERMS FROM THIS CHAPTER

Synovial joint
Cartilaginous joint
Hinge joint
Saddle joint
Gliding joint
Articular cartilage
Ligament
Posterior cruciate ligament (PCL)
Fibrous joint
Ball-and-socket joint
Pivot joint
Condyloid joint
Synovial fluid
Joint capsule
Anterior cruciate ligament (ACL)
Range of motion

CRITICAL THINKING QUESTIONS

1. **What type of joint allows for the greatest range of motion?**
   a. Hinge joint
   b. Ball-and-socket joint
   c. Pivot joint
   d. Fixed joint
2. **Ligaments connect:**
   a. Muscle to bone
   b. Bone to bone
   c. Muscle to muscle
   d. Cartilage to bone
3. **Which joint type is found between the bones of the skull?**
   a. Synovial joint
   b. Fibrous joint
   c. Cartilaginous joint
   d. Ball-and-socket joint
4. **The knee joint is an example of a:**
   a. Ball-and-socket joint
   b. Hinge joint
   c. Pivot joint
   d. Saddle joint
5. **What is the primary function of synovial fluid in joints?**
   a. To connect bones
   b. To absorb shock
   c. To lubricate and reduce friction
   d. To strengthen ligaments

Short Answer Questions

1. What are the three main types of joints based on their movement?
2. Describe the basic structural components of a typical synovial joint.
3. What are the different types of ligaments, and what roles do they play in joint stability?
4. How do joints and ligaments work together to facilitate movement and provide support?
5. Name two common injuries that affect joints and two that affect ligaments.
6. What symptoms are typically associated with ligament injuries?
7. Why is maintaining joint and ligament health important for overall mobility and function?

Answer to Critical Thinking Questions

1. (b); 2. (b); 3. (b); 4. (b); 5. (c)

REFERENCES

1. Chadwick, K. P., Regnault, S., Allen, V., & Hutchinson, J. R. (2014b). Three-dimensional anatomy of the ostrich (Struthio camelus) knee joint. *PeerJ*, *2*, e706. https://doi.org/10.7717/peerj.706Alivernini, S., & Kurowska-Stolarska, M. (2017). Synovial tissue macrophages: Friend or foe? https://core.ac.uk/download/143476600.pdf (accessed on 14th June 2025).
2. Alves, F. R., da Silva Moura, L., da Silva, A. B. S., de Jesus Rosa Pereira Alves, L., et al. (2017). Macroscopic anatomy, histopathology, and image diagnosis of joints and synovial cartilages. https://core.ac.uk/download/322432755.pdf (accessed on 14th June 2025).
3. Anandacoomarasamy, A., Christakou, A., Junge, A., Kaikkonen, A., Viladot, A., Pijnenburg, A. C., Marchi, A. G., et al. (2009). Understanding acute ankle ligamentous sprain injury in sports. https://core.ac.uk/download/pdf/8316580.pdf (accessed on 14th June 2025).
4. Badler, N. I., Lee, P., & Wong, S. (2025). *Strength Modeling Report.* https://core.ac.uk/download/pdf/42843112.pdf (accessed on 14th June 2025).
5. Baird, A., Bell, C., Burda, H., Dahmann, C., Feenstra, J., Fleischer, C., Goode, D., et al. (2013). Flexibility within the middle ears of vertebrates. https://core.ac.uk/download/17030984.pdf (accessed on 14th June 2025).
6. Barszcz, K., Czubaj, N., Janczyk, P., Kupczynska, M., et al. (2013). Morphology of the transverse ligament of the atlas and the alar ligaments in the silver fox (*Vulpes vulpes var*). https://core.ac.uk/download/288113943.pdf (accessed on 14th June 2025).
7. Batenhorst, E. Z. Y. (2020). *A Dancer's View: Analysis and Prevention of Common Dance Injuries.* https://core.ac.uk/download/352161862.pdf (accessed on 14th June 2025).
8. Borges, M. M. (2016). *Complications Associated with Closing Wedge Ostectomy Procedure for Treatment of Cranial Cruciate Ligament Rupture in Dogs: A Retrospective Study of 145 Cases.* https://core.ac.uk/download/61489983.pdf (accessed on 14th June 2025).
9. Bransby-Zachary, M., Condon, B., Gislason, M. K., Hems, T., et al. (2009). A three-dimensional finite element model of maximal grip loading in the human wrist. https://core.ac.uk/download/9025217.pdf (accessed on 14th June 2025).
10. Buchanan, G., Ma, M., & Rea, P. M. (2014). A multimedia package for patient understanding and rehabilitation of non-contact anterior cruciate ligament injuries. https://core.ac.uk/download/16461708.pdf (accessed on 14th June 2025).
11. Davis, M. A., Fernández Hernando, M., Flores, D. V., Mejía Gómez, C., et al. (2019). Adult acquired flatfoot deformity: Anatomy, biomechanics, staging, and imaging findings. https://core.ac.uk/download/231897567.pdf (accessed on 14th June 2025).
12. DePhillipo, N. N., Larson, C. M., O'Neill, O. R., & LaPrade, R. F. (2020). Guidelines for ambulatory surgery centers for the care of surgically necessary/time-sensitive orthopedic cases during the COVID-19 pandemic. *Journal of Bone and Joint Surgery, 102*, 933–936. https://doi.org/10.2106/jbjs.20.00489 (accessed on 14th June 2025).
13. Entius, C. A., Kleinrensink, G. J., Pool-Goudzwaard, A. L., Snijders, C. J., et al. (2001). The sacroiliac part of the iliolumbar ligament. https://core.ac.uk/download/18522857.pdf (accessed on 14th June 2025).

14. Esat, I. I., & Ozada, N. (2009). Articular human joint modelling. https://core.ac.uk/download/20089625.pdf (accessed on 14th June 2025).

15. Fabbri, M., Ferretti, A., Guzzini, M., Iorio, R., et al. (2016). Extra-articular tenodesis combined with an anterior cruciate ligament reconstruction in acute anterior cruciate ligament tear in elite female football players. https://core.ac.uk/download/74324720.pdf (accessed on 14th June 2025).

16. Gielen, I., van Bree, H., & Van Ryssen, B. (2012). Diagnostic imaging of the canine stifle. https://core.ac.uk/download/55823299.pdf (accessed on 14th June 2025).

17. Gillie, A. E. (2011). *Incidence and Prevention of Injury of The Anterior Cruciate Ligament in Females*. https://core.ac.uk/download/58823893.pdf (accessed on 14th June 2025).

18. Gislason, M. K., Nash, D. H., & Stansfield, B. W. (2010). Finite element model creation and stability considerations of complex biological articulation: The human wrist joint. https://core.ac.uk/download/9028028.pdf (accessed on 14th June 2025).

19. Harris, G. F., & Slavens, B. A. (2012). *Biomechanics*. https://core.ac.uk/download/213080657.pdf (accessed on 14th June 2025).

20. Hull, E., Kynkäänniemi, S. M., Niinimäki, S., Puolakka, K., et al. (2021). Tendons and ligaments of the *Rangifer tarandus* metapodial and hoof. https://core.ac.uk/download/628855975.pdf (accessed on 14th June 2025).

21. Inostroza Millas, F. (2018). *Common Sports Related Injuries with A Focus on The Ankle and Knee Joints*. https://core.ac.uk/download/217325149.pdf (accessed on 14th June 2025).

22. Krishna, P., Metan, S. S., & Mohankumar, G. C. (2014). FEM model an effective tool to evaluate Von Mises stresses in shoulder joint and muscles for adduction and abduction. https://core.ac.uk/download/pdf/81132706.pdf (accessed on 14th June 2025).

23. Marsden, R. S. (2019). *The Effects of Sacroiliac Manipulation and Pelvic Blocking on Active Gluteus Medius Trigger Points: A Randomized Clinical Trial*. https://core.ac.uk/download/323341134.pdf (accessed on 14th June 2025).

24. Mespreuve, M., Verstraete, K., & Waked, K. (2017). Imaging findings at the quadrangular joint in carpal boss. https://core.ac.uk/download/84595797.pdf (accessed on 14th June 2025).

25. Patil, R. K., & Jadhav, T. A. (2020). A critical review on Sandhi Sharir with special reference to Upasana Pramana. https://core.ac.uk/download/478521845.pdf (accessed on 14th June 2025).

26. Polanco, M. A. (2022). *Utilization of Finite Element Analysis Techniques for Adolescent Idiopathic Scoliosis Surgical Planning*. https://core.ac.uk/download/534831653.pdf (accessed on 14th June 2025).

27. Rosse, C. (2000). Terminologies Anatomica; considered from the perspective of next-generation knowledge sources. https://core.ac.uk/download/pdf/9412243.pdf (accessed on 14th June 2025).

28. Wallace, C. (2018). *Effects of Glucocorticoids on Chondrocytes and Cartilage*. https://open.bu.edu/bitstream/2144/31287/5/Wallace_bu_0017N_13687.pdf (accessed on 14th June 2025).

MUSCULAR SYSTEM: OVERVIEW

7

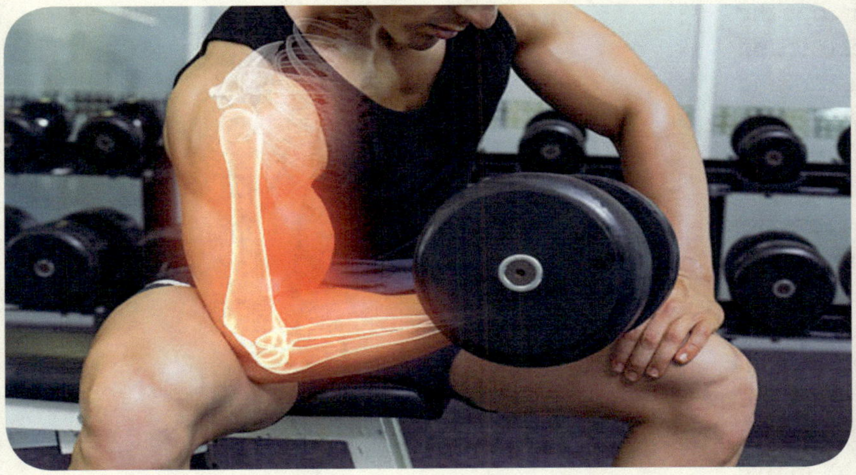

LEARNING OBJECTIVES

After studying this chapter, you will be able to:

1. Identify and differentiate between the types of muscles
2. Describe muscle structure and functions
3. Describe the process of muscle development
4. Identify frequent disorders of muscles, their signs and possible causes
5. Describe how muscles function to generate and control movement in the human body

Introduction

The musculature, a fascinating and intricate system of tissues, is an essential component of human locomotion and physiology. Composed of over 600 individual muscles, the system is primarily responsible for governing particular types of body movement, maintaining posture, and controlling necessary activities like circulation and digestion. The skeleton and muscles work together to form the musculoskeletal (MSK) system, which not only provides support structure but also enables a variety of activities, from simple gestures to complex athletic movements. Understanding the appreciation of how these structures work with other body systems to homeostasis and facilitate general well-being includes knowledge of the muscular system's components of the skeletal, smooth, and cardiac muscles. Besides their basic function in movement and equilibrium, muscles are part of many physiological processes that form the basis of our day-to-day lives. For example, voluntary movement is enabled by skeletal muscles and controlled by the central nervous system, with the ability to coordinate complex actions. Conversely, smooth muscles allow involuntary organ movements, including the digestive system, thus playing a central role in life's life-sustaining functions like digestion and circulation. Moreover, cardiac muscle, exclusive to the heart, illustrates how muscular tissue has adapted to serve special physiological needs. Such specialties reflect the intricacy of the muscular systems and the need for much research and understanding to maintain life. As one explores the details of the muscular system, it becomes clear that the system is not just crucial for physical action but is also intricately connected to mental and developmental states. It has been established through research that movement of the body can express emotion and psychological state, as well as affect our mental health. For example, the somatic theories illustrate the profound connection between movement and our mood and states of mind and suggest that the way we move can be a measure of our emotional health. This then opens up research into how the muscular system is not only a structural and mechanical component of us, but an active component of our whole experience and sense of self. By exploring these relationships, it is possible to observe the dynamic role of the muscular system in upholding an integrative vision of human health and well-being.

Definition of the Muscular System

The muscular system is an extensive network of tissues with significant roles in the human body, primarily movement, posture, and generating heat. The existence of muscle fibers characterizes it, and it allows for voluntary and involuntary function, with the ability to have reflexes as well as voluntary movement. The muscular system comprises three general categories of muscle tissues: skeletal, smooth, and cardiac. Skeletal muscles, which can be voluntarily controlled, are attached to bones and enable body movements such as walking and lifting. Smooth muscles in organs such as the intestines and arteries work involuntarily to regulate internal functions such as digestion and circulation. Cardiac muscle, unique to the heart, possesses four characteristics of both skeletal and smooth muscles, enabling rhythmic contraction for blood circulation.

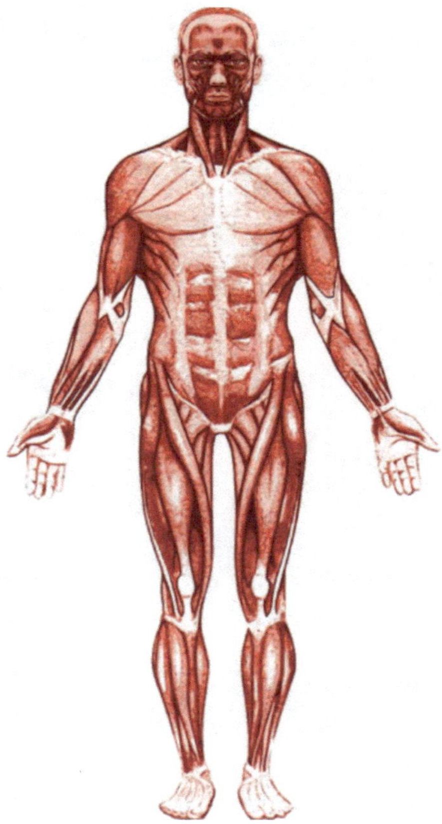

Figure 7.1. Full-body illustration of the human muscular system, showing the major muscle groups involved in movement and posture.

Source: https://science4fun.info/wp-content/uploads/2019/04/muscular-system.jpg.

Aside from facilitating motion, the muscular system also supports the maintenance of body posture and stability. The concurrent contraction of muscles aids in the sustenance of various postures while standing or sitting, reducing the chances of injury. Additionally, by producing heat, muscle fibers support an individual's metabolic rate, which is crucial for preserving a steady core body temperature throughout activity.

It is worth noting that muscle contraction is controlled by a highly complex interplay of neural impulses and biochemical processes, including the generation of energy from ATP. It is beneficial to comprehend these processes, especially in sports science and rehabilitation, where optimization of muscle function can play a significant role in performance and recovery (Figure 7.1). Through this, the muscular system is not only engaged in locomotion but also involved in postural control and thermoregulation. The relevance of the muscular system extends to other physiological and psychological aspects, affecting health and overall well-being. Muscle health also translates directly into metabolic health, with greater muscle mass indicating improved insulin sensitivity and reduced risk of metabolic disease. Conversely, an inactive life may lead to muscle atrophy that subsequently affects mobility and the likelihood of injury. The psychological benefits also arise from exercise that increases the output of endorphins and mood uplift. With the decline in physical activity today, understanding the definition and function of the muscular system is more vital than ever. The connection between muscle well-being and quality of life highlights the importance of physical activity in developing both physical and mental strength. Due to this, ongoing research on the muscular system remains a priority in addressing the challenges of contemporary health issues.

Importance of the Muscular System in Human Physiology

The muscle system is extremely vital in human physiology, primarily because it contributes to producing motions that facilitate day-to-day functioning and improved performance. Muscles are responsible for voluntary movements, such as walking, gripping, and talking, as well as involuntary movements like breathing and digestion. Muscle fibers contract when stimulated by the nervous system, converting biochemical energy to mechanical energy. This process indicates coordination between the nervous and muscular systems, emphasizing their dependence on each other in homeostasis and proper body functions. While people are physically active, the efficiency of the muscular systems directly determines their endurance, strength, and agility, and therefore is essential in athletic function and general health. Additionally, the muscular system plays a vital role in the body's metabolic process. Skeletal muscle, making up the bulk of the body's weight, plays a crucial role in glucose uptake, fatty acid oxidation, energy balance, and metabolic well-being. The dynamic existence of muscle cells enables them to adapt to varying physiological demands through hypertrophy and increased cardiovascular efficiency, thereby enhancing overall metabolic rate. Engagement in regular resistance exercise, for example, not only strengthens the muscle fibers but also induces endocrine responses that contribute to metabolic control. This underlines the significance of active life, as maintenance of muscle mass is essential for the prevention of the metabolic diseases of obesity and diabetes, indicating the varied functionality of the muscular system towards the promotion of body welfare and longevity. The intricate interaction between the muscular and nervous systems also equates to insight into neuromuscular diseases, which are paradigmatic illustrations of the consequences of muscular dysfunction on health. Research has demonstrated that contraction and muscle cell differentiation rely upon successful innervation, and the process is bedeviled with challenges when these mechanisms go awry. For instance, research has demonstrated that human primary muscle cells cultured without nerves exhibit limited capability for contraction. This parameter reflects substantial reliance on neural stimulation for maximally efficient function. The creation of co-cultures, including spinal cord explants, has proven a valuable model to investigate the neuromuscular interface and muscular disease. This research not only contributes to muscle physiology but also demonstrates potential in developing therapeutic methods in neuromuscular illnesses, thereby reaffirming the role of the muscular system in maintaining structural integrity as well as functional capability in human physiology (Arnold et al., 2012; Brenneman et al., 2016s).

7.1. Types of Muscles

Learning Outcome

1. Define skeletal muscle characteristics and cardiac muscle characteristics
2. Discuss smooth muscle characteristics

It is crucial to learn about the types of muscles within the human body to know how movement and stability are made possible. There are three main types of muscles: skeletal, smooth, and cardiac. Skeletal muscles, which are under voluntary control, play a significant role in facilitating movement as they attach bones through tendons. These contain striations and are also responsible for facilitating posture and producing heat through contractions. The ability of skeletal muscles to selectively adapt to various physical exercises through hypertrophy and atrophy is central to athletic training and recovery. Smooth muscles are involuntary and found in the walls of internal organs like the gastrointestinal tract and blood vessels. Smooth muscles are responsible for functions such as digestion and regulation of blood flow, and have a rhythmic and slow mode of contraction. In contrast to their skeletal siblings, smooth muscles are striation-free, allowing them to contract more smoothly and sustain longer durations of activity before tiring. Mechanisms for smooth muscle contraction are complex, with hormones and neurotransmitters that ensure body homeostasis. Cardiac muscle, as the sole cardiac muscle variety of the heart, possesses special characteristics that distinguish it from both skeletal and smooth muscles. It is striated like skeletal muscle but involuntarily acting, consisting of specialized cells called cardiomyocytes that are connected by intercalated discs. These discs are capable of rapid electrical conduction that enables synchronized contractions necessary for effective blood pumping. The cardiac muscle's ability to adapt to changing physiological demands, such as increased workload during exercise, ensures adequate blood circulation and supply of oxygen throughout the body. Understanding these differences among muscle types not only advances physiological knowledge but also aids in the treatment and diagnosis of numerous muscular and cardiovascular illnesses, particularly in subjects with metabolic syndromes (Oberbach et al., 2012) and in creating devices imitating human-like movement (Nakata et al., 2002) (Figure 7.2).

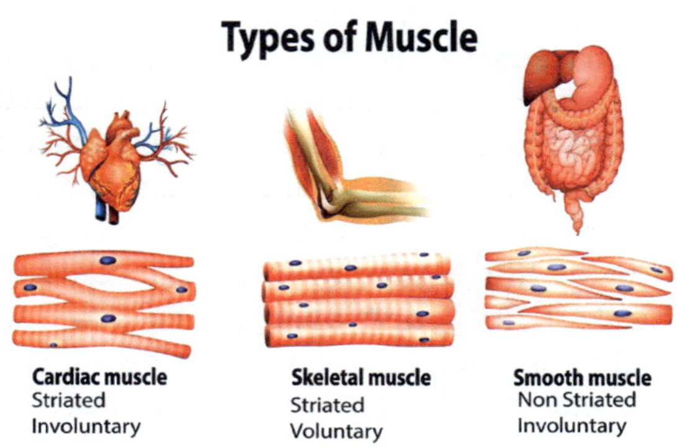

Figure 7.2. Types of muscle.

Source: https://external-content.duckduckgo.com/iu/?u=https%3A%2F%2Fi.pinimg.com%2Foriginals%2F43%2Fdf%2Fd4%2F43dfd403aadb4b906c0a6eaf66c71646.jpg&f=1&nofb=1&ipt=c5991c34fca844961247cd2a165f0a067617f6251738b1272ce2e9d60c49ca38.

7.1.1. Skeletal Muscle Characteristics

Skeletal muscle, the key member of the muscular system, possesses some unique features that distinguish it from the rest of the muscles.

Most importantly, skeletal muscle fibers are differentiated based on their rate of contraction and metabolic properties, existing as two types: slow-twitch (Type I) and fast-twitch (Type II) fibers.

The slow-twitch fibers are distinguished by their endurance properties, which allow for long-duration activities such as marathon running by using aerobic metabolism to provide energy. Whereas fast-twitch fibers are designed to perform short bursts of speed and power, relying primarily on anaerobic metabolism. This also reflects not just the functional adaptability of skeletal muscle but also the physiological importance for athletes, who can possess varying quantities of these types of fibers, influencing their efficiency and performance and resistance to fatigue while performing physical activity.

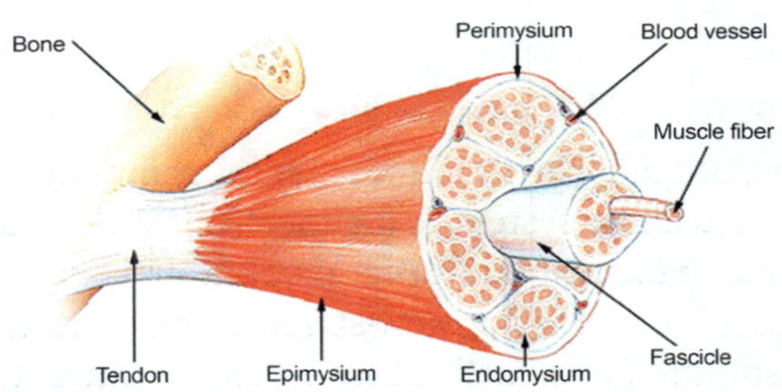

Figure 7.3. Structure of a skeletal muscle.

Source: https://study.com/cimages/multimages/16/b496a80f-6159-437e-8574-f50e67fa1e78_webp.net-resizeimage.jpg.

Moreover, the structural and functional integrity of skeletal muscle can also be significantly compromised by extrinsic factors.

The physiological deconditioning that occurs with prolonged bed rest, for example, causes a significant reduction in muscle volume, cross-sectional area, and overall strength, especially in antigravity muscles that must act against gravity while standing and moving. Reduced physical activity can result in negative adaptations, such as decreased plasma volume and cardiac output, that collectively compromise muscle function. This condition suggests the necessity of prolonged physical activity in maintaining muscular health and warns of the risks of sedentary lifestyles, particularly among populations such as the elderly or convalescents. Thus, early intervention with ambulation and resistive training is essential to negate these adverse effects and promote skeletal muscle preservation and regeneration (Drury et al., 2007) (Figure 7.3).

Additionally, the cellular composition of the skeletal muscle is critical when it comes to its adaptability and resistance to stress. Research has shown that acute muscle stress can influence the kinetics of the immunoproteasome, which is a dedicated unit for cellular remodeling and protein degradation. Following intense exercise, e.g., downhill running, the immunoproteasome activity is boosted to manage and ensure muscle homeostasis effectively. This adjustment explains the muscle's capacity to recover and maintain function after injury, suggesting that stressors, although challenging, condition skeletal muscle for improved performance. Cooperation between various proteasomal components during restoration phases accentuates the role of metabolic pathways in skeletal muscle characteristics. Also, it reinforces the notion that regular physical stressors can enhance muscle strength as well as functional competence overall (Baumann et al., 2017).

7.1.2. Cardiac Muscle Characteristics

The cardiac muscle, which is one of the most significant components of the muscular system, has distinct properties that set it apart from other muscles. Unlike the skeletal muscle, which is under voluntary control, cardiac muscle functions involuntarily, operating automatically to ensure the essential heart contractions that enable blood flow.

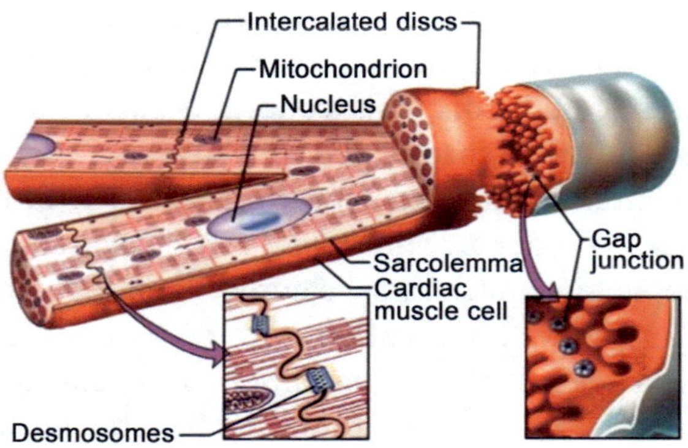

Figure 7.4. Structure of cardiac muscle cell.

Source: https://external-content.duckduckgo.com/iu/?u=https%3A%2F%2Fwww.online-sciences.com%2Fwp-content%2Fuploads%2F2021%2F04%2Ffeatures-of-cardiac-muscle-fibers-2.jpg&f=1&nofb=1&ipt=6f6619f125c2ea80d4ad4d93c0e95211e6a3c718e9f6175c938429c6d38f6aa3.

The individual muscle tissue is structurally striated, similar to skeletal muscle, which shows a highly organized pattern of sarcomeres. But the striations of cardiac muscle are less prominent, and the fibers are held together with intercalated disks. These are specialized junctions that are capable of rapid electrical transmission between cells, conferring synchrony in the hearts' contraction and thus making them an archetypal component of efficient cardiovascular operation. Metabolically, the cardiac muscle fibers possess a dense proliferation of mitochondria, which corresponds to their reliance on aerobic respiration to generate ATP (Figure 7.4). This reliance is crucial because cardiac muscle is constantly active even at rest, and thus energy efficiency is critical. In addition to this, the presence of myoglobin within the cardiac muscle cells facilitates the storage of oxygen to sustain an extended energy production by the incessant pumping action of the heart. This metabolic adaptation is crucial because the heart must undergo continuous stress without fatigue. These characteristics enable the cardiac muscle to meet the stringent demands of its function, contrasting with both skeletal and smooth muscles, which possess other energy-generating mechanisms. In addition, the flexibility of the cardiac muscles to varied physiological demands is crucial in overall health. For instance, regular exercise might lead to physiological hypertrophy such that the cardiac muscle becomes strengthened and enlarged secondary to increased workload and becomes more efficient. Pathological conditions, such as hypertension, on the other hand, lead to maladaptive remodeling with adverse effects. These events are crucial to recognize in the clinic since they indicate cardiovascular disease and health. The cardiac muscle's impressive attributes not only demonstrate its importance in the muscle system but also underscore the need for continued cardiovascular physiology and pathology studies to improve health results further.

7.1.3. Smooth Muscle Characteristics

Smooth muscle, the fundamental component of the muscular system, is distinct from skeletal and cardiac muscle due to its involuntary origin. It possesses a special, non-striated structure with a spindle form, facilitating efficient contraction and relaxation mechanisms necessary to sustain various body functions. Found most commonly in hollow organ walls—such as the intestines, blood vessels, and bladder—smooth muscle fibers act subconsciously, responding to autonomic nervous system or hormone stimuli. This one feature is essential for functions such as peristalsis in the digestive tract and blood pressure control through vasodilation and vasoconstriction, showing its absolute requirement in homeostasis. In the contractile component, smooth muscle employs a system distinct from its striated counterparts (Figure 7.5).

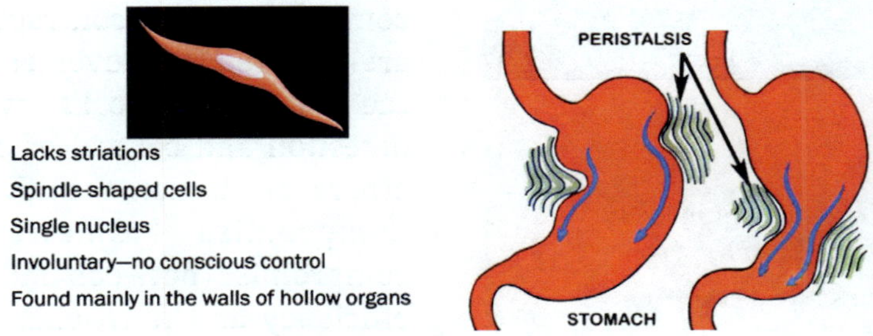

Figure 7.5. Smooth muscle characteristics.

Source: https://external-content.duckduckgo.com/iu/?u=https%3A%2F%2Fimage1.slideserve.com%2F2805208%2Fsmooth-muscle-characteristics-l.jpg&f=1&nofb=1&ipt=6e433f816dbfd9415d5b52705761effbdd559a7c9291c2b919744d46fc7596ee.

Smooth muscle contraction takes longer but lasts longer, and therefore, it is particularly adapted to activities involving persistent tension. This is because there exist myofilaments that are not aligned in any premised pattern, thereby producing a contractile network with the ability to continue exerting force over an extended duration of time. Smooth muscle also has the potential to undergo hyperplasia, which can allow cell growth and an increase in cell number upon stimulus such as mechanical stress. This adaptability indicates its significance in numerous physiological conditions, especially when there is a high demand, and also under pathological procedures that may require muscle remodeling, further solidifying its position within the entire muscular system. The interaction between smooth muscle and extracellular matrix (ECM) is a topic worthy of study, particularly in terms of muscle stability and function. The ECM, made up of proteins such as laminins and collagen, is responsible for structural support and communication between muscle cells and the environment diseases such as laminin-α2-deficientcongenital muscular dystrophy, the absence of proper matrix composition results in impaired muscle function and stability, illustrating the significance of extracellular interactions on smooth muscle integrity. An understanding of such relationships sheds light upon the therapies for muscle disease, in which promotion or reconstitution of matrix components could enhance functional deficit. Thus, the relationship between smooth muscle characteristics and ECM enclosing them is a complex but relevant aspect of the muscular system, where collaboration among scientists in muscle physiology and pathology is essential, especially in association with the mind-brain-body tripod, as evidenced by current studies (Tan et al., 2007; Meinen et al., 2005).

Test Your Knowledge

1. What are the distinguishing features of skeletal muscle tissue?
2. How does cardiac muscle differ from other muscle types in structure and function?

7.2. Muscle Structure and Function

Learning Outcome

1. Describe the general functions of muscles within the musculoskeletal (MSK) system
2. Explain the specific muscle function

Muscle is a specialized tissue of the body that creates movement, posture, and heat. Muscle tissue is made up of cells that are called muscle fibers and contract and relax when stimulated.

7.2.1. Muscle Structure

To appreciate the intricacies of muscle anatomy, one must understand the hierarchical design of muscle tissues. Fundamentally, the muscles consist of individual fibers referred to as myofibers, rod-shaped cells grouped in fascicles. The fibers contain myofibrils, the contractile elements where actin and myosin filaments intercross, enabling muscle contraction via sliding filament mechanisms. This structure provides both strength and flexibility, enabling muscles to adapt to various physical tasks. The encapsulating connective tissues, including the endomysium, perimysium, and epimysium, also play significant functions in keeping muscle fibers intact while enabling attachment to the bones and helping with overall structural support. Through the integration of these elements, the muscular design not only allows motion but also holds in it the complexities required for the diverse functions demanded of different activities by organisms. More than its basic anatomy is involved in the structure of muscle; it also encompasses the dynamics of how the structures move during motion. Complications arise when there is the presence of muscle composition, including not only skeletal muscle but also cardiac and smooth muscle, each adapted to unique requirements for operation. For instance, skeletal muscle is characterized by a high degree of voluntary control and rapid contraction capability, which are required for movement. Smooth muscle, on the other hand, works involuntarily, suited for digestion and control of blood vessels, among others. In addition, the novel Muscle-Mechanical Compromise Framework highlights the compromise between maximizing mechanical efficiency and functional versatility of human and animal locomotion. This perspective supports the analysis of how structure within muscles determines gait and posture, ultimately constituting the role of structural design in catching up with functional requirements (Richard et al., 2016). The diversity in muscle structures between different species is a reflection of evolutionary modifications under the needs and demands of the environment and survival. Importantly, research into muscular modularity and integration has revealed evolutionary mechanisms that direct muscle structure. Comparative investigation, using techniques like Anatomical Network investigation (AnNA), shows that, despite apparent functional similarities, skeletal and muscular networks differ in structure, particularly between the upper and lower limbs. These findings refute traditional notions of limb homology, emphasizing the need for an innovative conceptual framework that combines both evolutionary biology and functional anatomy. Clarifying muscle morphology-functional consequence relationships allows scientists to proceed towards general discourse on what variations in muscles mean for mobility, adaptation, and organismal success in changing environments (Goswami et al., 2015).

7.2.1.1. Muscle Fibers and Their Composition

Muscle fibers are also broadly classified into two categories: slow-twitch (Type I) and fast-twitch (Type II) fibers, each with distinctive structural and functional characteristics. Slow-twitch fibers have a high mitochondrial concentration and myoglobin, which allow for sustained aerobic respiration, a process highly utilized in endurance activities such as marathon running. The fibers are resistant to fatigue, allowing for sustained muscle contractions with lower energy expenditures. Conversely, fast-twitch muscle fibers are designed for momentary instances of power and strength and operate nearly all anaerobically. They contain more glycogen and fewer mitochondria than Type I fibers, favoring rapid contractions but short duration of energy provision. The mixed content of muscle fibers underscores the complexity of the muscular system because athletes have mixed muscle fiber content depending on the genetic aspect and individualized training regimens (Figure 7.6).

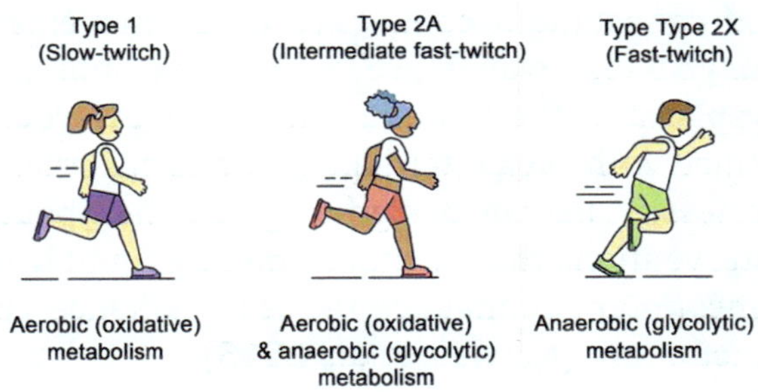

Figure 7.6. Muscle fiber types.

Source: https://bodyworksprime.com/wp-content/uploads/muscle-fiber-type-slow-vs-fast.jpg.webp.

The biochemical composition of muscle fibers has a significant influence on their functional properties and overall performance capacity. Structures such as myofibrils, made up of contractile proteins like actin and myosin, constitute the center stage of the contraction function of muscle fibers. Additionally, the presence of creatine plays a vital role in providing energy during intense muscle contractions, particularly in fast-twitch fibers. Creatine use not only enhances rapid ATP generation required for the speeding up of movements but also increases muscle strength and bulk in clinical groups. This association highlights the significance of nutritional interventions, such as creatine supplementation, which promotes positive changes in muscle composition and function, particularly helpful for patients with muscle wasting, including cancer patients. Furthermore, the dipeptide carnosine, in which the highest concentrations occur in fast-twitch fibers, is another vital constituent for optimal muscle performance. Carnosine serves as an internal pH buffer, preventing acidosis-induced fatigue and maintaining intramuscular cellular environmental balance during high-intensity anaerobic exercise. The synthesis of carnosine from beta-alanine and L-histidine is vital to athletes because its increase via supplementation was found to enhance performance in exercise with varying levels of intensity. It was particularly observed that individuals with a higher percentage of fast-twitch fibers have larger amounts of carnosine, showing an association of fiber type and physiological performance. The relationship between muscle fiber type, supplementation program, and exercise performance underscores the intricate interaction of biochemical units that are accountable for the operation of muscles, emphasizing the importance of ongoing research in this field towards optimal athletic performance and well-being.

7.2.1.2. Connective Tissues Associated with Muscles

Connective tissues are a significant component of the muscular form and function, and aside from support, they also facilitate movement. The tissues consist of numerous elements, including tendons, ligaments, and fascia, that contribute to overall muscle integrity and performance. Tendons, which connect muscles and bones, are structural elements that withstand tensile forces generated in muscle contractions. Ligaments do attach bone to bone, though, to stabilize joints and maintain alignment during movement. Fascia covers muscles, compartmentalizing them and allowing the gliding of one muscle against another freely.

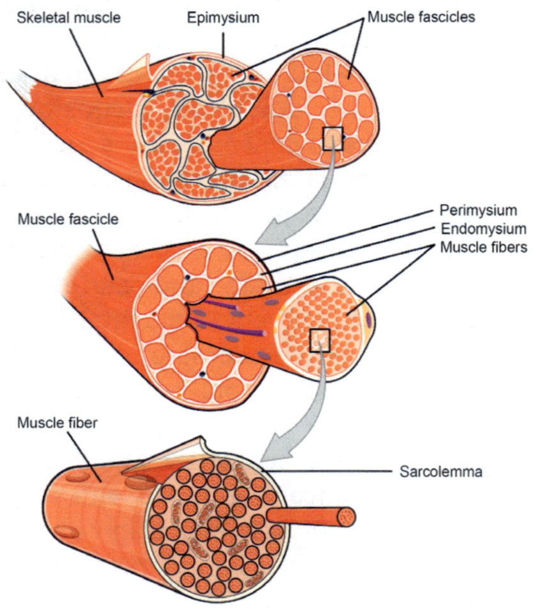

Figure 7.7. The three connective tissue layers of a skeletal muscle. The muscle is surrounded by a connective tissue sheath called epimysium.

Source: https://www.researchgate.net/figure/The-three-connective-tissue-layers-of-a-skeletal-muscle-The-muscle-is-surrounded-by-a_fig1_328713555.

This blending of connective tissue with muscle fiber allows a cohesive interaction that is necessary for good movement and force development within the body. Health and maintenance of such connective tissues play a critical role in optimal muscular performance. Connective tissues undergo various mechanical loads throughout the life of individuals, which influence their morphology as well as elasticity. Disruption of integrity in such tissues leads to injuries such as strain or sprain, which impair muscular performance. Moreover, the integrity of connective tissue may also be influenced by age, activity, and general health. It is crucial to diagnose and treat disorders of the connective tissue because understanding problems such as myofascial pelvic pain (MFPP) highlights this need. MFPP, with its trigger points in the pelvic floor muscles, showcases how connective tissue dysfunction can create widespread pain and discomfort, demonstrating the interrelatedness of connective and muscular systems (Katzman et al., 2012) (Figure 7.7). Emerging evidence highlights the interactive dynamic between muscle activity and connective tissue adaptability. During muscle contraction and the production of forces, muscles produce mechanical loading on tendons, ligaments, and fascia, which loads the cells in these connective tissues to adapt by remodeling and repair. Adapting to increased exercise levels or recovering from injuries requires this adaptation mechanism. Moreover, biomechanical considerations affecting muscle and concomitant connective tissue movement can go a long way in preventing developmental dysplasia of the hip and other MSK disorders. Armed with such interdependencies, healthcare professionals can design targeted therapeutic interventions that maximize muscles' and their concomitant connective tissues' resilience and functioning (Nowlan et al., 2015).

7.2.1.3. The Role of Tendons in Muscle Function

The role of tendons in muscle is intricate, with the crucial role of joining muscles and bones and, simultaneously, facilitating movement. Tendons are functional units of compact connective tissue that convey the force generated in muscle contractions to the skeleton to enable movement at joints. This process of transmission is necessary because muscles cannot generate movement independently; they must rely on tendons to cover the gap between muscle fibers and bone structures. The efficiency and strength of this coupling are particularly significant because tendons' ability to withstand tensile forces ultimately determines overall muscular performance. In addition, the elasticity of the tendons allows energy storage and release, which enhances the efficiency of motions, especially in motions such as running and jumping (Figure 7.8).

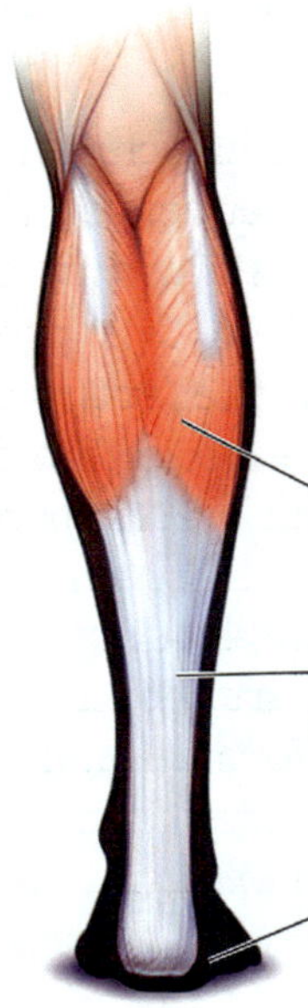

Figure 7.8. Tendons connect your muscles to your bones.

Source: https://my.clevelandclinic.org/health/body/21738-tendon.

Besides, the structural composition of the tendon is what makes it functionally effective. Tendons consist of collagen fibers arranged in a parallel manner that endows them with high tensile strength and the ability to withstand high mechanical loads. Like insect steering muscles, whose response is dynamic by nonlinear mechanisms during flight, mammalian tendons equally adapt to the mechanical demands imposed upon them. This adaptability is essential for joint stability and optimal muscle economy in a multitude of physical endeavors. The fine-tuning of muscle contractions and the operation of tendons not only optimize synergistic movement but also prevent injury by allowing controlled force transmission through joints. This highlights the tendon's important function in the larger context of the muscular system. Also, the emerging discipline of neuromechanics provides informative insights into the function of tendons from a systems perspective. This paradigm is concerned with the interaction between physical structure, mechanical needs, and neural control strategies for movement. Knowledge of such interactions can shed light on how tendons adapt to changing load and activity, lending support to the concept of tendons as active structures. For instance, the tendons' energy absorption and release mechanisms illustrate their basic significance in the optimization of movement patterns and the conservation of energy during repetitive activity. While scientists continue to develop their understanding of the complexities of tendon function, is worth noting how their function within the operation of the muscle is more than mere force transfer, making them a central component in the intricate system that comprises the muscular system as a whole (Santello et al., 2017; Wisser et al., 2014).

7.2.2. Muscle Function

Understanding how muscles work is essential for comprehending the muscular system's role in enabling movement and maintaining body stability. Muscles attain their main functions by contracting and converting nervous impulses into mechanical movements. There are three types of muscles: skeletal, cardiac, and smooth, each with special functions in the body. Skeletal muscles are in charge of voluntary movement and are under intense central nervous system control, while cardiac muscles work involuntarily to circulate blood throughout the body. Smooth muscles within the hollow organs also work involuntarily, synchronizing internal processes like digestion. This dynamic relationship between types of muscle emphasizes not only their specific functions, but also how their combined function supports the functions of the body, from movement to circulation, to describe the intricate balance of the muscular system. The deconditioning consequences of disuse, as induced by prolonged bed rest, demonstrate the susceptibility of the muscular system to diminished muscle function. Studies have illustrated that bed rest leads to profound muscular atrophy, with consequent decreases in skeletal muscle volume and force, specifically in antigravity muscles that are essential for posture and balance. Muscle force generation is further decreased by cardiovascular function reduction, influencing overall energy expenditure and physical performance.

Bed rest particularly alters the hydrostatic pressure gradients in the cardiovascular system and influences skeletal and muscle health. Patients and clinicians must be aware of these effects because early intervention with exercise can counteract the adverse effects of immobility and thereby preserve skeletal architecture and muscle function during immobilization (Drury et al., 2007). Oxidative stress also makes significant contributions to muscle function, notably in muscular dystrophies such as Duchenne muscular dystrophy (DMD). This condition illustrates the contribution of genetic causes to progressive muscle integrity breakdown, underpinned by chronic inflammation as well as oxidative damage. Evidence has shown that antioxidant response pathways, such as the NRF2 pathway, have significant contributions to protection against oxidative stress in affected muscle tissues. For instance, differences in enzymatic antioxidant responses between age groups of DMD patients reflect the significance of maintaining antioxidant capacity for preserving muscle function. Because inflammation biomarkers like IL-6 correlate with muscle degeneration, exploring therapeutic interventions aimed at oxidative stress may further our understanding of the nature of muscle function in health and disease (Petrillo et al., 2017). This emphasis on the biochemical milieu inside and outside of muscle fibers helps to highlight the sophistication involved in maintaining muscular health in a variety of pathological states.

7.2.2.1. Mechanism of Muscle Contraction

The physiology behind muscle contraction is a complex process of a sequence of biochemical and mechanical events within the cellular environment. Central to this process is the interaction between the actin and myosin filaments within the muscle fibers. When the signal from the nervous system is received by a muscle cell, calcium ions are released from the sarcoplasmic reticulum, leading to contraction. These calcium ions are bound to troponin, which causes a conformational change that moves tropomyosin away from actin binding sites. Myosin heads next bind to these sites, forming cross-bridges, and in the power stroke, the myosin heads pivot to pull on the actin filaments to move them towards the center of the sarcomere, shortening the muscle. This intricate coordination of proteins results in efficient and energetic contractions that are required for movement and other physical processes. Beyond calcium ion function, energy delivery plays a significant part in the process of muscle contraction. Adenosine triphosphate (ATP) is the primary source of energy, driving the motion of the myosin heads. The breakdown of ATP provides the mechanism for the myosin to alter its structure, integral to muscle contraction. Because each power stroke would require ATP to be replenished continuously, particularly with hard work, ATP sources would be from creatine phosphate and anaerobic glycolysis. However, aerobic respiration would be most effective in prolonged efforts. Surprisingly, it is found that high levels of carnosine, a dipeptide that is found in muscle tissue, enhance performance during high-intensity exercise by maintaining intracellular pH stability and buffering lactic acid, highlighting its role in muscle contraction energy regulation (Baguet et al., 2010) (Figure 7.9).

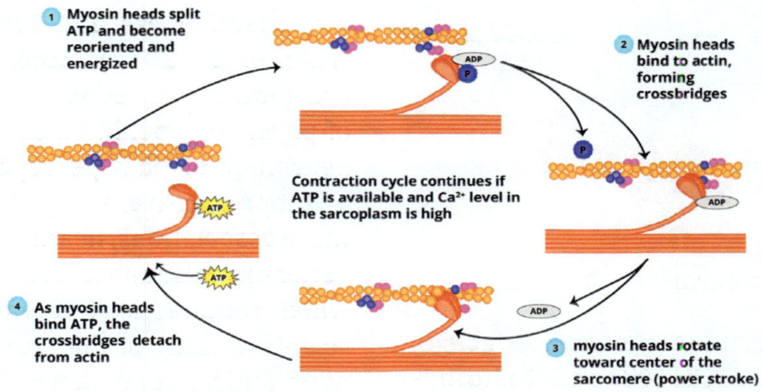

Figure 7.9. Muscle contraction mechanisms.

Source: https://www.vedantu.com/neet/mechanism-of-muscle-contraction-and-relaxation.

Recent findings have clarified the role of the immunoproteasome in muscle remodeling and suggested a new aspect to the contraction mechanism of muscle. The immunoproteasome, a variant of the standard proteasome, has been discovered to be regulated in atrophic muscle under stress, with the inference that it is involved in maintaining cellular homeostasis during contraction (Baumann et al., 2017). When challenged by novel exercise, like downhill running, there appears to be an upregulation of specific proteasome subunits crucial for muscle repair and adaptation. This indicates the relevance of proteasomal activity not merely in protein degradation but also the healing from stress-induced muscle damage. Appreciation for the variety of functions that these cellular components have increases our knowledge of the muscular system and its ability to adapt dynamically to a variety of physical requirements.

7.2.2.2. Role of the Nervous System in Muscle Activation

The intricate relationship between the nervous system and muscle stimulation is at the heart of the functioning of the muscular system. The primary method of muscle stimulation begins with the CNS processing and responding to sensory input. Motor neurons, which carry messages from the CNS to the muscle fibers, are an integral component of this intricate process. When stimulated, a motor neuron releases neurotransmitters at the neuromuscular junction to initiate an action potential in the muscle fiber. This initiates a chain of biochemical events that ultimately result in muscle contraction. This physiological process emphasizes the interconnectedness of sensory information, neural processing, and motor output, illustrating how the nervous system regulates muscle movement required for both voluntary and involuntary actions. This, in turn, assists in regulating homeostasis and interacting with the environment. Furthermore, the role of the nervous system is not merely that of activation; it is also vital in the coordination of smooth and precise muscle movement (Figure 7.10).

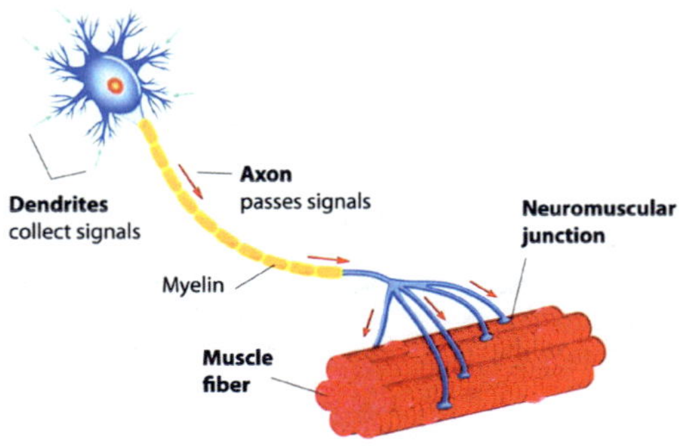

Figure 7.10. Motor neuron.

Source: https://external-content.duckduckgo.com/iu/?u=https%3A%2F%2Fbodybuilding-wizard.com%2Fwp-content%2Fuploads%2F2021%2F04%2Fnerve-muscle-connection-1024x768.jpg&f=1&nofb=1&ipt=3a176cf319a8fed912bdbe852b8881836a30e0cfc5991452ca9df381251f1a3b.

The brain is constantly integrating sensory input from proprioceptors, which signal body position and movement. Feedback within the loop enables instantaneous adjustment of muscle coordination and force production. For example, during walking or running, the nervous system must rapidly adjust muscle contractions to accommodate terrain modification or speed. The predictive control model demonstrates how verbal self-monitoring, as with muscle control, can influence movement patterns, as has been highlighted in research utilizing lip muscle activity in patients with schizophrenia during auditory verbal hallucinations (AVHs) (Dohen et al., 2013). These results illuminate the complexity of how the nervous system commands not only the muscle activation but also the quality and precision of the movement, as it plays a central role in the muscular system's function. Furthermore, understanding the interaction between muscle activation and pain perception again emphasizes the nervous system's role in muscle function. Pain neurophysiology puts equal emphasis on both nociception and motor control as two-way, with the potential for discomfort to affect muscle activation and movement patterns. Shoulder pain, for instance, can produce compensatory adaptations to muscle activation, influencing the effectiveness and efficacy of movement (Falla et al., 2014). Accordingly, practitioners are required to consider both the principles of physiology behind muscle activation and the neurology of pain perception. By establishing a comprehensive, integrated understanding of these associations, healthcare professionals can better diagnose and treat muscular abnormalities, which requires an integrated approach to the scientific study of the muscular system and its neurological dependency for optimal function.

7.2.2.3. Energy Sources for Muscle Activity

The muscular system employs a variety of energy sources to supply muscle activity, primarily via ATP production. ATP is the immediate energy currency of muscle contraction for dynamic movement and sustained activity. Energy for the synthesis of ATP arises from three main pathways: the phosphagen system, glycolysis, and aerobic metabolism. The phosphagen system utilizes stored creatine phosphate to drive brief intense periods of activity and is therefore a requirement for explosive movements like sprinting or weight training. For more than a few seconds' worth of activity, glycolysis is stimulated, which breaks down glucose anaerobically to produce ATP quickly but with lactic acid as waste. The system is required during low-level exercise, providing energy when stored instant fuel depletes. With sustained physical activity, the body adapts to aerobic metabolism, which utilizes predominantly carbohydrates and fats as sources of energy. Such a route is more sustainable and enables prolonged muscle activity through efficient production of ATP through oxidative phosphorylation. Aerobic metabolism not only permits endurance sports such as running or cycling but also enables muscle cells to efficiently use oxygen in a way that they are capable of metabolizing nutrients into energy in the long term. The muscle fiber adaptation, depending on the activity type, also demonstrates this energy sourcing (Figure 7.11).

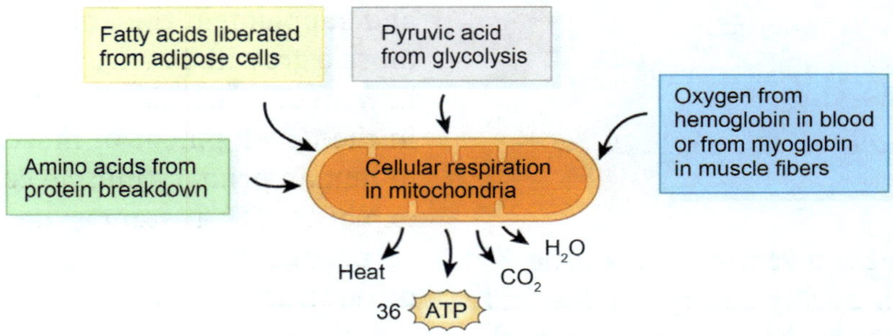

Figure 7.11. Source of muscle energy.

Source: https://external-content.duckduckgo.com/iu/?u=https%3A%2F%2Fimage2.slideserve.com%2F4691814%2Fsources-of-muscle-energy3-l.jpg&f=1&nofb=1&ipt=3190e50a34e4e26b597cf81c44969f9f1573407e41ebc236a6bf6bb343680ef9.

For instance, high levels of mitochondria make slow-twitch fibers suited for aerobic energy production, while fast-twitch fibers are suited for short bursts of anaerobic energy. In this manner, a well-balanced training program can enhance the muscle's capacity to utilize these various sources of energy in the best possible manner. Recent evidence places great significance on glycogen stores and nutrient availability in muscle functioning. For instance, research established significant differences in levels of blood glucose and glycogen between low vitality and normal vitality piglets, which established that the availability of energy has the most critical impact on motor execution and activity (Aerts et al., 2019). Knowledge of these processes is valuable, especially in contexts like space travel, where there exists an elevated demand for efficient use of energy due to altered physiological states (Altman et al., 1986). Optimal dietary regimens can enhance energy storage as glycogen as well as total energy economy, thereby optimizing muscular performance under various conditions of physical stress. Such information draws attention to the significance of adaptations in metabolism and dietary elements in maintaining proper muscle function and optimizing athletic performance.

Test Your Knowledge

1. What are the primary functions of muscles in the human body?
2. How do muscles contribute to posture and movement?

7.3. Muscle Development

Learning Outcome

1. Discuss the muscle growth and hypertrophy
2. Analyze the factors influencing muscle development
3. Identify the impact of exercise on muscle health

Muscle development is a very complex process that begins early on during embryonic life and extends throughout the life of an individual. Muscle fiber differentiation is primarily done through the proliferation and maturation of myoblasts, which are precursor cells for muscle lineage. As they fuse to form multinucleated myofibers, the type of muscle tissue and its function can contribute significantly to establishing one's physical capability. The role of innervation plays a critical role at this stage of differentiation; without adequate neural links, muscle fibers possess little ability to contract and develop normally. This influence illustrates the necessity for neuromuscular junction development in the maturation of functional muscle tissue, further emphasizing the observation that muscle development not only relies on intrinsic cellular processes but is also significantly influenced by extrinsic factors such as nerve stimulation. Investigation into muscular power and the mechanisms underlying it has brought with it the investigation of different training methods to maximize sports performance. In particular, power within a muscular context is characterized as the product of force and velocity, as opposed to strength or maximal force alone. Training methods such as isotonic, isometric, and plyometric exercises have been included in this research to find out how effective they are in increasing muscular power. Recent research has yielded conflicting results on the most appropriate velocities of contraction needed for maximal power development. Above all, the inclusion of newer training methods, such as inertial loading, requires more investigation as it pertains to muscle power adaptation. By advancing our understanding of these dynamics, researchers can develop advanced training regimes that optimize levels of athletic ability and supplement the knowledge gaps regarding muscle growth. In vitro studies have established how neuromuscular interactions are involved in the development of muscle cells. Co-culture of human primary muscle cells and spinal cord explants, for instance, has proven effective in producing proper innervation, leading to differentiation and functionalization of the muscle fibers. This new method more closely duplicates normal physiological conditions than standard monolayer cultures, enabling the study of muscle development at close range. The co-culture procedure not only supports the physical development of the muscle fibers but also enables the integrated study of neuromuscular junctions. These advances provide conclusive insight into muscle fiber behavior both in health and disease, making them extremely useful for the development of potentially therapeutic interventions. With the use of these findings, researchers can significantly enhance knowledge regarding muscle development and available interventions to fight neuromuscular diseases, and ultimately bridge the gap between basic science and clinical practice.

7.3.1. Muscle Growth and Hypertrophy

Muscle growth and hypertrophy are crucial components of the muscular system that reflect the body's capacity to adapt to physical stressors. Hypertrophy, or muscle fiber growth, is primarily a byproduct of resistance exercise, which induces micro-tears in the muscles. Micro-tears stimulate a physiological stimulus to turn on satellite cells for muscle repair and growth. The hormonal milieu, of course, is also essential, with the influence of hormones such as testosterone and growth hormone having an enormous effect on hypertrophic response. Furthermore, the protein synthesis to protein breakdown ratio has a role in determining muscle size and overall strength (Figure 7.12).

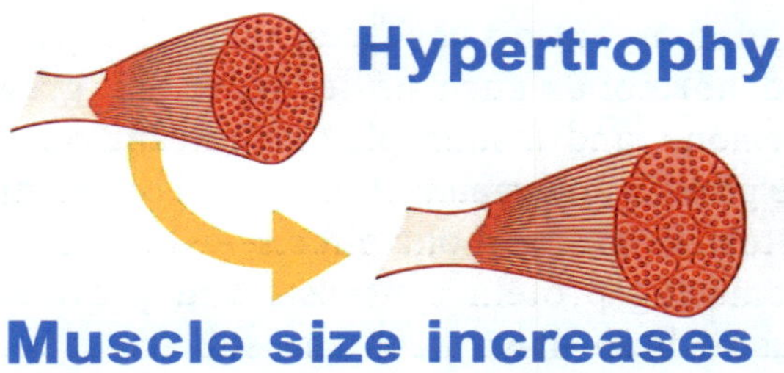

Figure 7.12. Hyperplasia growth is observed with an increase in muscle fiber numbers.

Source: https://workoutable.com/muscle-growth/.

Understanding this intricate interplay of factors offers profound insights into optimising growth and sports performance, thereby keeping the science of hypertrophy at the nucleus of broad disciplines from sport science to rehabilitation. What is more, the manifestations of hypertrophy do not end at muscle growth; they have a profound influence on functional performance and metabolic well-being. Enhanced muscle strength enhances sports performance and supports everyday functions, therefore reducing the risk of injury. In addition, greater muscle mass is associated with higher basal metabolic rates, which can be used to regulate weight and overall metabolic health. Resistance training not only increases hypertrophy but also has beneficial effects on insulin sensitivity and glucose metabolism, both of which are significant components in the prevention of conditions such as Type 2 diabetes. Thus, an understanding of muscle hypertrophy and growth mechanisms can be translated directly into training regimens and lifestyle habits to maximize health benefits across many populations. While resistance training is a key stimulus for muscle hypertrophy, muscle growth can be inhibited by numerous factors, including disuse and some physiological conditions. For instance, studies of muscle atrophy within new environments, such as space travel, reveal challenges faced in the maintenance of muscle mass within phases of reduced gravitational influence. Trials have proven that prolonged exposure to microgravity leads to severe muscle atrophy, not merely hindering strength but overall body function (Herbison et al., 2025). These findings emphasize the importance of investigating countermeasures to relieve muscle degeneration without the constant presence of mechanical stressors, which can be of relevance in a variety of settings, including injury recovery or fighting age-related muscle wasting. Lastly, understanding the complex dynamics of muscle growth and hypertrophy informs researchers and practitioners with procedures to encourage and enhance muscular health effectively (Herbison et al., 2025) (Figure 7.13).

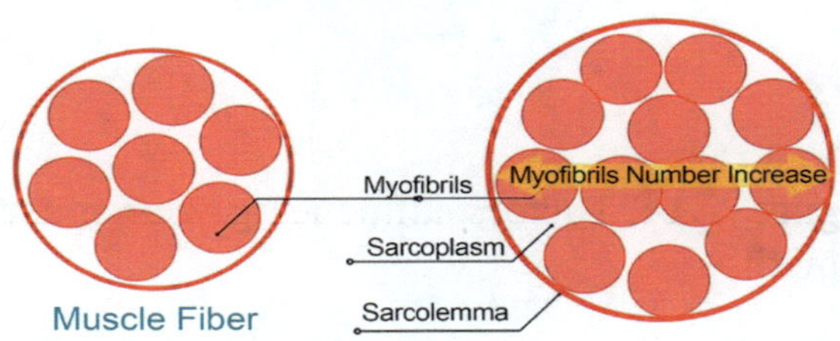

Figure 7.13. Sarcomere hypertrophy.

Source: https://workoutable.com/muscle-growth/.

7.3.2. Factors Influencing Muscle Development

Muscle hypertrophy is a complicated process governed by many internal and external factors, the major drivers among these being nutrition, exercise, and endocrine regulation. Nutrition plays a pivotal role, with the availability of macronutrients, and more so protein, being of paramount significance to facilitate muscle repair and hypertrophy. Adequate protein provides the building blocks for amino acid synthesis of muscle protein, which is critical in the hypertrophic process of resistance exercise. Further, nutrients like vitamins and minerals contribute to overall metabolism and energy generation, which optimize muscle performance and recovery. The period of nutrient intake, especially concerning exercise sessions, may also optimize muscle adaptation. Consequently, having an optimal nutrition plan that focuses on protein intake and a well-balanced diet significantly enhances muscle development, constituting a keystone element besides exercise (Figure 7.14).

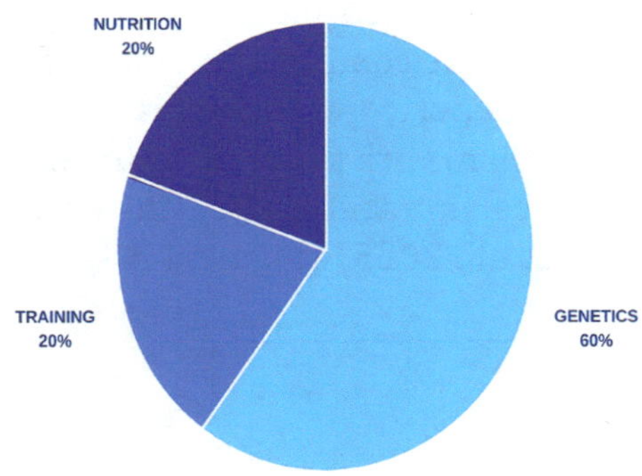

Figure 7.14. Factors influencing your muscle growth.

Source: https://progressivefitness101.com/wp-content/uploads/2021/02/Factors-Influencing-Your-Muscle-Growth-1024x1024.jpg.

Exercise, particularly resistance exercise, induces muscle hypertrophy through mechanical tension and metabolic stress, which elicit various cell responses. Progressive overload, which is a principle of successive increases in demands on the muscles, is necessary for continued growth. It involves not only weight increments but also variation in exercises and recruitment patterns, which stimulate muscle fibers differently and permit symmetrical growth. Additionally, recovery activities, like sound sleep and rest, allow for repair and adaptation activities in the muscles. Higher recovery also helps to support additional strength gain and performance. Hence, the union of equal, varied training and adequate recovery time enhances maximum muscle growth, highlighting the significance of a standard training regime based on personal need and performance level. Hormonal regulation is also a key factor in muscle growth, and hormones such as testosterone, growth hormone, and insulin play significant roles in the growth and repair of muscles. For example, testosterone's anabolic effects—which include promoting protein synthesis and preventing muscle loss—have been the subject of much researchSimilarly, growth hormone contributes to tissue growth and is a significant regulator of metabolism, affecting fat utilization and muscle sparing. Research has indicated that patients with disordered hormone levels tend to exhibit changes in muscle mass and strength outcomes. For instance, in cancer patients, decreased muscle mass correlates with poorer outcomes in cancer therapy and lower quality of life, which is an indicator of the importance of effective interventions, such as exercise and dietetic interventions that can enhance hormone levels and muscle function. Overall comprehension of these hormonal actions is critical for the development of targeted treatments that will optimize muscle mass and function across varied populations (Fairman et al., 2018; Carroll et al., 2015).

7.3.3. The Impact of Exercise on Muscle Health

Engaging in constant exercise has been shown to affect the muscle's health, which involves various physiological factors required to maintain muscular endurance and strength. Exercise guarantees that there is an increase in muscle fibers, thereby increasing their dimensions, thus supporting the development of strength. It is the result of mechanical stress developed during physical training, leading to the growth of muscle tissue through repair. Moreover, different training modalities, such as resistance training and plyometric training, have specifically been designed to develop muscle power and endurance for overall sport performance. Notably, power training, characterized by high-velocity movement, presents a unique stimulus that has the potential to achieve even superior performance compared to strength training. Thus, the inclusion of varied exercises in one's training program is critical to achieve maximal muscular adaptation and to enhance even muscle health, as supported by scientific evidence on how different velocities of training contribute to maximizing maximal power in a sports context (Brenneman et al., 2016).

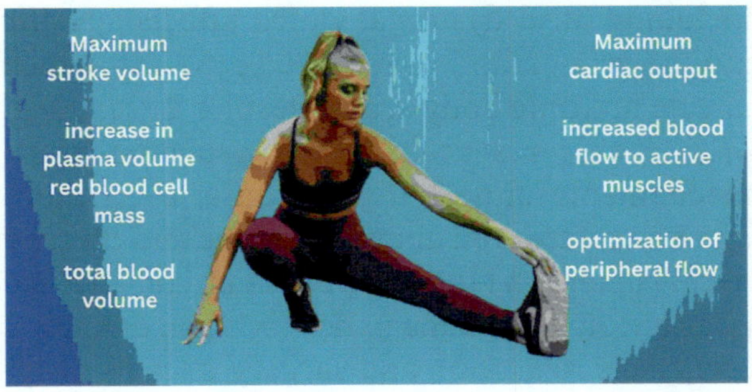
Maximum stroke volume
increase in plasma volume red blood cell mass
total blood volume
Maximum cardiac output
increased blood flow to active muscles
optimization of peripheral flow

Figure 7.15. Effects of physical exercise on muscle health.

Source: https://www.sportzyogi.com/wp-content/uploads/2024/07/EFFECTS-OF-PHYSICAL-EXERCISES-ON-THE-MUSCULAR-SYSTEM-scaled.jpg.

Moreover, exercise is also a critical intervention for the prevention of muscle atrophy due to aging, or sarcopenia, and the management of muscle mass loss in patient groups. Resistance training, in particular, has proven to be effective in preserving and even augmenting muscle mass among older adults and patients with diseases that predispose them to wasting of muscle mass, such as cancer. For patients receiving cancer treatment, preservation of muscle status can likewise significantly impact their quality of life and treatment outcome. Research has demonstrated that incorporating exercise into treatment protocols has a positive effect on muscle mass and strength, ultimately improving function and resistance to the adverse effects of treatment. This goes a long way in illuminating the therapeutic potential of exercise both as an adjunct and as part of the overall management of cancer patients, further suggesting the need for research into the combination of exercise and diet (Fairman et al., 2018) (Figure 7.15). In essence, the varied benefits of exercise to muscle health extend far beyond physical enhancement to include higher-order implications for health and well-being. Frequent engagement in physical activity provides a foundation for long-term muscle function, facilitating composite mobility and self-maintenance, particularly within older populations. Moreover, the coupling of exercise and diet, such as creatine supplementation, may indeed add to gains from exercise training, particularly within the clinical setting where atrophy is an all too frequent occurrence. The intricate interrelationship between muscle health and exercise highlights the need for intervention strategies that focus explicitly on both exercise interventions and nutritional regimens. Future research should continue to explore these dynamics and investigate how individualized exercise programs can be effectively integrated into various healthcare models to optimize muscle health and overall well-being (Fairman et al., 2018).

Test Your Knowledge

1. What is the difference between muscle growth and hypertrophy?
2. Name two key factors that influence muscle development.

7.4. Common Muscle Disorders

Learning Outcome

1. Understand the overview of muscular dystrophies
2. Identify the impact of injuries on muscle function
3. Discus the conditions affecting muscle tone and strength

Muscle disorders represent a wide variety of conditions that significantly impair muscle function, causing significant mobility and everyday activity problems. Some of the most common muscle disorders include muscular dystrophies, a condition of hereditary disorders involving progressive weakening and degeneration of skeletal muscle. DMD is the most prevalent form, occurring predominantly in males and appearing at an early age. The condition is linked with mutations in the dystrophin gene, a central component in maintaining muscle cell integrity. Patients progress to be more severely affected in motor function and ultimately wheelchair-bound by early adolescence. Understanding the genetic etiology of muscular dystrophies not only enhances diagnosis but also provides an entry into potential therapeutic interventions to delay or halt the progression of these debilitating diseases. A second significant group among muscle disorders is myopathy, which can develop because of a range of reasons, such as inflammatory, metabolic, and genetic. Inflammatory myopathies, such as polymyositis and dermatomyositis, are the aftermath of autoimmune reactions characterized by inflammation and muscle weakness. The signs can be heterogeneous, but are prone to include progressive weakness in the muscles, fatigue, and, in some cases, a rash. These conditions are not only characterized by muscular symptoms but also by the fact that they possess the capability of affecting overall health, so early identification and treatment are crucial. New therapies are also focusing on immunosuppressive treatments targeting the autoimmune response and thereby reducing muscle damage. Further studies are ongoing to investigate more sophisticated treatment techniques, including biological drugs that can heal and restore function in damaged muscles. Dystonia, another well-known muscle disorder, is defined by spasmodic muscle contractions resulting in twisting or repetitive movement. Although often misdiagnosed due to its complex presentation, dystonia has the potential to affect daily life and functional capacity significantly. The disorder is subdivided into some forms, including focal dystonia, which affects specific muscle groups, and generalized dystonia, which affects multiple body areas. Despite a great deal of scientific research on the neurobiological mechanisms underlying dystonia, even more must be discovered about the cause and therapy of this disorder. Modern treatment may include pharmacological management with an emphasis on muscle relaxation and surgery, such as deep-brain stimulation. The interrelation of dystonia with other movement disorders also compels more comprehensive care, strategies aimed at controlling symptoms and improving the quality of life in patients who are affected (Albanese et al., 2015; Dohen et al., 2013).

7.4.1. Overview of Muscular Dystrophies

Muscular dystrophies are a group of inherited conditions of progressive muscle degeneration and weakness. Muscular dystrophies affect the skeletal muscles, responsible for movement, and can also involve cardiac and smooth muscles. The pathogenesis of muscular dystrophies includes mutations in genes that are responsible for synthesizing proteins required to maintain muscle structure. These mutations are responsible for both muscle weakness and progressive loss of muscle tissue, which compromises mobility and overall functional ability. Each type of muscular dystrophy has specific characteristics and severity, and these can be influenced by onset age and the interventions that are accessible. Thus, an understanding of classifications and presentation of muscular dystrophies is valuable in the organization of successful management and to optimize patient quality of life. Laminin-α2-deficient congenital muscular dystrophy, an MDC1A type, is one of the more severe types of muscular dystrophies. It is caused by mutations in the lama2 gene, which codes for the laminin-α2 chain, a structural component of the ECM that provides structural strength to the muscle fiber. Loss of laminin-α2 results in a loose connection between the muscle fiber membrane and the overlying ECM, leading to degeneration and irreversible muscle loss. Research has indicated that in diseases like MDC1A, the application of new therapeutic strategies like gene therapy and delivery of miniaturized forms of ECM proteins is highly effective in reducing symptoms. Through the restoration of structure to muscle fibers, these forms of treatment hold the potential for restoring muscle function and preventing the progression of this debilitating disease (Meinen et al., 2005) (Figure 7.16).

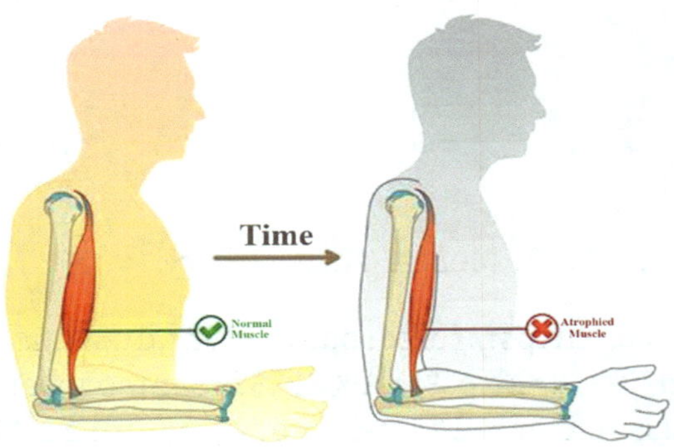

Figure 7.16. Muscular dystrophy.

Source: https://external-content.duckduckgo.com/iu/?u=https%3A%2F%2Ftse3.mm.bing.net% 2Fth%2Fid%2FOIP.4Jt4l6aB4CWKGhtUevYUOgHaFt%3 Fcb%3Diwc2%26pid%3DApi&f=1&ipt=4d5bac926a7e6d25b1478f9d4361b8efe0f08fe6cec908cfc78eaed78661cf35.

In efforts to combat muscular dystrophies' offered challenges, diagnostic innovation is of utmost significance. New approaches, particularly those involving machine learning, have been under assessment for their potential in diagnosing congenital muscular dystrophies from image examination. The systems utilize convolutional neural networks to dissect confocal microscopy images to facilitate independent patch classification of muscle tissue and identify regions of interest. This approach not only facilitates earlier and more accurate diagnosis but also enables clinicians to monitor disease evolution and treatment efficacy to a greater extent. As the application of these new technologies continues to increase, they have the potential to expand our understanding and management of muscular dystrophies, leading eventually to improved therapeutic outcomes and quality of life for individuals with these disorders (Badosa et al., 2019).

7.4.2. Impact of Injuries on Muscle Function

Injuries greatly restrict muscle function and can have lasting implications that transcend the resulting physical restriction. When a muscle is injured, say by a tear or strain, it has a complex healing process in which its form and function are altered. Early inflammation serves the purpose of repairing damaged tissue, but ongoing inflammation results in delayed recovery and muscle atrophy. This atrophy not only occurs within the injured muscle but also radiates to affect neighboring muscle groups since they must compensate by restoring lost strength or range of motion (ROM). The functional implications of such trauma can severely restrict athletic performance and activity, and therefore, significant and functional rehabilitation should follow in a timely fashion to restore the muscle to its prior state of function. Also, muscle injuries are inherently related to the neuromuscular controlling procedures that manage movement and coordination. Injured muscles will often experience an influence known as neuromuscular inhibition, in which the brain restricts the activation of the damaged muscle as protection against further injury. This reduction in muscle recruitment can lead to a decrease in strength, proprioception, and overall muscle function despite physical therapy interventions. Thus, rehabilitation of muscle function is not merely a question of fixing the physical damage; it involves an integrated approach that incorporates neuromuscular exercise and motor coordination training. These training methods are vital for athletes, particularly with advancing age, as newer evidence indicates injury risk may not always increase with increasing age, but along with diminished muscle function and neuromuscular control, particularly among those engaged in frequent competitive sports (Baker et al., 2015). Furthermore, it is crucial to consider the kind of training one does to recover from a muscle injury. Eccentric training, with an emphasis on controlled lengthening of the muscle, has shown promise for enhancing outcomes with muscle injury rehabilitation. Research has identified that the incorporation of eccentric training can increase strength, power, and resistive qualities of a muscle, particularly in youthful athletes. While muscles are being rehabilitated, both of these modalities not only aid in recovery but also address the force absorption properties required to maximize athletic function and prevent injury. To that end, appreciation of the intricate relationship between injury, training, and muscle function is key to the development of effective recovery regimes that reverse the negative impact of injury on overall muscular health (Berg et al., 2019).

7.4.3. Conditions affecting muscle tone and strength

The muscle systems' function in stability and movement is highly reliant on many of the conditions of muscle strength and tone. Bed rest of extended duration is one of the significant causes of muscle deconditioning. When bed rest is warranted by medical illness in patients, there is a substantial reduction in the volume and strength of muscles, particularly antigravity muscles, which are required for the maintenance of posture and movement. Research has established that such immobilization decreases muscle force production and reduces overall energy expenditure, ultimately impairing physical function and general health.

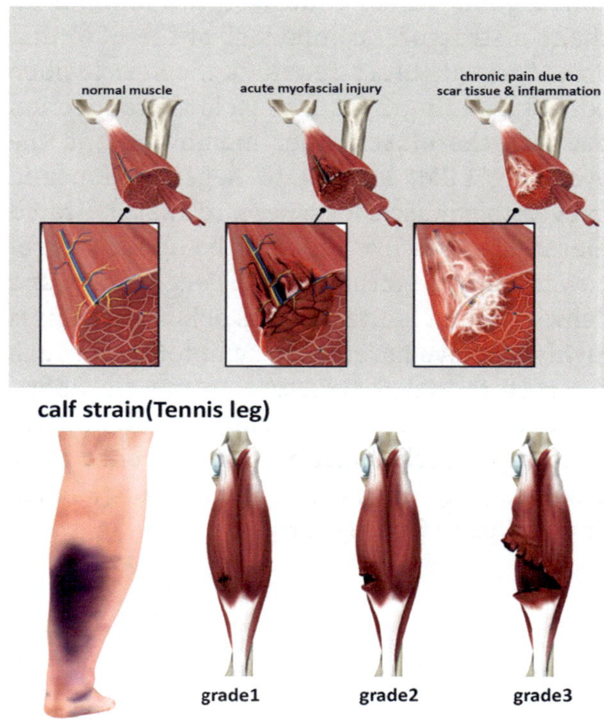

Figure 7.17. Muscle strain injury.

Source: https://external-content.duckduckgo.com/iu/?u=https%3A%2F%2Fsantabarbaradeeptissue.com%2Fwp-content%2Fuploads%2F2021%2F08%2FMuscle-Strains.jpg&f=1&nofb=1&ipt=89987d10532a3757ea897bacf9048d1e916ad9f359e6fe6b7cff3de0c8901ef3.

The loss of muscle strength that ensues can cause falls and subsequent injury, thus highlighting the need for early ambulation and exercise to reverse these negative consequences of immobility and maintain muscle integrity (Drury et al., 2007).

Apart from immobilization, the mechanical circumstances under which movement occurs also cause muscle tone and strength. For instance, the surroundings that a developing fetus experiences, such as amniotic fluid volume and womb space, significantly influence muscle development. This biomechanical property is one of the reasons that restricted movement is shown to inhibit adequate development of the skeleton, which leads to many MSK conditions. Reduced fetal movements, for example, are linked with conditions including developmental dysplasia of the hip and arthrogryposis, highlighting the critical role of dynamic and unencumbered movement to regular muscular and skeletal health (Nowlan et al., 2015) (Figure 7.17). Therefore, such observations illustrate the intimate interaction among environmental factors, opportunity for movement, and the resulting muscle strength and tone. Moreover, neurological conditions such as cerebral palsy also significantly affect muscle tone and strength throughout life. The condition can potentially lead to hypertonia or hypotonia, which is manifested as abnormally tight (spasticity) or loose (flaccidity) muscles, respectively, significantly altering an individual's ability to execute tasks requiring strength and coordination. Muscle tone fluctuation that comes with cerebral palsy can not only present challenges in mobility but also in the execution of fine motor skills needed by activities of daily living. Intervention methods like physical therapy and muscle strengthening are necessary in early intervention to enhance muscle tone and functional capabilities. Such methods aim to improve the muscle strength and overall motor function of affected individuals, thereby facilitating more effective movement and quality of life.

Test Your Knowledge

1. What are muscular dystrophies, and how do they generally affect the muscles?
2. How can muscle injuries impact overall muscle function and mobility?

7.5. The Role of Muscles in Movement

Learning Outcome

1. Explain the agonist and antagonist muscle pairs
2. Understand the importance of coordination in movement
3. Discus the relationship between muscles and joints

Muscles play a critical role in the facilitation of motion through contraction and force development. The three types of muscle tissue within the muscular system are skeletal, smooth, and cardiac. Skeletal muscles, which are connected to bones through the assistance of tendons, are primarily engaged in voluntary motions, facilitating coordination and execution of complex motor functions. Smooth muscles, found within internal organs, function involuntarily to regulate activities such as digestion and blood flow, facilitating general body movement less mechanically. Cardiac muscle, found only in the heart, functions continuously to pump blood throughout the entire body, which is required for the supply of oxygen and nutrients to contracting muscles during exercise. This cooperative function of the different muscles demonstrates the complexity of the muscular system and how it plays a central role in every type of movement and activity. Movement mechanics involve not just muscle contraction but also the integration of various systems, including the skeleton and nervous system. When contracting, a muscle becomes tense on bones to create levers that allow movement at joints. This interaction forms the basis of activities, ranging from simple movements like lifting an object to advanced sporting performances that require degrees of agility and speed. The nervous system also has a fundamental role in controlling muscular contraction through motor neurons, which transmit messages from the brain to muscle tissues. An example of such an intricate relationship is discussed in sports science, where the knowledge of muscular power is fundamental to ensuring maximum performance.

Muscle power, or the product of force and velocity, is often more important than raw strength in athletic outcomes, demonstrating the necessity of efficient muscle function in motion (Brenneman et al., 2016). Moreover, the role of muscles in movement also applies to isolated physiological responses under specific circumstances, including AVHs in schizophrenic patients. Research has indicated that inner speech may take the form of the very subtle activation of lip muscles without any articulation taking place, proving that cognitive function is linked with the activation of muscles. The condition identifies the complexity of muscle control and its relevance outside the context of bodily movement. With such knowledge, it is possible to design effective therapy in the management of disorders that involve both MSK and neurology functions. With further advancement of muscle dynamic studies, it is increasingly essential to narrow knowledge gaps and maximize training and rehabilitation techniques, thus enhancing overall movement economy and well-being (Dohen et al., 2013).

7.5.1. Agonist and Antagonist Muscle Pairs

The MSK system operates on a synergistic combination of muscle groups, the agonist and antagonist sets, working in opposition to allow movement and offer stability. Agonist muscles are responsible primarily for creating movement, contracting to produce force in a single direction. Antagonist muscles work instead to impede this movement, offering balance and control through counter-action to that of the agonists. This is important for coordinated movement.

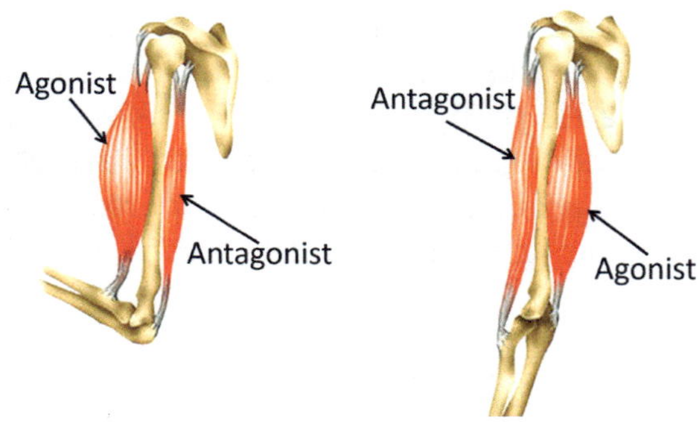

Figure 7.18. Agonist and antagonistic muscles.

Source: https://external-content.duckduckgo.com/iu/?u=https%3A%2F%2Fkeystagewiki.com%2Fimages%2Fthumb%2Ff%2Ff1%2FAntagonisticPair.png%2F1200px-AntagonisticPair.png&f=1&nofb=1&ipt=cf8cf89ef61455581a82070cf36fcdd9b5df257560089883ddbc8cd525414cc1.

For example, upon elbow flexion, the biceps brachii is the agonist and the triceps brachii is the antagonist. This coordinated effort enables effortless and accurate movement without running the risk of injury that an unrestrained or excessive contraction of one muscle group could bring. Understanding the agonist-antagonist relationship sheds light on the neural processes that govern motor behavior as well. Each muscle pair is linked by sensory feedback neural mechanisms that are necessary for modulating the muscle contractions in the instant. For instance, in a study with patients with essential tremor, researchers have found that motor units of agonist-antagonist muscle pairs have apparent phase differences during contraction of the muscles. This suggests that the central nervous system continuously monitors and adjusts muscle function as a function of sensory input, necessary for operations that generate precise movement. The cooperativity of agonist and antagonist pairs not only controls smooth motion but also plays a crucial role in posture stability and tremor avoidance, illustrating the extensive influence of muscle dynamics on general motor function (Puttaraksa et al., 2023) (Figure 7.18). Beyond their intrinsic role in movement, agonist and antagonist muscle groups also play a role in rehabilitative interventions and movement disorder knowledge. As an example, dysfunction in agonist-antagonist interaction can lead to imbalances that may be a causative factor for chronic pain or diminished mobility. Research into muscle activation patterns, particularly as they apply to disorders such as essential tremor, highlights the importance of attending to these muscle groups within the treatment setting. Electrical stimulation methods that exploit the phase interaction of antagonist muscle pairs hold promise for decreasing tremor-related symptoms, demonstrating how advanced knowledge of muscle dynamics can be employed to define beneficial treatment regimens (Steinacker et al., 1972). As knowledge of agonist and antagonist pair function increases, it has the potential to enhance treatment for restoring normal movement patterns and improving results in many MSK disorders.

7.5.2. The Importance of Coordination in Movement

Coordination is also involved in facilitating efficient movement since it involves the intricate functioning of various body systems, primarily the muscular system. The ability to perform complex motor activities relies heavily on the neuromuscular circuits that control how muscles contract and function. When a person conducts a bodily task, such as throwing a ball or a dance move, various groups of muscles must work together to achieve the intended effect. By working together, one gets smooth movement, minimizing injury risks, and enhancing performance in general.

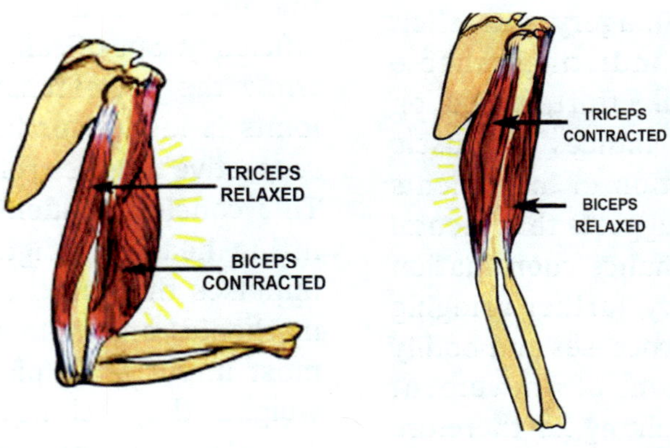

Figure 7.19. Coordination movement.

Source: https://images.slideplayer.com/41/11176983/slides/slide_2.jpg.

Thus, studying coordination mechanics helps with the development of appropriate training programs for improving sporting performance and functional movement in different populations.

Practitioners, by emphasizing coordination, are better positioned to help their clients' MSK health and design skill acquisition for a broad spectrum of physical tasks. Coordination gains even more significance when it is used about maturation, especially among children. With increasing maturity, coordination improves, and significant differences exist in the quality and sophistication of movement. These differences in physical, injury, and performance outcomes among various maturational groups emphasize the necessity of specific interventions that are directed towards these differences. For example, specific coaching methods can maximize motor potential and minimize the chances of injury by enhancing coordination ability specific to each level of maturity. This approach, as guided by existing research, can direct practitioners on when and how to include training exercises optimally. This consideration is in support of the larger goal of promoting adaptive movement and enabling physical literacy in populations aged for school, thereby the success of programs for development among young people (Berger et al., 2019) (Figure 7.19).There is also evidence supporting the role of imagery and rehearsal in the coordination of movements, supporting its role as part of training programs. Experiments have shown that mental imagery can elicit physiological responses indistinguishable from those of real physical effort, based on electromyographical (EMG) indices of muscle contraction during imagination of movements (Bakker et al., 1996). This suggests that mental practice of activities can enhance coordination and facilitate muscle memory, further bridging the gap between cognitive processes and bodily movement. The integration of movement imagery with coordination training can therefore improve learning outcomes and performance effectiveness in varied contexts. The implications of these findings stress the inclusion of both physical and mental coordination exercises within training programs to ensure the full utilization of the muscular system and its contribution to movement.

7.5.3. The Relationship Between Muscles and Joints

The intricate interplay of muscles and joints is what makes the MSK system work, and each component is integral to movement and support. Tendons transmit muscle force to the bones to create movement at joints where the bones cross. The combined leverage provides a range of movement, which any physical function requires, ranging from everyday activities to complex athletic acts. It not only facilitates movement but also provides a cushion to the joints from overloading and damage, as muscles act as shock absorbers when in motion. With this appreciation of the relationship, it is easier to understand biomechanics and overall mechanics of human body performance, and how one can maintain healthy joints while optimizing muscle effectiveness. The effectiveness of the muscle-joint relationship is further demonstrated when it is used within structured activities, such as weightlifting, where efficient muscle activation is vital for optimal function. As evidenced in experiments on weightlifting dynamics, the interplay between muscle-specific practical mechanical advantage (EMA) and joint impulse plays a key role when one considers the effect of diverse loads on movement efficiency. Specifically, evidence indicates that while the net extensor impulse generated at joints is higher for heavier loads, the EMA of respective muscles remains virtually unaltered. This conclusion identifies that the motion of lifting heavier weights relies more on joint impulses than on the manipulation of muscle mechanics, and that joint structure and function most importantly play a key role in efficient weightlifting techniques (Harris et al., 2016). Therefore, the understanding of these concepts can significantly enhance training programs and injury prevention in athletes. Furthermore, the adoption of somatic theories into the analysis of muscle and joint function opens avenues for the development of artificial movement systems with human movement. Research into automatic choreography methods indicates that the principles of somatics can enhance realistic movement generation in robotics and computer graphics. By their discussion of human movement from both the psychological and developmental perspectives, these theories provide frameworks for the study of how muscle action and joint mechanics cooperate to produce coordinated patterns of movement. By this interdisciplinary approach, not only is more known about human biomechanics, but practical application is also delivered in working on responsive robotic systems that can interact meaningfully with their world (Nakata et al., 2002). Collectively, the relationship between joints and muscles not only lies at the heart of human movement but also serves as a vital reference for technological development in robotics and rehabilitation.

Test Your Knowledge

1. What is the role of agonist and antagonist muscle pairs during movement?
2. How do muscles and joints work together to produce movement?

SUMMARY

The morphology of the muscular system is essential to respect its functional purpose in making movement and posture possible, as well as playing a role in the functions of the body. The intricate group of muscles not only offers support to the skeleton but also communicates with the nervous system to produce coordinated movement that is essential for day-to-day functioning. The interface of the energy cost of muscle activity is of profound importance to comprehend body performance and the state of health. Significantly, advances in techniques such as surface electromyography (sEMG) have facilitated our understanding of being able to more accurately measure muscle activity toto screen for ergonomic utilization properly. Findings of experiments with sEMG indicate its potentiality, with restrictions still in place, that it needs to act to complement existing machinery in measuring overall analysis (Ašić et al., 2010). In addition, the nuances of muscular power point towards its significance as a measure of athletic ability above mere strength measurement. It is necessary to make a distinction between strength and power since the former involves both force and speed of movement, thus playing a vital role in competitive sport achievement. Research suggests that various training methodologies, including isotonic and plyometric techniques, can influence muscular power outcomes significantly. However, current literature reveals inconsistencies concerning the most effective training velocities and loads required to maximize power gains. Furthermore, the introduction of inertial load training paradigms represents an uncharted yet promising avenue for enhancing muscular power adaptation, warranting further investigation. This study advocates for the necessity of well-designed studies to establish best training programs that will ultimately aid in sports performance (Brenneman et al., 2016). In summary, knowledge of the muscular system encompasses diverse aspects, such as its basic functions and the complexity of training muscles. The use of sophisticated technology, such as sEMG, provides an enhanced understanding of muscle activity monitoring, facilitating the development of ergonomic practices and training regimens for athletes. The study of muscular power training procedures continues to progress, revealing gaps that researchers must close to optimize training outcomes for athletes. As the field evolves, it is imperative to relate theory to practice so that knowledge garnered from research has expression in tangible gains for both health and performance. Therefore, ongoing research on the muscular system remains paramount to optimizing our understanding of human physiology and optimizing physical potential in a wide range of venues.

The muscular system is a fundamental component of human physiology, enabling movement, maintenance of posture, and generation of heat. It is composed of three basic categories of muscles: skeletal, cardiac, and smooth. Each has distinctive functions and structural characteristics that enable it to carry out its function effectively. Skeletal muscles, which are attached to bones with the use of tendons, perform voluntary movements, whereas cardiac muscle lines the walls of the heart to enable involuntary rhythmical contractions. Smooth muscle encircles internal organs and vessels, which regulate involuntary actions such as digestion and vascular regulation. It is necessary to understand this fundamental information in grasping more complex interactions and accommodations that may occur with the muscular system, particularly in sport performance, as well as training techniques. Research on muscular power highlights its significant role in sporting performance, specifically in the formula of force and speed. This aspect of muscular capacity is more important in performance outcomes than clean strength. Current literature examining varying contraction speeds shows that there is a need for more research on training methods for enhancing muscular power. While traditional modalities such as isotonic, isokinetic, isometric, and plyometric training provide evidence for improving performance, not much emphasis has been put on the potential efficacy of inertial load training. Closing the gaps in this field of research could have widespread implications for enhancing the training of athletes and optimizing their muscular power, aligning methods of training with maximum performance requirements (Brenneman et al., 2016). Additionally, technological innovations, particularly in machine learning for diagnosis, are also revolutionizing our understanding and management of muscular diseases. Their application, especially of systems using Convolutional Neural Networks, demonstrates the potential of high-resolution image analysis in the diagnosis of congenital muscular dystrophies. They scan patches of confocal microscopy images to develop an overall understanding, thus enhancing therapeutic efficacy monitoring and the accuracy of diagnoses. The integration of such technology in MSK research not only assists clinicians in making timely decisions but also helps create patient-specific treatment plans, resulting in improved patient outcomes in muscular health (Badosa et al., 2019).

KEY TERMS FROM THIS CHAPTER

- Skeletal muscle
- Smooth muscle
- Myofibril
- Actin
- Tropomyosin
- Neuromuscular junction
- Muscle contraction
- Tendon
- Cardiac muscle
- Muscle fiber
- Sarcomere
- Myosin
- Troponin
- Motor unit
- Muscle tone
- Origin

CRITICAL THINKING QUESTIONS

1. **What is the primary function of the muscular system?**
   a. To produce hormones
   b. To facilitate movement
   c. To protect internal organs
   d. To store minerals
2. **Which type of muscle tissue is under voluntary control?**
   a. Cardiac muscle
   b. Smooth muscle
   c. Skeletal muscle
   d. Involuntary muscle
3. **Which muscle type is found only in the heart?**
   a. Skeletal muscle
   b. Smooth muscle
   c. Cardiac muscle
   d. Voluntary muscle
4. **Smooth muscle is primarily found in:**
   a. The walls of blood vessels and organs
   b. The bones
   c. The heart
   d. The skin
5. **Which protein is responsible for muscle contraction?**
   a. Collagen
   b. Myosin
   c. Keratin
   d. Elastin

Short Answer Questions

1. What are the three main types of muscles in the human body?
2. Describe the basic structure of a skeletal muscle fiber.
3. How do muscles generate force and enable movement?
4. What are the key stages in muscle development from infancy to adulthood?
5. Name two common muscle disorders and their typical symptoms.
6. How do muscles work together with the skeletal system to produce movement?
7. Why is muscle health important for overall physical function and mobility?

Answer to Critical Thinking Questions

1. (b); 2. (c); 3. (c); 4. (a); 5. (b)

References

1. Vanden Hole, C., Ayuso, M., Aerts, P., Prims, S., Van Cruchten, S., & Van Ginneken, C. (2019). Glucose and glycogen levels in piglets that differ in birth weight and vitality. *Heliyon*, *5*(9), e02510. https://doi.org/10.1016/j.heliyon.2019.e02510Albanese, A., Alongi, A., Altenmüller, E., Argyelan, M., Baird, A., Baizabal-Carvallo, J. F., Berardelli, A., et al. (2015). Dystonia and paroxysmal dyskinesias: Under-recognized movement disorders in domestic animals? A comparison with human dystonia/paroxysmal dyskinesias. https://core.ac.uk/download/36778981.pdf (accessed on 14th June 2025).
2. Altman, P. L., & Fisher, K. D. (1986). *Research Opportunities in Nutrition and Metabolism in Space*. https://core.ac.uk/download/pdf/10458014.pdf (accessed on 14th June 2025).
3. Arnold, A. S., Christe, M., & Handschin, C. (2012). A functional motor unit in the culture dish: Co-culture of spinal cord explants and muscle cells. https://core.ac.uk/download/18254851.pdf (accessed on 14th June 2025).
4. Badosa, C., Bazaga, A., Jiménez-Mallebrera, C., Porta, S., et al. (2019). A convolutional neural network for the automatic diagnosis of collagen VI-related muscular dystrophies. http://arxiv.org/abs/1901.11074 (accessed on 14th June 2025).
5. Baguet, A., Beeckman, S., Derave, W., Everaert, I., et al. (2010). Muscle carnosine metabolism and β-alanine supplementation in relation to exercise and training. https://core.ac.uk/download/55837517.pdf (accessed on 14th June 2025).
6. Baker, J. R. (2015). The prevalence and risks of injury for masters' athletes: Current findings. https://core.ac.uk/download/211331646.pdf (accessed on 14th June 2025).
7. Bakker, F. C., Boschker, M. S. J., & Chung, T. (1996). Changes in muscular activity while imagining weight lifting using stimulus or response propositions. https://core.ac.uk/download/pdf/18453505.pdf (accessed on 14th June 2025).
8. Baumann, C. W., Ferrington, D. A., Kwak, D., Thompson, L. V., et al. (2017). Downhill exercise alters immunoproteasome content in mouse skeletal muscle. https://open.bu.edu/bitstream/2144/40890/8/Downhill%20Exercise....accepted%20files.pdf (accessed on 14th June 2025).
9. Berg, H. E., Boling, M. C., Buchanan, P., Dolezal, B. A., Drury, D. G., Eston, R., Frizziero, A., et al. (2019). Eccentric resistance training in youth: Perspectives for long-term athletic development. https://core.ac.uk/download/304335131.pdf (accessed on 14th June 2025).
10. Berger, N., Best, R., Maulder, P. S., Standing, R. J., et al. (2019). An investigation into the impact of coaching strategies with respect to physical and performance characteristics of male youth of varying biological maturation. https://core.ac.uk/download/287723710.pdf (accessed on 14th June 2025).
11. Brenneman, M. T. (2016). *Training for Muscular Power Adaptations: The Role of Contraction Type and Velocity*. https://core.ac.uk/download/211333301.pdf (accessed on 14th June 2025).
12. Carroll, L., Cordero, J., & Naszai, M. (2015). Intestinal stem cell proliferation and epithelial homeostasis in the adult *Drosophila* midgut. https://core.ac.uk/download/42368228.pdf (accessed on 14th June 2025).
13. Dohen, M., Loevenbruck, H., Perrier, P., Polosan, M., et al. (2013). An EMG study of the lip muscles during covert auditory verbal hallucinations in schizophrenia. https://core.ac.uk/download/47281309.pdf (accessed on 14th June 2025).

14. Drury, D. G., & Stuempfle, K. J. (2007). The physiological consequences of bed rest. https://cupola.gettysburg.edu/cgi/viewcontent.cgi?article=1029&context=healthfac (accessed on 14th June 2025).

15. Fairman, C. M., Galvao, D. A., Hart, N. H., Kendall, S., et al. (2018). The potential therapeutic effects of creatine supplementation on body composition and muscle function in cancer. https://core.ac.uk/download/213607833.pdf (accessed on 14th June 2025).

16. Falla, D., Lluch, E., Meeus, M., Nijs, J., et al. (2014). Influence of shoulder pain on muscle function: Implications for the assessment and therapy of shoulder disorders. https://core.ac.uk/download/55799562.pdf (accessed on 14th June 2025).

17. Gartner, W. B., & Murphy, M. R. (2025). Pilot workload and fatigue: A critical survey of concepts and assessment techniques. https://core.ac.uk/download/pdf/42880558.pdf (accessed on 14th June 2025).

18. Goswami, A., Porto, A., Porto, A., Leroi, A. M., Esteve-Altava, B., Esteve-Altava, B., Esteve-Altava, B., et al. (2015). Anatomical network comparison of human upper and lower, newborn and adult, and normal and abnormal limbs, with notes on development, pathology and limb serial homology vs. homoplasy. https://core.ac.uk/download/36779022.pdf (accessed on 14th June 2025).

19. Harris, C., & Kipp, K. (2016). Muscle-specific effective mechanical advantage and joint impulse in weightlifting. https://core.ac.uk/download/213075289.pdf (accessed on 14th June 2025).

20. Herbison, G. J., & Talbot, J. M. (2025). Research opportunities in muscle atrophy. https://core.ac.uk/download/pdf/42848744.pdf (accessed on 14th June 2025).

21. Katzman, W. B., & Pastore, E. A. (2012). Recognizing myofascial pelvic pain in the female patient with chronic pelvic pain. https://core.ac.uk/download/305124272.pdf (accessed on 14th June 2025).

22. Kucuk, S., Mickle, M. H., Vogt, W. G., Zipf, R., et al. (2025). Computer simulation of a pilot in V/STOL aircraft control loops. https://core.ac.uk/download/pdf/42828496.pdf (accessed on 14th June 2025).

23. Meinen, S. (2005). Artificial restoration of the linkage between laminin and dystroglycan ameliorates the disease progression of MDC1A muscular dystrophy at all stages. https://core.ac.uk/download/18233984.pdf (accessed on 14th June 2025).

24. N/A. (2025). *Aerospace Medicine and Biology: A Continuing Bibliography (Supplement 221).* https://core.ac.uk/download/pdf/42859695.pdf (accessed on 14th June 2025).

25. N/A. (2025). *Aerospace Medicine and Biology: A Continuing Bibliography with Indexes (Supplement 309).* https://core.ac.uk/download/pdf/42832898.pdf (accessed on 14th June 2025).

26. Nakata, T. (2002). Generation of whole-body expressive movement based on somatically theories. https://core.ac.uk/download/pdf/85265.pdf (accessed on 14th June 2025).

27. Nowlan, N. C. (2015). Biomechanics of fetal movement. https://core.ac.uk/download/76995826.pdf (accessed on 14th June 2025).

28. Oberbach, A., Buchwalow, I., Punkt, K., Kandt, K., Blueher, M., & Adams, V. (2012). Nitric oxide synthase in skeletal muscle fibers of patients with type 2 diabetes. https://core.ac.uk/download/pdf/1570004.pdf (accessed on 14th June 2025).

29. Petrillo, S., Pelosi, L., Piemonte, F., Travaglini, L., et al. (2017). Oxidative stress in Duchenne muscular dystrophy: Focus on the NRF2 redox pathway. https://core.ac.uk/download/pdf/98345141.pdf (accessed on 14th June 2025).

30. Puttaraksa, G. (2023). Modeling the neurophysiology of tremor to develop a peripheral neuroprosthesis for tremor suppression. https://core.ac.uk/download/554493102.pdf (accessed on 14th June 2025).

31. Richard, J., & Usherwood, J. R. (2016). The muscle-mechanical compromise framework: Implications for the scaling of gait and posture. https://core.ac.uk/download/76980897.pdf (accessed on 14th June 2025).

32. Santello, M., & Valero-Cuevas, F. J. (2017). On neuromechanical approaches for the study of biological grasp and manipulation. http://arxiv.org/abs/1710.08557 (accessed on 14th June 2025).

33. Steinacker, A. (1972). Aspects of the oculomotor system of *Callinectes sapidus*. https://core.ac.uk/download/303901256.pdf (accessed on 14th June 2025).

34. Sušić, A., Veljović, F., & Jurčević Lulić, T. (2010). Ergonomic evaluation of task execution: Surface electromyography in muscular activity screening. https://core.ac.uk/download/14423699.pdf (accessed on 14th June 2025).

35. Tan, Ü. (2007). The psychomotor theory of human mind. https://core.ac.uk/download/pdf/86857.pdf (accessed on 14th June 2025).

36. Wisser, A., Biewener, A. A., Hedenström, A., Ennos, A. R., Henke, B. L., Balint, C. N., Balint, C. N., et al. (2014). *In vivo* time-resolved microtomography reveals the mechanics of the blowfly flight motor. https://core.ac.uk/download/36777697.pdf (accessed on 14th June 2025).

MUSCLES OF THE HEAD AND NECK

8

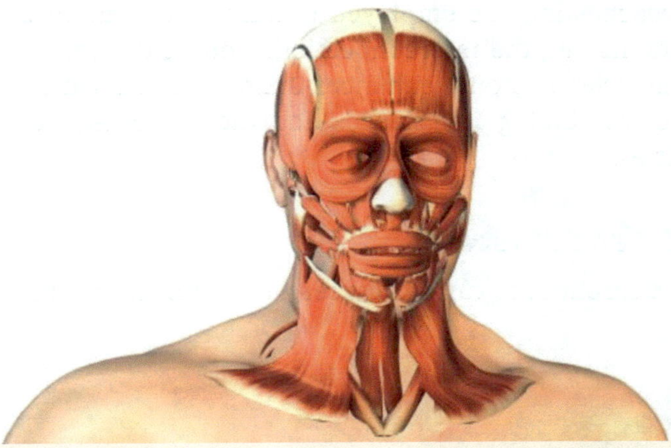

LEARNING OBJECTIVES

After studying this chapter, you will be able to:

1. Describe the anatomy of the head muscles
2. Identify the muscles of mastication
3. Provide an overview of the major muscles of the neck
4. Identify the muscles involved in facial expression
5. Explain the functions of key neck muscles
6. Discuss the clinical relevance of head and neck muscles

Introduction

The muscles of the head and neck play a vital role in movement and expression, reflecting the intricate relationship between structure and function within the human body. The muscle groups in the head and neck are of varying types, including the facial expression muscles, mastication muscles, and neck movement muscles. Understanding these muscles is essential in various fields, from medicine and physical therapy to aesthetics and speech pathology. Detailed exploration of such muscle groups not only maximizes our knowledge of human anatomy but also serves to render apparent the dynamic interplay involved in the processes of everyday activity, such as eating, speech, and emotional expression. Studies in such muscles provide insight into how their integration functions and how this integrates into broader issues of health and well-being. Beyond their basic function, head and neck muscles have been of considerable scientific interest, particularly in how they influence neurological function and physiological responses. Syncretism of practices such as acupuncture suggests there is more to the complexity of these muscle groups. By way of illustration, observational data from Traditional Chinese Medicine detail that some acupoints, maybe equivalent to muscular or nervous tissue, would be able to have a profound effect on body functions (Dorsher, 2009). This relationship is an ostensible link between knowledge garnered in ancient times and contemporary scientific inquiry, relating further research into how these groups of muscles are not simply anatomical structures but also part of systemic networks within the body. Understanding these relations is crucial for future health therapy research and rehabilitation methods. Continuing examination of muscles of the head and neck illustrates their importance in both functional and anatomical teaching. A study of these groups of muscles builds an initial requirement in knowledge for more specialized areas of surgery and neurology. As most diagnostic and treatment procedures rely on accurate anatomical information, acquiring dissection and anatomical visualization technique skills is essential. Analogous to honey bee anatomy courses placing high priority on dissection as a method of examination of complex systems, similar approaches may be employed to human musculature studies (Casagrande-Jaloretto et al., 2013). In establishing the interconnections among the varied disciplines, the research on the head and neck muscles not only enhances anatomical education but also indicates the multidisciplinary nature of the biological sciences and their relevance to health care and the efficacy of treatment modalities.

Importance of Understanding Head and Neck Muscles

Understanding the muscles of the head and neck is essential to various careers, including medicine, physical therapy, and speech pathology.

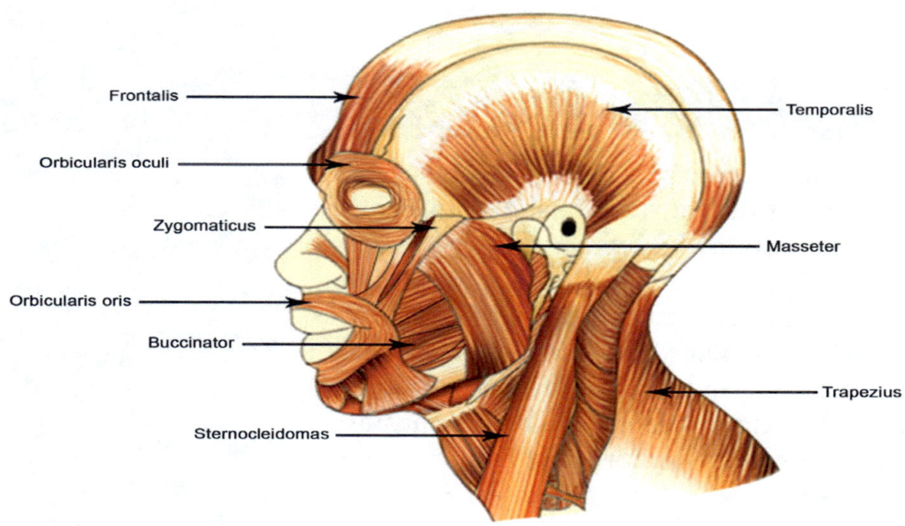

Figure 8.1. Muscles of the head and neck.

Source: https://training.seer.cancer.gov/anatomy/muscular/groups/head_neck.html.

Not only do these muscles play essential roles in fundamental human functions like jaw movement, facial expression, and swallowing, but they also influence higher-order processes of cognition and communication. For instance, the intricate coordination of facial muscles is primarily responsible for non-verbal communication, expressing emotions as strongly as verbal messages. The identification of the anatomical organization of muscles allows health professionals to effectively treat temporomandibular joint (TMJ) disease and speech disorders (Figure 8.1). Thus, an appropriate understanding of the musculature of the head and neck brings not only improved clinical results but also serves to enhance therapeutic processes aimed at improving the quality of life of patients. Head and neck muscles are also significant for study to comprehend the evolutionary areas of human anatomy. Recent research based on anatomical network analysis (AnNA) illustrates how the musculoskeletal (MSK) structure of the head and neck evolved during evolution, particularly in primates and their close relatives. Based on the analysis, increased complexity within human muscles, particularly within facial regions, affects facial communication as well as social interaction behavior. Specifically, the presence of distinct facial modules suggests an enormous evolutionary advantage in being able to express emotions more effectively. The study suggests a selective pressure toward more complex facial expressions, which underpin social bonding and communication strategies, accounting for the deep connection between muscle evolution and cognitive development (Goswami et al., 2018). Besides, understanding head and neck musculature complexities may prove to be highly advantageous in clinical rehabilitation planning and diagnosis. Familiarity with anatomy can enable professionals to notice symptoms of dysfunction that are not noticeable otherwise. For example, weakness or imbalance in specific muscle groups can lead to voice production disorders, swallowing disorders, and even respiratory compromise. This is particularly relevant in the voice disorder therapeutic situation, whereby understanding the muscular dynamics of the phonation process is essential to addressing the condition. Additionally, understanding the interconnectedness of head and neck muscles can inform surgical treatments and rehabilitative treatments so that general care can be given to trauma- or disease-related conditions. Ultimately, the relevance of head and neck muscle knowledge extends beyond anatomical specificity; it encompasses a whole worldview of how they contribute to health, well-being, and communication (Aspden et al., 2014).

Overview of Muscle Functions in the Head and Neck

The head and neck muscles play a crucial role not only in facilitating movement but also in enabling vital functions such as communication and swallowing. Facial muscles, for example, are very organized in their construction to provide space for a variety of facial expressions that allow human beings to convey emotions without verbal language. Such a capacity is particularly significant during social interactions where the cues trigger increased understanding and empathy among individuals. Moreover, the facial and neck muscles that facilitate mastication are pivotal to the processes of eating and speaking. Both highlight muscular coordination as crucial to both physiological and social operations, attesting to an evolved integration of body parts honed across the ages to accomplish the tasks of communication and nourishment in human life. Neuroscience has increasingly elucidated the interplay between these functions of head and neck muscles and the neural mechanisms that drive them. As dynamic interfaces between our motor outputs and sensory inputs, the head and neck muscles respond to varied stimuli to facilitate rapid behavior adjustments. For example, the excitation and inhibition of muscles in speech are coordinated with the processing of auditory information, and this allows for effective information exchange. Recent findings of genetic and molecular mechanisms influencing information flow within sensory-motor circuits further clarify these interactions, specifically describing how certain neuron classes integrate and transfer signals. Such observations can not only enhance our knowledge of human anatomy but also of the evolutionary changes that have shaped our ability to respond to environmental stimuli through complex muscular movement, as would be evident in primates' development of structures for communication (Goswami et al., 2018). Understanding the complexity of stratified patterns found in the head and neck muscle functions also entails consideration of the implications of MSK evolution over long periods. The variation in muscular arrangements reflects both environmental adaptations and social pressures on individuals. Additional head and neck muscles have been found to appear in primate evolution, particularly human evolution, resulting in subtle differences like a reduction in network density and complexity in human beings (Goswami et al., 2018). These anatomical transformations not only support more intricate facial expressions but also enhance speech capabilities. This evolution raises fascinating questions regarding the mechanisms by which muscular and neural systems coordinate to facilitate survival and social interaction behaviors, hence illustrating the profound interlacings between anatomy, physiology, and behavioral outputs over human evolutionary history.

8.1. Anatomy of the Head Muscles

Learning Outcome

1. Explain the major muscle groups in the head
2. Define the location and structure of facial muscles
3. Describe the role of head muscles in expression and communication

The head muscle anatomy is not only vital to the comprehension of human physiology but also vital for application in rehabilitation and sports medicine. Such muscles, including the temporalis, masseter, and facial expression muscles, play a critical role in processes such as mastication and communication. For instance, the temporalis muscle is used to elevate and retract the mandible for effective chewing. Similarly, the masseter muscle, one of the strongest muscles in the human body, enables firm clenching that is necessary for food breakdown. Understanding of the intricate interplay of these muscles provides insight into their function and ability to resist varied conditions, especially in sporting activities involving repeated impact, necessitating adequate muscle conditioning to maintain head and neck stability. Recent research has indicated that strengthening cervical musculature reduces the risk of concussion during sports, according to anatomical relationships and mechanisms between head muscles. Although research has not definitively proven a direct relationship between muscle size and the prevention of concussions, studies indicate that neck strength is the key to reducing impact forces. Specifically, research also indicates that not only general neck muscle strength but also stiffness and activation during impact are vital for force dissipation. Therefore, even though athletes can undergo various programs of training to reinforce such muscles, one must understand the biomechanical realities that govern head and neck interactions during collision as well as how muscle architecture can contribute to the prevention of injury (Bull et al., 2015). The latest technological advances, particularly in multi-body dynamics analysis (MDA), have significantly enhanced our knowledge of head muscle anatomy. With this technique, one can create accurate three-dimensional representations of muscle structures, which enable a more advanced appreciation of their functions and correlations. In animals like Sphenodon, researchers employ MDA to see muscles' locations, attachment spots, and orientation that are difficult for traditional imaging to depict. Such in-depth modeling not only benefits academic research but also has practical applications in the design of rehabilitation schemes and maximizing sport performance through the identification of primary anatomical structures dictating muscle function (Curtis et al., 2009). Such an innovative framework highlights the importance of integrating new analytical techniques in the study of head muscle anatomy and thereby serving theoretical knowledge and practical applications in both sporting and clinical settings (Figure 8.2).

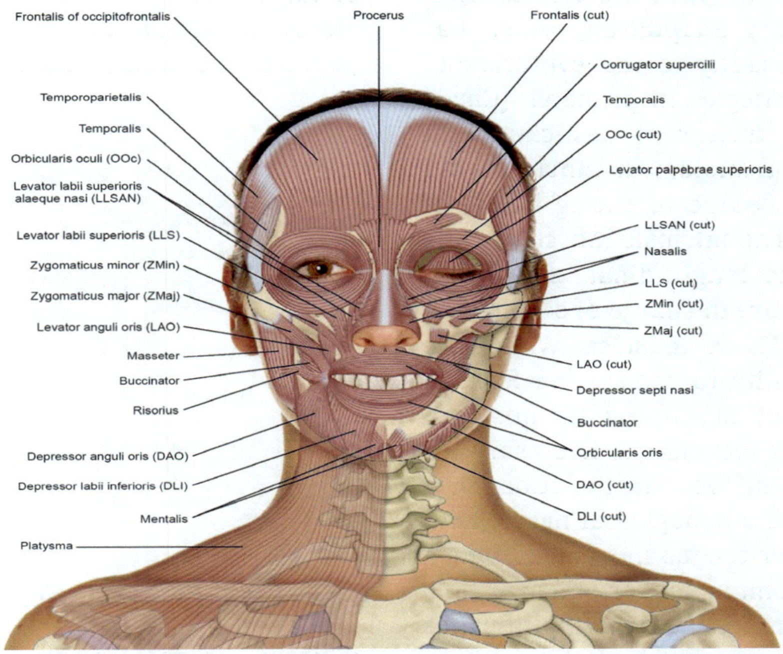

Figure 8.2. The muscles of head.

Source: https://external-content.duckduckgo.com/iu/?u=http%3A%2F%2Fmusculoskeletalkey.com%2Fwp-content%2Fuploads%2F2016%2F08%2FF500157f09-02-9780323086844.jpg&f=1&nofb=1&ipt=dfc11dbbb4ffbeed5bf7927f031cd81525d00db58249d19947d02f4d8029ee0d.

8.1.1. Major Muscle Groups in the Head

Of the major groups of muscles of the head, facial expression muscles are most significant for non-verbal communication and emotional expression. Facial expression muscles are innervated by the facial nerve and facilitate a richly varied movement that distorts the face. The orbicularis oculi muscle is especially notable in that it encircles the eyes, allowing for blinking and expression of mood states like happiness or sadness by variation in expression. Similarly, the minor and major zygomaticus muscles lift the corners of the mouth which assist in smiling. Anatomical network analysis hypotheses that modularity and integration of such facial muscles are evolutionary adaptations that enhance social interactions because, as evidenced by their independent left and right modules, they enable the ability to express subtlety and asymmetry (Goswami et al., 2018). Therefore, such muscles form a vital component of human emotional life and interpersonal communication. The masticatory masseter, temporalis, and pterygoid muscles significantly contribute to the complex mechanics of chewing. The masseter muscle, one of the strongest muscles in the human body, elevates the mandible vertically upwards, facilitating forceful biting. With the temporalis, used to elevate and retract the jaw, these muscles aid in the grinding action needed to crush food. Pterygoid muscles also assist lateral and medial mandibular movements to allow more functional movement when masticating. Surprisingly, the evolutionary history of such muscles testifies to long-term dietary adaptation, which has contributed significantly to the evolution of diverse feeding strategies in primates (Christ et al., 2010). Thus, muscles of mastication not only carry essential biological functions but also illustrate the course of eating habits of human ancestors. The intrinsic muscles of the tongue, namely the longitudinal, transverse, and vertical fibers, are in charge of swallowing and articulation. These muscles, which are unique in their ability to change the form of the tongue without modifying its position, enable the complex movements necessary for speech production and food manipulation. They are innervated by the hypoglossal nerve, with delicate control over tongue movement, which is fundamental to communication and digestion. Recent research underlines the significance of these intrinsic muscles in the evolution of human beings, since speech mechanisms adaptations most probably occur alongside enlargement of such muscular characteristics (Goswami et al., 2018). Furthermore, their developmental origins are distinct from those of neck muscles, indicating that head muscles have more specialized functions compared to those in the trunk (Christ et al., 2010). Therefore, the intrinsic muscles of the tongue demonstrate the intricate relationship between musculature and the functional requirement of human action.

8.1.2. Location and Structure of Facial Muscles

The muscles of the face, which essentially have the responsibility of expressing feelings, are placed relatively high under the skin and allow for a wide range of movements. The facial muscles are referred to as the muscles of facial expression and are generally derived from the second branchial arch during embryogenesis. Spread throughout the facial region, they intertwine, overlap, and adhere to the skin rather than bones, allowing them to store tension that is translated into facial expressions. Of importance, the musculature surrounding the eyes, mouth, and forehead is pivotal to nonverbal communication.

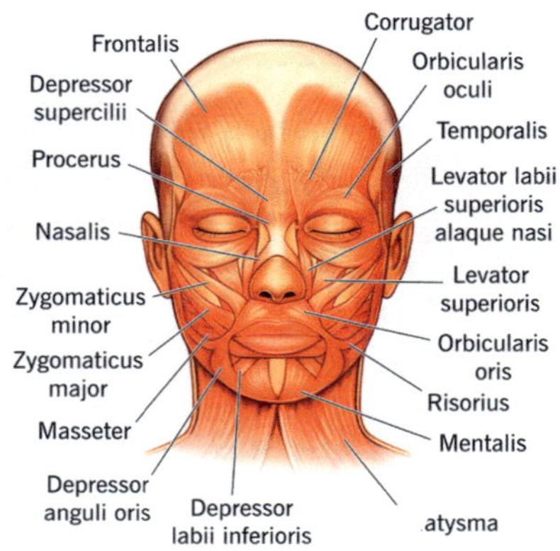

Figure 8.3. Facial muscles.

Source: https://my.clevelandclinic.org/-/scassets/images/org/health/articles/facial-muscles.

Their strategic location, combined with their direct access to the skin, provides them with a unique ability to express an enormous variety of feelings, proving the evolutionary significance of facial musculature in interpersonal attachment and social interaction. Facial muscles are organized by their flat, slender, and often oval structures, reflecting their evolved function in fine motor control. As opposed to other bony-attached skeletal muscles, facial muscles possess a unique fibrous, membranous structure, which enables them to be more elastic. They are capable of contracting and relaxing exactly, allowing them to perform smooth and subtle movements (Figure 8.3). For instance, the orbicularis oculi muscle encircles the eye and can blink and squint, while the zygomaticus major muscle is responsible for smiling and elevating the corners of the mouth. Their incorporation into the facial skeleton, along with their associated actions, emphasizes their contribution to both functional attributes such as mastication and expressive ones, marrying neuroanatomical functions with socio-emotional communication. The embryonic origin of facial muscles also reveals essential information on their location and associated functions. Cranial neural crest mesenchyme, which is involved in the patterning and formation of facial muscles, influences their form and function during embryogenesis. Aberrations from this developmental process lead to congenital abnormalities, underscoring the significance of these tissues in clinical and evolutionary contexts. Faced with the dissimilar biomechanical demands, the divergence in muscle structure and location has allowed for adaptation through evolutionary history. Face muscles are highly specialized, allowing for a dynamic balance between structural integrity and expression potential due to the interaction of mechanical loads and molecular processes. This information is key to the learning of facial rehabilitation techniques and the management of facial musculature disorders, revealing the profound underpinnings of anatomical structure in determining human wellness (N/A, 2018; Abzhanov et al., 2019).

8.1.3. Role of Head Muscles in Expression and Communication

The role of muscles in the head in expression and communication is multifaceted and essential, aiding in the nuances of human communication. Facial muscles, under various categories such as the orbicularis oris and zygomaticus major, are responsible for conveying a wide range of emotions from joy to pain.

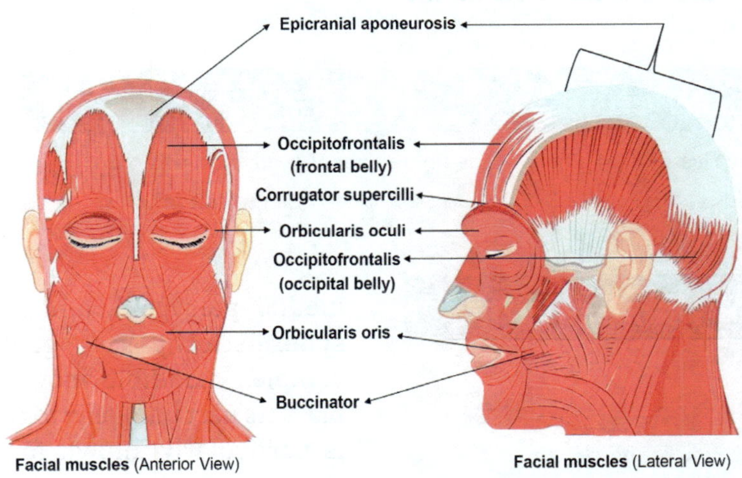

Figure 8.4. Muscles of facial expression.

Source: https://external-content.duckduckgo.com/iu/?u=https%3A%2F%2Fwww.slideteam.net%2Fmedia%2Fcatalog%2Fproduct%2Fcache%2F960x720%2F0%2F5%2F0514_front_and_side_views_of_the_muscles_of_facial_expressions_medical_images_for_powerpoint_Slide01.jpg&f=1&nofb=1&ipt=3951db574cde500aef6f0dfb2fe000ba18828b9270754fb0633031a2bf7f0de7.

The muscles aid in expressing non-verbal communication, which has a more pronounced impact than verbal words, therefore enhancing the communication process among people. Their evolutionary development was traced back to the expansion of human social complexity, which made more evolved forms of expression possible. Notably, anatomical network analysis research has explained how facial muscle modularity and integration make this expressive possibility feasible, and how primates have dramatically transformed their facial morphologies better to convey emotion and vocal signaling in social interactions (Goswami et al., 2018) (Figure 8.4). Besides, the influence of head musculature extends beyond expression proper to affect vocalization and laughter, both of which are significant aspects of social bonding. Head muscle use is also core in controlling tone, pitch, and emotional content within speech. Laughter ability, a half-voluntary behavior, is an extension of the same, as it relies upon delicate interaction among several groups of muscles, such as laryngeal and neck muscles. Advanced tools such as surface electromyography (sEMG) have been proposed to study these muscle activations more effectively, to provide a better insight into laughter's social functions. This device can provide insights into the coordination of the movements of the muscles employed in creating facial expressions and voice, demonstrating the multi-aspectual role of head muscles in social communication (Bianchi-Berthouze et al., 2015). In summary, head muscles play an unavoidable role in non-verbal and verbal communication as key mediators in transmitting emotional and social information. Multidisciplinary exploration of the integration of networks in these muscles reveals adaptive changes in primate lineages, particularly with facial expressions involving complex social interactions. As human evolutionary trends demonstrate a balance between muscle complexity and functional adequacy, the evolutionary development of such muscular patterns is pivotal to demarcating patterns of communication. Thus, understanding the intricate anatomy as well as function of muscles in the head not only facilitates an understanding of human behavior but also sheds light on the underlying evolutionary dynamics of social communication (Goswami et al., 2018).

Test Your Knowledge

1. Where are facial muscles located, and what is unique about their structure?
2. How do head muscles contribute to facial expression and communication?

8.2. Muscles of Mastication

Learning Outcome

1. Understand the overview of the chewing muscles
2. Identify the key muscles involved in mastication
3. Explain the importance of mastication for digestion

The masticatory muscles are components of the overall head and neck musculature, tasked with the complex task of grinding and chewing food. These muscles, namely the masseter, temporalis, medial pterygoid, and lateral pterygoid, act synergistically as a group to facilitate the complex mandible movements. Every muscle plays its part uniquely; for example, the masseter is particularly known for its power, enabling strong jaw closure, while the temporalis helps elevate and retract the mandible. Pterygoid muscles, owing to their unique orientation, deliver the lateral movements necessary for food manipulation. These synergistic interactions among muscles are not only critical for adequate mastication but also for speech and swallowing, underlining the interconnectedness of these functions in the oral cavity's anatomy, a barrier vital to various physiological functions (Burgess et al., 2017). Anatomical evidence proves the significance of muscles of mastication beyond mere mechanical effect. For example, the lateral pterygoid plays a crucial role in lateral jaw excursion enabling the grinding motion that reduces food particles. Their effectiveness is backed by the fact that they are involved with the TMJ, a critical pivot point. Malfunctions or disorders of the muscles or TMJ can cause mastication disorders that interrupt mastication to produce pain, restrictions in jaw movement, or even headaches. Because the oral cavity is essential in the process of digestion and communication, the health of the muscles that are involved in mastication plays a significant part in maintaining overall well-being and quality of life (Burgess et al., 2017) (Figure 8.5).

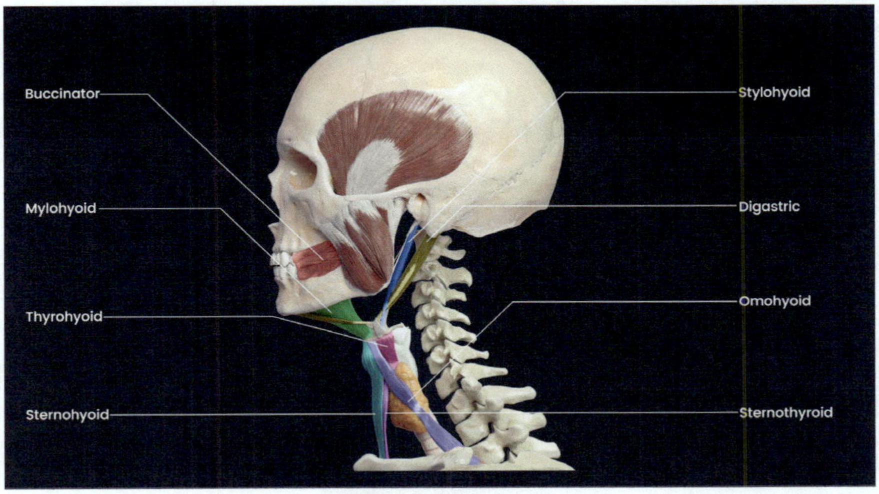

Figure 8.5. Accessory muscles of mastication.

Source: https://admin.anatomy.app/Media/images/9b584553-dd30-4935-86f6-158046b4fc82_large.jpg.

Research on the evolution of mastication muscle adaptations presents a fascinating trajectory under dietary and communication pressures. Modularity in anatomy can be used to understand how the muscular system of the head and neck evolved to accommodate different environments. Experiments conducted on the anatomical network analysis have shown that while early primates possessed more rudimentary muscular integration, the later anthropoids possessed asymmetrical facial modules, which allowed for complex facial expressions, likely to be associated with social and communicative complexity. This enhanced muscular organization reflects a shift towards a higher number of muscles of the head and neck, which, paradoxically, translated to reduced network density and complexity in humans. These findings highlight the subtle distinction between structural modifications and functional demands placed on the muscles of mastication.

8.2.1. Overview of Chewing Muscles

The muscles of mastication, which are responsible for the mastication process, include the masseter, temporalis, and pterygoid muscles. The masseter muscle, regarded by most as the strongest muscle despite its size, originates from the zygomatic arch and is inserted on the mandible to enable effective elevation and retrusion of the jaw. The muscle significantly contributes to the anatomical organization of the jaw to allow effective grinding and tearing of food. Besides these, the fan-shaped temporalis muscle lateral to the head is also synchronized with the masseter in mastication. Thanks to its particular location, it can assist in elevating the mandible and retracting the jaw, which underscores the importance of such muscles in dynamic masticatory functions essential for effective digestion and nutrition. The pterygoid muscles, which include the medial and lateral components, are significant in the complex chewing biomechanics. The medial pterygoid muscle, located on the medial side of the mandible, primarily helps in jaw elevation, similar to the masseter. But the lateral pterygoid muscle allows for protrusion of the mandible forward, a crucial component of the grinding process in mastication. These muscles act synergistically to produce a smooth force, allowing for the minute movements involved in mastication of diverse foods (Figure 8.6).

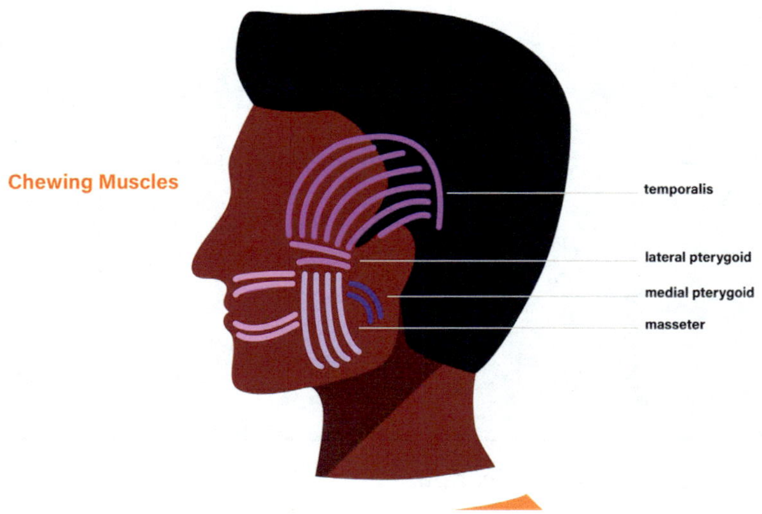

Figure 8.6. Chewing muscles.

Source: https://external-content.duckduckgo.com/iu/?u=https%3A%2F%2Fwww.eatingwell.com%2Fthmb%2FA20DMzX8UOsNdGeG2HaaiDt_Dq8%3D%2F1500x0%2Ffilters%3Ano_upscale()%3Amax_bytes(150000)%3Astrip_icc()%2Fchewing-muscles-2000-ffa0eee911c549bcb777b9582ca4ccf5.jpg&f=1&nofb=1&ipt=597e4fbe401e55b85e1fb2ae5dd90492d70accf7d26fada68c6faa9a6c7f4d77.

Their integration reflects the evolutionary specialization of the human jaw to deal with omnivorous diets, displaying a remarkable amount of specialization that allows both functional proficiency and dietary variability. Dysfunction in the muscles of chewing can potentially lead to significant functional impairment, both in oral and overall health. For instance, conditions such as bruxism, TMJ dysfunction, and other muscular imbalances can disrupt proper masticatory function, leading to pain and diminished quality of life. Additionally, there is evidence of the existence of a high correlation between swallowing dysfunctions and the muscular dynamics of chewing; children who had such dysfunctions showed measurable differences in orofacial muscle activity with the application of orthodontic treatments, affirming the relatedness of chewing and swallowing (Giustino et al., 2019). Additionally, studies indicate varying cranial bone stress during feeding among species and suggest that chewing muscles are not only involved in food processing but also drive cranial form and plasticity according to diets (Evans et al., 2014). Such an overlap between anatomy and function highlights the significance of chewing muscles in terms of health and concerning medicine and dentistry.

8.2.2. Key Muscles Involved in Mastication

Mastication, or chewing, is a complex process involving the coordinated movement of multiple muscle groups in the head and neck. The four main muscles working for this intention are the masseter, temporalis, lateral pterygoid, and medial pterygoid. The masseter muscle, a powerfully built muscle located at the angle of the jaw, elevates the mandible to shut the teeth and crush food. Its powerful composition aids forceful movement and is thus crucial for adequate mastication. The temporalis, located on the side of the head, primarily helps draw the mandible up and backwards, thereby aiding the overall process. This intricate interplay between the muscles not only facilitates the mechanical breakdown of food but also accentuates the evolutionary adaptation of these structures so that they can optimize the processing of the diet, as is evident through the anatomical intricacy observed among species (Burgess et al., 2017) (Figure 8.7).

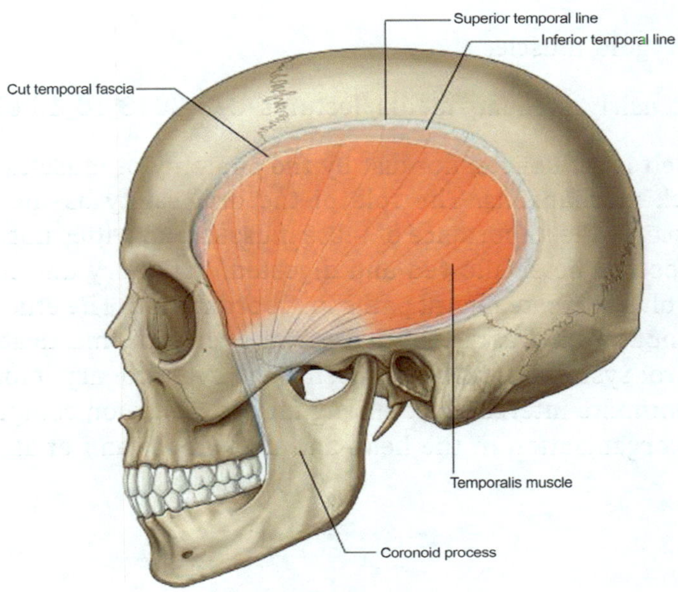

Figure 8.7. Temporalis muscle (muscle of mastication).

Source: https://uomustansiriyah.edu.iq/media/lectures/2/2_2018_10_16!07_54_34_AM.pdf.

Besides these large muscles, the medial and lateral pterygoids play an important role in the mastication process. The lateral pterygoid is unique in that it allows for protraction and lateral mandibular movement and thus can allow side-to-side motion—vital to grinding and crushing food between the molars. Conversely, the medial pterygoid elevates the mandible and assists the masseter to provide the compressive force for adequate mastication. The precise coordination of the four muscles not only ensures mechanistically optimal food processing but also aids in the optimization of mandible motion, proving the functional significance of coordination of muscles in mastication (Burgess et al., 2017) (Figure 8.8).

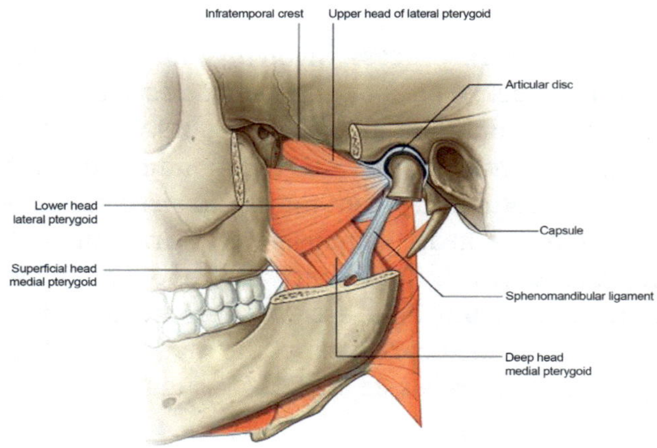

Figure 8.8. Lateral pterygoid muscle.

Source: https://uomustansiriyah.edu.iq/media/lectures/2/2_2018_10_16!07_54_34_AM.pdf.

Further, mastication itself is influenced not just by the anatomy of muscles but also by neurologic regulation and feedback mechanisms. The role of the oral cavity as the initial segment of the digestive system underscores the importance of these muscular activities not only in food breakdown but also in preparing food to be swallowed and digested. Voluntary and involuntary masticatory muscle contractions involve intricate neural paths for coordination. The efficiency of chewing is also augmented by sensory input from oral tissues that permits real-time masticatory compensation. This multi-dimensional control system ultimately presents the evolutionary importance of mastication, suggesting there is an intimate interconnect among dietary behavior, compliance of structure, and musculoskeletal (MSK) organization in the head and neck (Goswami et al., 2018) (Figure 8.9).

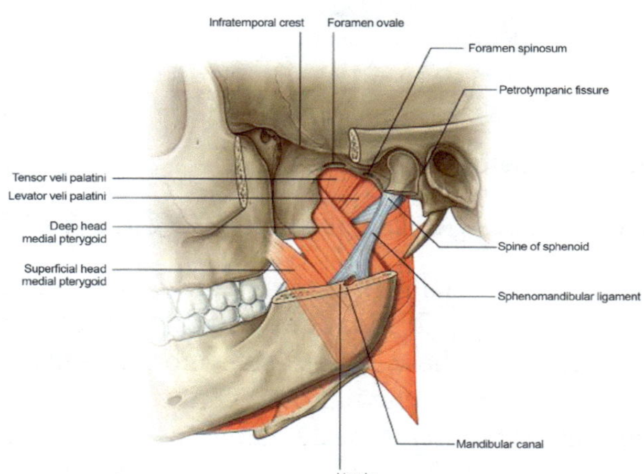

Figure 8.9. Medial pterygoid muscle.

Source: https://uomustansiriyah.edu.iq/media/lectures/2/2_2018_10_16!07_54_34_AM.pdf.

8.2.3. Importance of Mastication for Digestion

Mastication, or chewing, is essential in food digestion via mechanical disintegration of solid food particles and presentation of large surface areas for enzymatic action. The process is a complicated one that involves the coordinated action of various muscles in the head and neck, including the masseter, temporalis, and pterygoid muscles. As they close, they create the grinding movement that is necessary to fragment food into small pieces, which not only aids in swallowing but also enhances the efficiency of the digestive enzymes secreted in the stomach. Moreover, physical fragmentation of food initiates the process of digestion by stimulating the excretion of saliva rich in essential enzymes such as amylase, which is crucial for the digestion of carbohydrates. Therefore, proper mastication is vital for maximizing digestion, such that food is adequately prepared for further biochemical degradation and nutrient uptake, especially. Mastication is also associated with the overall health of the gastrointestinal tract, especially concerning dietary fiber. Studies show that food containing dietary fiber has a considerable impact on oral and gastric secretions and upper gastrointestinal tract motility. This modulation is particularly fitting as fiber physically alters the physicochemical properties of the luminal contents and affects the efficiency with which the stomach can continue digestion. Foods high in fiber require more effective mastication, which yields greater salivary production with the stimulation of digestive enzymes and hence makes the process of digestion a more effective one. By allowing for an adequate shearing of fiber-containing foods during mastication, individuals can effectively support their gastrointestinal health, and in doing so, potentially shield themselves from several upper GI pathology as revealed by emerging evidence (Brownlee et al., 2014). Further, functional characteristics of the masticatory apparatus are capable of profoundly affecting its efficiency, as detailed by studies that examined the musculature's morphology and activity. Varying muscle thickness and integrity in the strength of bite force are essential parameters in the evaluation of masticatory efficiency and, consequently, digestion. Research has shown that temporomandibular dysfunction can result in a decrease in bite force in subjects, which can compromise their performance in chewing and digesting food (Pereira et al., 2018). In addition, factors such as dentition stage and age can influence these characteristics, notably the transition from mixed to permanent dentition, which is associated with an increase in bite force due to enhanced masticatory efficiency. Overall, the interaction between mastication and digestion identifies the importance of the masticatory muscles in both nutrient assimilation and gastrointestinal well-being.

Test Your Knowledge

1. What is the primary function of the chewing muscles?
2. Why is mastication important for the digestive process?

8.3. Neck Muscles Overview

Learning Outcome

1. Understand the major muscle groups in the neck
2. Describe the functions of neck muscles
3. Explain the relationship between neck muscles and head movement

The neck muscles play a crucial role in enabling a range of movement and structural support within the head and neck area. Composed of several separate groups of muscles, the muscles can be generally categorized as extrinsic and intrinsic muscle groups. Extrinsic muscles, such as the trapezius and sternocleidomastoid (SCM), are predominantly responsible for gross movement, including flexion of the head and rotation of the head. Conversely, intrinsic muscles like the scalenes and the longus capitis play a vital role in fine postural adjustment and preservation of respiratory function. Both the anatomy of these muscle groups and their functional study are essential to appreciate their contribution to medical disorders of the head and neck. The anatomical significance of these muscles merely underlines the necessity for complete evaluation of neck muscles to understand their contribution towards MSK well-being. The evolutionary aspects of neck musculature contribute to their morphological and functional sophistication. Recent research in using network theory to investigate skull and neck anatomy demonstrates that the MSK system has evolved to accommodate more sophisticated modes of communication, particularly in the case of primates. The study proves that the facial module asymmetrical growth in anthropoids is linked with the ability to express more intricate, subtle emotions and thus highlights the functional value of those muscles to social living. Moreover, higher counts of head and neck muscles accompanying human evolution are linked with reduced network density and structural complexity in humans, and this suggests that there exists a trade-off between muscular expansion and structural efficiency. These findings require a critical analysis of how anatomical adaptation influences both evolutionary biology and clinical practice in respect to the head and neck. With technology in medical imaging evolving, the need to be familiar with the musculature of the neck compared to pathologies like perineural spread (PNS) of tumors is crucial. The intricate plexus of cranial nerves that innervates the muscles of the neck is often involved in malignancies located at head and neck locations. Of specific interest, tumors of the trigeminal and facial nerves are often engaged in neural pathway dissemination, which can improve prognoses and complicate treatment regimens. The implications of recognizing PNS are of the highest priority; it calls for an activist approach in imaging diagnosis, wherein familiarity with the anatomy of neck muscles assists in accurate evaluation and treatment. Therefore, it is essential to have a thorough understanding of neck musculature not only to comprehend its normal physiology but also to combat the intricacies emerging due to pathological processes within this vulnerable zone of the body (Goswami et al., 2018; Ciurea et al., 2021).

8.3.1. Major Muscle Groups in the Neck

The neck also holds numerous essential muscle groups that are at the core of a range of functions, including movement, stabilization, and support of head and neck structures. Some of the most prominent muscles found in the neck is the SCM muscle, which plays a vital role in the rotation and flexion of the head. Its unique position allows it to perform motions such as bending the head to the shoulder or turning it to look in different directions. The trapezius muscle, extending from the occipital bone to the center of the back, also assists in lateral flexion and extension of the neck, along with motion of the shoulder. All these muscles are involved in dynamic head mobility, allowing free movement that is essential in day-to-day activities as well as in complex physical exertion (Figure 8.10).

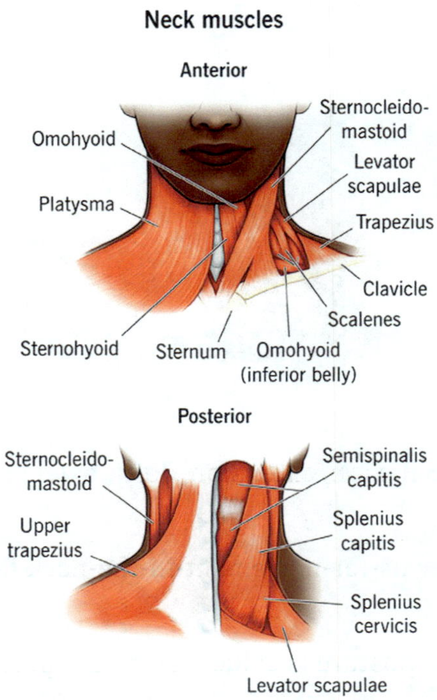

Figure 8.10. Your neck muscles are part of a complex musculoskeletal system that connects the base of your skull to your torso.

Source: https://my.clevelandclinic.org/-/scassets/images/org/health/articles/neck-muscles.

The second large group of neck muscles is the scalene muscles, which include the anterior, middle, and posterior scalene. They are primarily responsible for lateral flexion of the neck and assist in elevation of the first and second ribs during inspiration, and therefore their function in respiratory mechanics. The scalene muscles also serve a vital protective role in guarding the brachial plexus and large vessels, as these structures course from the neck downward into the upper limbs. Such a design is made possible for a functional correlation between respiration and movement of the upper limb, demonstrating how intertwined the muscle groups are. Understanding the anatomy and function of the scalene muscles is crucial to clinicians and students, particularly in diagnosing and treating MSK disorders of the neck and shoulder region. Furthermore, deeper layers of the muscles of the neck, including the longus colli and the longus capitis, have a significant role to play in the stability and mobility of the cervical spine. These muscles perform essential functions such as sustaining the head's posture and allowing the finest of movements of the neck. Latest studies using anatomical network analysis (AnNA) have found evolutionary specializations of these groups of muscles, particularly their integration and modularity within the head and neck MSK system (Goswami et al., 2018). The evolutionary significance of these muscles is reinforced through this research, as it points out how increases in muscular complexity can affect overall functional ability globally. The relationship between anatomy and muscle organization is particularly emphasized, with modifications in the neck muscles having far-reaching effects beyond the fundamental aspects of posture to encompass such sophisticated evolutionary attributes as vocalization and facial expression in primates.

8.3.2. Functions of Neck Muscles

Neck muscle movements are critical to several movements and postures and facilitate both head mobility and stability. They include primarily the SCM and trapezius muscles and contribute crucially to several activities such as nodding, turning, and tilting. The SCM, for instance, contracts bilaterally to flex the neck and on one side to rotate and laterally flex the head to the opposite side. This exceptional capability allows for dynamic movements required in everyday activities, from driving to reading. The trapezius also supports significantly by stabilizing both the cervical spine and the shoulder girdle, thus contributing to general upper body posture and power. The interdependence of these muscles on one another emphasizes their capacity to provide an even and effective MSK system, revealing the complexity of neck muscle activity in the human body. Aside from facilitating movement, muscles in the neck make substantial contributions to postural stability and the integration of stability with other human functioning systems, particularly locomotion and complex action (Figure 8.11).

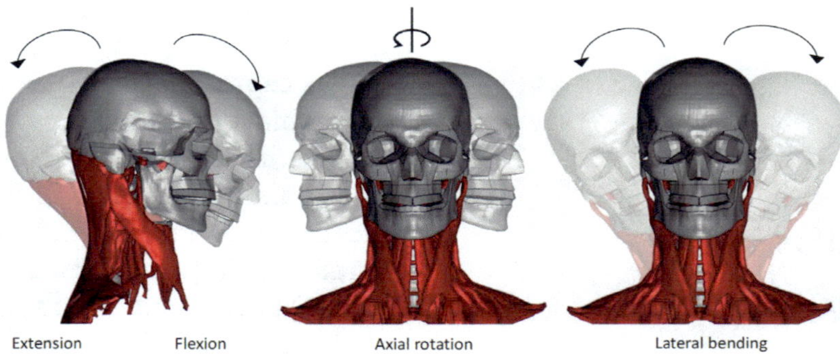

Figure 8.11. Anatomical terms for movement in the neck: flexion/extension [left], axial rotation [middle], lateral bending [right].

Source: https://www.researchgate.net/figure/Anatomical-terms-for-movement-in-the-neck-flexion-extension-left-axial-rotation_fig1_350823152.

The intricate relationship between neck muscle function and posture is evidenced by the possibility that tension and coordination variations may influence overall head and neck alignment. For instance, strengths or abnormalities of the muscles of the neck can lead to secondary adaptations in the remaining muscles that may hurt gait and balance. These relations are especially crucial to realize, especially about certain medical conditions. Treatment to enhance the functioning of such muscles has a significant impact on postural alignment and stability,. It hence reinforces their role not just in the process of movement but in locomotor capacity and in overall biomechanical health, as indicated when explaining complex sensory systems which guarantee stable locomotion (Gurfinkel, 2025). Moreover, the neck muscles also exhibit a remarkable correlation with structural structures such as the hyoid bone, which is responsible for the maintenance of posture and enabling appropriate airway mechanics. The hyoid bone unique suspensory apparatus, supported frombone's unique suspensory apparatus, supported by muscles in the neck, allows essential functions of the cervix, such as breathing and swallowing. Surgical interventions such as hyoid suspension highlight the importance of integrity in the neck muscles; surgical interventions illustrate how movements within the suprahyoid and infrahyoid musculature impact overall posture and movement kinematics. In post-operative evaluation, changes in postural stability portray the interdependency between neck muscle function and optimal hyoid mechanics, and persistent adaptive mechanisms reasserting the body's ability to change over time for structural changes. These results emphasize the significance of neck muscle functions not only in mobility but also in the maintenance of physiological balance. Hence, coordination between the skeletal systems and the neck muscles is a dominant element in the efficiency of human movement and well-being (Battaglia et al., 2017).

8.3.3. Relationship Between Neck Muscles and Head Movement

The intricate relationship between the neck muscles and head movement is the direct cause of the effortless execution of a multitude of motions required for daily functions and activities. The neck has numerous muscles, like the SCM, trapezius, and splenius, that collectively manage head orientation and posture. Muscles work synergistically to execute complex movements such as rotation, flexion, and extension. Dysfunction of any of these muscles may lead to limited mobility and pain in the head. Moreover, conditions like forward head posture (FHP) can exacerbate these, leading to alterations in both musculature and associated ROM. Current studies reveal that FHP subjects display heightened mechanosensitivity of the cervical tissue, which means reduced pain threshold and ROM, such as extension and right rotation, disclosing the connection between muscle mechanics and head movement efficiency (Ochoa et al., 2020). Understanding the functions of neck muscles in head movement steps into the domain of evolutionary anatomy, particularly when primates and their communication adaptations are taken into account. An AnNA study reveals how the head and neck MSK complex developed to support more sophisticated features of facial expression and vocalization. The evolution of asymmetrical facial modules in anthropoids illustrates a shift towards evolved expression, facilitated by the intricate interaction of neck musculature. This evolutionary perspective points out that while the number of head and neck muscles has grown overall, it has paradoxically led to a decrease in network complexity and density in humans (Goswami et al., 2018). This means that the functional needs of head movement and expression have shaped the anatomical organization of neck muscles so that they emphasize their flexibility following communicative needs. The clinical uses of understanding the connection between head movement and neck muscles are particularly valuable in the clinic. Conditions such as MSK pain and cervical spine pathology are closely related to neck muscle function and are frequently examined through physical therapy. Interventions that strengthen or stretch specific muscles of the neck can lead to better head movement and decreased pain. Furthermore, recognition of the impact of posture, and specifically FHP, allows for targeted treatment focused on the preservation of MSK balance. This not only enhances patients' quality of life but also highlights the importance of efficient functioning of neck muscles in the context of moving the head. With ongoing research further specifying these interactions, more therapeutic interventions can be tailored to provide a counteracting effect of the negative impact of MSK dysfunction of the neck.

Test Your Knowledge

1. What are the primary functions of neck muscles?
2. How do neck muscles contribute to head movement and stability?

8.4. Muscles Involved in Facial Expression

Learning Outcome

1. Identification of key facial expression muscles
2. Define mechanisms of facial expression
3. Understand the impact of facial muscles on non-verbal communication

The intricate network of muscles involved in the expression of the face is mainly composed of the mimetic muscles, which are specifically charged with expressing emotional states and social signals. Unlike the other skeletal muscles, which are primarily responsible for the movement of the skeleton, these muscles can alter the face's skin, permitting the function of smiling, frowning, and elevation of the eyebrows. This ability to produce subtle expressions has profound implications for non-verbal interaction, as the display of facial features can play a decisive role in determining interpersonal relationships and social association. From primate evolution comes an understanding of the divergence and asymmetry in facial muscles that express an adaptation for the display of more subtle emotions, demonstrating how anatomical variation is linked to behavioral potential in social contexts, highlighting the significance of facial expressiveness in human behavior and evolution (Goswami et al., 2018). Development of the facial expression muscles is even more fascinating when viewed in the context of anatomical variation across species. The study reveals how embryonic lineage is responsible for variance between such muscles, reflecting an intricate pattern of evolutionary experience. One of the enduring significances is the involvement of cranial neural crest mesenchyme in patterning the development and integration of skin, muscle, and connective tissue of the face. Disruptions at this stage of development can lead to a range of defects or variations impacting performance and expression in various species. Not only does this help highlight the importance of genetic and environmental input into development, but it also illustrates the forces of evolution that are active upon facial morphology and function (Abzhanov et al., 2019). These factors enhance the comprehension of how intricate control of facial expressions has evolved to enhance the capabilities of communication. Additionally, the evolution of the face muscles employed in facial expression mirrors the utmost adaptability and complexity of the MSK system. In humans, the increase in the number of such muscles corresponds with a reduced network density, which signifies a transition towards more evolved control over facial expressiveness. This evolution enables the expression of a broader range of emotions and nuances, crucial for effective communication in social groups. Additionally, while the overall organization of facial muscles is preserved across primates, human beings possess unique asymmetrical facial modules that highlight our capacity for complex expressions. The investigation of this muscle growth reveals a robust correlation between anatomical form and functional capacity, underscoring the adaptive role of facial expression to refine social interaction and emotional nuance (Goswami et al., 2018; Abzhanov et al., 2019).

8.4.1. Identification of Key Facial Expression Muscles

It is essential to acknowledge the dominant facial expression muscles in the quest to know the manner in which emotions are expressed and perceived. The intricate network of facial muscles enables the expression of a vast array of emotions, ranging from smiles to tears. Two critical muscles are the zygomaticus major and minor, which are responsible for lifting the outer corners of the mouth to form smiles. In addition, the orbicularis oculi muscle plays a very significant role in the display of happiness in that it enables the skin around the eyes to crinkle, more commonly referred to as "crow's feet." Learning these muscles reveals not only the biological basis of emotional expression but also emphasizes just how significant they are in the context of social interaction and communication. The intricate analysis of such facial muscles is also helpful in fields such as psychology, anthropology, and robotics, wherein identification and simulation of human expressions is crucial (193825 et al., 2018) (Figure 8.12).

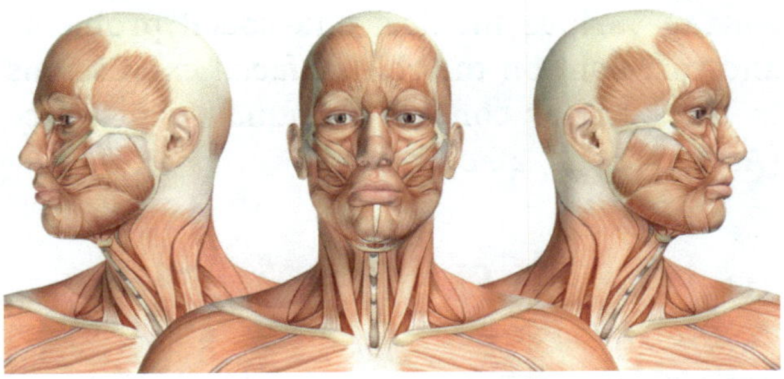

Figure 8.12. Anatomical illustration of facial and neck muscles from multiple angles, showing muscle structure involved in expression and movement.

Source: https://revisedental.com/wp-content/uploads/2020/05/shutterstock_326899520-scaled.jpg.

Moreover, the platysma and corrugator supercilii muscles make it possible for more developed facial expressions. The platysma, from jaw to neck, is used in expressions of sorrow or shock, and the corrugator supercilii, located above the eyebrows, is used in frowning or worry. All this diversity in the muscular structure allows for minute variations in facial expression, enabling human social life and emotional experience. Besides, studies have shown that the correct interpretation of facial expressions is essential for effective communication; observation has particular importance in cases such as therapy and robotics, wherein identification of emotions can be utilized towards smoother interactions. The mechanisms through which these muscles work are a very impressive coming together of biological functioning and emotional psychology (Blow et al., 2009). Besides, the study of facial expression muscles holds significant consequences in several applied fields, including robotics and artificial intelligence. The development of robots like KASPAR demonstrates the potential for the development of machines that can carry out human-like social interactions via facial expression articulation. By simulating human facial musculature, robots can respond emotionally aptly, thus resulting in more natural human-machine interactions. This multidisciplinary answer, one that combines understanding from anatomy, psychology, and design, is a true step forward in the field of human-robot interaction studies. As we examine muscle expression mechanisms, the ability to simulate or read these feelings will soon lead to profound changes in therapeutic practices, educational practices, and machinery interfaces (193825 et al., 2018).

8.4.2. Mechanisms of Facial Expression

Facial expression physiology is directly related to the head and neck muscles in a complicated interaction of anatomical configuration and physiological regulation. The facial muscles are the primary facial expression muscles, which are innervated primarily by the facial nerve (cranial nerve VII). These muscles, including the orbicularis oculi and zygomaticus major, enable fine control over facial expressions, allowing humans to express a wide range of emotions. Each muscle contributes its share towards overall coordination of expression through coordinated contractions that may be modulated in intensity and duration. Drawing on this information can be crucial for appreciating not only the underlying mechanisms of human emotion but also their implications for communication, social bonding, and even the management of disease states involving facial musculature and expression (Figure 8.13).

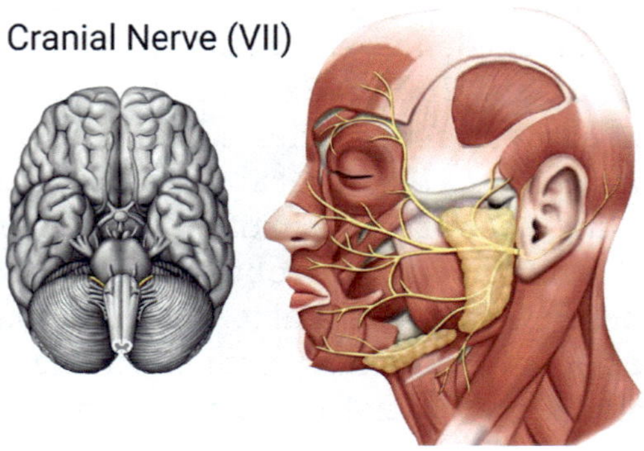

Figure 8.13. cranial nerve VII.

Source: https://media.allaboutvision.com/cms/caas/v1/media/406904/data/picture/056a4e2e01f26e30b4490898da6bfc09.jpg.

Recent research has highlighted how processes of development that control these facial muscles can influence their functional efficacy. The cranial neural crest mesenchyme plays a key role in jaw- and face-associated muscle organization and patterning, as seen in most species, including humans. Abnormalities within these developmental processes could lead to alterations in muscle development, like facial asymmetry, or influence the ability to express emotions. Studies on the molecular and cellular mechanisms of muscle development provide important insights into the evolutionary adaptations of facial and jaw musculature and their connections to social and communicative behaviors. These considerations imply the salience of facial expressions not only as biological functions but also as adaptive traits that have optimized human adaptability within social environments, a sign of complex evolutionary brocade constructed through anatomy and behavior (Abzhanov et al., 2019). Furthermore, the biomechanics inherent in facial expressions further delineate their salience in human relationships. The dynamic nature of such expressions—along with the intricate organization of connective tissues and nerves—allows rapid and robust signals to be communicated in social situations. Such complexity has high relevance in fields such as psychology and artificial intelligence, where human facial expressions can be deciphered to ease interpersonal communication and enhance interface designs. Additionally, understanding these mechanisms is necessary for intervention in cosmetic and reconstructive surgery, in which the restoration of muscular function and expression plays a crucial role in improving patient results. With an increasing number of studies continuing to unveil the nuances of muscular movement and expression in the head and neck, the increased awareness will aid in solving various medical and social problems and cast light on the role of facial expressions in the broader context of human experience (Aspden et al., 2014).

8.4.3. Impact of Facial Muscles on Non-Verbal Communication

Active movements of the facial muscles significantly impact the non-verbal language complexities. These muscles play a critical role in the expression of emotions and intentions without verbal language. Facial expressions, formed through the contraction and, in turn, relaxation of muscles, allow individuals to convey nuanced emotional states, thus allowing for interpersonal connections. Research has shown that specific facial expressions, such as smiles or frowns, can produce respective emotional responses in observers, signifying the broader role of facial musculature in social interaction. This means the general importance of facial expressions in communication and points to the significance of the interaction between anatomy and emotion. Understanding of the mechanisms enhances our comprehension of human interaction, particularly within environments such as those of therapists or social gatherings. The interaction between facial muscles and emotional expression extends beyond dyadic interaction and permeates different fields of professionalism. In customer service interactions, for instance, the service staff members' facial expressions can mimic those of customers, thereby influencing the emotional temper of the interaction. An experiment to validate the impact of facial expressions in service failure recognized that service employees had facial expressions mirroring the angry consumer's emotional state, hence inducing emotional contagion in the service encounter (Butcher et al., 2007). The importance of facial muscles in determining reactions and outcomes in service contexts, where the sensitivity and awareness of emotions have the power to enhance customer satisfaction, is thus accentuated. By gaining insight into their facial expressions, experts can handle complex emotional areas like a pro, with the result being more productive communication and resolution strategies. Furthermore, the implications of non-verbal communication from facial muscles extend into humanoid robot design aimed at social interaction. A prime example of this is the minimally expressive robot KASPAR, which uses facial musculature design to enhance human-robot interaction research (Blow et al., 2009). This robot design is aimed at delivering emotional expression and understanding, reflecting the necessity of non-verbal communication within successful interactions. By mimicking human facial expressions, KASPAR is capable of interacting with users in a manner that provides support for therapeutic and interactive sessions, particularly for users with social impairments. These developments reflect the use of facial muscles not only within biological interaction but also in technological development directed towards human-like interaction and imitation. Therefore, research into the function of facial muscles in non-verbal communication connects biology and technology, molding the future of the model of interpersonal interactions.

Test Your Knowledge

1. Which muscles are primarily responsible for facial expressions like smiling or frowning?
2. How do facial muscles create different expressions?

8.5. Muscles of the Neck and Their Functions

Learning Outcome

1. Describe the major muscles of the neck and their functional roles
2. Explain the significance of neck muscles in supporting and maintaining posture
3. Analyze the contribution of neck muscles to head stability and controlled movement

The neck muscles are of extreme importance in supporting different functionalities and motions necessary for everyday activity. They can be classified into two large groups based on their position: anterior and posterior muscles. The anterior muscles, the major one being the SCM, are essential for rotation of the head as well as flexion, enabling people to tilt and turn their heads in diverse directions. This asymmetrical orientation of this muscle allows for it to play a double role, both as a flexor and rotator of the neck. The opposing muscles, for example, the trapezius and the splenius group, are responsible for extending and stabilizing the neck. Suppose one is familiar with the anatomical and functional features of these muscle groups. In that case, one can gain an appreciation for how they all contribute to bigger movements and posture alignment as part of the overall neck and head musculature. After their initial movement, the neck muscles contribute significantly to posture support, which is essential to physical health. Poor posture over time is a cause of muscular strain and discomfort, and could be caused by tight or overly developed neck muscles. Muscle weakness of these muscles can also be a cause of instability and lack of support for the cervical spine. The trapezius, running from the back to the neck, is a muscle that has several functions, aiding in shoulder elevation and contributing to the strength of the neck. Also, the deep cervical flexors play a role in improving posture by resisting head weight. It is essential to have a complete concept of the interaction between the muscles since it can dictate therapeutic interventions in neck pain and postural correction, as well as quality of life. Higher learning has highlighted that the effect of neck muscle function is greater than simplistic mechanical movements. To illustrate, research in complementary and alternative medicine using scientific studies reveals correlations between nervous representation in muscular pathways and acupuncture points. Such a holistic knowledge suggests that acupuncture may engage neck muscles as well as associated nervous coordination in therapeutic applications to enhance muscular function and overall health. Such findings indicate how practices going back thousands of years could add to current anatomical knowledge, possibly bridging the gap between traditional knowledge and contemporary medical applications. Therefore, it is possible for a multidimensional review of the neck muscles and their complex inter-relationships to give valuable information, informing clinical procedures and expanding our knowledge of the complex interactions of the musculature of the body (Dorsher, 2009; Casagrande-Jaloretto et al., 2013).

8.5.1. Major Muscles of the Neck and Their Roles

The neck houses a series of essential muscles used for the movement and fixation of the head. The key player in this respect is the SCM muscle, which originates from the sternum and clavicle and attaches to the mastoid process of the temporal bone. It permits a variety of movements, including rotation and flexion of the neck, thereby allowing one to look sideways or nod. It is also essential in the maintenance of posture, effectively resisting weight transmission during movement of the head. Beyond its functional importance, the SCM serves as a landmark during clinical assessment and treatment, outlining anatomical regions of importance to clinicians.

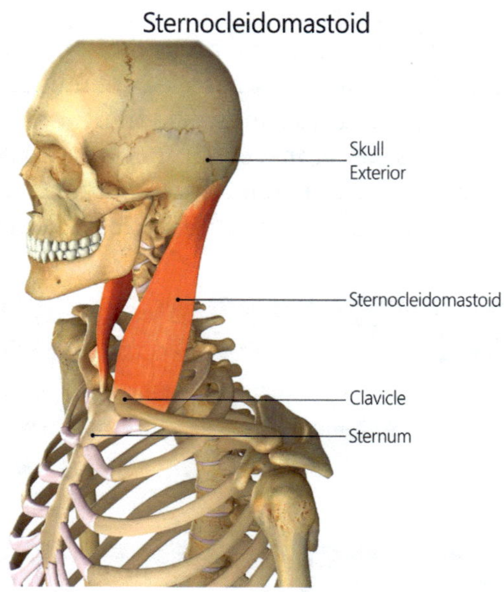

Figure 8.14. Sternocleidomastoid (SCM) muscle.

Source: https://www.rehabmypatient.com/media/uploads/articles/Sternocleidomastoid.jpg.

Thus, understanding the function of the SCM provides essential observations on anatomical and functional features of cranial movement. Another key muscle of the neck is the trapezius, a big kite-shaped muscle that extends from the occipital bone to the thoracic vertebrae. This versatile muscle has upper, middle, and lower fibers, each serving a distinct function in the motion of the head and shoulders. The upper fibers are used for shrugging the shoulders and elevating the scapula, while the middle fibers assist in retracting the scapula. Notably, the lower fibers contribute to depression of the scapula, further identifying the trapezius as vital for mobility and stability of the upper limb. Its extensive coverage and multifunctional actions render it necessary in athletic performance and daily function. Additionally, the trapezius role crosses into the area of postural support, in that it helps in dissuading disorders related to tension of the neck and shoulder region, which signifies its importance regarding health and function (Figure 8.14). The levator scapulae is another vital muscle of the neck that deserves mention because it is involved in shoulder and neck mechanics. The muscle arises from the transverse processes of cervical vertebrae I, II, III, and IV and attaches to the scapula, particularly the superior angle. Elevation of the scapula is the central role of the levator scapulae, helping in movements like shrugging and lateral bending of the neck. In addition, it also assists the trapezius in stabilizing the shoulder girdle during arm movement. Surprisingly, levator scapulae dysfunction or tightness may also result in neck pain and irritation, especially in patients with poor posture or repetitive strain syndromes. The significance of this muscle stretch extends beyond simple movement, as it relates to daily activities and demonstrates the interaction between neck muscles and general physical well-being. This is particularly evident in disorders such as chronic Otitis media, where muscle function can impact ear health (Baldini et al., 2014).

8.5.2. Importance of Neck Muscles in Posture

Neck muscles play a key role in maintaining proper posture, given that they stabilize the head and cervical spine. These muscles, including SCM, trapezius, and splenius capitis, are responsible for controlling head movements and orienting the head so that it is in line with the spine. When such muscles function well, they assist in the maintenance of neutral spine alignment, minimizing excessive loading on the vertebrae and associated structures. However, the majority of individuals cannot maintain ideal posture due to improper ergonomic habits or lifestyle, thereby inducing muscle strength imbalances in the muscles of the neck. Consequently, the unusual posture may generate pain and increased susceptibility to cervical spine pathology, which can complicate one's overall health and mobility (Kavounoudias et al., 2008). The role of neck muscle fatigue in affecting posture is indicative of the complexity involved in maintaining the body's stability and balance. Experiments have discovered that during muscle fatigue of the neck, compensation is sought through alterations in postural strategies, leading to larger center of pressure displacements and heightened reliance on vestibular and somatosensory input for balance (Kavounoudias et al., 2008) (Figure 8.15).

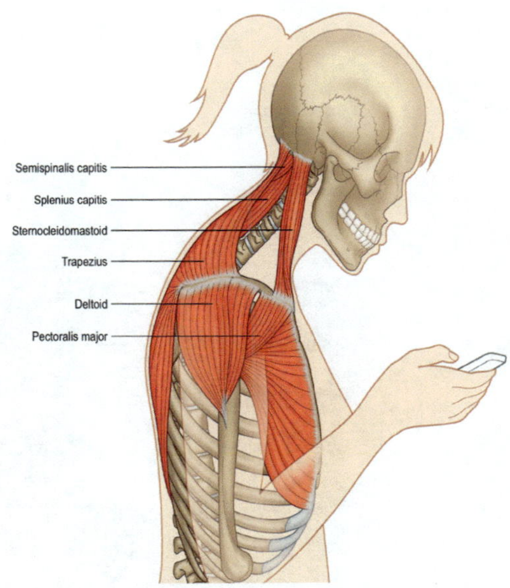

Figure 8.15. Forward head position.

Source: https://images.squarespace-cdn.com/content/v1/5b4e58369d5abb9d6adac232/1551109596558-R7IT939ML9RYM50C7JTT/Figure_18.4.png.

As a result, an inclined head position can exaggerate instability, making it more difficult for individuals to remain standing. This is a classic example of how much the neck muscles play a role in postural control; their fatigue can have a cascading effect on the entire body. Thus, enhancing the strength and endurance of these muscles through specific exercises may improve overall postural stability, leading to better alignment and a reduced risk of postural-related issues. The well-being and working of the muscles of the neck are important, not only for static posture, but also for dynamic movements. A conditioned and strong neck facilitates easy changes in postures, whether sitting, standing, or transitioning. Besides, muscles in the neck contribute significantly to many activities requiring coordination and strength, such as sports and exercise. However, modern lifestyles tend to induce poor posture and muscle imbalance due to prolonged periods of sedentary behavior and poor movement. These challenges are overcome through preventive measures, such as regular physical activity and ergonomic inspections, making them essential. Employing methods such as physiotherapy and exercises will assist in significantly enhancing the strength of the muscles of the neck, ultimately enhancing posture and quality of life for individuals, particularly those with a predisposition to neck and spinal disorders (Ahmad et al., 2015).

8.5.3. Neck Muscles and Their Contribution to Head Stability

The muscles of the neck are essential to the stability of the head, supporting static and dynamic postural control. The SCM, the splenius capitis, and the suboccipital muscles, among others, work in concert to support the weight of the head and allow a range of movement without compromising the integrity of the cervical spine.

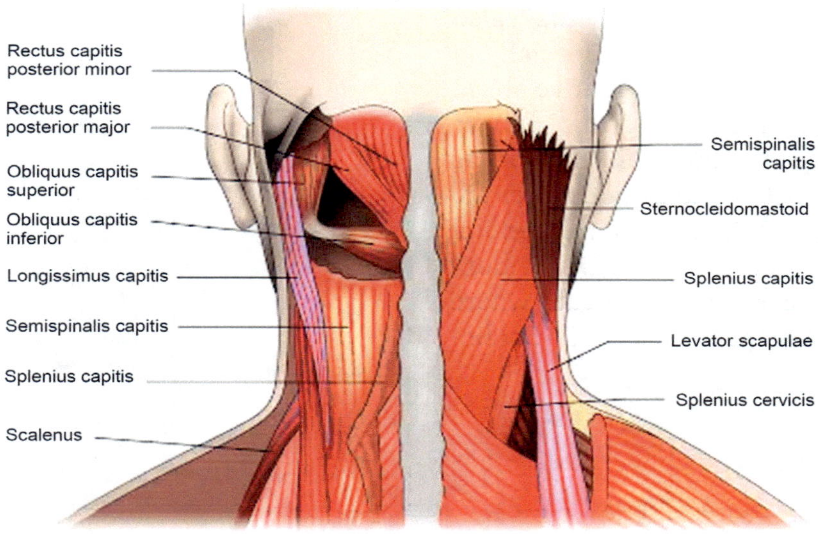

Figure 8.16. This intricate system of muscles is responsible for a variety of functions, making them indispensable for maintaining both stability and mobility in the neck region.

Source: https://centenoschultz.com/wp-content/uploads/csc-neck-muscles.png.webp.

By stabilizing the head during various activities, these muscles play a significant role in maintaining a person's balance and overall functional capacity. Research indicates that neck muscle fatigue can lead to altered performance of balance, which underscores the critical relationship between stability of the head and neck musculature. When neck muscles are fatigued, alterations in sway velocity and perceived stability are noted, which underscores their critical function in the performance of postural control across various conditions (Fagan et al., 2014). Apart from providing static support, the role of neck muscles also includes dynamic proprioception and vestibular integration. Neck muscle mechanoreceptors provide essential feedback to the central nervous system regarding head position and movement. This feedback is crucial for eye and head coordination and stability with static and dynamic tasks. Research shows that muscle fatigue of the neck increases the reliance on vestibular and neck somatosensory information in postural control. The compensation process can cause an increased destabilizing effect when the head is in specific orientations, as reported in situations where subjects performed tasks involving head tilts (Kavounoudias et al., 2008) (Figure 8.16).

These observations highlight the significance of optimal neck muscle function for adequate postural stability. Both in clinical practice and in sport, knowledge of the contribution of neck muscles to head stability is increasingly important. Contact sports players are potentially at greater risk for neck trauma with subsequent influence on stability and balance. Such injury has a cascade of effects, including alterations in proprioceptive feedback and increased use of compensatory mechanisms that place subjects at risk for further injury. Rehabilitation protocols are likely to focus on the strengthening of neck musculature to reinstitute stability and prevent repetition of injury. With consideration of both strength and endurance of the muscles within the neck, practitioners are then able to promote head stability, and subsequently, functional capacity and quality of life in patients rehabilitating from neck injury (Fagan et al., 2014). Last but not least, an integrated view of muscle dynamics in the neck must be used to promote resilience and function in the athletic and non-athletic populations.

Test Your Knowledge

1. What are two major muscles of the neck and what are their primary roles?
2. How do neck muscles help maintain proper posture?

8.6. Clinical Relevance of Head and Neck Muscles

Learning Outcome

1. Discuss the common disorders affecting the head and neck muscles
2. Identify the impact of muscle dysfunction on daily activities
3. Define treatment options for muscle-related issues

The clinical importance of head and neck muscles is much greater than their simple anatomical location; these muscles are pivotal in many physiological processes that are critical to survival and increased quality of life. Understanding the dynamics of these muscles is essential in a wide range of medical situations, particularly in diagnosing and managing conditions such as dysphagia and temporomandibular disorders (TMD). The masticatory and swallowing muscles, including the masseter and the suprahyoid group, can exhibit dysfunction that compromises oral and pharyngeal function. Treatment of such muscular dysfunctions is essential to the restoration of regular eating, speaking, and breathing function, all of which play a large part in an individual's general state of health and well-being. The interactive dynamics of function with structure in these muscles are a reflection of the importance of these muscles in therapy and of the necessity for clinicians to be mindful of such mechanisms in both surgical and rehab therapies (Aspden et al., 2014). In the act of swallowing, structural components of the head and neck work together to facilitate this complex process. The suprahyoid muscles, for instance, are necessary for the hyolaryngeal complex to be raised, a movement which must occur for food passage from the oral cavity to the esophagus to be secure. They can cause dysphagia upon dysfunction, which is the inability to swallow and potential aspiration and associated respiratory issues. The two-sling mechanism of hyolaryngeal elevation has been explored in recent research with emphasis on the coordinated contraction of these muscles for airway protection and safe swallowing. This anatomy knowledge is essential for clinicians working with patients with swallowing disorders and who require measures to optimize muscle function and, as a result, swallowing safety (Pearson et al., 2012). Moreover, assessment of muscle function of the head and neck is of great clinical relevance in the treatment of several medical disorders. For instance, muscle functional MRI and dynamic imaging techniques are crucial elements in the evaluation of contribution of these muscles during the act of swallowing. Understanding how the head and neck muscles are engaged in normal and abnormal swallowing can be utilized to direct targeted interventions such as therapeutic maneuvers and diet modifications. Furthermore, the accurate knowledge of the anatomical and functional interaction among these muscles allows clinicians to develop individualized rehabilitation programs that are capable of reversing the possible risks of dysphagia. In summary, the integrated knowledge of head and neck muscle function and disease proves to illustrate their strong clinical relevance, a fact that continues to drive research unabated as well as new approaches in diagnosis and treatment (Pearson et al., 2012; Aspden et al., 2014).

8.6.1. Common Disorders Affecting Head and Neck Muscles

Head and neck muscle disorders may significantly change the quality of life of a patient, most often leading to chronic pain and disability. Tension-type headache, TMJ disorder, and cervical dystonia are frequently encountered in clinical settings. Muscle contractions in the scalp and neck, secondary to tension or bad posture, often accompany tension-type headache. Likewise, TMJ disorders may also result from tension in the muscles associated with jaw clenching or grinding, causing pain and restricted jaw movement. These disorders not only cause MSK pain but also could cause secondary symptoms such as tiredness, anxiety, and impaired activities of daily living, highlighting the intricate interconnection between physical and psychological well-being among those affected by these disorders.

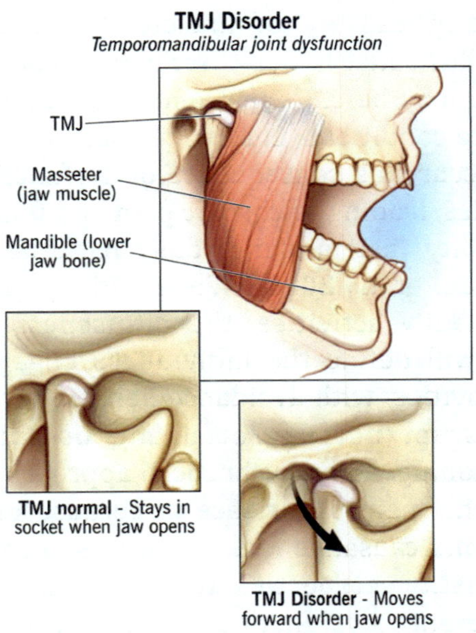

Figure 8.17. Temporomandibular joint (TMJ) disorders are a group of over 30 conditions that affect your jaw joint and surrounding muscles.

Source: https://my.clevelandclinic.org/health/diseases/15066-temporomandibular-disorders-tmd-overview.

Cervical dystonia, which is another common condition, is caused by involuntary muscle contractions in the neck that result in abnormal head positions. This movement disorder involves the SCM and other muscles of the neck, creating severe discomfort and functional impairment for the affected individuals. Patients describe a feeling of tension or pain that can be made worse with activities that demand prolonged head position. Additionally, studies indicated that muscle fatigue in the neck might influence balance as observed in studies of the impact of neck fatigue on sway velocity and subjective stability in active adults (Fagan et al., 2014) (Figure 8.17). Thus, the comprehension of the interaction between muscle function and stability is most crucial in developing effective management plans for cervical dystonia and other allied disorders. Further, management and treatment of these diseases of the head and neck muscles are highly complex and typically need an interdisciplinary approach. Resolution of symptoms mainly relies on physiotherapy, pharmacotherapy, and ergonomic adjustments. For instance, specific exercises and manual treatment can contribute to the restoration of muscle imbalances and the relaxation of hypertonic muscles. Drugs such as muscle relaxants or anti-inflammatory medications may be helpful in offering symptomatic relief, but are often associated with side effects. In addition, patient education regarding posture, stress-controlling measures, and lifestyle modifications may empower individuals to take an active role in their treatment and ultimately improve their results. The requirement to alleviate pain and restore functional capacity is in alignment with current research aimed at optimizing treatment outcomes and quality of life for patients, reiterating the importance of integrative care as it relates to head and neck muscle disorders (Vassallo et al., 2008).

8.6.2. Impact of Muscle Dysfunction on Daily Activities

Head and neck muscles have a significant role not just in simple physiological processes but also in influencing daily routines. Dysfunction in the head and neck muscles can significantly hinder one's ability to accomplish specific tasks that are usually taken for granted. For example, muscle weakness or coordination failure may cause problems with chewing and swallowing, turning mealtime into a fearful prospect. These issues are not just about nutritional intake, but may also lead to social withdrawal due to embarrassment or fear on eating occasions. Because such muscles are essential to communication, any impairment of these muscles will result in speech difficulties, further ostracizing individuals and impacting their social integration. Thus, the effect of head and neck region muscle dysfunction extends beyond physical limitations to include severe emotional and psychological consequences as well. Also, the outcomes of dysfunction of muscles are typically compounded in the process of treatment of head and neck cancer. Patients undergoing such treatments tend to have MSK issues that lead to compromised function. Their treatment protocols, which are typically developed by multidisciplinary teams, aim to correct the same through the inclusion of guidelines for supportive care to avert the harmful impact of muscle dysfunction (David et al., 2020) (Figure 8.18).

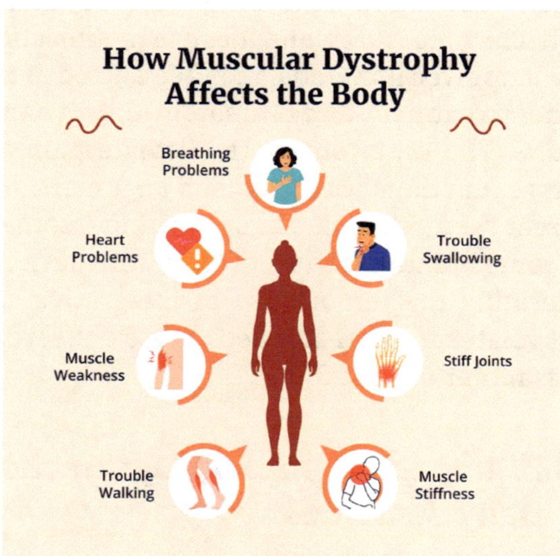

Figure 8.18. Effects of muscular dystrophy on the body, highlighting common symptoms and complications.

Source: https://images.everydayhealth.com/images/seo-graphic-content-initiative/eh-how-muscular-dystrophy-affects-the-body-seo-graphics.png?sfvrsn=8ef8f666_3.

For example, physical therapy and occupational therapy may be started to improve the strength and coordination of the involved muscle groups. Therefore, focused interventions not only aid in the rehabilitation of activities of daily living but also have a significant effect on quality of life as patients deal with treatment and rehabilitation issues. Therefore, the recognition of interaction between muscle dysfunction and everyday functioning supports holistic care methods. The applicability of muscle dysfunction is also illustrated under chronic pain conditions, which may be classified under head and neck muscle conditions. Chronic primary pain (CPP) can occur as a consequence of dysfunctions in muscles, leading to chronic pain and functional disability that influence daily patterns of life (Michael et al., 2018). While patients perform their daily activities, the diffuseness of the pain will define the individual's engagement in activities, with avoidance behaviors tending to disrupt normal social and occupational functioning. A biopsychosocial approach values that this pain experience is because of more than one causative factor, and this encourages a holistic perspective toward management. Addressing dysfunction of the muscles and their subsequent pain, clinicians are able to enhance functional recovery in line with this, empowering patients to resume their daily lives in spite of muscle-related dysfunction issues.

8.6.3. Treatment Options for Muscle-Related Issues

Management of muscle issues in the head and neck is a multi-modal form of solution, addressing various therapeutic avenues unique to the condition at hand. The series of treatments ranges from non-invasive forms, such as physical therapy and exercise protocols, to more invasive treatments such as surgery. Physical therapy tends to be the first line of treatment, consisting of strengthening exercises particular to the head and neck muscles. This rehabilitation can minimize pain and maximize function, especially if the etiology is tension or strain of the muscle. Also, modalities such as ultrasound and electrical stimulation can further promote healing by maximizing circulation and minimizing spasms. Through these combined therapies, practitioners aim to restore normal muscle function with minimal pain, insisting on the importance of an individualized treatment regimen. In addition to physical therapy, pharmacological treatment may also be performed to address muscle issues. Nonsteroidal anti-inflammatory agents (NSAIDs) are usually the first choice in reducing inflammation and pain, should there be muscle damage or TMJ disorder. When over-the-counter medications are deemed insufficient, physicians may prescribe muscle relaxants to treat spasticity and pain more effectively. Moreover, botulinum toxin injections have also become increasingly popular as a form of treatment for certain muscular disorders, particularly those related to chronic tension or pain. Interestingly, such injections can be of great value and contribute significantly to the quality of life, but must be precisely dosed and monitored to avoid side effects. Strategic use of these pharmacologic therapies in conjunction with physical therapy can potentially optimize outcomes, requiring that health care professionals assess each patient's individual needs. For more severe muscle disorders, interdisciplinary therapy may also be beneficial, blending alternative therapy with conventional therapy. Therapy modalities like massage and acupuncture are increasingly popular for their symptomatic relief and overall muscle health value. Literature also endorses the application of these unconventional therapies as a method to relieve muscle tension, enhance recovery, and even improve sleep quality in chronic muscle pain patients, i.e., obstructive sleep apnea (Nelson et al., 2022). The psychological aspects of chronic pain, anxiety, and depression can also be managed by cognitive-behavioral therapy and mindfulness training, encouraging an overall treatment regimen. Multidisciplinary teamwork among various healthcare providers—e.g., physiotherapists, doctors, and complementary practitioners—is capable of offering patients overall care tailored specifically to their respective muscular challenges, ultimately enhancing their recovery process and life quality (Mohiuddin, 2019).

Test Your Knowledge

1. How can muscle dysfunction affect a person's ability to perform daily activities?
2. What are two treatment options commonly used to manage muscle dysfunction?

SUMMARY

Understanding the head and neck muscles is vital in both clinical and anatomical studies. The muscles in the head and neck coordinate several functions, such as movement, posture, and breathing, as well as being involved in complex functions involving neuromuscular regulation. The complex musculature facilitates smooth motion of the head and maintains essential functions like swallowing and speech. Additionally, appreciation of various muscle groups, for example, SCM and trapezius, provides understanding of how an imbalance of the muscles can lead to dysfunction or pain. This has important implications for MSK health and rehabilitation practice practitioners. Research in the neck muscles shows that structural properties are not the sole determining factors, but rather functional capabilities significantly influence proprioceptive accuracy, particularly among patients with neck tension or pain. The findings show that recent muscle contraction history influences head repositioning accuracy, as demonstrated in one study where active posterior neck muscle contraction caused measurable errors in target positioning. The findings indicate the complexity of the interplay between neck muscles and their relevance to clinical procedures, where accurate measurements of muscle function are crucial. Therefore, clinicians must consider historical muscle activity in their evaluation and treatment protocols for cervical-related issues, fostering more personalized and effective intervention approaches (Gudavalli et al., 2006). Advancements in imaging and analysis techniques, such as ultrasound and deep learning algorithms, are revolutionizing our understanding of cervical muscle dynamics. By providing objective visualization of muscle borders, researchers are now able to classify conditions like cervical dystonia more accurately, to distinguish them from normative conditions. Empiric methodology allows for closer monitoring of muscle function and more selective intervention. Such methodologies increase the accuracy of treatment plans and enhance understanding of the pathological mechanisms that control neck disorders. As research continues to explore the link between muscle structure and function, clinicians will be more equipped to enhance diagnostic and therapeutic outcomes in head and neck health (Cunningham et al., 2019).

Head and neck muscles play a major role in several physiological functions, including speech-related movements, swallowing, and facial expressions. A thorough analysis of the groups of muscles begins with their classification anatomically. The muscles belong to two general categories: the facial muscles that control expression, and the muscles of the neck that control movement of the head and neck. This anatomical difference highlights the relationship between form and function, demonstrating how specific muscle configurations enable coordinated action. For example, the SCM muscle is critical for rotation and flexion of the neck, highlighting the role of such muscles in everyday tasks such as the turning of the head to face varying directions. These facts are priceless in the acquisition of a comprehensive view of the biomechanics and functional anatomy of muscles in this region (Aspden et al., 2014). About developmental biology, one has to appreciate that head and neck muscle development differs from trunk muscle development. Studies demonstrate that the head muscles derive primarily from cranial mesoderm, whereas neck muscles originate from a separate lineage, which is referred to as the occipital lateral plate mesoderm. Importantly, research shows that these neck muscles not only have distinct origins but also exhibit separate developmental times, suggesting an onset following other muscle groups. These findings imply that there is a complex evolutionary accommodation since these muscles share similar characteristics to head musculature and do not conform to the typical patterns of development of trunk muscles (Christ et al., 2010). The variation of this diversity illuminates the occurrence of muscle development in different areas of the body, and further research is needed for the evolutionary and genetic origins of these anatomical structures (Aspden et al., 2014). Moreover, the functional importance of this muscle differentiation goes beyond mere movement; it influences the production of speech, breathing, and even emotion. For example, coordination between varying head and neck muscles allows for the fine movements necessary in articulation, which is so vital to human communication. The clinical importance of these groups of muscles is also underscored in that malfunctioning thereof can be a harbinger to speech disorders and other deficits. Exploration of interactions between muscle structure, origin, and function enhances our knowledge of not only human anatomy but also evolutionary biology and genetics, paving the way for revolutionary therapeutic interventions. By incorporating outcomes from developmental biology and functional anatomy, scientists can identify more effective treatments for head and neck musculature pathologies (Christ et al., 2010).

KEY TERMS FROM THIS CHAPTER

- Orbicularis oculi
- Orbicularis oris
- Zygomaticus major
- Zygomaticus minor
- Masseter
- Temporalis
- Platysma
- Sternocleidomastoid
- Scalenes
- Semispinalis capitis
- Digastric
- Levator scapulae
- Splenius capitis
- Acupoints
- Neurology
- Non-verbal communication

CRITICAL THINKING QUESTIONS

1. **Which muscle is primarily responsible for closing the jaw during chewing?**
   a. Temporalis
   b. Sternocleidomastoid
   c. Orbicularis Oris
   d. Platysma
2. **The sternocleidomastoid muscle is involved in:**
   a. Smiling
   b. Rotating and flexing the neck
   c. Closing the eyes
   d. Elevating the shoulders
3. **Which muscle allows you to raise your eyebrows and wrinkle your forehead?**
   a. Masseter
   b. Frontalis
   c. Buccinator
   d. Orbicularis oculi
4. **The orbicularis Oris muscle functions to:**
   a. Blink and close the eyes
   b. Open the jaw
   c. Close and pucker the lips
   d. Rotate the head
5. **Which muscle is an essential one for chewing and is located on the side of the jaw?**
   a. Platysma
   b. Masseter
   c. Zygomaticus
   d. Occipitalis

Short Answer Questions

1. What are the basic principles in the anatomical organization of the head muscles?
2. Name the major muscles of mastication and describe their primary functions.
3. Which key muscles are found in the neck, and what general functions do they serve?
4. List three muscles involved in facial expression and the actions they produce.
5. What are the main functions of the sternocleidomastoid and trapezius muscles in the neck?
6. How do head and neck muscles contribute to daily activities such as speaking, chewing, and swallowing?
7. Why is knowledge of head and neck muscle anatomy clinically significant in healthcare practice?

Answer to Critical Thinking Questions

1. (a); 2. (b); 3. (b); 4. (c); 5. (b)

REFERENCES

1. Woronowicz, K. C., & Schneider, R. A. (2019b). Molecular and cellular mechanisms underlying the evolution of form and function in the amniote jaw. *EvoDevo, 10*(1). https://doi.org/10.1186/s13227-019-0131-8Achalandabaso Ochoa, A., Fernández Matías, R., Gallego Izquierdo, T., Martínez Merinero, R., et al. (2020). Relationship between forward head posture and tissue mechanosensitive: A cross-sectional study. https://core.ac.uk/download/641599489.pdf (accessed on 14th June 2025).
2. Ahmad, A., Ravisankaran, K., Singh, S., Seena, S., et al. (2015). A clinical study to evaluate the effect of Karpasasthyadi Taila Nasya, physiotherapy and a combination of both in cervical spondylosis. https://core.ac.uk/download/333819322.pdf (accessed on 14th June 2025).
3. Aspden, R. M., Gilbert, F. J., Gregory, J., Miller, S., et al. (2014). Using active shape modeling based on MRI to study morphologic and pitch-related functional changes affecting vocal structures and the airway. https://core.ac.uk/download/30435772.pdf (accessed on 14th June 2025).
4. Baldini, A., Fuchs, J. C., Linden, J. F., Tucker, A. S., et al. (2014). A defect in early myogenesis causes otitis media in two mouse models of 22q11.2 deletion syndrome. https://core.ac.uk/download/29410931.pdf (accessed on 14th June 2025).
5. Battaglia, A., Dispenza, F., Gallina, S., Lorusso, F., et al. (2017). Postural changes in patients undergoing hyoid surgery for OSAS. https://core.ac.uk/download/146519220.pdf (accessed on 14th June 2025).
6. Beer, R. D., Izquierdo, E. J., & Williams, P. L. (2015). Information flow through a model of the *C. elegans* klinotaxis circuit. http://arxiv.org/abs/1502.04262 (accessed on 14th June 2025).
7. Bianchi-Berthouze, N. L., Cosentino, S., Kong, W., Sessa, S., et al. (2015). Automatic discrimination of laughter using distributed sEMG. https://core.ac.uk/download/79499855.pdf (accessed on 14th June 2025).
8. Blow, M., Dautenhahn, K., Kose-Bagci, H., Mirza, R., et al. (2009). KASPAR–A minimally expressive humanoid robot for human-robot interaction research. https://core.ac.uk/download/9553210.pdf (accessed on 14th June 2025).
9. Brownlee, I. A. (2014). The impact of dietary fiber intake on the physiology and health of the stomach and upper gastrointestinal tract. https://core.ac.uk/download/237199484.pdf (accessed on 14th June 2025).
10. Bull, N. D. (2015). Will strengthening the cervical muscles of the neck diminish the risk of concussions? https://core.ac.uk/download/233575738.pdf (accessed on 14th June 2025).
11. Burgess, J., Eisen, D., Lynch, D. P., Nordlund, J. J., et al. (2017). Oral examination. https://core.ac.uk/download/213072873.pdf (accessed on 14th June 2025).
12. Butcher, K., Dallimore, K., & Sparks, B. (2007). The influence of angry customer outbursts on service providers' facial displays and affective states. https://core.ac.uk/download/11036908.pdf (accessed on 14th June 2025).
13. Casagrande-Jalorettto, D. C., Brent, C. S., van Englesdorp, D., Cox-Foster, D., Hatjina, F., Dade, H. A., Hatjina, F., et al. (2013). Standard methods for *Apis mellifera* anatomy and dissection. https://core.ac.uk/download/18548084.pdf (accessed on 14th June 2025).

14. Christ, B., Harel, I., Huang, R., Otto, A., et al. (2010). The occipital lateral plate mesoderm is a novel source for vertebrate neck musculature. https://core.ac.uk/download/107913.pdf (accessed on 14th June 2025).

15. Ciurea, A., Csutak, C., Dinu, C., Hedesiu, M., et al. (2021). Perineural spread in head and neck malignancies: Imaging findings–An updated literature review. https://core.ac.uk/download/644449258.pdf (accessed on 14th June 2025).

16. Cunningham, R. J., Harding, P., Kobylecki, C., Loram, I. D., et al. (2019). Objective analysis of neck muscle boundaries for cervical dystonia using ultrasound imaging and deep learning. https://core.ac.uk/download/286351179.pdf (accessed on 14th June 2025).

17. Curtis, N., Evans, S. E., Fagan, M. J., Jones, M. E., et al. (2009). Visualizing muscle anatomy using three-dimensional computer models–An example using the head and neck muscles of *Sphenodon*. https://core.ac.uk/download/1876869.pdf (accessed on 14th June 2025).

18. Dorsher, P. (2009). The neuroanatomic basis of the acupuncture principal meridians. https://core.ac.uk/download/pdf/288827.pdf (accessed on 14th June 2025).

19. Evans, S. E., Fagan, M. J., Iriarte-Diaz, J., O'Reilly, J. C., et al. (2014). *In vivo* cranial bone strain and bite force in the agamid lizard *Uromastyx geyri*. https://core.ac.uk/download/151156686.pdf (accessed on 14th June 2025).

20. Fagan, M. J., & Gosselin, G. (2014). The effects of cervical muscle fatigue on balance–A study with elite amateur rugby league players. https://core.ac.uk/download/151157050.pdf (accessed on 14th June 2025).

21. Giustino, V., Martines, F., Messina, G., Pirino, A., et al. (2019). Orofacial muscles activity in children with swallowing dysfunction and removable functional appliances. https://core.ac.uk/download/286528435.pdf (accessed on 14th June 2025).

22. Goswami, A., Porto, A., Porto, A., Burrows, A. M., Esteve-Altava, B., Esteve-Altava, B., Esteve-Altava, B., et al. (2018). Primate modularity and evolution: First anatomical network analysis of primate head and neck musculoskeletal system. https://core.ac.uk/download/151211716.pdf (accessed on 14th June 2025).

23. Gudavalli, M. R., Henderson, C. N. R., Owens, E. F., Pickar, J. G., et al. (2006). Head repositioning errors in normal student volunteers: A possible tool to assess the neck's neuromuscular system. https://core.ac.uk/download/pdf/3945610.pdf (accessed on 14th June 2025).

24. Gurfinkel, V. S. (2025). Significance of vestibular and proprioceptive afforestation in the regulation of human posture. https://core.ac.uk/download/pdf/42862097.pdf (accessed on 14th June 2025).

25. Kavounoudias, A., Nardone, A., Straube, A., Tagaki, A., Davidson, B. S., Hassan, B. S., Hlavacka, F., et al. (2008). Differential postural effects of plantar-flexor muscles fatigue under normal, altered and improved vestibular and neck somatosensory conditions. http://arxiv.org/abs/0807.3608 (accessed on 14th June 2025).

26. Mohiuddin, A. K. (2019). Issues behind choosing alternative measures to cancer care & cure. *International Research in Medical and Health Science.* https://www.semanticscholar.org/paper/58bdc8c9e869dda6c09a41719901a6b5cc748e3c (accessed on 14th June 2025).

27. N/A. (2018). Branchial cleft cysts: A pictorial review. https://core.ac.uk/download/160736713.pdf (accessed on 14th June 2025).

28. Nelson, B., & Wiles, A. (2022). A more expansive approach to obstructive sleep apnea. *Cancer Cytopathology, 130.* https://www.semanticscholar.org/paper/706a30c1500032ac3419b423ff24167283097356 (accessed on 14th June 2025).

29. Nicholas, M. K., Vlaeyen, J. W. S., Rief, W., Barke, A., Aziz, Q., Benoliel, R., Cohen, M., et al. (2018). The IASP classification of chronic pain for ICD-11: Chronic primary pain. *Pain, 160*, 28–37. https://doi.org/10.1097/j.pain.0000000000001390 (accessed on 14th June 2025).

30. Pearson, W. G. (2012). A two-sling mechanism of hyolaryngeal elevation in the pharyngeal phase of swallowing. https://open.bu.edu/bitstream/2144/12585/11/Pearson_William_2012_nosig_nocv.pdf (accessed on 14th June 2025).

31. Pereira, L. J. (2018). Avaliação morfologica, funcional e sensorial do sistema mastigatorio. https://core.ac.uk/download/296839914.pdf (accessed on 14th June 2025).

32. Pfister, D. G., Spencer, S., Adelstein, D. J., Adkins, D. R., Anzai, Y., Brizel, D. M., Bruce, J. Y., et al. (2020). Head and neck cancers, version 2.2020, NCCN clinical practice guidelines in oncology. *Journal of the National Comprehensive Cancer Network, 18*, 873–898. https://doi.org/10.6004/jnccn.2020.0031 (accessed on 14th June 2025).

33. Taylor, M. P., & Wedel, M. J. (2012). Why sauropods had long necks; and why giraffes have short necks. https://core.ac.uk/download/29026739.pdf (accessed on 14th June 2025).

34. Vassallo, K. (2008). Shoulder pain in general practice. https://core.ac.uk/download/46602184.pdf (accessed on 14th June 2025).

MUSCLES OF THE THORAX AND ABDOMEN

9

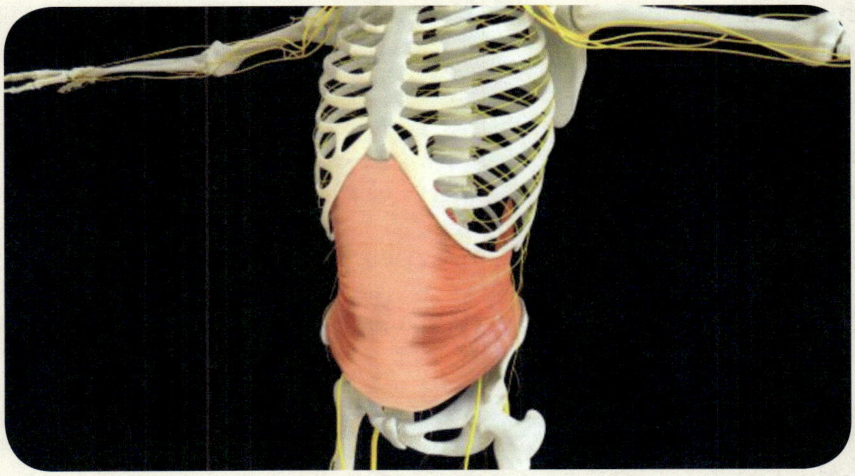

Introduction

The abdominal and thoracic muscles play a significant role in the general operation and overall structure of the human body. The two groups of muscles are primarily responsible for basic functions such as breathing, posture maintenance, and trunk movements. Understanding the anatomy and physiological processes of these muscles allows for complete comprehension of how they are involved in critical processes, such as the opening and closing of the chest cavity to allow or restrict breathing. It is imperative to recognize that voluntary and involuntary muscle functions are related, thus making the body's dynamic capability optimal. This interrelatedness is also an indication of the importance of learning about these groups of muscle, as their operation extends beyond particular movements to involve systemic physiological functions essential for survival and everyday living. In addition to their roles in respiration and walking, the thoracic and abdominal muscles also have tasks in protecting internal organs and serving as points of origin and insertion for various structures. The

LEARNING OBJECTIVES

After studying this chapter, you will be able to:

1. Describe the anatomy of the thoracic muscles
2. Identify the anatomical structure of the abdominal muscles
3. Describe the structure and function of the intercostal muscles
4. Describe the structure and function of the diaphragm
5. Identify the rectus abdominis muscle
6. Describe the oblique muscles

thoracic muscles, including the diaphragm and intercostals, work together to facilitate adequate breathing patterns, while the abdominal muscles support core stabilization. Such stabilization is necessary in physical activities requiring strength or accuracy, such as lifting or twisting. In addition, familiarization with the functional anatomy of the muscles will help to provide insight into common pathological conditions, such as hernias or lung disease, with even greater focus on their clinical significance. Study of the structural characteristics and functions of these muscles leads the way to innovation in therapies and rehabilitation programs aimed at restoring normal function. Research on thoracic and abdominal musculature also assists us in enhancing our knowledge of locomotion and body mechanics. A case in point is the way motor branch coordination, as discussed in median nerve research, prescribes the role of the muscles in facilitating movement while maintaining homeostasis within the organism. This information points to the intricate relationship between nervous system regulation and muscular function. To that end, the awareness that results from studying such muscle groups not only adds to intellectual knowledge but also informs practice in departments ranging from sport science to physiotherapy, where tailor-made interventions can be designed for improved performance and recovery. Lastly, thorough analysis of the thorax and abdominal muscles has the promise to contribute both to scholarly studies and practical applications in health and exercise, yielding a foundation for continued exploration in biomedical studies as well as clinical applications.

Definition of Thoracic and Abdominal Muscles

The thoracic and abdominal muscles are a complex system of muscles crucial to most functions of the body, particularly those related to respiration, stabilization, and walking. The majority of thoracic muscles, including the intercostal muscles and the diaphragm, work together to facilitate breathing. The intercostal muscles, between the ribs, are responsible for much of the expanding and contracting of the chest cavity with breathing, and the diaphragm is the chief breathing muscle, contracting during inspiration to suck air into the lungs. These muscles act together to produce the pressure gradient required for adequate ventilation.

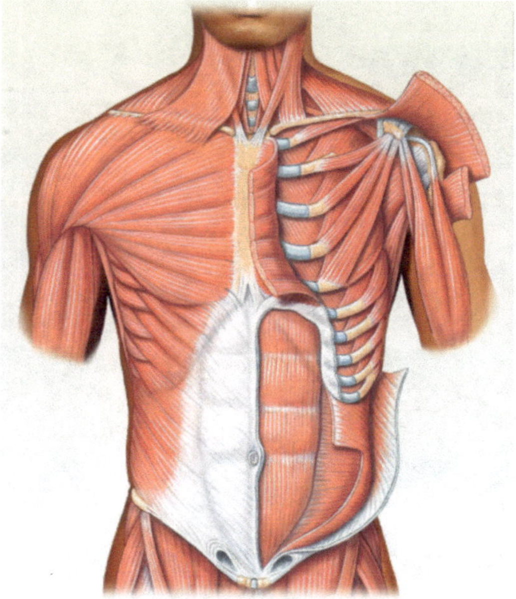

Figure 9.1. Anatomical illustration of the upper body muscles, showing the layered structure of the chest, shoulder, and abdominal muscle groups.

Source: https://external-content.duckduckgo.com/iu/?u=https%3A%2F%2Fo.quizlet.com%2FEZPBvQ.4VdIU3WEqxgCQKw_b.png&f=1&nofb=1&ipt=f5283bdd8b6531e983310279a72ca25e38cfc38ef16208b5f53940a593f1cd73.

This organizational pattern is central to comprehending numerous medical examinations and interventions, in this case, prioritizing the intrinsic connection between muscle function and respiratory health. In contrast, the abdominal muscles describe a unique but significant set of functions associated with core support and guarding internal organs. Primary muscle groups in this region include the rectus abdominis, external obliques, internal obliques, and the transverse abdominis. These muscles work synergistically to provide additional support to the spine, enabling a degree of motion such as flexion, rotation, and lateral bending of the trunk. Additionally, abdominal muscles play a significant role in the upkeep of intra-abdominal pressure, necessary for functions such as urination, defecation, and childbirth. This intricate relationship of muscles exhibits an advanced understanding of anatomy and physiology, illustrating the significance of accuracy when using anatomical terms to guarantee accurate communication between the medical community (Casagrande-Jaloretto et al., 2013) (Figure 9.1).

The structural integrity and functional efficacy of thoracic and abdominal muscles are more than just respiratory and core stability functions; they are also essential for athletic performance and rehabilitation. The thoracic and abdominal muscles are often utilized to carry out complex movements that require strength, flexibility, and endurance. Exercise protocols used to build these muscle groups can lead to improved athletic performance, injury prevention, and effectiveness in rehabilitation. Furthermore, advances in anatomical knowledge, as debated within texts like Terminologia Anatomica, improve our understanding of such musculoskeletal (MSK) relationships and how they relate to clinical practice (Rosse et al., 2000). By developing a greater awareness of thorax and abdominal anatomy, medical practitioners are able to address issues of dysfunction of the muscle better and optimize treatments for affected patients.

Importance of These Muscles in Human Anatomy

The abdominal and thoracic muscles play a crucial role in supporting core functions within the human body, such as breathing and movement. The muscles that exist between the ribs are critical in facilitating the process of breathing. They contract in the act of inhaling to expand the chest cavity and enable the lungs to draw in air, which is a testament to their importance in the proper breathing process. In addition, the diaphragm, that dome-shaped muscle at the base of the thoracic cavity, is the primary inspiratory force. The coordinated action of these muscles not only makes ventilation effective but also serves to maintain intrathoracic pressure, essential to cardiovascular integrity. Hence, a better understanding of these muscles enhances our admiration for these vital functions in sustaining life through respiration and homeostasis of the body. In addition to their tasks in breathing, muscles of the thorax and abdomen supply a lot of the core stability and posture required for physical performance as well as health. The abdominal muscles, including the rectus abdominis, obliques, and transverse abdominis, work together to stabilize the spine and pelvis to produce movements such as twisting, bending, and lifting. Stability of this nature is required for activities ranging from everyday chores to sports. Moreover, having a solid core can prevent one from being injured and reduce stress on the back as well. In educational environments, such as anatomy class, the emphasis put on these groups of muscles enforces their relevance not just for clinical use, but for overall physical fitness as well. Based on recent studies, newly adopted methods of teaching that involve such functions of muscles can significantly improve the learning process among medical students and how they understand human anatomy (Gomar et al., 2019; Albanese et al., 2018). Thoracic and abdominal muscles also contribute significantly to surgical procedures and interventions. A deep anatomical knowledge of the muscles is required for doctors, especially surgeons, as it directs them on how to carry out operations such as abdominal or thoracotomy surgery. Accurate recognition of muscle layers and understanding of how they correspond to other structures minimizes risks and contributes to better patient outcomes during operations. Additionally, with the new educational environment—most institutions no longer teaching classical dissection courses—applying replacement methods, i.e., simulation or prosection, comes more to the foreground. These new approaches not only facilitate today's educational requirements but also maintain high levels of anatomical knowledge so that future healthcare professionals are well-placed to handle the intricacies associated with the thoracic and abdominal regions of the human body (Albanese et al., 2018).

9.1. Anatomy of the Thoracic Muscles

Learning Outcome

1. Explain the major muscles of the thorax
2. Describe the functions of thoracic muscles
3. Understand the relationship between thoracic muscles and respiration

Thoracic muscles play a critical role in the mechanics of respiration, both in the movement and in supporting the rib cage. The most recognized among these muscles are the intercostal muscles, which lie between the ribs and branch into three layers of external, internal, and innermost intercostals. The external intercostals contract during inhalation to assist in opening the thoracic cavity, and the internal intercostals assist in exhalation, particularly with forceful exhalation. The two muscles collectively contribute not only to lung capacity but also add more stability and structure in general throughout the thoracic region. Understanding the intricate anatomy of these muscles is vital for an appreciation of the mechanism of respiration and physical work demanded by the thorax in performing various activities. The diaphragm is also the primary muscle of respiration, separating the thoracic and abdominal cavities. The dome-shaped diaphragm is fixed to the lower ribs, sternum, and lumbar vertebrae, which become smaller and thinner when the individual takes a breath in, developing a negative pressure to pull air into the lungs. When the diaphragm relaxes, it bulges upward, which helps in exhalation. The coordination between the diaphragm and intercostal muscles is a demonstration of the complex relationships among thoracic muscles to ensure practical respiratory function. Furthermore, the differences in muscle strength or trauma in these areas can significantly influence the mechanics of breathing, as a testament to the function of the diaphragm in thoracic anatomy for health and execution of physical activities. Thoracic muscles also assist with upper body postural alignment and movement beyond respiration. Other muscles, such as the pectoralis major and serratus anterior, are crucial in facilitating movement and shoulder stabilization. The serratus anterior assists with scapular protraction and upward rotation, which is significant in elevating the arm. The pectoralis major, however, assists with arm rotation and adduction, enabling a range of upper-body movements. As these muscles become part of the surrounding musculature, their normal function becomes essential in upper limb strength and endurance activities. Therefore, good knowledge of thoracic musculature is vital not only in clinical assessment of respiratory disease but also in optimizing body performance in various sporting and daily activities.

9.1.1. Major Muscles of the Thorax

The thoracic cavity houses a variety of important muscles essential to the mechanics of respiration and movement of the upper extremities. The pectoralis major and minor, serratus anterior, and intercostal muscles are the major muscles of the thorax, and each plays a vital role in thoracic function. The pectoralis major, by its broad origin on the clavicle and sternum, is primarily tasked with arm flexion, adduction, and internal rotation. Contrasted with this is the pectoralis minor below, which stabilizes the scapula and indirectly contributes to breath dynamics by elevating the ribs during maximal inspiration. Recognition of these muscles records their inter-relationship not only in movement, but in respiratory physiology. It emphasizes the importance of thoracic musculature in facilitating posture and movement within a range of activities. Intercostal muscles, located between the ribs, play a critical role in the respiratory process (Figure 9.2).

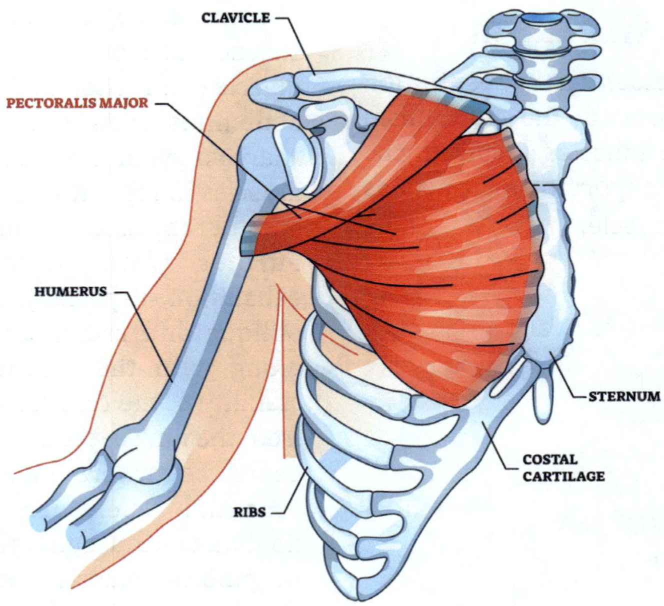

Figure 9.2. The pectoralis major muscle.

Source: https://images.squarespace-cdn.com/content/v1/60c12e7694bedc06ee36c972/1030105d-51f2-4326-9b42-ae4a56b8361d/Pectoralis+major+muscle.jpg.

They are divided into external and internal layers, with external intercostals primarily responsible for inhalation, while internal intercostals assist in exhalation. Such coordination emphasizes the dynamic nature of thoracic musculature, particularly during exercise. Combined with the serratus anterior, which is connected to the upper eight or nine ribs, the thoracic muscles facilitate arm movement and stabilize the scapula, critical for lifting and reaching tasks. This muscle arrangement demonstrates the flexibility of the muscles, contributing to overall upper body strength and ROM. In addition, the singular positioning of these muscles renders energy transfer effective in movement, rendering the thorax a functional region for respiratory and upper limb movement. Further scrutiny of thoracic muscle function reveals a complex association with physical exercise and the effects on respiratory efficiency. Improved muscular development in this region enhances vital capacity, illustrating the significance of thoracic strength to athletic ability. For instance, athletes' endurance and strength increase in sports that rely heavily on these muscles because of increased oxygen demand for supply and usage. Furthermore, flexibility in these muscles can be observed even in various training programs, which help make them stronger, as well as thoracic function in general. Thus, a precise knowledge of the thoracic major muscles underpins broader discourse about physical conditioning, respiratory health, and sports training. Such comprehension is central to an understanding of how muscle structure, mechanics of respiration, and performance are related, highlighting the sophisticated engineering of the thoracic region in terms of worldwide musculoskeletal (MSK) health.

9.1.2. Functions of Thoracic Muscles

Thoracic muscles are essential in respiration as they form integral parts of the mechanism of breathing. Of all the muscles involved, the diaphragm is the most important as it acts as the major inspiratory muscle.

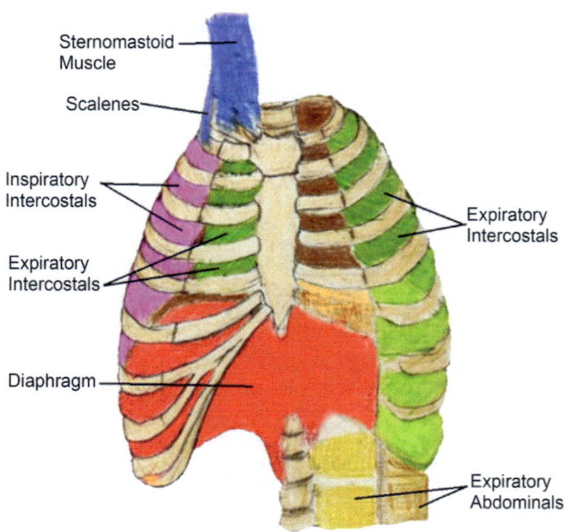

Figure 9.3. Muscles of respiration.

Source: https://ars.els-cdn.com/content/image/3-s2.0-B9780323900508000017-f01-11-9780323900508.jpg.

Muscles such as the pectoralis major and minor and the serratus anterior contribute significantly to arm and shoulder movement. They are involved in activities such as lifting, pushing, and pulling, all of which are necessary in daily life as well as sports. The dynamic interaction of these muscles not only helps to facilitate upper limb movement but also assists with the stabilization of posture. Along with their complementary movements, thoracic muscles allow for an entire ROMs simultaneously while guarding against the integrity of nearby anatomical structures, thereby affirming their multi-functional state in human anatomy. Thoracic muscles also serve a crucial purpose in allowing for a multitude of actions other than respiration and structural support, including motion present in the abdominal region. Expirations like coughs, sneezes, and even speech rely on coordinated muscle contraction in the thorax. The transverse abdominis, even though an abdominal muscle, shares a synergistic function with the thoracic muscles in regulating intra-abdominal pressure and thereby assisting in respiratory mechanics. Further, while performing activities like exhalation, especially forceful exhalation, the oblique and rectus abdominis muscles work along with the thoracic muscles to ensure stability at the core for efficient expulsion of air from the lungs. It is imperative during strenuous exercises, where maximum performance is essential. Therefore, the thoracic muscles demonstrate a synergistic arrangement with neighboring muscle groups in emphasizing their multifunctional role in various physiological processes (Flack et al., 1921; Sanusi et al., 1986).

9.1.3. Relationship Between Thoracic Muscles and Respiration

Thoracic muscles play an essential role in facilitating respiration by way of the mechanical action required for exhalation and inhalation. Of the thoracic muscles, the most significant is the diaphragm, the principal muscle used during inspiration. When the diaphragm contracts, it flattens and moves downward, expanding the volume of the thoracic cavity and decreasing intrathoracic pressure. This negative pressure allows air to flow into the lungs. Intercostal muscles, located intercostally between the ribs, also contribute to respiratory mechanics by providing support and stability to the rib cage and assisting in expanding and contracting the thoracic cavity. With this concerted effort, these muscles ensure effective respiration, with modifications for varied physical needs, such as during exercise or rest, ultimately facilitating cellular metabolism and the exchange of gases. Moreover, the correlation between thoracic muscles and respiration also holds true for their role in postural support and posture maintenance during the act of respiration. The scalenes and sternocleidomastoid (SCM) muscles of the thoracic cavity help in the elevation of the first two ribs, further increasing the volume of the thoracic cavity with the act of deep breathing. Thoracic muscles have a high interrelationship, with the best posture ensuring maximum respiratory efficiency; slouching or misalignment may reduce lung volume and airflow. Furthermore, the thoracic region is immediately connected with the abdominal muscles that help in respiration by modulating intra-abdominal pressure. This is crucial for efficient diaphragm action as well as for coughing or sneezing actions that are based on synchronized thoracic and abdominal muscle contraction. Finally, studies of insect flight mechanics offer a fascinating perspective on evolutionary solutions of thoracic muscles for breathing. For instance, the indirect flight muscle of the fruit fly exhibits typical patterns of strain in activity that correlate to optimization for energy efficiency as well as muscle action within thoracic volume. The relation between muscle strain and respiratory function illustrates how thoracic musculature not only enables locomotion but also controls the respiratory process in a complex way. As established in research, maintaining precise strain levels in muscle fibers is necessary to effect successful cycles of contraction and relaxation. This physiological relationship emphasizes the complexity and variety of thoracic muscles and their intrinsic role in both respiration and locomotion, thereby indicating an evolutionary relationship between respiratory efficiency, energy efficiency, and muscle function (Chan et al., 1996; Sivaprasad et al., 2010).

Test Your Knowledge

1. What are the major muscles of the thorax, and where are they located?
2. What are the primary functions of the thoracic muscles in relation to posture and movement?

9.2. Anatomy of the Abdominal Muscles

Learning Outcome

1. Define the major muscles of the abdomen
2. Discuss the functions of abdominal muscles
3. Describe the role of abdominal muscles in posture and movement

The anatomy of the abdominal muscles is crucial to an understanding of the overall MSK design of the human body. The abdominal muscles are primarily classified into four groups: the rectus abdominis, the external oblique, the internal oblique, and the transversus abdominis. Each muscle of these groups plays a distinct function in core stability, movement, and respiration. The rectus abdominis, or six-pack, courses along the front of the abdomen and is used to flex the lumbar spine. The external obliques and internal obliques, which sit on either side of the abdomen, assist in trunk rotation and lateral flexion. Finally, the transversus abdominis acts as a natural corset by stabilizing the abdominal organs and maintaining intra-abdominal pressure, which helps with many bodily functions. Understanding the anatomical interplay between the muscles reveals their functional contribution to everyday activities as well as sporting performance. For instance, coordination between the oblique muscles and the rectus abdominis is essential during rotation, such as in tennis or baseball, where twisting is constant and powerful. Coordination between these muscles also helps maintain posture, which is necessary for preventing injuries related to improper body mechanics. The stabilizing aspect of the transversus abdominis affects the pelvis and the spine. In combination, abdominal muscles could not only improve physical performance but also assist in protecting internal organs when test subjects perform tasks with high impact (Figure 9.4).

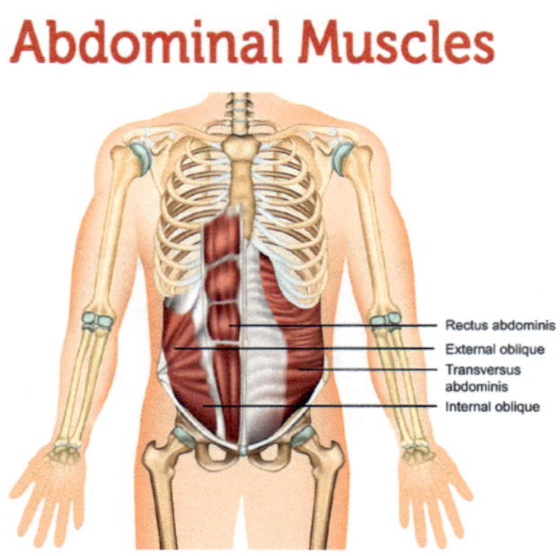

Figure 9.4. Abdominal muscles.

Source: https://assets.lybrate.com/imgs/tic/enadp/image-of-the-abdominal-muscles.jpg.

Studies of abdominal muscle anatomy extend beyond its basic structure; it also encompasses its interface with thoracic musculature. The diaphragm, as an exhalatory muscle, closely interacts with the abdominal muscles during activities such as exhalation and carrying heavy weights. A well-efficient abdominal wall optimizes the performance of the diaphragm, which leads to improved efficiency in breathing. Also, as with studies of other organisms, such as the honey bee *Apis mellifera*, anatomical information is essential to thorough biomechanical analysis. Cross-species comparison highlights the importance of muscle anatomy within different organisms and can propel human MSK science further, offering insight into functional adaptations and therapeutic approaches (Casagrande-Jaloretto et al., 2013; Rucker et al., 1901).

9.2.1. Major Muscles of the Abdomen

The abdomen houses several large muscle groups that are critical to many aspects of body function, including movement, posture, and even breathing. Of these, the rectus abdominis is perhaps most visible, colloquially referred to as the six-pack muscle due to its visually prominent segments.

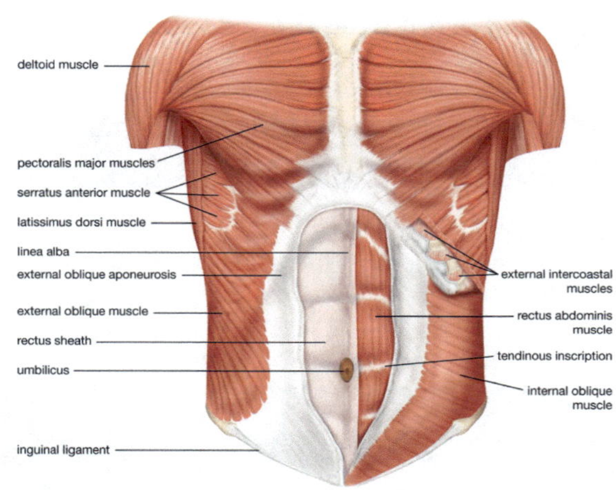

Figure 9.5. Muscles of the abdominal wall.

Source: https://www.britannica.com/science/abdominal-muscle.

This two-sided muscle runs vertically on the front abdomen from the pubic symphysis to the xiphoid process. It plays a significant role in lumbar spine flexion and, therefore, assists in sitting up and lifting the trunk from the floor.

Therefore, the rectus abdominis not only plays the core stability function but also has a vital function in functional movement, demonstrating its contribution to sport performance and activities of daily living. These intrinsic functions highlight the importance of the rectus abdominis in understanding the overall musculature involved with the abdominal region. In addition to the rectus abdominis, the external oblique muscles are integral components of the abdominal wall. They are positioned on either side of the abdomen and run from the lower ribs to the pelvis diagonally, allowing for twisting and lateral flexion of the trunk (Figure 9.5).

They are also tasked with compressing the abdominal cavity, which comes in handy in functions such as forced expiration and stabilization of the trunk during complex movements. Notably, the location and structure of external obliques enable them to function synergistically with other abdominal muscles to enhance overall core strength and stability. Their role is also to stabilize posture, therefore illustrating their integral function in stabilizing posture, thereby illustrating their integral role in the abdominal musculature and the biomechanics of the whole body. Lastly, the internal oblique muscles are found beneath the external obliques and perform similar functions except that the direction of their fibers differs. These muscles begin from the iliac crest and inguinal ligament, travel upwards and forward to attach to the lower ribs. This design allows the internal obliques to facilitate trunk rotation and lateral flexion and help with abdominal pressure. Like their external counterparts, internal obliques are very effective in stabilizing the spine in motion. They are also extremely vital in protective mechanisms against injury when participating in athletic activities. Understanding the individual yet complementary functions of abdominal muscles, such as the internal and external obliques, sets the sophistication of the abdominal wall and its utility in structural stability and movement effectiveness in the human body (Casagrande-Jaloretto et al., 2013; Gill et al., 1972).

9.2.2. Functions of Abdominal Muscles

The abdominal muscles have several essential functions that play a significant role in general body mechanics and stability. There are many layers of the abdominal muscles, which include the rectus abdominis, transverse abdominis, and the obliques, with each having a different role in movement and support. They help and control flexion of the spine by being actively used in rotation, lateral bending, and flexion. The coordination of this is key in the upkeep of posture and balance throughout daily function, as well as athletic performance. The abdominal muscles also aid in compressing the abdominal cavity, which is vital in numerous physiological functions. Stabilization of these muscles is crucial during lifting, twisting, and turning, making them key elements of the kinetic chain that stabilize the thorax and abdomen. Moreover, abdominal muscles play a vital role in respiration as well as maintaining intra-abdominal pressure. When the breath is expelled, particularly during more forceful breathing, abdominal muscles contract to push the diaphragm upward and thereby enable air to exit the lungs. The functional interdependence of both muscular and respiratory systems is thus expressed through this contribution of abdominal muscles to respiratory mechanics. Apart from compressing the abdominal cavity, these muscles assist in functions like defecation, urination, and childbirth, demonstrating their role in core stability and overall body function. Their influence thus extends beyond movement and into fundamental body functions that sustain life. Activation and strength of these muscles lie at the core of sports performance, but no less so for bodily health and integrity. In physical fitness and rehabilitation settings, knowledge of abdominal muscle functions is necessary to develop effective exercise programs. These muscles can be strengthened in a way that will help to prevent injury, enhance stability and balance, and increase athletic performance through facilitating the ability to produce more force and control in movement. In contrast, weakness of the abdominal muscles can contribute to an array of problems, such as poor posture, back strain, and reduced capacity for functional movement in daily living. Thus, certain exercises specific to all levels of the abdominal muscles are prescribed regularly to those individuals recovering from injury or looking to improve their functional movement patterns. The overall understanding of these muscles' functions validates their role in the context of the overall muscular system of the thorax and abdomen, illustrating the reciprocal relationship between muscular function and physical health (Casagrande-Jaloretto et al., 2013). It is essential for the further examination of these muscles to develop rehabilitating techniques and enhance sports training techniques (Rucker et al., 1901).

9.2.3. Role of Abdominal Muscles in Posture and Movement

The abdominal muscles have a fundamental role in aiding in posture maintenance, providing a stabilizing influence for the torso and aiding in the positioning of the spine. The abdominal muscles, comprising the rectus abdominis, obliques, and transversus abdominis, all function during static and dynamic postural maintenance. When sitting or standing to carry out daily tasks, the abdominal muscles are activated to support the spine, preventing injury and allowing for effective movement. They also play a part in the overall balance and stability of the body because they synergize with the thoracic muscles. With age, changes in the strength and elasticity of these muscles can lead to postural imbalances, a reason why some strengthening exercises need to be incorporated into exercise programs so that healthy movement and posture can be maintained (Casagrande-Jaloretto et al., 2013) (Figure 9.6).

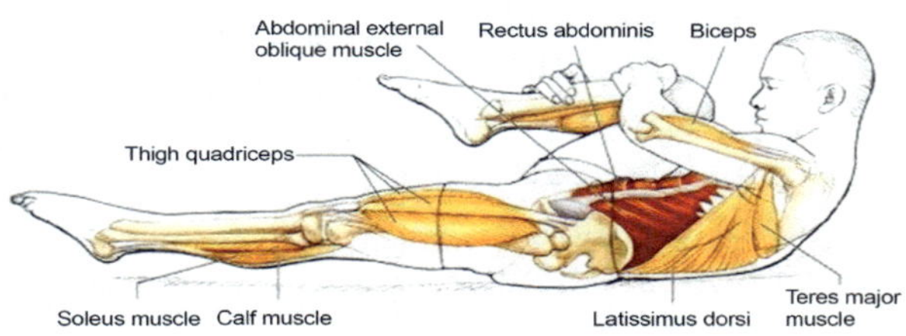

Figure 9.6. The exercises focus particularly on strengthening the abdominals in their action of spinal flexion.

Source: https://i.pinimg.com/1200x/1f/30/2b/1f302b87749a5cfeed5b0ff13ef97757.jpg.

Besides their roles in posture, abdominal muscles contribute significantly to moving various physical activities. Abdominal muscles are the primary movers when the trunk flexes, rotates, or laterally bends, enabling individuals to perform tasks requiring strength and agility. For instance, with movements such as lifting or throwing, activation of the core muscles facilitates good transfer of force from the lower to the upper body. The abdominal muscles also act as protective support for visceral organs, stabilizing the thoracic and pelvic regions during movement. This coordination is also essential in sports performance, as the core is a foundation for the creation of power and general efficacy in dynamic motion. Thus, the prolonged activation of the abdominal muscles has a direct influence on one's capacity to participate in various forms of physical movement (Joshua et al., 2014). Coordination of the abdominal muscles with the thoracic region is significant in the context of breathing and general functional capability. In the process of inhalation and exhalation, the diaphragm collaborates with abdominal muscles to produce pressure changes that enable the flow of air. Such a delicate synergy is best experienced in activities such as singing or weight lifting, where there is a need for specific breathing techniques. A stable core further enables effective diaphragmatic breathing by stabilizing the rib cage and facilitating lung inflation. Contrary to this, an impaired muscle in the abdomen can lead to inefficient breathing and postural issues. Via muscle coordination, the abdominal region, besides influencing postures related to exercise, contributes to vital physiological activities, referencing its intrinsic contribution to posture in addition to general movement mechanics (Casagranda-Jaloretto et al., 2013).

Test Your Knowledge

1. What are the major muscles of the abdomen, and where are they located?
2. How do abdominal muscles contribute to maintaining posture and enabling movement?

9.3. Intercostal Muscles

Learning Outcome

1. Explain the location and structure of the intercostal muscles
2. Define the role in breathing mechanics
3. Discuss the clinical significance of the intercostal muscles

The intercostal muscles are all significant in the process of breathing and play important roles within the thoracic cavity. The intercostal muscles are found between the ribs and are classified into three categories, namely the external intercostals, internal intercostals, and innermost intercostals. The external intercostal muscles help to draw in air by elevating the ribs during breathing in, hence increasing the volume within the thoracic cavity. In contrast, the intercostals internally are primarily responsible for assisting forced exhalation by protruding the ribs, reducing thoracic volume. This cooperation by intercostal muscles not only assists respiration but also helps stabilize the ribcage, allowing controlled air flow during bodily motion, such as exercise or high-level activity. In addition to their respiratory importance, intercostal muscles also contribute to overall trunk stability and posture. Their interaction with the diaphragm is essential to ventilation, with their contraction securing the stability of intrathoracic pressure during various phases of the respiratory cycle. Recent evidence illustrates the anatomical and functional interrelationships among the intercostal muscles and other thoracic units, emphasizing their relevance in clinical as well as educational environments. The incorporation of dynamic anatomical studies within medical training curricula will assist in making students more sensitive to the impact of these muscles on respiratory mechanics. This sensitivity aligns with the trend towards integrated curricula, which emphasize the interrelatedness of various body systems, as highlighted in the controversy surrounding cadaver dissection and the anatomical approach to thoracic training (Bolender et al., 2015). Despite their importance, the intercostal muscles are underrated in anatomical instruction as compared to large muscle groups. Contemporary teaching strategies underscore the need for a comprehensive approach to learning these muscles, particularly within combined medical curricula that combine thoracic anatomy with other systems' functions, such as the renal system. The dissected specimens preserved for teaching purposes not only illuminate the anatomical detail of intercostal muscles but also their functional implications in various physiological situations. Through exposure to the physiological functions and anatomical detail of intercostal muscles, medical students can appreciate interrelations in the thoracic region (Flack et al., 1921). This knowledge is vital for future practitioners who will be relying on a solid understanding of respiratory mechanics to inform their clinical practice.

9.3.1. Location and Structure of Intercostal Muscles

The intercostal muscles are critical components of the thoracic musculature that reside between each pair of ribs.

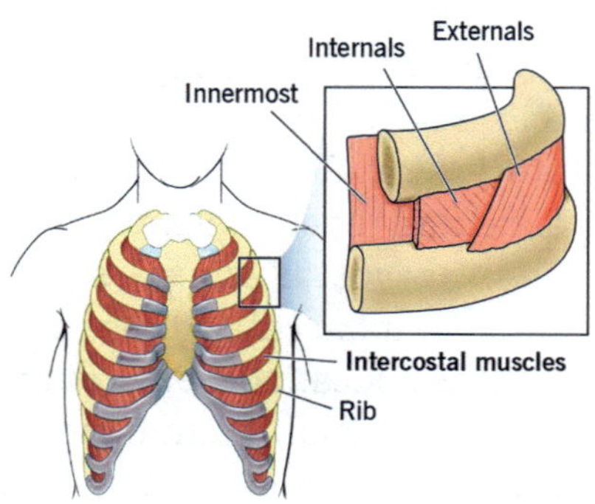

Figure 9.7. Intercoastal muscles: Between your ribs are intercostal muscles, with the externals up front, internals in the middle and innermost at the back.

Source: https://my.clevelandclinic.org/-/scassets/images/org/health/articles/intercostal-muscles.jpg

They play a strong role in respiratory mechanics by facilitating expansion of the thoracic cavity on inhalation and contraction of the thoracic cavity on exhalation. The muscles are classified into three distinct layers, including external intercostals, internal intercostals, and innermost intercostals. The external intercostals, obliquely inclined downward and forward, contribute to the inhalation process by elevating the ribs and thereby increasing the thoracic capacity. The internal intercostals, positioned at right angles to the external layer, are responsible primarily for forced expiration, tugging the ribs downwards. The innermost intercostals, with the same function as that of the internal intercostals, also contribute during forceful respiratory effort (Figure 9.7).

Therefore, proper organization and function of these muscles are essential to practical respiratory mechanics, making them central to the thoracic musculature. In addition to primary respiration, intercostal muscles are essential in maintaining the structural integrity of the thoracic cavity. Not only do their locations between the ribs help with breathing, but they also aid in rib cage stabilization with concomitant movements, including physical activity and changes in posture. Such stability is significant because the thoracic cage houses other essential organs such as the heart and lungs. Moreover, coordination of intercostal muscle activity facilitates the effortless transition between inhalation and exhalation, raising the efficiency of respiratory function as a whole. Such synergy is necessary during rest as well as exercise, assisting oxygen transport to tissues and carbon dioxide removal. Thus, the anatomy and location of the intercostal muscles demonstrate their complicated role in the thoracic dynamics, merging muscular action with crucial physiological functions. The anatomical complexity of the intercostal muscles corresponds with the intricacy of the muscular systems pertinent to respiratory mechanisms. The intercostal muscles are supplied by the intercostal nerves derived from the thoracic spinal nerves, which enables the coordinated and precise control of breathing efforts. Astonishingly, research has illuminated the coordination between numerous muscles employed during breathing and revealed the contribution of other muscles, such as the diaphragm and accessory muscles, to the various phases of breathing. Studies on activation patterns of muscles indicate that intercostal muscles activate in a very advanced manner, as they react to varying physical activities. As discussed in Holstege et al. (2009), the muscular activation is influenced by several controls of a neurological nature and can vary according to, say, posture or intensity of physical activity. This dynamic cooperation is representative of the importance of the intercostal muscles in the broader context of thoracic and abdominal muscles, as is showcased in academic articles such as those found in Bumeister et al. (2016).

9.3.2. Role in Breathing Mechanics

Thoracic muscles are involved in the mechanics of breathing directly, as they are the primary ventilatory drivers. The diaphragm contracts when the body inhales, increasing the thoracic volume. Intrapleural pressure is lowered with the contraction of the diaphragm, creating a vacuum into which air flows into the lungs. In addition, accessory muscles such as the intercostal and scalene muscles contribute to rib cage widening, further augmenting lung capacity during deep breathing. These muscles respond to the metabolic demands of the body, enhancing respiratory effort with exercise while enhancing the quantity of air introduced into the lungs. Effective coordination between these groups of muscles is required since their dysfunction will result in decreased respiratory efficiency, testifying to their role in maintaining adequate oxygenation and carbon dioxide removal in the body. Research now acknowledges the complex interplays between upper-body exercise (UBE) and respiratory mechanics and how these affect breathing efficiency. Studies have shown that, during UBE, mechanical-ventilatory responses also vary from what is known during lower-body exercise (Figure 9.8).

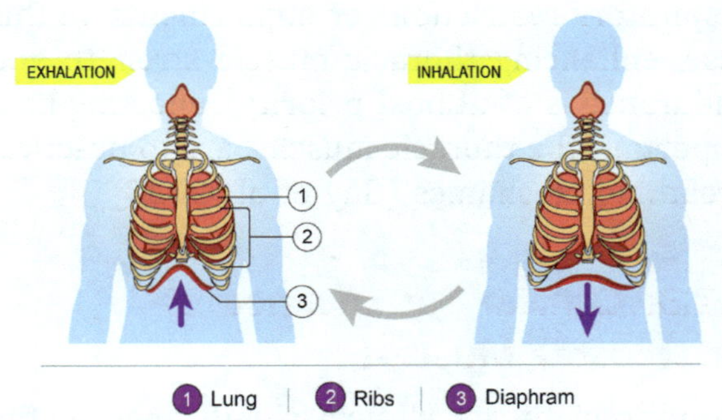

Figure 9.8. Mechanism of breathing.

Source: https://cdn1.byjus.com/wp-content/uploads/2019/04/Cellular-Respiration-RESPIRATION1.png.

Specifically, UBE is likely to leave a small tidal volume with a requirement for augmented respiratory frequency to maintain metabolic demand. This adjustment is expected to enhance thoracic muscle recruitment, with resulting increased central neural drive being required to achieve optimal ventilation. Breathing becomes harder due to the double load of physical work and mechanical limitations on the thoracic structure. Having such dynamics in mind, one understands the pivotal contribution of thoracic musculature to breathing mechanics, particularly under various forms of physical stress, and emphasizes the need for targeted approaches in managing exercise-induced challenges in breathing (Tiller et al., 2014). Moreover, the intricate interaction of chest wall mechanics and recruitment of breathing muscles is imperative to optimal functioning of breathing. With high activity levels, the mechanical demand on respiratory muscles may induce over-reliance on diaphragmatic and accessory muscle use, potentially leading to fatigue. Clinically, patients have been observed to show breathlessness or reduced exercise tolerance when the respiratory muscles are overloaded. Fatigue subsequently affects lung function, further impairing oxygen delivery throughout the body. An understanding of the mechanical-ventilatory interface can thus be relevant to rehabilitation in patients with respiratory restrictions or impairments. In this case, enhancing thoracic muscle strength and endurance is of utmost priority, reflecting how important the thoracic muscles are to practical breathing mechanics (Guy et al., 2025).

9.3.3. Clinical Significance of Intercostal Muscles

To appreciate the clinical significance of the intercostal muscles is to realize their essential contribution towards the mechanics of respiration and thoracic function in general. The intercostal muscles, found between the ribs, allow for ribcage expansion and contraction during inspiration and expiration. The external intercostal muscles, for example, contribute to the process of inhalation through the elevation of the ribs, while the internal intercostal muscles contribute to forced exhalation. Dysfunction of these muscles plays a vital role in respiratory efficiency and may result in hypoventilation or respiratory distress. These are crucial beyond the level of mechanics; effective breathing is essential to maintain proper gas exchange in the lungs, influencing cardiovascular status and overall physical functioning. The clinical relevance of the intercostal muscles in respiratory therapy and training is also remarkable, as they can be addressed to enhance lung capacity in patients with restrictive lung diseases, indicating their relevance to both rehabilitative and surgical applications. Intercostal muscles also hold importance when taking into account thoracic trauma and surgery assessment. Knowledge of these muscles is of utmost importance to surgeons performing procedures such as rib resections or thoracotomies, since iatrogenic damage can result in complications such as pneumothorax or impaired respiratory status. The intercostal muscles may further provide insight into the degree of injury and potential for complications, such as hemothorax, with trauma and rib fractures. Awareness of their body location is helpful in planning appropriate surgical techniques and for implementing appropriate pain relief strategies. Furthermore, radiologists should understand variations in intercostal muscle anatomy, such as the presence of the rectus sternalis muscle, that may impact diagnostic imaging reports and surgical planning (Abraham et al., 2016). Therefore, intercostal muscles play essential functions in preventive medicine and surgery within the thoracic cavity. Beyond their mechanical functions, intercostal muscles participate in the overall processes of phonation and vocalization, especially in some areas such as singing. Different research has established that coordinated action among these muscles is essential to sustaining breath control and generating sound, with variability in muscle activation affecting overall vocal performance (Pettersen et al., 2005). For classical vocalists, intercostal muscles are engaged in the control of respiratory phases during high-intensity vocalization, pointing to their importance not only in everyday functions but in professional artistic performances. Their pattern of activity demonstrates which muscle activation supports expiration as well as phonation and signifies a complicated interaction that underscores the intercostal muscles' multidimensional role. Lastly, an understanding of the clinical significance of these muscles extends beyond typical respiratory functions to indicate their implication in vocal health, performing capacity in the performing arts, and rehabilitation techniques for maximizing respiratory and voice capacities.

Test Your Knowledge

1. Where are the intercostal muscles located, and what is their structural arrangement?
2. How do the intercostal muscles contribute to the mechanics of breathing?

9.4. Diaphragm

Learning Outcome

1. Define the anatomy of the diaphragm
2. Explain the function of respiration
3. Identify the impact of the diaphragm on abdominal pressure

The diaphragm is a major muscle of the thorax and is the prime mover of respiration. It is located between the thoracic and abdominal cavities and takes a dome shape when at rest, but flattens when active, thus increasing the volume of the thoracic cavity. The change in volume causes air to be drawn into the lungs, which increases gas exchange necessary for sustaining life. The phrenic nerve supplies the diaphragm, and practical function is required for adequate ventilation. Dysfunction or paralysis of the muscle leads to severe respiratory distress, illustrating its essential role in normal physiological function. Moreover, the diaphragm works in association with accessory respiratory muscles during strenuous effort, thereby increasing its effectiveness in supplying the oxygen demands of the body during exercise, and this demonstrates its adaptability in various situations of respiratory mechanics. Under abdominal interaction, the diaphragm plays a vital role outside its respiratory function. During inspiration, the diaphragm descends as the abdominal muscles descend, allowing the abdominal cavity to accommodate the thoracic cavity's excess volume. This symmetrical motion not only helps with breathing but also with stabilizing abdominal pressure and is necessary during heavy lifting or straining. The attachment of the diaphragm to the pelvic floor emphasizes its involvement in core stability as well. As such, any derangement of the diaphragm is likely to create a variety of complications, possibly affecting posture and neuromuscular effectiveness of the torso. In addition, the function of the diaphragm in regulating intra-abdominal pressure forms the basis for systemic processes, such as digestion and circulation, further emphasizing its significance in the overall musculature of the thorax and the abdomen. Recent findings suggest that a healthy diaphragm significantly enhances endurance and exercise-induced power production, thereby improving sporting performance. The strength of the diaphragm and sporting competence, particularly in endurance sporting endeavors, have been examined in many studies. Specifically, rapid and efficient recruitment of fibers in the diaphragm, as in fast-twitch fibers in specific muscles, can promote ventilatory efficiency, an observation noted in research on other animals such as bottlenose dolphins. Such animals utilize muscles in a way that demonstrates a biomechanical coupling between movement and respiration, akin to the functional dynamics of human physiology. Understanding the diaphragm's intricate role in respiratory and muscular processes not only makes visible its position at the center of health and well-being but also opens the way for rehabilitation and training techniques aimed at optimizing its operation in thoracic and abdominal function.

9.4.1. Anatomy of the Diaphragm

The diaphragm is a significant thoracic muscular organ of the body that serves as the primary respiratory muscle. It is a dome-shaped septum that separates the thoracic cavity from the abdominal cavity, and it forms a significant boundary for the organs within those cavities. Composed of skeletal muscle, the diaphragm has the ability to both contract and relax, allowing inhalation and exhalation. During inhalation, the diaphragm contracts, dropping the dome, thereby increasing thoracic volume and introducing air into the lungs. During exhalation, the diaphragm relaxes, and the lung volume decreases, thereby expelling air. This recurring action strengthens the diaphragm's critical role in managing respiratory mechanics and facilitating oxygenation in the lungs.

Anatomically, the diaphragm is divided into three principal regions: the sternal, costal, and lumbar components, all of which work synergistically towards its total function. The sternal component is formed from the xiphoid process of the sternum, while the costal component merges with the cartilages of the lower six ribs. The lumbar component is formed from the lumbar vertebrae, where it becomes the crus – strong tendinous structures that anchor the diaphragm posteriorly. The central tendon is a thin, fibrous sheet that functions as the site of convergence for these regions, providing structural integrity and allowing for effective contraction of the muscles. These subdivisions are essential to understanding the functional dynamics of the diaphragm, particularly when one takes into account interactions with adjacent muscles and the processes involved in altering thoracic pressure with respiration (Figure 9.9).

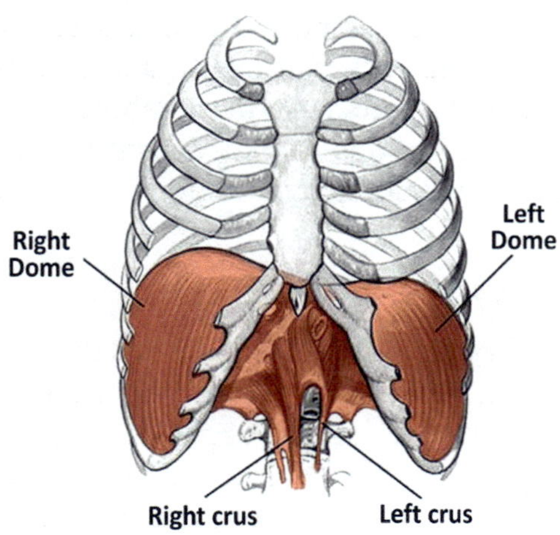

Figure 9.9. The diaphragm is split into two lobes, left and right.

Source: https://teachmeanatomy.info/wp-content/uploads/Structure-of-the-Diaphragm.jpg.

Besides, the diaphragm is innervated by the phrenic nerve, originating from cervical nerves C3 to C5. Innervation is vital as it helps to coordinate the contraction and relaxation of the muscle in respiration. Furthermore, the efficacy of the diaphragms can also be influenced by various factors like posture, body fitness, and the presence of some respiratory disorders. For instance, patients with lung dysfunction are likely to have varying diaphragm mechanics, which may lead to inefficiency of respiration. Practitioners and researchers need to understand these nuances to be able to comprehend respiratory pathophysiology and therapy. In the end, a precise knowledge of the anatomy and function of the diaphragm contributes to a broader understanding of the thoracic and abdominal muscular system, underlining its significance in physiology and medicine.

9.4.2. Function in Respiration

The thoracic and abdominal muscles play an essential role in efficient respiration, in the sense that they control the breathing dynamics through synchronized movements. Respiration is based on the contraction and relaxation of these muscles, which work to change the volume of the thoracic cavity and, therefore, the intrathoracic pressure. Key muscles are the diaphragm, the primary muscle of respiration; external intercostals, which lift the rib cage with inspiration; and internal intercostals, which contribute to forced expiration. This balance creates a pressure gradient that allows breathing to be comfortable for air to move in and out of the lungs. Not only are they essential for oxygen utilization, but also for carbon dioxide expulsion, thereby maintaining homeostasis in the body, a process required for general metabolic health. Furthermore, respiration is supported by abdominal muscles, which assist in supplementing respiratory function during heightened exertion. Rectus abdominis, transversus abdominis, and oblique muscles play an essential role during forced expiration. In contraction, these muscles increase abdominal pressure, which compels the diaphragm upward and reduces the thoracic cavity volume, and this proves helpful in expelling air. This is particularly a serious event during strenuous exercise when the body must eliminate carbon dioxide rapidly and let in more oxygen (Figure 9.10).

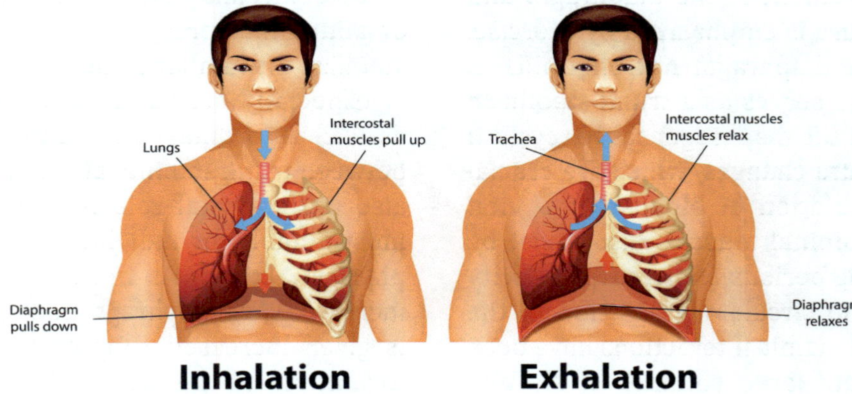

Figure 9.10. The diaphragm functions in breathing.

Source: https://www.freepik.com/free-vector/diaphragm-functions-breathing_13374446.htm#fromView=keyword&page=1&position=0&uuid=b01a75a3-83bb-4e7e-a7f2-8b8302b040ed&query=Diaphragm+Anatomy.

The coordinated function of both the abdominal and thoracic muscles defines the interconnected nature of the two muscle groups. With their coordinated functions, they not only facilitate the basic act of breathing but also enable the body to respond to increased respiratory demands during exercise. The function of the thoracic and abdominal muscles in breathing is also clarified through their neural control and physiological adaptability. The central nervous system regulates the timing and magnitude of muscle contraction, a crucial aspect in the coordination of inhalation and exhalation. Additionally, studies have proven that when these muscles are undercompensated, either through trauma or disease, respiratory efficiency is considerably lowered, leading to probable hypoxia or other pathology. Knowledge of these muscles' functional role, then, is greater than anatomy; it illuminates the state of respiratory well-being and disease management. The complex interconnection of the diaphragm, ribcage, and abdominal muscles demonstrates how critical such structures are to normal respiration and bodily function, with ramifications extending into fields like physical therapy and rehabilitation methods of optimal respiratory function (Rucker et al., 1901; Sivaprasad et al., 2010).

9.4.3. Impact of Diaphragm on Abdominal Pressure

The diaphragm regulates abdominal pressure, and it has important impacts on respiratory mechanics and cardiovascular function. During inspiration, the contraction of the diaphragm muscle creates a negative pressure within the thoracic cavity, which in turn sucks air into the lungs. The downward movement of the diaphragm, produced by this contraction, compresses the abdominal cavity, thereby increasing intra-abdominal pressure. Thus, this pressure increase stimulates venous return from the lower limbs to the heart to create improved blood flow. Increased venous return is particularly crucial in activities requiring more vigorous efforts, when abdominal pressure with the aid of the diaphragm is even more potent. Synergistic actions of the diaphragm and abdominal muscles combined optimize this pressure regulation for effective respiratory and circulatory processes. Further, the relationship between the movement of the diaphragm and abdominal pressure is emphasized by exercise. During work, the diaphragm not only aids in breathing but also serves as a trunk stabilizer. Cyclical motion of the diaphragm causes cyclical abdominal pressure changes, which are crucial for effective circulation of blood to the vital organs. The abdominal muscles also assist by contracting during periods of increased activity to supplement the circulatory function of the diaphragm. The dynamic interactions have been shown to facilitate large volumes of shifting blood between the limbs and trunk, highlighting the diaphragm's contribution to hemodynamic stability during exercise. As coordination of the diaphragm and abdominal muscles increases, the efficiency of all body functions, such as oxygenation and waste elimination, also benefits from these adjustments (Andrea et al., 2016).

Beyond its contribution to respiration and circulation, the influence of the diaphragm on abdominal pressure also extends to supporting core stability and posture. Through the generation of abdominal pressure, the diaphragm helps stabilize the lumbar spine during motion, which is especially crucial to athletic performance as well as ordinary activities. The connection between trunk stability and abdominal pressure also plays a vital role in preventing injuries, most notably for individuals engaged in heavy physical activity. As intra-abdominal pressure increases with diaphragm contraction, the spine is given increased support for a more stable formation of the trunk. This biomechanical advantage not only enhances performance but also reduces the dangers of injury by efficiently managing forces that are encountered during exercise. The diaphragm is thus not a passive participant but an essential muscle with a critical role in spinal integrity and abdominal pressure (Aliverti et al., 2015).

Test Your Knowledge

1. How does the diaphragm function during respiration?
2. In what way does the diaphragm influence intra-abdominal pressure, and why is this important?

9.5. Rectus Abdominis

Learning Outcome

1. Discuss the structure and location of the rectus abdominis
2. Describe the role in flexion and stabilization of the torso
3. Understand the importance of athletic performance and core strength

The rectus abdominis, one of the larger muscles of the abdomen, plays a critical role in core stability and enables a myriad of physiological functions. This paired muscle courses vertically on the abdominal front from the pubic symphysis to the xiphoid process, and to the fifth, sixth, and seventh costal cartilages of the ribs. look, also referred to as the six-pack, due to tendinous intersections crossing the muscle. Its primary actions include lumbar spine flexion, stabilization of the pelvis, and aiding in respiration, underlining its value. The rectus abdominis plays a significant role in various tasks, from sporting performance to everyday movements, underlining its contribution to MSK health. Aside from its anatomical relevance, the rectus abdominis also plays a role in certain conditions and exercises involved with general health and rehabilitation. One prominent condition of this muscle is diastasis rectus abdominis (DRA), which happens when the rectus abdominis splits and creates a visible gap between the two muscle bellies. Herrgård et al. (2025) further indicate that DRA is particularly prevalent in postpartum women, with an estimated one-third experiencing long-term effects after pregnancy. Identifying the impact of this condition is vital to healthcare providers as successful rehab is primarily determined by particular exercises for rehabilitating core strength and stability. Because evidence suggests a conservative physiotherapy intervention for DRA is beneficial, tailored exercise programs become the focus in recovery protocols. The effect of the rectus abdominis is not only physical movement, but also has a significant impact on voice performance and breathing control. A study of how the movement of abdominal muscles is connected with vocalization indicated that the sound was more intense, and the EMG activity in the rectus abdominis and other abdominal muscles was more pronounced. Huravitch et al. (2003) maintain that understanding this correlation is critical to singers and those rehabilitating vocal impairments, in that combined abdominal control can enhance vocal ability. The correlation illustrates the multiple-muscle functions of the rectus abdominis, stressing its importance not only in the support of posture and physical activity but also in vocal well-being, thereby showing the diverse functions this muscle serves in the human body's overall function.

9.5.1. Structure and Location of the Rectus Abdominis

The rectus abdominis is a large, paired muscle of the anterior abdominal wall that descends vertically from the pubic symphysis inferiorly to the xiphoid process and fifth through seventh ribs superiorly. This muscle is critical for flexion of the trunk as well as core stability. Structurally, the rectus abdominis is enveloped by the rectus sheath, a fibrous sheath formed by the aponeuroses of the external and internal oblique and transverse abdominal muscles. Structurally, it provides support while facilitating functional movement by securing the rectus abdominis, enabling effective contraction for tasks like bending and twisting. One of the major identifying features of the rectus abdominis is its fragmented shape, typically split into three or more bellies by tendinous intersections. The intersections are what give the muscle its strength and leverage, enabling the rapid and forceful movements. The function of the rectus abdominis extends far beyond mere flexion; it also plays a vital role in controlling intra-abdominal pressure, supporting posture, and respiratory mechanics, particularly during exhalation. Appreciation of muscle structure and its connection with the surrounding musculature is significant in determining its function in the framework of rehabilitation, especially concerning conditions that impact both its integrity and function, such as DRA (Figure 9.11).

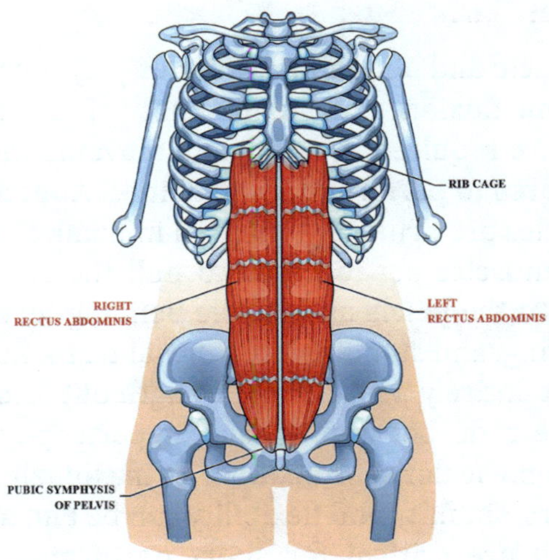

Figure 9.11. Rectus abdominis.

Source: https://external-content.duckduckgo.com/iu/?u=https%3A%2F%2Fi.pinimg.com%2Foriginals%2Fda%2F7c%2F8d%2Fda7c8df1d75c35dded3bbfe2d3069b9c.jpg&f=1&nofb=1&ip

t=d1d550870693be9649d5cdaf56ccd13a11aa097d5b3263227e0ec35fe4489dd5.

The anatomical significance of the rectus abdominis is highlighted in several scenarios, including its response to the stresses of the body and the impact when pregnant. As discussed, the rectus abdominis is susceptible to an event known as DRA that is characterized by a separation of the muscle bellies along the midline due to increased tension from increasing intra-abdominal pressure, particularly during pregnancy (Herrgård et al., 2025). This is a prevalent condition among postpartum women, thereby indicating the sheer need for rehabilitative measures that allow for recovery and restoration of function (Sharma et al., 2023). Furthermore, a clear insight into the rectus abdominis, its anatomy, situs, and vulnerability to injury, promotes a greater appreciation for the complexity of abdominal musculature and its place in the larger scheme of thoracic and abdominal physiology.

9.5.2. Role in Flexion and Stabilization of the Torso

Thoracic and abdominal muscles play a crucial role in flexion and stabilization of the torso and are required in a range of movements and postures to perform daily activities. Abdominal muscles are primarily engaged in trunk flexion. The muscles act together to pull the rib cage toward the pelvis and enable bending forward, twisting, and standing up. Normal trunk flexion is not entirely a matter of strength but also one of the ratio between muscle hypertrophy and neuromuscular coordination. By maximizing the factors, stability and flexibility can be enhanced, which are critical for sport performance as well as for protection against injury. This symbiotic relationship between stability and flexion is brought to the fore by their function in fundamental movements, proving to require functional abdominal musculature to uphold general torso integrity. Stabilization of posture, particularly during movement, is another essential function performed by thoracic and abdominal muscles. The muscles provide a continuous feedback mechanism, responding to alterations in body position and to external forces to achieve balance. Abdominal muscles, for example, must work together with the muscles in the back during bodily movements such as lifting or carrying to redistribute loads and support posture. This collaboration helps minimize the risk of injury, particularly in the lumbar region, which is vulnerable to strains. Newer models have shown the suitability of using three-dimensional computer-based techniques to calculate vibrations passing through the seated human body and describe the mechanics of postural stabilization mechanisms working hand in glove (Desai et al., 2024) (Figure 9.12).

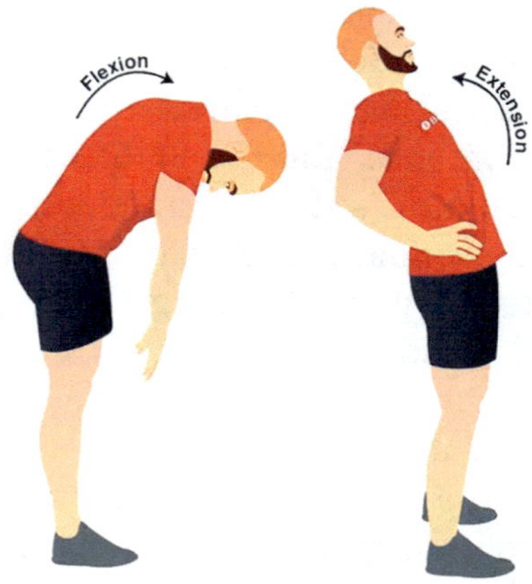

Figure 9.12. Trunk flexion.

Source: https://external-content.duckduckgo.com/iu/?u=https%3A%2F%2Fbodyworksprime.com%2Fwp-content%2Fuploads%2Ftrunk-flexion.jpg.webp&f=1&nofb=1&ipt=5772a1ac002ed261a7415749be3d55613ffda775432e705c4ae234fb86dc99ae.

Stabilization is an active process and not a passive process; it requires active recruitment of the core muscles, underlining the requirement for specific strength training to facilitate stability against destructive forces. Muscular performance in trunk stabilization and flexion activities has also been found to be influenced by variables such as sex and fitness level, research has found. A study of isometric trunk flexion maximal voluntary contractions discovered that males had greater torque, although in extended postures, while there were no differences seen in sitting upright postures (Deering et al., 2017). This shows that the level of strength may vary between the sexes, but that stabilization of the torso through flexion is comparable in both. Furthermore, lean body mass and activity levels were both positively correlated with the strength of the trunk flexors, emphasizing the functional significance of active living to the support of abdominal muscle strength. These findings justify the necessity of abdominal conditioning not only for strength but also for a decrease in fatigability during long-term postural maintenance. Through understanding these dynamics, one is more effectively able to modify training regimens to enhance trunk stability and overall bodily functioning.

9.5.3. Importance in Athletic Performance and Core Strength

The thoracic and abdominal core muscles are the center of enhancing sporting capability through their influence on core strength. The abdominal muscles and the diaphragm together form a strong core, which is at the center of nearly all bodily actions. Core strength stabilizes the pelvis and spine in dynamic movement, in addition to improving balance and coordination, which are crucial for individuals in sports. The addition of diaphragm training, highlighted in recent studies, has become more and more recognized among exercise trainers. The strengthening of diaphragm function can further increase performance as a whole by providing increased oxygen consumption and reduced muscle tension, which is equivalent to improved movement patterns (Foltz et al., 2016) (Figure 9.13).

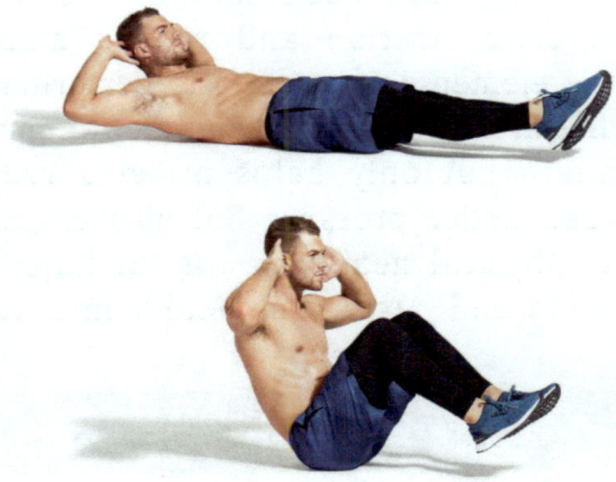

Figure 9.13. Demonstration of a V-sit crunch exercise, targeting the abdominal muscles to improve core strength and stability.

Source: https://hips.hearstapps.com/hmg-prod/images/v-sit-crunch-1585734647.jpg?resize=980:*.

Hence, the abdominal and thoracic muscles are critical components in achieving the structural stability needed for optimal athletic performance. Furthermore, core strength obtained through the use of thoracic and abdominal muscles also assists in injury prevention, a critical aspect in sports training. Efficiently conditioned core muscles effectively absorb shock and reduce the stress on the lower back and hips during collision sports. By building up such muscle groups, athletes are capable of developing resistance against common injuries such as sprains and strains, thus enabling a longer sporting career. A study shows that athletes with strong core muscles are less at risk of injury and better able to play at greater intensities due to their enhanced stability and endurance (Middlemas et al., 1999). This symbiotic relationship of core strength to injury prevention is crucial for those athletes wishing to maximize their performance while minimizing downtime in the form of injury. Even more, the physical and psychological benefits of core training extend beyond the strictly physical, influencing global athletic condition and focus. Practices such as yoga, which promote core engagement and control of breathing, have been shown to enhance mental concentration and reduce anxiety, essential elements of top sports performance. Engaging in practices involving diaphragmatic respiration not only helps athletes remain composed under pressure but also enhances general physical health by way of improved respiration and circulation (Middlemas et al., 1999). This fusion of brain and body training cultivates a more complete understanding that incorporates the interdependence of mind and body throughout athletic activity. Thus, the importance of thoracic and abdominal muscles transfers to psychological domains, confirming their worth in optimizing overall athletic ability.

Test Your Knowledge

1. How does the rectus abdominis contribute to torso flexion and core stabilization?
2. Why is the rectus abdominis necessary for athletic performance and overall core strength?

9.6. Oblique Muscles

Learning Outcome

1. Discuss the types of oblique muscles (external and internal)
2. Explain the functions in trunk rotation and lateral flexion
3. Define relevance in injury prevention and rehabilitation

The obliques, the external and the internal obliques, play a crucial role in the dynamic organization of the thoracic and abdominal compartments.

They are located laterally on the trunk and perform functions like flexion of the trunk, lateral flexion, and rotation. The external obliques are the largest of the abdominal musculature. They are attached to the lower ribs and descend medially to attach to the Linea alba, pubic tubercle, and anterior portion of the iliac crest.

Their shape is such that they can bring about a wide range of movements, thus contributing to the overall stability of the thorax as well as facilitating the intricate movements required for respiration and locomotion (Figure 9.14).

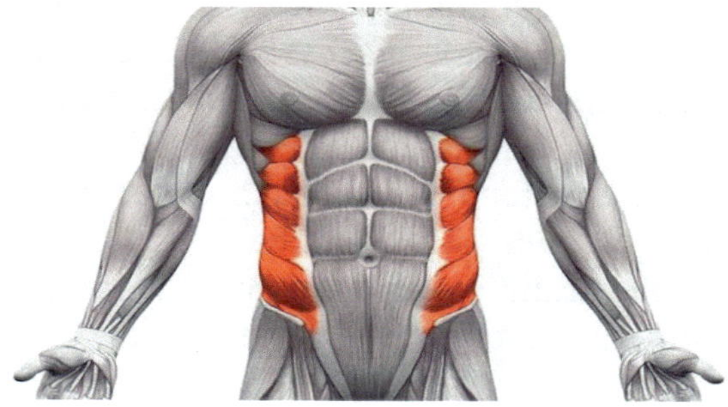

Figure 9.14. Anatomical illustration highlighting the abdominal oblique muscles, essential for trunk rotation, lateral flexion, and core stabilization.

Source: https://external-content.duckduckgo.com/iu/?u=https%3A%2F%2Fbodybuilding-wizard.com%2Fwp-content%2Fuploads%2F2018%2F09%2Fabdominal-oblique-muscles-functional-anatomy-guide-1.jpg&f=1&nofb=1&ipt=168d87b79ce029faa2cb3caadab25503c267c78595194f585cdc2148588bf81c.

Importantly, coordination of these muscles demonstrates how compound motion involves the use of various groups of muscles to enable more streamlined physical movement, thus stressing the importance of muscle function about integral movement mechanics. Internal oblique muscles, located beneath the surface layer, also contribute to the complex musculature of the torsos by adding extra strength and capability for movement. These muscles are derived from the iliac crest, thoracolumbar fascia, and inguinal ligament, inserting on the inferior ribs and Linea alba. They have fibers that are at right angles to those of the external obliques. They thus are able to assist in trunk rotation and lateral flexion, emphasizing the synergistic relationship of the two. Such concurrent interaction is crucial for bending and twisting exercises, underlining the significance of both layers of muscle in sporting activities. Furthermore, the internal obliques play a crucial role in stabilizing the pelvis, which is critical for maintaining healthy posture and exercise. This makes them indispensable for functional movement and injury prevention. The oblique muscles' significance extends beyond mere movement; they also play an essential role in promoting core stability. A stable core, aided by strong oblique muscles, is necessary for balance, sound posture, and efficient transmission of force during movement. The relationship of the obliques with the other abdominal muscles, transversus abdominis and rectus abdominis, exhibits a model of cooperation required for effective movement, especially in complex usage like athletic training or rehab. Interestingly, symptoms like DRA can have a radical impact on the function of these muscles by altering the stability of the abdominal wall architecture, leading to potential core instability and strength issues (Herrgård et al., 2025). Rehabilitation of such symptoms through appropriate rehabilitation can assist in achieving effective function, thereby improving overall physical well-being and functioning.

9.6.1. Types of Oblique Muscles (External and Internal)

The oblique muscles, constituents of the structural matrix of the abdominal wall, are two principal layers: the internal oblique muscles and the external oblique muscle.

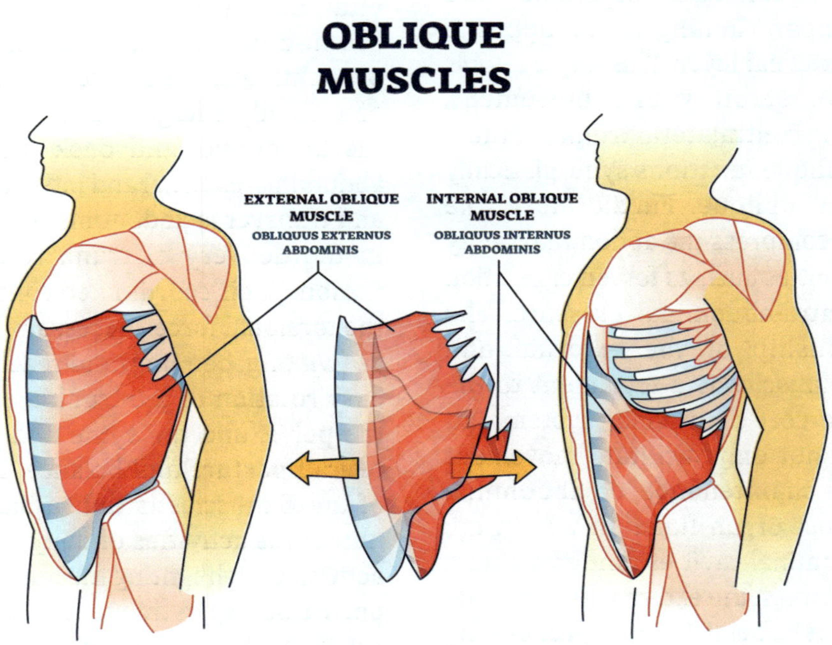

Figure 9.15. Internal and external obliques.

Source: https://steelsupplements.com/blogs/steel-blog/how-to-do-oblique-crunches-form-benefits.

The more superficial of these two muscles, the external oblique, originates from the lower eight ribs and runs obliquely downward and medially. It interdigitates with the latissimus dorsi and the serratus anterior, and this again emphasizes its role in maintaining abdominal integrity and also the mechanics of respiration. Structurally, the external oblique muscle has the significant function of trunk rotation and lateral flexion, bilaterally, to assist in flexing the vertebral column. The layer of the muscle assists in producing support during lifting and twisting through force distribution, thereby safeguarding internal organs within the thorax and abdomen. The significance of the external oblique muscle is also evident by its effect on posture and stability within the core musculature. Contrary to the external obliques, internal oblique muscles are positioned beneath the external obliques and exhibit a varied functional behavior (Figure 9.15).

The origin of the internal oblique is from the iliac crest, ligamentum inguinale, and fascia thoracolumbar, running in the opposite diagonal to the external layer. This angle allows for synergism of stability and movement, particularly during contralateral trunk rotation, as the internal oblique functions synergistically with the external oblique. Furthermore, the internal obliques compress the abdominal cavity to assist with activities such as forced expiration and control of intra-abdominal pressure. The dynamic relationship of the external and internal oblique muscles is a testament to the complexity of the core's muscular system and their capacity to not only facilitate movement but support the maintenance of abdominal pressure and assist organ function within the thoracic and abdominal cavities. Understanding the interaction between the external and internal oblique muscles is crucial for comprehending MSK health and injury rehabilitation. For instance, muscle disorders like DRA affect these muscles, leading to functional impairments that interfere with mobility and general quality of life. DRA, a frequent finding in postpartum women, is an abdominal muscle wall separation of the rectus abdominis muscle that can be the consequence of weakened oblique muscles and the discrepancy in abdominal pressure dynamics (Herrgård et al., 2025). Improvement of such issues using specific rehabilitation training can significantly enhance core stability and physical function. Current evidence informs a multidimensional approach to training the oblique muscles, emphasizing the necessity of exercise regimens that are specific to the individual and include both internal and external obliques. Enhanced knowledge of the two forms of muscle heralds improved clinical practice, exercise, and rehabilitation methods, having a direct impact on thoracic and abdominal health outcomes (Muralimohan et al., 2009).

9.6.2. Functions in Trunk Rotation and Lateral Flexion

Lateral flexion and trunk rotation are vital components of thorax and abdomen biomechanics. These movements are predominantly executed with the assistance of a highly integrated set of muscles within the abdominal and back regions. The rectus abdominis, external and internal oblique muscles, and transverse abdominis play a significant role in the delivery of trunk rotation and lateral flexion. Their coordinated contraction generates the torsional forces necessary for activities such as twisting, bending, and reaching. Additionally, easy rotation of the trunk assists in stabilizing the pelvis and the spine and consequently the overall posture and balance. Synergistic action of these muscles is thus a basic component of numerous activities of daily living and sporting activities, highlighting the importance of strength and flexibility in this sector. Lateral flexion with rotation of the trunk is critical in providing a degree of movement that is favorable for daily usage. Quadratus lumborum is a deep abdominal muscle that has a special function in lateral flexion by drawing the pelvis and spine towards each other when they move. This allows the body to flex sideways without compromising the position, hence preventing injury. Moreover, the synchronization of obliques and erector spinae muscles ensures that the trunk is stabilized while moving laterally. The synchronized action of the muscles is significant in sports involving bending actions or lateral movements, such as tennis or basketball. Through their role in lateral flexion, these muscles contribute to dynamic torso stabilization, enhancing general sport performance and functional movement patterns in competitive sports as well as daily functioning. The understanding of trunk rotation and lateral flexion is not only relevant to the athlete but also to physical rehabilitation and assessment practice. Manual muscle testing, a serious physical therapy evaluation instrument, assesses the strength and function of such muscles under varying positions. Accurate evaluation distinguishes between muscle imbalances or weakness that predispose to injury. Research indicates marked differences in muscular strength between the sexes, namely, in the capacity for maximal voluntary contractions with trunk motion, indicating the need for targeted rehabilitation interventions. Proper strengthening and conditioning of the trunk muscles help minimize fatigability, therefore, performance and endurance. Thus, interventions for muscles involved in the activities of trunk rotation and lateral flexion play a key role in prevention against injury as well as improving functional outcomes, making them significant in the bigger picture of MSK functioning and athletic performance (DiDonna et al., 2005; Deering et al., 2017).

9.6.3. Relevance in Injury Prevention and Rehabilitation

In the area of injury prevention and recovery, it is crucial to understand specifically the muscles of the thorax and the abdomen. These muscle groups play a vital role in core stability, facilitating movement, and maintaining overall function within the body. Trauma to these areas has the potential to significantly jeopardize not only sports performance but also overall activities, thereby creating a rippling effect on the overall quality of life of a subject. The incorporation of appropriate rehabilitation programs to rehabilitate these muscle groups can assist in regaining functional movement with less potential for re-injury. The use of muscle strength training cannot be overemphasized, as optimal thoracic and abdominal musculature integrity is the basis for good biomechanics and economy of movement, which is essential in sporting as well as rehabilitation situations. Also, the addition of diaphragm training in rehabilitation protocols indicates the shifting ways of injury prevention. The latest research indicates that athletic trainers (AT) are increasingly recognizing the need to include breathing mechanisms in their rehabilitation protocols, thus focusing on comprehensive rehabilitation methods. The diaphragm, as an essential muscle in breathing and core stability, is a perfect example of the relationship between breath control and total muscular performance of the thoracic and abdominal cavities. According to AT specialists' observations, the addition of diaphragm training can enhance physical performance and improve respiration habits, both of which are foundational for optimal recovery from injury. Systematic use of these techniques underscores their value in rehabilitation treatment, generating more overall understanding of how muscle interaction influences recovery outcomes (Foltz et al., 2016). The field of biomechanics also emphasizes the importance of knowing about thoracic and abdominal muscles in preventing injury and rehabilitation. It is an interdisciplinary science that draws knowledge from the fields of engineering and physiology in understanding how these kinds of muscles function across various movements. Through the continued evolution of the science of biomechanics, investigators employ more advanced modeling techniques in simulating human motion, offering new insights into mechanisms of injury and the efficiency of rehabilitation. By reviewing the adaptation of thoracic and abdominal muscles to movement and stress, practitioners can formulate more effective prevention strategies and rehabilitation programs. This evidence-based practice not only results in improved recovery but also enhances optimal athletic performance and longevity of healthy motion (Harris et al., 2012). The interplay dynamic among these muscle groups emphasizes the need for ongoing research and education within the field so that practitioners are well-equipped to guide optimal recovery trajectories for their patients.

Test Your Knowledge

1. What are the differences between the external and internal oblique muscles in terms of structure and location?
2. How do the oblique muscles contribute to trunk rotation and lateral flexion?

SUMMARY

A study of the thoracic and abdominal muscles gives necessary insight into their anatomical and functional significance, particularly in the context of heterogeneous age populations. As the existing studies illustrate, trunk muscle function, particularly in the older population, is critical not only to maintain mobility but also to guarantee stability during varied activities. This emphasizes the need for the application of exercises that are tailored to the changes in muscle function in older adults. The accommodation facilitates older adults' ability to engage in physical activity safely and effectively and reduces injury risk. The findings emphasize the need to prioritize trunk muscle strength training with utmost priority across all age groups, particularly among ageing populations, underscoring the crucial roles of these muscles in stability and mobility. Moreover, assessment of trunk muscle function through electromyographic monitoring emphasizes an understanding of interindividual variation in muscle activation patterns. Elderly subjects also demonstrated capacity for effective activation of their abdominal muscles during stability exercises, in which activation percentages were noted to be higher than typically reported within younger groups of subjects. This implies that age does not merely relate to reduced muscle capability but that elderly individuals are capable of demonstrating significant activation of trunk muscles when stimulated in the proper manner. Such findings from more recent research, including assessment of functional muscle activation, serve to enlighten our understanding of the broader relevance to rehabilitation and prevention efforts in enhancing pelvic and spinal stability required to improve overall quality of life in older individuals (Burden et al., 2008). Finally, the interconnection between trunk muscle strength, stability, and overall health underscores the essential value of such muscles beyond mere structure. Thoracic and abdominal musculature form a foundation for the functional quality of movement that facilitates the required activities of daily living. Trunk stability, as described in the literature, is essential in ensuring not only physical independence but also psychological and social well-being, and particularly as an individual continues to increase in age. It is thus imperative that continuous research continues to explore new rehabilitation methods in maintaining and maximizing trunk muscle function. Lastly, developing an appreciation of the function of thorax and abdomen muscles creates an avenue for a complete model of health, evoking their reciprocal roles in encouraging an active and healthy existence in all populations (Milani et al., 2015).

Anatomy and functional significance of the thoracic and abdominal muscles are significant areas of study that yield considerable information about their anatomical organization and functional significance. The muscles play a role in basic functions of respiration, movement, and trunk stability. The diaphragm is the primary muscle of respiration, executing inhalation and exhalation by adjusting thoracic volume. The intercostal muscles help by expanding and contracting the rib cage to facilitate respiration. The abdominal muscles, rectus abdominis, and obliques provide structural support besides assisting in generating movements such as flexion, rotation, and stabilization of the thorax and pelvis. In concert, their synchronized action is necessary for maintaining correct posture and facilitating the movements used for everyday activities and sporting performance. Furthermore, neural processes have a significant function in controlling thoracic and abdominal movements. The observation of these muscles' activation provokes a pattern of complex motor unit interaction under the direction of specific neural pathways. Current studies show the central nervous system controls timing and force of muscle contractions, noting the variability of these muscles to adapt to various physical demands. For example, during vigorous physical activity, as documented in locomotion research, there is considerable recruitment of abdominal muscles for stabilizing the core and allowing more unrestricted movement of limbs. This adaptability is vital for maximizing mobility as well as stability, proving the importance of coordination of muscles in the thoracic and abdominal regions (Dickinson et al., 1996). In addition, awareness of the biomechanics of thoracic and abdominal muscles accounts for various clinical conditions of these areas. Dysfunction or weakness of muscles can lead to respiratory illnesses, postural disorders, and limitations in mobility. Rehabilitation could thus focus on improving muscle strength to attain restoration of function. In addition, research has revealed that increased coordination of the muscles of the thorax and abdomen enhances sporting performance and daily functioning. It is essential to acknowledge that the concerted activity of these muscles under the direction of neural organization and mechanical properties is vital in healthy and diseased conditions (Wosnitza et al., 2013). Continued research into these systems enhances human anatomy and physiology knowledge, which in the long term helps enhance clinical practice and athletic training methods.

KEY TERMS FROM THIS CHAPTER

- Pectoralis major
- Pectoralis minor
- Serratus anterior
- Intercostal muscles
- Diaphragm
- Rectus abdominis
- External oblique
- Internal oblique
- Transversus abdominis
- Linea alba
- Subclavius
- External intercostals
- Internal intercostals
- Innermost intercostals
- Quadratus lumborum

CRITICAL THINKING QUESTIONS

1. **Which muscle is primarily responsible for breathing by expanding the thoracic cavity?**
   a. External oblique
   b. Diaphragm
   c. Rectus abdominis
   d. Pectoralis major
2. **The rectus abdominis muscle is commonly known as the:**
   a. Chest muscle
   b. Side muscle
   c. Six-pack muscle
   d. Shoulder muscle
3. **Which muscle assists in forced exhalation and rotates the trunk?**
   a. Internal oblique
   b. Diaphragm
   c. Transversus abdominis
   d. Trapezius
4. **The pectoralis major muscle is located in the:**
   a. Abdomen
   b. Back
   c. Chest
   d. Neck
5. **Which abdominal muscle lies deepest and helps compress the abdominal contents?**
   a. External oblique
   b. Internal oblique
   c. Transversus abdominis
   d. Rectus abdominis

Short Answer Questions

1. What are the main thoracic muscles, and what roles do they play in respiration and posture?
2. Describe the general structure and function of the abdominal muscles.
3. What are the intercostal muscles, and how do they assist in the breathing process?
4. What is the anatomical structure of the diaphragm, and what is its primary function?
5. Where is the rectus abdominis located, and what is its role in trunk movement and stability?
6. Differentiate between the external and internal oblique muscles in terms of location and function.
7. How do the thoracic and abdominal muscles work together during respiration and core stabilization?

Answer to Critical Thinking Questions

1. (b); 2. (c); 3. (a); 4. (c); 5. (c)

REFERENCES

1. JP, J., KV, A., & Abraham, J. (2016). Unilateral left rectus sternalis muscle: a case report. *International Journal of Research in Medical Sciences*, 3042–3044. https://doi.org/10.18203/2320-6012.ijrms20162001Albanese, A., Arroyo-Jimenez, M. del, Attardi, G., Azer, S., Benninger, B., Bergman, R., et al. (2018). Experience from an optional dissection course in a clinically-orientated concept to complement system-based anatomy in a reformed curriculum. https://core.ac.uk/download/154767350.pdf (accessed on 14th June 2025).
2. Aliverti, A., Bovio, D., Kayser, B., Uva, B., et al. (2015). The "Abdominal Circulatory Pump": An auxiliary heart during exercise? https://core.ac.uk/download/77194317.pdf (accessed on 14th June 2025).
3. Aliverti, A., Uva, B., Uva, B., Kayser, B., & Bovio, D. (2016). The "Abdominal Circulatory Pump": An auxiliary heart during exercise? https://core.ac.uk/download/80335400.pdf (accessed on 14th June 2025).
4. Almorza Gomar, D., Carrasco Molinillo, M. del C., Prada Oliveira, J. A., Pérez Arana, E., et al. (2019). Enseñanza de Anatomía de Superficie Mediante la Pintura Corporal. https://core.ac.uk/download/228073327.pdf (accessed on 14th June 2025).
5. Bolender, D. L., Daly, F. J., Hoagland, T. M., Jain, S., et al. (2015). Posterior approach to kidney dissection: An old surgical approach for integrated medical curricula. https://core.ac.uk/download/146516999.pdf (accessed on 14th June 2025).
6. Bumeister, V. I., Prykhodko, O. O., Sulym, L. H., Yarmolenko, A. V., et al. (2016). *Splanchnology: Cardiovascular and Immune Systems*. https://core.ac.uk/download/141452995.pdf (accessed on 14th June 2025).
7. Burden, A., Radebold, A., Richardson, C., Hubley-Kozey, C. L., Hubley-Kozey, C. L., Hubley-Kozey, C. L., Hubley-Kozey, C. L., et al. (2008). The feasibility of measuring the activation of the trunk muscles in healthy older adults during trunk stability exercises. https://core.ac.uk/download/pdf/8265374.pdf (accessed on 14th June 2025).
8. Casagrande-Jaloretto, D. C., Brent, C. S., van Englesdorp, D., Cox-Foster, D., Hatjina, F., Dade, H. A., Hatjina, F., et al. (2013). Standard methods for *Apis mellifera* anatomy and dissection. https://core.ac.uk/download/18548084.pdf (accessed on 14th June 2025).
9. Chan, W. P., & Dickinson, M. H. (1996). *In vivo* length oscillations of indirect flight muscles in the fruit fly *Drosophila virilis*. https://core.ac.uk/download/4880664.pdf (accessed on 14th June 2025).
10. Cotten, P. B. (2009). The gross morphology and histochemistry of respiratory muscles in bottlenose dolphins (*Tursiops truncatus*). https://core.ac.uk/download/149230384.pdf (accessed on 14th June 2025).
11. Deering, R., Hunter, S. K., Neumann, D. A., Pashibin, M., et al. (2017). Muscle function and fatigability of trunk flexors in males and females. https://core.ac.uk/download/213081937.pdf (accessed on 14th June 2025).
12. Desai, R., Happee, R., & Papaioannou, G. (2024). Vibration transmission through the seated human body captured with a computationally efficient multibody model. https://core.ac.uk/download/616666834.pdf (accessed on 14th June 2025).

13. Dickinson, M. H., & Götz, K. G. (1996). The wake dynamics and flight forces of the fruit fly *Drosophila melanogaster*. https://core.ac.uk/download/4893666.pdf (accessed on 14th June 2025).

14. DiDonna, A. (2005). Instructional guidebook for manual muscle testing. https://core.ac.uk/download/643693730.pdf (accessed on 14th June 2025).

15. Flack, M. (1921). The Milroy Lectures on respiratory efficiency in relation to health and disease. https://core.ac.uk/download/pdf/211978526.pdf (accessed on 14th June 2025).

16. Foltz, M. R. (2016). Diaphragm training and evaluation as a therapeutic tool by athletic trainers in orthopedic rehabilitation. https://core.ac.uk/download/233949873.pdf (accessed on 14th June 2025).

17. Gill, D. R. (1972). A study of thoracic skeletomuscular in Peracarid (Crustacea). https://core.ac.uk/download/217166514.pdf (accessed on 14th June 2025).

18. Greene, J. B. (1968). Approaches to breath support and control. https://core.ac.uk/download/33363079.pdf (accessed on 14th June 2025).

19. Guy, H. J. B., & Prisk, G. K. (2025). Heart-lung interactions in aerospace medicine. https://core.ac.uk/download/pdf/42817596.pdf (accessed on 14th June 2025).

20. Harris, G. F., & Slavens, B. A. (2012). *Biomechanics*. https://core.ac.uk/download/213080657.pdf (accessed on 14th June 2025).

21. Herrgård, K. (2025). Rehabilitation of postpartum diastasis rectus abdominis: A patient guide for the Wellbeing Services County of Ostrobothnia (OVPH). https://core.ac.uk/download/638726603.pdf (accessed on 14th June 2025).

22. Holstege, G., & Subramanian, H. H. (2009). The nucleus retroambiguus control of respiration. https://core.ac.uk/download/17041438.pdf (accessed on 14th June 2025).

23. Huravitch, C., Relay, N., & Schulte, K. (2003). An electromyographic analysis of the abdominal musculature in the production of vocalization intensity during singing. https://core.ac.uk/download/235074023.pdf (accessed on 14th June 2025).

24. Joshua, A., Pare, V., & Shetty, L. (2014). Variations in dimensions and shape of thoracic cage with aging: An anatomical review. https://core.ac.uk/download/478454162.pdf (accessed on 14th June 2025).

25. Middlemas, S. J. (1999). *Yoga and the Athlete: A Building Block for Success: An Honors Thesis (HONRS 499)*. https://core.ac.uk/download/5010047.pdf (accessed on 14th June 2025).

26. Milani, A., Bezuidenhout, A. J., Yates, A. M., Farke, A. A., King, A. S., King, A. S., Müller, B., et al. (2015). Osteological and soft-tissue evidence for pneumatization in the cervical column of the ostrich (*Struthio camelus*) and observations on the vertebral columns of non-volant, semi-volant and semi-aquatic birds. https://core.ac.uk/download/80683151.pdf (accessed on 14th June 2025).

27. Muralimohan, P., & Sivaprasad, S. (2009). Neuromuscular systems in the fifth instar larva of silkworm *Bombyx mori* (Lepidoptera: Bombycidae): II–Abdominal musculature and its innervation. https://core.ac.uk/download/158352322.pdf (accessed on 14th June 2025).

28. Pettersen, V. (2005). From muscles to singing–The activity of accessory breathing muscles and thorax movement in classical singing. https://core.ac.uk/download/646167103.pdf (accessed on 14th June 2025).

29. Rosse, C. (2000). Terminologies Anatomica; considered from the perspective of next-generation knowledge sources. https://core.ac.uk/download/pdf/9412243.pdf (accessed on 14th June 2025).
30. Rucker, A. (1901). The Texan *Koenenia*. https://core.ac.uk/download/211338452.pdf (accessed on 14th June 2025).
31. Sanusi, J. B. (1986). Studies on the thoracic stretch receptor organ of *Manduca sexta* and effects of octopamine and demethylchlordimeform on the activity of the stretch receptor. https://core.ac.uk/download/33361106.pdf (accessed on 14th June 2025).
32. Sharma, G. B., & Lakhani, R. A. (2023). Anatomical exploration of Halasana. https://core.ac.uk/download/617189671.pdf (accessed on 14th June 2025).
33. Sillar, K. T. (2012). Neural events underlying escape swimming behavior in the squat lobster *Galathea strigosa* (Crustacea, Anomura). https://core.ac.uk/download/9045109.pdf (accessed on 14th June 2025).
34. Sivaprasad, S. (2010). Origin and peripheral distribution of the thoracic and abdominal median nerves in the fifth instar larva of the silkworm, *Bombyx mori* (Lepidoptera: Bombycidae). https://core.ac.uk/download/158352389.pdf (accessed on 14th June 2025).
35. Tautz, D. (2014). One size does not fit all. https://core.ac.uk/download/19842969.pdf (accessed on 14th June 2025).
36. Tiller, N. (2014). Respiratory mechanics during upper body exercise in healthy humans. https://core.ac.uk/download/30339777.pdf (accessed on 14th June 2025).
37. Wosnitza, A. (2013). Leg coordination during walking in insects. https://core.ac.uk/download/18524670.pdf (accessed on 14th June 2025).

MUSCLES OF THE LOWER LIMB

10

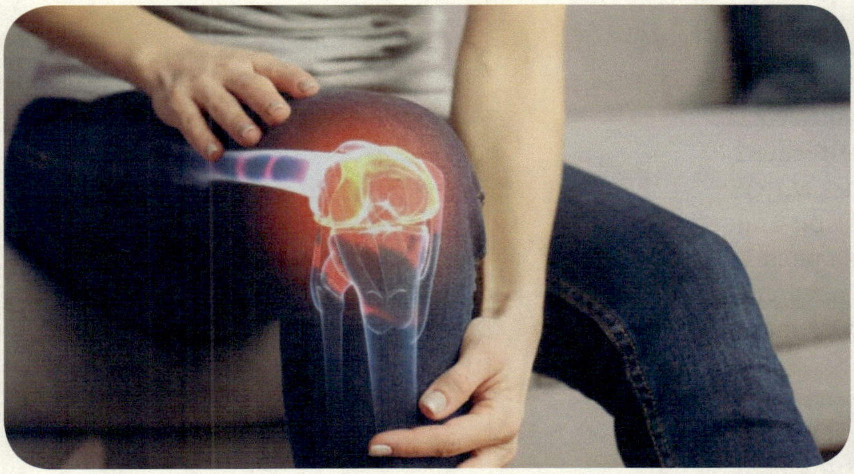

LEARNING OBJECTIVES

After studying this chapter, you will be able to:

1. Describe the anatomy of the lower limb
2. Identify the hip muscles
3. Describe the thigh muscles
4. Identify the major muscles of the leg
5. Describe the muscles of the foot
6. Explain the functional importance of lower limb muscles

Introduction

Lower limb muscles serve a fundamental role in the locomotion and stability of human beings, enabling walking, running, and jumping. Not only do the muscles assist in the support of the body's weight but also the intricate biomechanics involved in walking, which is bipedal locomotion. The anatomy and function of the lower limb muscles have much to do with human evolutionary characteristics, particularly when it comes to comparison with our primate relatives. Knowledge of lower extremity muscle architecture teaches us about the evolutionary processes behind the development of the human body and its successful bipedalism. The importance of lower limb muscles is further demonstrated by their impact on human movement in general, which highlights the need of muscular economy for both performance and injury prevention. As a result, their anatomy and physiology require careful examination. When muscles of the lower limb are under investigation, distinction is typically made between the major muscle groups like the quadriceps, hamstrings, glutes, and calf muscles. Each of these groups plays a distinct role in locomotor functions and postural control. Quadriceps, for instance, are essential for knee extension and are held accountable for important activities like climbing stairs and standing up from a sitting position. Similarly, hamstrings are involved in the flexion of the knee and the movement of the hip and counteract the action of the quadriceps during dynamic movement phases. Gluteal muscles are vital in stabilizing the pelvis as well as in providing mobility to the hip. Closer observation of the muscle groups discloses the anatomical complexity and functional interdependence, suggesting that there is a sophisticated system behind the energetic cost of lower limb functioning. This is reiterated by comparative MSK study findings, which make inferences about muscular evolution and functional adaptation between various species, such as the analysis of integration patterns in human anatomy compared to our primate relatives (Esteve-Altava et al., 2018). Also, inferences made from comparative anatomy between species can benefit the understanding of lower limb muscular structure. Studies in MSK architecture indicate the way differences in locomotory styles, such as running and climbing, influence the development of muscles and their organization. For example, it is established that larger animals, such as felids, exhibit a more conservative MSK organization. Still, the functional demands of human bipedality lead to a singular complexity of hindlimb muscles for autonomous mobility and support (Adams et al., 2016). Through exploration of the evolutionary history of these adaptations, the fine cooperation of muscle function and structure may be appreciated, laying the foundation for clinical assessment of MSK disease and advancement in sports training. A study of the muscles of the lower limb, thus, reveals not only the unique contribution of each to motion but also illuminates broad evolutionary concepts of relevance to human biomechanics.

Importance of Lower Limb Muscles

The lower limb muscles are a significant component of mobility, stability, and physical function. They are the key muscles that assist in various movements such as walking, running, jumping, and balance. The lower limb muscles are sophisticated groups delineated into the hip, thigh, leg, and foot regions, each having a unique contribution towards locomotion and postural control.

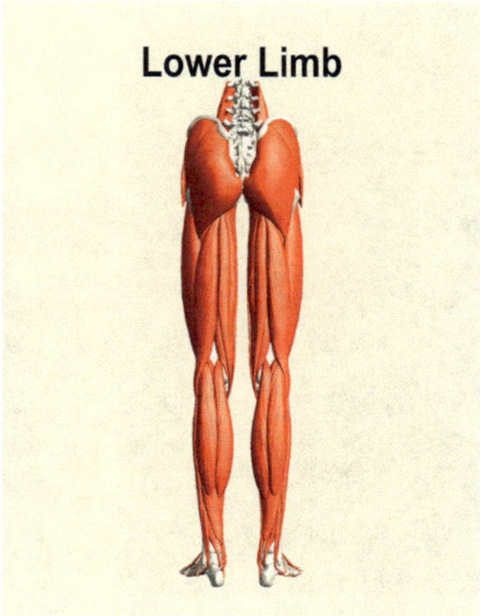

Figure 10.1. Posterior view of the lower limb muscles, illustrating major muscle groups involved in movement and support.

Source: https://external-content.duckduckgo.com/iu/?u=https%3A%2F%2Fwww.muscle-atlas.org%2Fassets%2Fimages%2Fmuscles%2Fpng%2FLowerLimb-5.png&f=1&nofb=1&ipt=427ace43deff0cd665d08a924011e8e26e16623c3170779419afe52221b665a2.

For instance, gluteal muscles not only stabilize the pelvis while walking but also assist in hip movements and serve as forceful propulsion motors. The group of quadriceps also plays an integral part in knee extension, an action needed during activities like standing up or walking upstairs. The variation of these muscle groups indicates the importance of lower limb muscles in maintaining successful movement patterns and minimizing the risk for weakness or imbalance-related injury. Further, lower limb muscle changes can be illustrated using evidence from evolution, such as extinct sthenurine kangaroos. Evidence indicates that these giant kangaroos adapted their muscle morphology to enable a bipedal striding gait rather than the usual hopping, which is energetically costly at big body sizes. The derived musculature and limb size suggest that such animals employed powerful lower limbs for stability and locomotion economy, confirming the biomechanical influence of muscle morphology on locomotion capacities (Figueirido et al., 2014) (Figure 10.1). Exploration of such adaptations reveals a previously unimaginable insight into evolutionary significance of lower limb muscles, proving the degree to which functional demands shape muscular growth through the ages. Understanding these adaptations can imply more universal principles applied to living structures, including conclusions that will benefit rehabilitation after injury or surgery. Apart from their functional significance, muscles of the lower limb are also crucial in maintaining musculoskeletal (MSK) system integrity. Muscle weakness, especially among older individuals or inactive persons, may trigger a cascade of mobility losses and therefore set the individual up for falls and fractures. Stability provided by well-conditioned lower limb muscles is necessary in joint stabilization as well as in preventing injury such as sprain and tears. For instance, the knee joint, with its advanced system of ligaments and muscles, depends entirely on assisted muscle strength to function optimally (Abourachid et al., 2014). Lower limb muscle interactions and anatomy can provide the platform upon which effective exercise programs for the development of muscle strength and joint stability can be produced. Lastly, the significance of lower limb muscles extends beyond movement alone, as they preserve quality of life and functional independence in various populations.

Overview of Muscle Groups

It is vital to understand the lower limb's muscle groups for the examination of body mechanics and movement. The lower limb has several essential muscle groups, which all serve for mobility, stability, and force production in activities like walking, running, and jumping. Key muscle groups are the quadriceps, hamstrings, gluteal muscles, and calf muscles. The quadriceps, which are four muscles at the front part of the thigh, are primarily responsible for knee extension and have a vital role to play in activities related to the movement of the leg. The hamstrings, located at the back of the thigh, enable knee flexion and contribute to hip extension, facilitating various movements essential for both sports activities and everyday tasks. The gluteal muscles play an important role in lower limb strength and the stability of the hip. The muscle group consists of three muscles—the gluteus maximus, gluteus Medius, and gluteus minimus—that have distinct yet complementary functions. The gluteus maximus, the most prominent muscle in the group, plays a vital role in hip extension and external rotation, especially in activities involving thrust and force. Conversely, the gluteus Medius and minimus are responsible for stabilizing the pelvis during walking and running to prevent excessive lateral movement. The stabilization is of utmost importance in ensuring balance and guarding the lower limb against injury, especially in sports environments where there is dynamic movement. All the muscles together present a firm platform of the lower body's kinetic chain, allowing functional and coordinated motion. Other than facilitating movement, the calf muscles, including the gastrocnemius and soleus, are significant in propulsion and posture work. The gastrocnemius, a large, two-joint muscle that crosses the knee and ankle joints, contributes primarily to knee flexion and ankle plantarflexion. Sprinting and jumping mainly use this muscle. The soleus muscle, though lesser in prominence, is also tasked with posture maintenance during standing and walking by supporting the ankle. The synergy between these muscles indicates good locomotion and balance, further emphasizing the importance of lower limb muscle groups. Understanding these muscle dynamics is critical to developing rehabilitation plans, particularly in cases of disuse or atrophy, as determined by studies showing the difference in muscle adaptation under disparate conditions, such as exposure to microgravity (Aerts et al., 2019) and prolonged disuse (Blottner et al., 2017).

10.1. Anatomy of the Lower Limb

Learning Outcome

1. Define the major bones involved
2. Discuss the muscle compartments
3. Explain the joint structures

The lower limb anatomy consists of a highly complex interaction of joints, bones, and muscles that all contribute to its mobility and functionality overall. The lower limb is primarily divided into four regions: hip, thigh, leg, and foot, each of which has a particular group of muscles responsible for diverse movements. In considering the muscles of the lower limb, it is essential to look at the agonist and antagonist groups, for example, the quadriceps and hamstrings, which act together to facilitate movement such as walking, running, and jumping. They are not just essential for walking but also have important roles in stabilizing the pelvis and balance in dynamic movements. Knowledge of these anatomical structures provides a basic foundation to study biomechanics and physical therapy, highlighting the synergy of structure and function in the human body. The muscles of the lower limb can be grouped into three large compartments: the anterior, posterior, and medial thigh compartments, as well as the anterior and posterior leg compartments. Each of these compartments is filled with muscular structures that will move the body in specific ways and is innervated with individual nerves. Such is the case of the anterior compartment of the thigh with its powerful quadriceps femoris that extends the knee. In contrast, the posterior compartment has the hamstring group flexing the knee and extending the hip.

Similarly, compartmental muscles of the leg provide dorsiflexion and plantarflexion of the foot, essential in walking and running. Understanding the compartmentalization of these muscles is crucial for the diagnosis and treatment of injuries, and it is a critical consideration for surgical planning and rehabilitation protocols. The precise examination of these compartments underscores the need to delineate functional anatomy in sports medicine as well as in clinical settings. Proper analysis of the lower limb muscles would not be feasible without the identification of their anatomical relationship with other structures, such as tendons, ligaments, and associated fascia. The anatomical relationship between these structures contributes to movement economy and injury resistance. For instance, tendons are fixed points of attachment where muscles can transmit forces across joints, and ligaments support the joint during dynamic movements. Fascial compartments that envelop these muscles enable them to move and cover vascular components. Muscle type differences in morphology, like slow-twitch and fast-twitch fibers, dictate performance and endurance in physical activities. Looking at the anatomy of the lower limb within this holistic context better equips researchers and practitioners to comprehend the advanced engineering of the human body and its ability to respond to a wide range of physical requirements (Cozart et al., 2017; Nichols et al., 2019) (Figure 10.2).

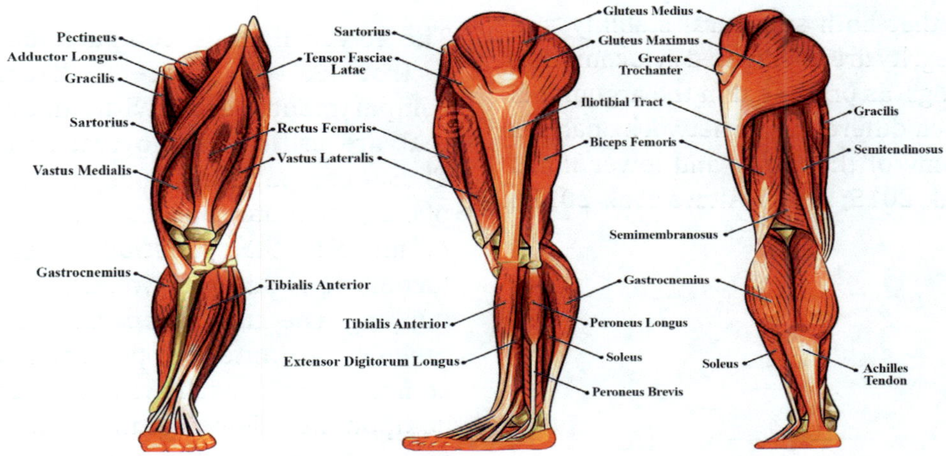

Figure 10.2. The lower limb muscles (anterior, posterior and lateral view).

Source: https://www.researchgate.net/figure/The-lower-limb-muscles-anterior-posterior-and-lateral-view-14_fig1_348955981.

10.1.1. Major Bones Involved

The bony skeleton of the lower limb is primarily composed of a series of significant bones that play basic functions in locomotion and load-bearing.

The femur, the longest and strongest bone in the human body, serves as the primary support for standing and walking, connecting the hip to the knee joint. Tibia and fibula, positioned in the lower leg, complement the femur with support and enable complex movements. The shinbone or tibia is the prominent bone for passing weight from the femur to the foot, with the fibula in a parallel position, offering lateral support and a point of attachment for muscles. These large bones collectively form the framework on which the lower limb muscles operate, supporting all kinds of movements from walking to running and jumping. Moreover, the pelvis's special anatomy greatly influences lower limb function. The ilium, ischium, and pubis constitute the pelvis and fuse with the sacrum to produce the pelvic girdle, a solid base for the lower limbs. This bony structure supports the weight of the body when it is moving and is part of bipedal walking. The acetabulum, the cup-like pelvis socket, encloses the head of the femur and creates the hip joint, which provides a dynamic range of motion (ROM) (Figure 10.3).

The pelvis and its correlated bone structure highlight the importance of structural disposition in facilitating effective muscle action within the lower limb, as any alteration or abnormality of bone shape can influence total mobility as well as stability, particularly in locomotion activities such as running or jumping. The lower limbs' complex structure is also illustrated via the bones of the foot, including the tarsals, metatarsals, and phalanges. The tarsal bones, i.e., the calcaneus and talus, bear the weight and absorb the shock in movement. The phalanges and metatarsals, forming the forefoot, bear the balance and push-off in gait cycles. All of these participate in the foot arch structure, which absorbs shock, accommodates different terrains, and provides a stable base for muscle function and attachment. The connectivity of such skeleton components, apart from highlighting the complex biomechanics of the lower limb, reveals the evolutionary adaptation to guarantee that both structural stability and functional integrity are highlighted in locomotion in human beings, as presented in the arguments by the observed differences in network analyses of MSK anatomy of the upper and lower limbs (Goswami et al., 2015; Esteve-Altava et al., 2018).

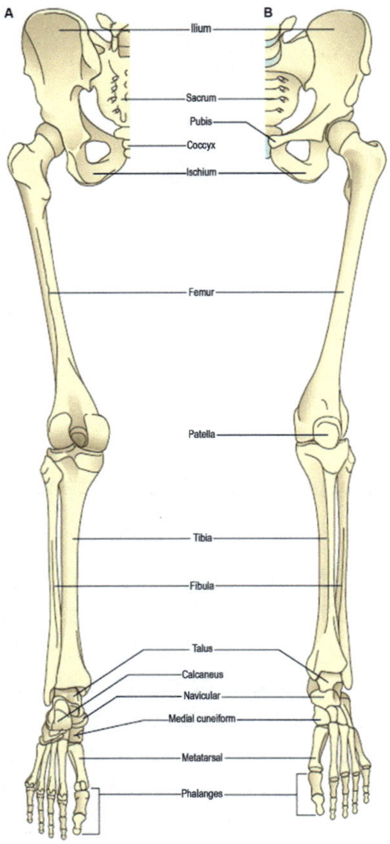

Figure 10.3. Lower limb skeletal anatomy.

Source: https://external-content.duckduckgo.com/iu/?u=https%3A%2F%2Fwww.researchgate.net%2Fprofile%2FChristian-Von-Scheidt%2Fpublication%2F339843670%2Ffigure%2Ffig1%2FAS%3A867848528343041%401583922621468%2FOn-the-Left-A-posterior-view-of-the-of-the-bones-of-the-lower-limb-On-the-right-B.ppm&f=1&nofb=1&ipt=985822c1f9f0d82aeb382bc3c41c5b5dfd478aeaa879d635d68ea9a0435b74fe.

10.1.2. Muscle Compartments

The lower limb is compartmentalized into a trochlea of different discrete muscle compartments, each with unique functions that are critical to movement and stability. These compartments, separated by fascial planes, facilitate coordination between groups of muscles that function synergistically in locomotion, such as walking, running, and jumping. The main compartments in the thigh include the anterior, posterior, and medial compartments, each with discrete muscular components. For instance, the quadriceps femoris group in the anterior compartment extends the knee. Compartmentalization not only aids functional movement but also protects the muscles and nerves within, reducing the likelihood of traumatic injury during training. It is vital to understand these muscle groups and their corresponding compartments to diagnose and manage lower limb injuries and effectively formulate rehabilitation programs. Also, the lower leg contains compartments of higher complexity, with the anterior, lateral, and posterior compartments further emphasizing the functional specialization of the lower limb musculature. The anterior compartment of the lower leg contains muscles such as the tibialis anterior, which is highly important for dorsiflexion as well as inversion of the foot. The posterior compartment, in contrast, is primarily responsible for plantarflexion, emphasizing the inherent specialization of these compartments. In addition, the lateral compartment has muscles that contribute to eversion and foot stability in bipedal walking. Compartmentalization enables the forces generated by one group of muscles to support another group's forces effectively, resulting in better overall limb functioning. As shown by several studies of locomotion mechanics, this compartmental organization is a key component of the biomechanical efficacy of the lower limb during different actions. It has a key evolutionary significance in tetrapod limb development (Abbasi et al., 2018). Examining the interaction between muscle compartments and their evolutionary history provides insights into lower limb adaptations over time. Terrestrial locomotion transitioned from aquatic required intrinsic changes in muscle organization, and early tetrapods developed modular limbs to offer accommodation of terrestrial habitats. Gradual compartmentalization of muscle groups resulted in an advanced ability to generate diverse movements that allowed survival and adaptability. This evolutionary process produced a highly developed integration of muscular and skeletal structures that not only enabled locomotion but also enhanced agility and stability. It appears that as the appendages evolved, functional capacities of muscle compartments differentiated so a wide range of movements, not available in their fish ancestors, could be achieved. It offers a more nuanced appreciation of the roles of the contemporary muscle compartments and informs therapeutic interventions in lower limb strengthening and rehabilitation (Henry et al., 2014).

10.1.3. Joint Structures

The intricate structure of joint architectures is centrally located in the functional biomechanics of the lower limb, particularly with regard to muscle actions. Joints represent key interfaces where bones converge, enabling movement along with stability through a variety of connective tissues such as ligaments and tendons. In the lower limb, synovial joints such as the hip, knee, and ankle provide a quintessential example of such intricacy. The presence of cartilage in the joint surfaces decreases friction and enables smooth motion, which is essential for activities like walking and running. The structure of these joints is also related to specific muscular adaptations. For instance, muscles with origin from the pelvis, such as the gluteal group, are essential in hip stabilization and movement initiation, hence evidence of joint structure and muscle function interrelation in lower limb biomechanics. The study of joint structure is more than anatomy; it encompasses understanding mechanical properties and how these affect muscle function. Evidence indicates that variations in joint architecture can lead to differences in functionality. For instance, the detail of the femorotibial joint in animals such as mice demonstrates adaptations favorable for high levels of contraction speed and joint control, crucial for locomotion stability and performance (Cappellari et al., 2016) (Figure 10.4).

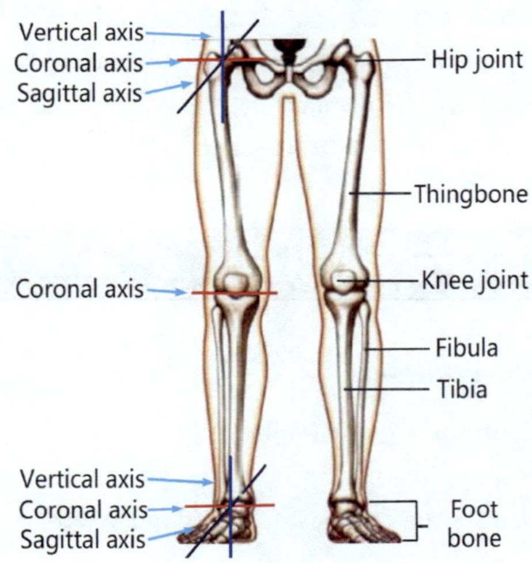

Figure 10.4. Bones, joints and muscle diagram of human lower limbs.

Source: https://www.researchgate.net/figure/Bones-joints-and-muscle-diagram-of-human-lower-limbs_fig1_364256760.

By studying the MSK geometry and muscle architecture, researchers become sensitive to the geometry of joint structures best adapted to enhance athletic function and reduce the risks of injury. Thus, biomechanical properties of joint structures must be considered when evaluating the lower limb muscles, with emphasis on the dynamic relationship of structure and function. Furthermore, biochemical adaptations in various species signify the plasticity of joint structures and their relevance in evolution. For example, the ostrich knee joint has an unusual anatomical configuration with double patellae that have specific biomechanical functions during locomotion (Abourachid et al., 2014). Such a unique structural conformity points to the evolutionary forces that have shaped joint configurations to function best. The interplay between joint structure and muscle function heralds the importance of contextual anatomy and biomechanics in the comprehension of locomotion. By analyzing these correlations, researchers can formulate hypotheses regarding the evolutionary origin of limb bone morphology, along with their implications for muscle function across species. Identifying structures of joints is not only useful in terms of better understanding human lower limb anatomy, but also assumes broader implications in the field of evolutionary biology.

Test Your Knowledge

1. What are the major bones that form the lower limb, and how are they connected?
2. What are the primary muscle compartments of the lower limb, and which movements do they control?

10.2. Hip Muscles

Learning Outcome

1. Identify the gluteal muscles
2. Describe the hip flexors
3. Identify the muscles of the adductor group

The hip muscles play a crucial role in lower limb mechanics, facilitating the movement necessary for ambulation and stability. The primary muscles involved are the gluteal muscles, the iliopsoas, and the adductors, all of which have unique contributions to hip function. Gluteus maximus, for instance, plays the most significant role in hip extension and external rotation and is most engaged in exercises that require power, including sprinting and climbing. In addition, the iliopsoas, made up of the psoas major and the iliacus, is critical for elevation of the thigh and hip flexion, which is significant during walking and running. Collectively, these muscles support locomotion as well as influence alignment and stability at the pelvis, qualifying the hip as a lower limb biomechanical "key joint." Research on animal locomotion provides data relevant to hip muscle function, emphasizing efficiency adaptations. For instance, ostrich gait studies have revealed that their hip muscle arrangement gives them excellent metabolic economy during their rapid movements. Ostriches are cursorial-adapted animals, and their hip-based mechanisms involve bi-articular muscles contributing towards stance phases. Observations indicate that the muscles are utilized predominantly during specific stages of gait to generate the force needed to propel the body along with energy absorption by knee extensor brakes. Implications highlight the degree of specialization of the hip muscles and how such adaptation may contribute to a better appreciation of human lower limb dynamics (et al., 2016). Musculature examination across species, including in mice, has revealed a proximodistal gradient between hip muscles that magnifies architectural differences. Proximal muscles closer to the hip exhibit characteristics better suited for high speeds of contraction and joint control, whereas more distal functional groups possess higher physiological cross-sectional areas (PCSAs) for generating force and economy of energy. This form of structural divergence translates the functional demands placed on these muscles in motion, and suggests a stability-optimal design for a set of activities. As the mouse hindlimb is an exemplary model system for neuromuscular research, awareness of these specializations brings a paradigm to the study of muscle design's applicability both during health and disease states, augmenting discussion further of hip musculature in lower limb research (Cappellari et al., 2016).

10.2.1. Gluteal Muscles

The gluteal muscles, such as the gluteus maximus, gluteus Medius, and gluteus minimus, are the focal point of the lower limb anatomy and physiology. The gluteus maximus, the largest and strongest muscle in the group, is primarily involved in hip extension, external rotation, and thigh abduction.

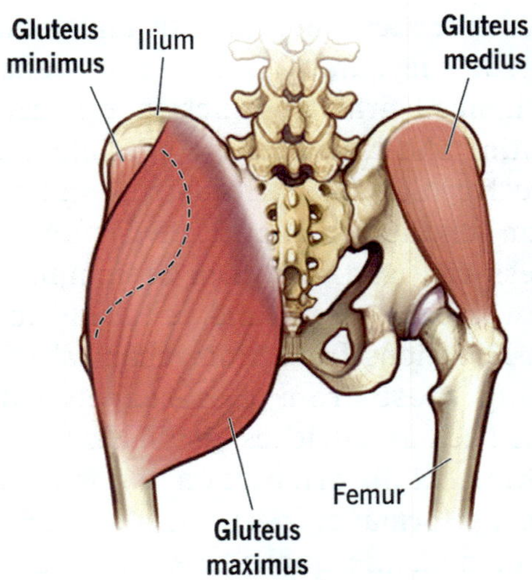

Figure 10.5. Three gluteal muscles (glutes): gluteus maximus, gluteus Medius and gluteus minimus.

Source: https://my.clevelandclinic.org/-/scassets/images/org/health/articles/gluteal-muscles-glutes.

The endurance of this muscle is essential not just for walking and running but also for holding an upright posture. Placement and orientation of these muscles allow effective production of force during locomotion, stabilizing the pelvis during gait cycles. They are thus a key element to activities that contain explosive power and endurance, which are equally essential in sports performance and daily movement. Inefficient working of these muscles could lead to malfunction and injury, demonstrating their significance in maintaining lower limb biomechanics intact (Figure 10.5). Other than the gluteus maximus, the gluteus Medius and minimus play significant roles in the movement and stability of the hip. Gluteus Medius is involved in hip abduction and stabilization of the pelvis during single-leg stance, which is crucial in running and walking. The gluteus minimus assists in hip abduction and internal rotation. Their location enables them to counteract the force of the body and pelvis' downward movement during walking. The coordination between these muscles is not only critical for proper movement but also for injury prevention, particularly among athletes who can be exposed to overuse injury. Understanding the functional anatomy of such muscles is vital to the development of rehabilitation protocols and sport training programs capable of enhancing lower limb performance as well as lessening risks of MSK injury. Recent studies have also thrown more light on the anatomical complexity of gluteal muscles through comparative anatomy among different species, casting further light on their evolutionary adaptations. For example, studies on marsupial locomotion, like that of the koala, demonstrate how muscular structure and function differ greatly among taxa and how this affects ecological niche and mobility. Differences in muscular identification from previous anatomical studies have proved variation and plasticity of gluteal musculature between and within species (Anetai et al., 2022). Such comparative analysis not only enhances our understanding of gluteal muscle function but also prescribes rehabilitation for human lower limb trauma. Such information can, in turn, be utilized towards differentiation of training methods emphasizing the growth of strength and stability of these significant muscle groups, ensuring enhanced performance in sporting activities alongside everyday function (Figueirido et al., 2014).

10.2.2. Hip Flexors

The hip flexors, which are made up of muscles on the anterior aspect of the hip joint, are of great value to lower extremity movement, particularly with ambulation, running, and climbing stairs. The iliopsoas muscle is the primary muscle and consists of the iliacus and the psoas major. These muscles play a crucial role in lifting the thigh towards the abdomen and also play a vital role in balance and posture during various physical actions. Their unique structure and biomechanical properties allow them to generate significant force while providing stability to the hip joint. The function of hip flexors is not just movement but also permits proper energy transfer during exercise, which is important in terms of athletic performance and recovery from rehabilitation (Figure 10.6).

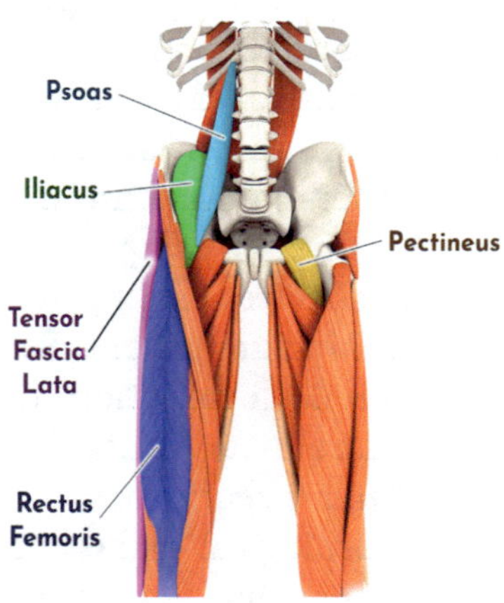

Figure 10.6. Hip flexors.

Source: https://cdn.gethypervisual.com/images/shopify/31636c67-11a7-49a9-a8bc-199c10d66a24/w1200_1cc3_hip-flexors-musculos.jpg.

Furthermore, the functional role of hip flexors can be described based on their anatomical characteristics, specifically their architecture. Research indicates that the organization of muscle fiber types and the PCSA of the muscles contribute to the capacity to contract speed and generate force. Muscle architecture research in related species, as outlined in the study of mouse hindlimb musculature, illustrates that differences between various groups of muscles, such as hip flexors, are key to optimizing motion and stability. These modifications allow for a proximal-distal gradient of muscular design, which reveals that proximal muscles like the hip flexors are optimized for rapid contractions and control of joints, in contrast to their distal counterparts, which have more roles to do with force generation and energy economy (Cappellari et al., 2016). This type of information is paramount in understanding how hip flexors cooperate with other muscles of the lower limb in effecting intricate movements. Understanding hip flexor mechanics is not only beneficial for enhanced athletic function but also for preventing and rehabilitating possible injuries. Inasmuch as they have a stabilizing and moving function for the hip, hip flexor dysfunction or tightness can lead to a host of complications like lower-back strain and reduced mobility. The observations from biomechanical models, including those from research on existing animals such as ostriches, emphasize the need for optimal limb orientation for maximizing muscle performance (Delp et al., 2015). The study of dynamic qualities of hip flexors in various settings—biomechanical constraints, muscle-tendon interactions, and adaptive responses—can reveal the basic principles controlling their function. As research continues to teach us about the intricate relationships between muscle structure, biomechanics, and control, techniques to optimize hip flexor function in athletic and clinical populations will continue to evolve to encourage mobility and overall lower limb well-being more optimally.

10.2.3. Adductor Group

The adductor group of muscles, which is located in the medial compartment of the thigh, plays a very significant role in the movement and stability of the lower limb. This group of muscles primarily comprises the adductor magnus, adductor longus, adductor brevis, pectineus, and gracilis muscles. These muscles are involved in producing the adduction of the hip joint, allowing one to cross the legs. In addition to their functional use, the adductors also stabilize the pelvis when walking or running, as needed to maintain balance and normal gait mechanics. Understanding the function and anatomy of the adductor group is an essential in order to understand their function in various sporting activities and daily movement, and their function in rehabilitation and prevention programs for injury.

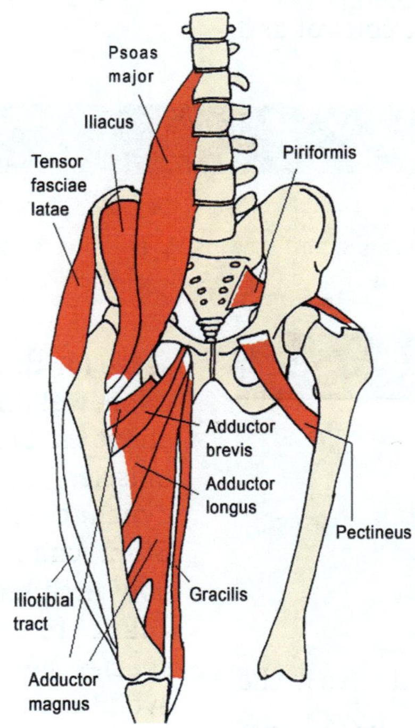

Figure 10.7. Adductor muscles of the hip.

Source: https://en.wikipedia.org/wiki/Adductor_muscles_of_the_hip#/media/File:Anterior_Hip_Muscles_2.PNG.

The anatomical design of the adductor muscles reflects their different specializations for various functional demands. They possess a sequence of arrangements of fibers and cross-sectional diameters, which impinges on force generation and contraction velocities. The parallel and pennate fibers form the architecture of the adductor group that accommodates both for quick movements and substantial strength generation. For instance, the adductor magnus has a unique structure where it possesses both the adductor and extensor functions at the hip and receives innervations by different nerves for its differing functions. This anatomical diversity enables the adductor group to function suitably in the provided tasks, allowing for both dynamic functions, such as sprinting or sidestepping, and stabilizing movements in various physical activities. These adaptations underscore the critical role of the adductor group in functional versatility and mechanical efficiency. During locomotion, the adductor muscles are crucial for lower limb movement efficiency and stability. A comparative analysis of the anatomy of the mouse hindlimb illustrates how these muscles are anatomically specialized for rapid contraction velocities to aid locomotor stability and efficiency (Cappellari et al., 2016) (Figure 10.7). The proximodistal gradient of muscle architecture found throughout similar functional groups emphasizes the functional relevance of the adductor muscles in both joint control and force generation. The architectural specialization afforded by the adductor group allows the group to effectively respond to the nuances of movement patterns presented throughout the bipedal gait pattern. Further, the interfusion of the adductor muscles with adjacent groups demonstrates the harmonious coordination necessary for maximal athletic potential and avoidance of injury. All these results on the functional anatomy of the adductor groups thus prove their vital role in maintaining both mobility and stability throughout activities.

Test Your Knowledge

1. What are the major gluteal muscles, and what roles do they play in movement and posture?
2. Which muscles are considered hip flexors, and what is their primary function?

10.3. Thigh Muscles

Learning Outcome

1. Define the quadriceps group and the hamstring group
2. Discuss the sartorius muscle

The thigh muscles are the functional ones in the lower limb and possess a range of movements utilized in day-to-day activities such as walking, running, and jumping. Primarily subdivided into three groups—anterior, posterior, and medial—the thigh muscles possess characteristic architectural structures respective of their specific roles. The anterior compartment, dominated by the quadriceps group, is the one involved in knee extension and aiding in hip flexion, with architecture conducive to forceful, rapid movement. The posterior compartment, made up of the hamstrings, is primarily responsible for hip extension and knee flexion to facilitate strength and agility activities. Lastly, adductor muscles in the medial compartment serve for thigh adduction to stabilize the pelvis upon walking. This intricacy speaks volumes about the biomechanical specificity of the thigh muscles, highlighting their crucial role in the dynamics of lower limbs and motor control. Biomechanical studies have demonstrated how architectural structures of thigh muscles adapt to the requirements that various species have been subjected to during their evolutionary history. In birds, for instance, the study of ostrich limb mechanics revealed the means through which muscle angles optimize locomotion efficiency. These findings highlight that animals like ostriches do not necessarily use limb postures that utilize the highest moment-generating capacities of the limbs, but instead prefer dynamic muscular characteristics that are effective in supporting body weight and stability during locomotion. Similarly, the musculature of the hindlimb in mice, as characterized in recent anatomical studies, has a proximal-to-distal gradient in muscle morphology to optimize locomotor stability and economy. These observations are a key evolutionary compromise in muscle organization, optimizing performance through different species and accentuating the complex functionality of thigh muscles as vital components in the locomotor mechanism of many animals (Delp et al., 2015; Cappellari et al., 2016) (Figure 10.8).

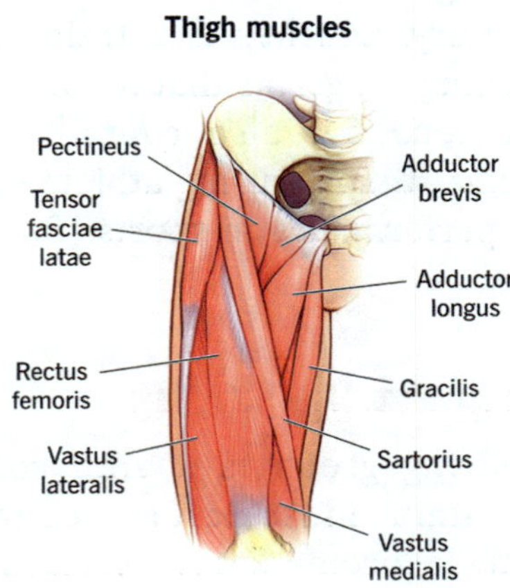

Figure 10.8. Your thighs contain some of the largest muscles in your body. You use them to bend, flex and rotate your lower body.

Source: https://my.clevelandclinic.org/-/scassets/images/org/health/articles/thigh-muscles.

The functional significance of thigh muscles extends beyond mere locomotion and also affects athletic performance and injury susceptibility. Architectural variations among such muscles decide their force generation capacity as well as their modes of contraction, both of which are crucial to various physical activities. Thus, for example, sportspersons have specialized training courses to develop quadriceps and hamstrings to improve performance in sports involving explosiveness in movement. Moreover, a thorough understanding of thigh muscle architecture forms the basis of rehabilitation procedures for individuals who have recovered from injury. A sense of the specific properties and functions of these muscles may provide focused therapies to not only facilitate recovery but also enhance the general stability and competency of the lower limb. Therefore, the physiology of the thigh muscles not only describes their biomechanical roles but also highlights their importance in the health, fitness, and rehabilitation environments.

10.3.1. Quadriceps Group

The quadriceps group of four muscles—rectus femoris, vastus lateralis, vastus medialis, and vastus intermedius—is an essential factor in the activity of the lower limb, particularly in the extension of the knee joint.

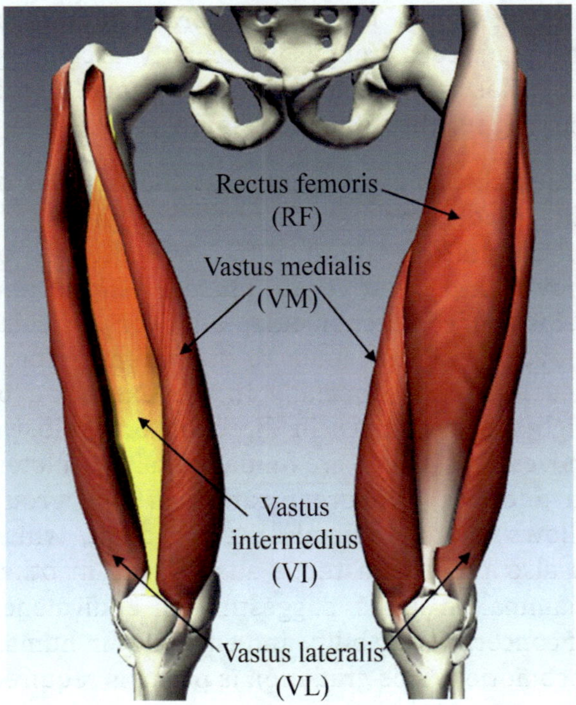

Figure 10.9. Anatomy of quadriceps femoris muscle group, which includes rectus femoris, vastus lateralis, vastus medialis and vastus intermedius.

Source: https://bod-blog-assets.prod.cd.beachbodyondemand.com/bod-blog/wp-content/uploads/2018/06/quad-muscles-thigh-anatomy-NEW.jpg.

The muscle group plays a vital role not only in activities like walking and running, but also in performing everyday tasks such as climbing stairs and standing up from a seated position. The rectus femoris, while it contributes to extension of the knee, is also involved in hip flexion, indicating its dual role that is necessary for total mobility. Moreover, the Vasti muscles are structurally formed to generate a high amount of force that is needed for powerful movement and body stabilization during dynamic activity. As its function becomes increasingly prominent during high-impact activities, understanding the intricate biomechanics of the quadriceps is necessary to develop effective strength-training protocols to improve athletic function and prevent injury. The architectural structure of the quadriceps group is particularly fascinating, as it has evolved to function optimally with varying functional loads (Figure 10.9).

Research has established that the muscles of the quadriceps demonstrate a high degree of adaptation about different patterns of movement, relative to muscle length and velocity of contraction. Adaptation for particular movements can lead to heightened force development, especially in the execution of high-speed changes in direction or explosive movements, which are fundamental to athletes. In addition, the organization of this group allows for a proximal-distal gradient, which is also present in those adaptations in other mammalian limbs, suggesting an equivalence of concern for stability and efficiency in human locomotion. This gradation is perhaps required not only in function but also in protection from harm, especially in dangerous sport environments in which the risk for knee injury is more pronounced. The applicability of the quadriceps groups extends to both sporting function and clinical relevance, particularly in the context of knee injuries, such as tears in the anterior cruciate ligament (ACL). It has been proven that quadriceps strength imbalances relate to increased vulnerability to such injury, which underscores the importance of the muscle group in the prevention of injury. More particularly, the strengthening and coordination of the quadriceps and hamstrings are vital in dynamic movements such as landing and cutting. Adequate rehabilitation exercises should therefore incorporate exercises to strengthen these muscles, assuring stability of the knee and reducing the biomechanical risk factors for ACL injury. Coaches and trainers should create training programs that not only address the quadriceps but also overall functional biomechanics, thus assuring athlete safety and sustained performance in sports (Boden et al., 2014).

10.3.2. Hamstring Group

The hamstring group is a vital component of lower limb musculature, contributing significantly to locomotion and various sporting exercises. Hamstrings consist of three primary muscles—semimembranosus, semitendinosus, and biceps femoris—that run from the pelvis's ischial tuberosity to the tibia and fibula in the lower leg.

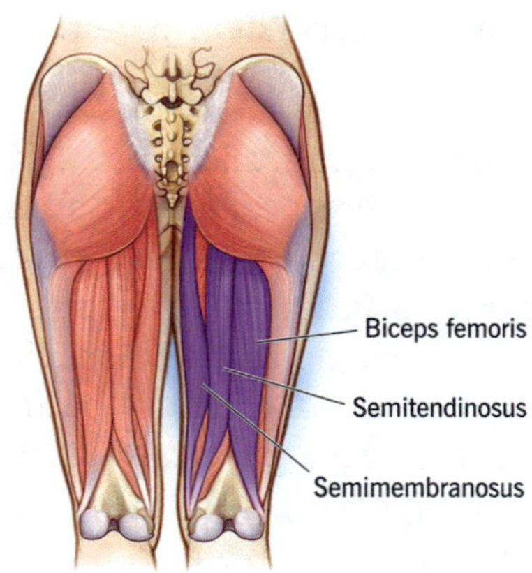

Figure 10.10. The three hamstring muscles are the biceps femoris, semitendinosus and semimembranosus.

*Source:*https://my.clevelandclinic.org/-/scassets/images/org/health/articles/hamstring-muscles.

Hamstrings are more or less exclusively responsible for knee flexion and hip extension, which are fundamental functions of running, jumping, and squatting. The functional anatomy of the hamstring group enables synergistic movement, where muscle contractions are able to allow complicated actions like deceleration and stabilization in activities involving high impact. Therefore, understanding the functional anatomy of these muscles is necessary for designing specific training and rehabilitation programs, especially in sports with sudden directional changes or explosive movements. Furthermore, the function of the hamstrings extends beyond the muscle to include a substantive relationship with injury prevention, particularly in relation to the ACL (Figure 10.10).

Increased hamstrings strength and flexibility have been associated with a reduced risk of ACL injury, especially for landing or cutting activity in sports. As witnessed in various studies, improved hamstrings muscle force during dynamic movements can attenuate biomechanical risk factors of non-contact ACL injuries. Specifically, strengthening the hamstrings and utilization of training on active trunk flexion during jumping and cutting can significantly impact landing biomechanics to generate a lower rate of injuries. This relationship highlights the importance of hamstring conditioning in integrated athletic training programs to maintain athletes' strength and uninjured. Notably, functional impairment of the hamstring group can significantly impair the sporting capacity and mobility in general of the individuals involved. Hamstring injuries, including strains or tears, are frequent among athletes and can lead to protracted recovery that hinders training and performance. Rehabilitation regimens tend to focus on recovery of strength, flexibility, and coordination of the hamstrings with specific concentration on their essential role in leg function. Furthermore, given that hamstring muscles also have a critical role in maintaining optimal posture and gait, their strengthening is crucial for overall lower limb stability and efficacy. These aspects thus highlight the need for in-depth evaluations of the functionality of the hamstring muscles within clinical and sports contexts, with the ultimate view of targeted interventions that not only address injuries but also help improve performance results among athletes who engage in various sports disciplines.

10.3.3. Sartorius Muscle

The sartorius muscle, also known as the longest muscle of the human body, has a significant role in the functional anatomy of the lower limb. It is situated between the anterior superior iliac spine (ASIS) and passes diagonally down the thigh to insert upon the proximal part of the tibia.

As a key contributor to hip and knee movement, the sartorius helps in hip joint flexion, abduction, and lateral rotation as well as in flexion of the knee. Its longitudinal direction ensures that it synergizes with other muscles in movements with complexities like squatting, running, and kicking. Furthermore, the sartorius also possesses clinical importance; damage or impairment to this muscle could lead to complications to the biomechanics of the lower limb, impacting overall mobility and athletic potential. The anatomical position of the sartorius muscle indicates an integration that is vital to the musculature that it surrounds, namely, allowing for the preservation of stability during dynamic movement. This muscle is closely associated with the quadriceps group, a chief extension of the knee, and with the iliopsoas, another significant hip flexor. Functional interdependence among these muscles is necessary in sports involving fast and complicated movements. A deeper understanding of the relationship between them provides insights into rehabilitation methods for recovery from lower limb injuries (Figure 10.11).

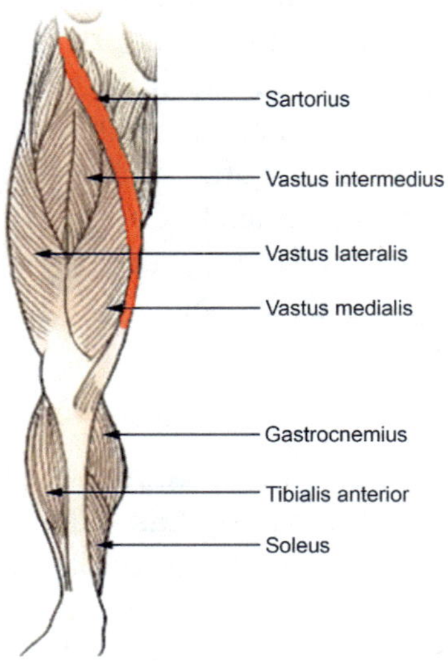

Figure 10.11. Sartorius muscle.

Source: https://en.wikipedia.org/wiki/Sartorius_muscle#/media/File:Sartorius.png.

Moreover, sophisticated imaging technology has, over the past few years, revealed complex information regarding muscle structure and function, which can elucidate the often overlooked soft tissue dynamics of the sartorius muscle (Ahn et al., 2017). The new information is crucial to maximizing therapeutic interventions as well as athletic performance through dedicated training protocols. The sartorius muscle is a key biomechanical element in the lower limb, a paradigm of muscular integration essential for movement coordination. By methods like Anatomical Network Analysis (AnNA), researchers have now begun to reveal the sophisticated relationships among muscles affecting both the normal and pathological status of the limb. These analyses conclude that despite sharing a common interface, the sartorius and the involved muscles have their own discrete roles for the integrated modularity of the lower limb MSK system (Goswami et al., 2015). Understanding this modularity is vital in assessing movement efficiency as well as preventing injury. Moreover, with further developments in scientific research, the function of the sartorius muscle in sports and ordinary movements dictates the necessity of more study and clinical attention, expanding our knowledge of its role in human locomotion.

Test Your Knowledge

1. What muscles make up the quadriceps group, and what is their primary function?
2. Which muscles are included in the hamstring group, and what movements do they facilitate?

10.4. Leg Muscles

Learning Outcome

1. Identify the anterior compartment muscles and the lateral compartment muscles
2. Discuss the posterior compartment muscles

Muscles in the lower limb are essential to facilitate movement, stability, and overall function required for everyday life and sports. Lower limb muscles are classified into several groups, some of which are the quadriceps, hamstrings, gastrocnemius, and soleus, all functioning differently to assist in lower extremity mechanics. Quadriceps are composed of four distinct muscles and are primarily responsible for knee extension, facilitating movements such as standing, walking, and jumping. Conversely, the hamstrings, located posterior to the thigh, permit flexion of the knee and play a significant role in running and cycling. Such anatomical diversity within leg muscles demonstrates the complexity of human movement and bears witness to the adaptation that facilitates effective patterns of movement applicable to different sporting activities. An understanding of the neurophysiological basis of coordination of the leg muscles explains some aspects of rehabilitation and prosthetic device development. The intricacy of muscle interactions reflects the need for elaborate control systems, particularly for mobility-disabled patients. New technologies, such as functional neuromuscular stimulation (FNS), hold out the promise to restore lost functions of mobility by electrically exciting paralyzed muscles, with tremendous promise in rehab centers. For instance, control methods like feedforward and feedback systems are beneficial in the reconstruction of limb motion with an emphasis on attainment of naturally perceived goals rather than adherence to stiff joint angle trajectories. These personalized approaches reflect growing recognition of the value of tailoring rehabilitation protocols to unique patients, thereby maximizing their quality of life as they counter the challenges of muscle fatigue and performance variability in functional activity (Abbas et al., 1996) (Figure 10.12).

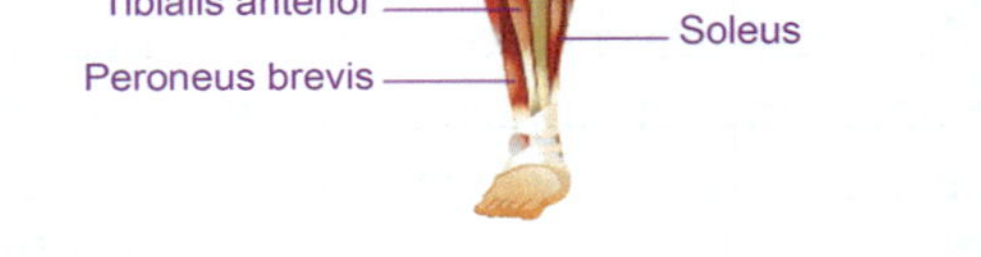

Figure 10.12. Parts of leg muscles.

Source: https://cdn1.byjus.com/wp-content/uploads/2022/08/Leg-muscles.png.

The increasing number of amputations also underscored the value of advances in muscle function of the leg and the design of the prosthesis. Approximately 2 million people in the United States are amputees, leading to a substantial change in their mobility and lifestyle. The progression from crude prosthetics to high-technology biomechanical devices is the far-reaching advancement of technology in its pursuit of a better outcome for amputees. Multidisciplinary care teams of doctors, physical therapists, and orthotists ensure that individuals who lose limbs can lead their usual lives and specialize in various activities. The use of advanced muscle control systems not only minimizes the loss of mobility but also enables the user to interact with the world naturally and more effectively, thereby enhancing their overall well-being and independence (Ramos et al., 2015).

10.4.1. Anterior Compartment Muscles

The muscles of the lower limb's anterior compartment play a significant role in supplying movement as well as stability in physical motion. The quadriceps femoris group dominates the anterior compartment, and it is made up of four distinct muscles: rectus femoris, vastus lateralis, vastus medialis, and the vastus intermedius. The four muscles combined contribute to extending the knee joint and supply movements such as walking, running, and jumping. The rectus femoris also has the unique function of hip flexion due to its origin from the ilium, once more emphasizing the versatility and importance of these muscles. Due to their significant function in activities involving lower limb stabilization and extension, any damage or dysfunction of this compartment can affect overall mobility and sports performance. Injury to the anterior compartmental muscles typically requires high-technology rehabilitation efforts for the process of healing and recovery of function. Strikingly, strains or tears may be brought on by overuse, direct trauma, or instability, particularly in high-level sports. In order to return to full function, rehabilitation involves strengthening and increasing flexibility. Most importantly, patient education regarding the anatomy and mechanism of the anterior compartment is essential to their healing. New educational tools, such as multimedia packages combining anatomical dissection, 3D modules, and animation, enhance patients' comprehension of their injury and rehabilitation procedures. With intensive insight into their bodily state, patients may show increased adherence to rehabilitation regimens, thereby leading to better functional outcomes (Buchanan et al., 2014) (Figure 10.13).

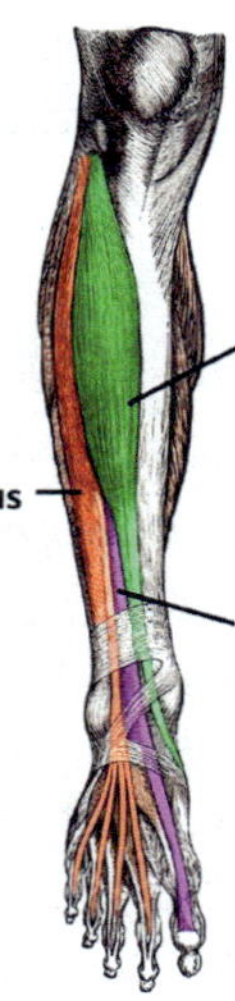

Figure 10.13. Muscles of the anterior leg.

Source: https://teachmeanatomy.info/wp-content/uploads/Muscles-of-the-Anterior-Leg-925x1024.jpg.

Apart from the mere movement, the biomechanical role of the anterior compartment muscles extends to stabilizing the knee joint as well as helping maintain good balance and posture. Weakness or dysfunction of the quadriceps will lead to instability of the knee and predispose the knee to injuries such as tears of the ACL. With the anatomical complexity and functional significance of this muscle group, ongoing research into interactions between the anterior compartment and other lower limb muscle groups continues to develop. This is particularly relevant regarding the development of effective interventions for the prevention of injury and optimal sporting performance. Further understanding of how such muscles operate together in conjunction with one another by advanced imaging technology can potentially refine clinical practice and athletic training methodologies (Ahn et al., 2017).

10.4.2. Lateral Compartment Muscles

The lateral compartment of the lower limb is responsible for stability and motion, primarily by its main muscles: the fibularis longus and fibularis brevis. Both of these muscles contribute primarily to eversion of the foot, an action essential for balance on uneven surfaces and with active movements such as running or jumping. Functionally, eversion stabilizes the ankle joint against sprains, which are a frequent occurrence in sporting activities. Along with other muscles, the lateral compartment also assists in the process of plantarflexion and thereby the general mobility of the foot. An understanding of the anatomy and potential weaknesses of this compartment is central to any rehabilitation strategy, especially within the context of the rising incidence of injury related to sports and exercise involving lateral movement. Injuries to lateral compartment muscles have a significant impact on the capacity of an individual to perform minimal movements, and thus demonstrate the role of these muscles in lower limb function. Injuries such as tendinitis or tears can be caused by overuse or acute trauma and typically demand serious rehabilitation to allow full function. Literature emphasizes that patient education and knowledge regarding such injuries are paramount for proper recovery. Unfortunately, most patients struggle to follow prescribed rehabilitation measures due to a lack of understanding of their conditions and the recovery process procedures. The clinicians therefore benefit by employing advanced learning tools that incorporate anatomical training to encompass clinical information on rehabilitation processes to enhance patient compliance as well as enhance recovery outcomes (Buchanan et al., 2014) (Figure 10.14).

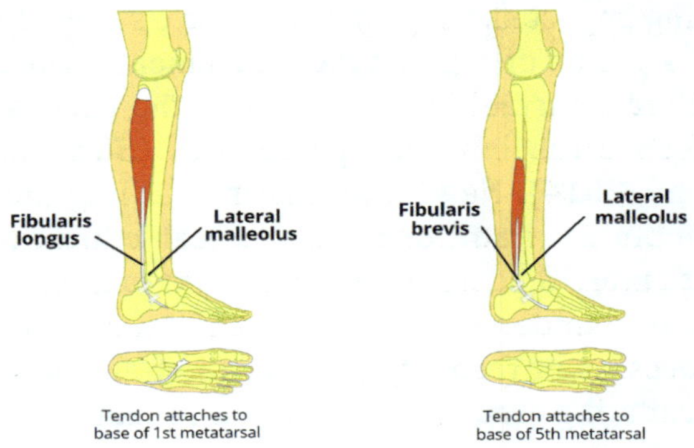

Figure 10.14. Muscles in the lateral compartment of the leg.

Source: https://teachmeanatomy.info/wp-content/uploads/Muscles-in-the-Lateral-Compartment-of-the-Leg-1024x702.png.

Improved care and communication of recovery for patients with lateral compartment injury can translate into improved long-term outcomes. Further, with progress in imaging and modeling techniques, our appreciation of the lateral compartment muscles has been completely revolutionized. Current methods, such as contrast-enhanced computed tomography (CT), provide accurate visualization of muscle anatomy and dynamics and allow a greater understanding of the role of each within the lower limb. This enhanced anatomical knowledge offers priceless benefits not only to medical professionals but also to educators and researchers studying the biomechanics of gait and motion. The intricate dynamics of the lateral compartment muscles and their associations with the surrounding structures indicate the necessity for comprehensive anatomical manuals in academia and clinical settings (Ahn et al., 2017). By leveraging contemporary technology to expand our understanding of these muscles, we can enhance injury prevention and rehabilitation measures, ultimately leading to improved outcomes for individuals participating in physical activity.

10.4.3. Posterior Compartment Muscles

The posterior compartment muscles are essential in the lower limb biomechanics, primarily dedicated to movement involving the ankle and the knee.

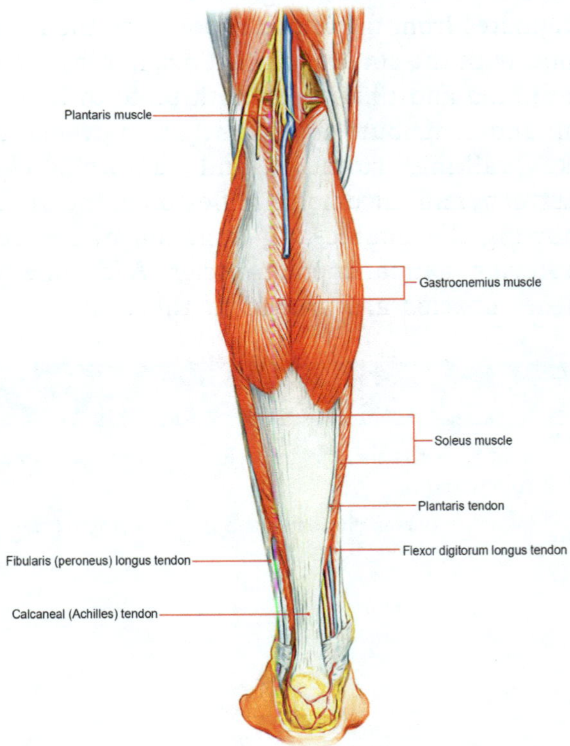

Figure 10.15. Posterior compartment of the leg.

Source: https://www.earthslab.com/wp-content/uploads/2017/07/posterior-compartment-of-leg.jpg.

The compartment predominantly consists of the hamstring muscles, which comprise the semimembranosus, semitendinosus, and the biceps femoris. The muscles originate at the ischial tuberosity and insert at different locations on the tibia and fibula and are thus capable of facilitating knee flexion and hip extension. Their role is essential not only in jumping and running but also in stabilizing during movement. Coordination of the posterior compartment muscles is also essential as failure in this would have a significant impact on the mobility of an individual as well as the lower limb function overall. In addition to the hamstrings, the posterior compartment also consists of the gastrocnemius and soleus muscles, which are vital in plantar flexion of the ankle. The two-headed gastrocnemius muscle originates from the femur superior to the knee joint, with the soleus below it originating from the fibula and tibia. They both unite to be the calf and contribute significantly to movements like walking, running, and jumping. The gastrocnemius also helps in flexion of the knee, showing the double-duty function of several posterior compartment muscles. Additionally, these muscles are crucial in those activities that demand explosive power and endurance, which underlines their significance in sporting and daily life activities (Figure 10.15).

Understanding the significance of posterior compartment muscles goes well beyond mere anatomy; it encompasses the function of injury and rehabilitation. Injuries to the muscles, particularly in athletes, can result in extended recovery periods as well as levels of performance being impacted. For instance, muscle strain may be a result of high-impact movements, which generate instability and reaffirm the need for effective rehabilitation procedures (Buchanan et al., 2014). New advances in teaching aids, combining traditional anatomical education with more modern approaches, aim to improve patient understanding of such injuries and processes of recovery (Buchanan et al., 2014). Facilitating greater adherence to rehabilitation programs, it is hoped that outcomes will be improved, allowing individuals to recover function successfully. Thus, it is essential to know the anatomy and function of posterior compartment muscles both for clinical reasons and for enhanced sports performance.

Test Your Knowledge

1. What are the primary muscles found in the anterior compartment of the leg, and what are their primary functions?
2. Which muscles comprise the lateral compartment of the leg, and what roles do they play in foot movement?

10.5. Foot Muscles

Learning Outcome

1. Discuss the intrinsic muscles of the foot
2. Define extrinsic muscles and their functions
3. Identify the role in balance and movement

The foot, a complex anatomy composed of numerous muscles, is charged with locomotion and balance. The intrinsic muscles of the foot, which are entirely within it, allow the various movements and arch support.

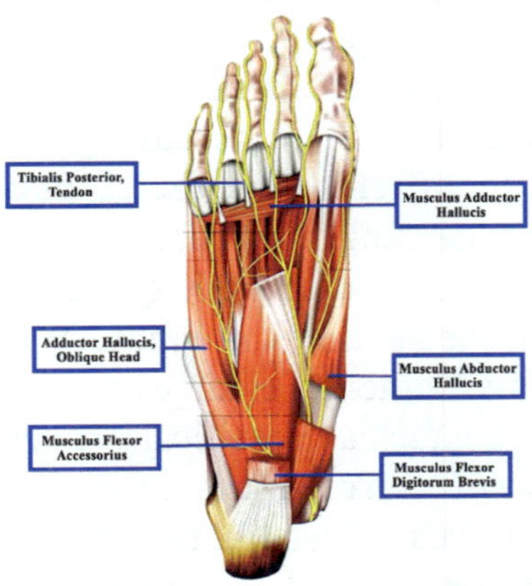

Figure 10.16. Muscles in the foot.

Source: https://www.joionline.net/wp-content/uploads/2020/07/Foot-Muscle-Label.jpg.

These intrinsic muscles, including the abductor hallucis, flexor digitorum brevis, and the quadratus plantae, are critical to balance as well as the facilitation of precise movement necessary for running and walking. Moreover, extrinsic muscles like gastrocnemius and tibialis anterior, those originating in the lower leg and inserting into the foot, assist these intrinsic muscles in obtaining synchronized motion. Understanding the muscular anatomy of the foot is essential since it has tangible implications not only for sporting function but also for lower limb biomechanical health, describing the coordination of musculature of the foot in function of human ambulation. The evolutionary significance of foot muscles is displayed by their adjustment to varying locomotor challenges across species. For example, the extinct adaptations of sthenurine kangaroos show limb musculature alterations between their bipedalism and gigantic body sizes, which affect their mode of locomotion and land stability (Figueirido et al., 2014) (Figure 10.16).

This difference highlights how the structure of the foot muscles can vary as a reaction to locomotor strategy and environmental stress, upholding the argument that form is function. In the contemporary human, foot musculature has evolved similarly to address bipedal walking requirements as well as the specific demands of competitive athletics. Such evolutionary insight not only enhances our knowledge of human anatomy but also offers possibilities for research into how variations in the muscle composition of the foot could affect mobility and injury susceptibility. Research has increasingly highlighted the intricate interrelations between muscle action and anatomical integration in the lower limb, and significant developments in the mechanics of the foot have been reported. Experiments using techniques like Anatomical Network Analysis (AnNA) illustrate how the anatomy of foot muscles interacts with the skeletal structure to provide stability and effective movement (Goswami et al., 2015). Coordination between groups of muscles enables the foot to perform a wide range of activities, including propulsion and nuanced balance compensation. Hence, knowledge of this muscle architecture and its association with the skeletal components becomes critical to fields such as rehabilitation, sports science, and orthopedics. Knowledge of foot muscle dynamics will help formulate targeted therapies and interventions, ultimately leading to enhanced mobility and quality of life in subjects suffering from MSK disorders.

10.5.1. Intrinsic Muscles of the Foot

The intrinsic foot muscles play a fundamental role in supporting stability as well as the facility of movement and thus form a crucial component of the muscular apparatus of the lower limb. They are entirely contained within the foot and are only involved with the finer motor activities of the toes.

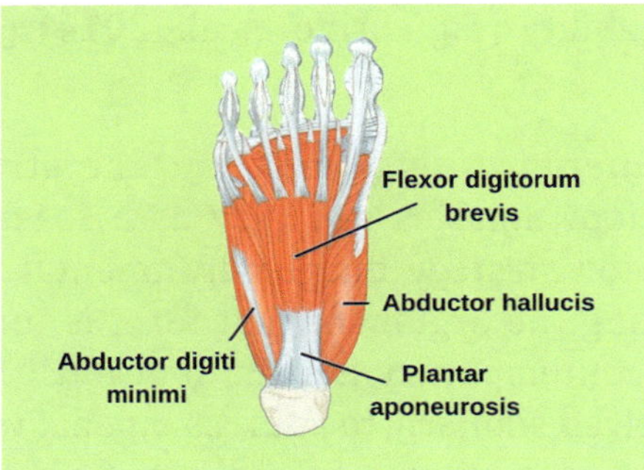

Figure 10.17. Intrinsic foot muscles.

Source: https://images.squarespace-cdn.com/content/5ef1c230f61f1932e94d317d/1661492338318-GOQAOGBDS01VCNBZUSZG/Intrinsic+Foot+Muscles.jpg?content-type=image%2Fjpeg.

They participate in functions such as grasping the ground, accommodating different ground surfaces, and shock absorption while walking. The positioning of these muscles allows them to work in a coordinated manner that encourages balance and supports the foot arch, a necessary characteristic for walking, running, and jumping. Apart from their functional significance, it also illuminates how foot mechanics disruption might influence overall lower limb biomechanics and cause potential injury, and thereby reveals the intrinsic muscles' function in postural control and walking economy. The intrinsic foot muscles are further separated into two groups, the dorsal and plantar muscles, according to the anatomical classification. The dorsal group consists of extensor hallucis brevis and extensor digitorum brevis, whereas the plantar group contains diverse layers like the abductor hallucis, quadratus plantae, and flexor digitorum brevis, etc. The intrinsic muscles have specific functions; e.g., abductor hallucis stabilizes the great toe, whereas flexor digitorum brevis is responsible for flexion of the middle phalanges of the lateral four toes (Figure 10.17). Furthermore, these muscles are synergistic with the extrinsic muscles of the lower limb, which provide for complex movement and adjustments necessary to manage varying surfaces, a quality that is significant for locomotion efficiency and injury prevention. Their intricate interaction sheds light on the biomechanical principles of lower limb movement and provides an avenue for understanding sports performance and rehabilitative designs. As a result of the terrain-based variation in movement, the role of intrinsic foot muscles becomes increasingly crucial in response to different obstacles and terrain. Current biomechanical research suggests that these muscles alter their activity based on visual sensory input so that anticipatory responses occur to environmental changes, such as uneven terrain or obstacles. Specifically, during travel across uneven terrain, the intrinsic muscles provide for ready readjustment to maintain balance and prevent falls, defining their essential role in locomotion control. Such a capability again testifies to the complexity of human gait mechanics and to therapeutic techniques for the promotion of balance and the prevention of injury in sport and older subjects. These results can lead to the development of improved training programs and rehabilitation exercises that are better tailored to the dynamic nature of foot function within the broader framework of lower limb biomechanics (Harris et al., 2012; Akaike et al., 2025).

10.5.2. Extrinsic Muscles and Their Functions

The extrinsic lower limb muscles play a fundamental role in facilitating movement and stability within the region. The muscles are derived outside the lower limb but end on the bones of the leg and foot, illustrating their crucial role in controlling a range of movements, including walking, running, and jumping. The primary extrinsic muscles include the gastrocnemius, soleus, and tibialis anterior, each serving different functional components of locomotion. For instance, the combination of gastrocnemius and soleus produces plantarflexion at the ankle, which allows for powerful propulsion during activities like sprinting or jumping. Dorsiflexion, on the other hand, is produced by the tibialis anterior and enables the foot to be elevated and provides for secure clearance during the walking swing phase. Understanding the interaction of these muscles is expressed in total lower limb dynamics and locomotor efficiency. Through a study of the biomechanical properties of extrinsic muscles, it is evident that their functions are most intimately related to the neural control mechanisms of movement. Recent research identifies that premotor cortices such as PMd and PMv possess tuning characteristics that correspond with the biomechanic properties of extrinsic muscle groups, suggesting a more intimate relation to motor performance compared to what was previously believed (Hatsopoulos et al., 2015) (Figure 10.18).

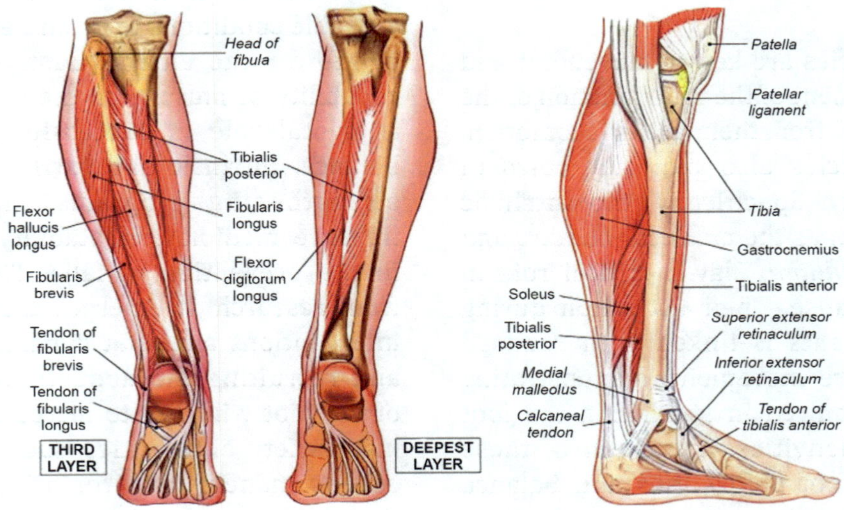

Figure 10.18. Extrinsic muscles that move the foot and toes.

Source: https://ik.imagekit.io/02fmeo4exvw/expert-articles/2018/04/2018-04-05-How-strong-is-your-foot-01.jpg.

This neural adaptation is reflective of how the brain optimizes movement strategies according to the mechanical feedback from muscles and joints. Such dynamic interaction becomes significant with complex movements, highlighting the necessity of extrinsic muscle coordination in achieving optimal mobility. Besides, the ability of these muscles to conform to various biomechanical demands demonstrates their applicability to sports performance as well as rehabilitation and their importance in the functional architecture of the lower limbs. Additionally, the anatomical complexity of extrinsic muscles is evident through their multifaceted morphological adaptation within species, ultimately advancing our understanding regarding human evolution and functional capacity. Network analysis of MSK system anatomy shows extensive forelimb to hindlimb structural differentiation, with emergent patterns of integration and modularity (Esteve-Altava et al., 2018). While the forelimb achieves some degrees of complexity in manipulation, hindlimb evolution has led to specialization for bipedal walking and extrinsic muscles that play a key role in this process. For humans, the integrity of these muscle groups is crucial for balance and the generation of locomotor force. Last but not least, studying the relationship between the structural anatomy and the functional capacity of the extrinsic muscles deepens our understanding of human movement and underscores their indispensable function in everyday activities as well as in specialized sports activities.

10.5.3. Role in Balance and Movement

Lower limb muscles are key to movement and balance, a constituent of the total function of the human body. Aside from their role in locomotion, lower limb muscles also play key roles in postural stability. Specifically, the intrinsic foot muscles, such as the *abductor hallucis* and *abductor digiti minimi*, play a critical role in mediolateral balance. Their activation during dynamic movements is linked with reduced center of pressure movement, demonstrating that they are required in stabilizing the foot during various activities. Activation of these muscles avoids foot deformities and balance disorders, especially in populations such as the elderly or diabetic patients, improving overall mobility and reducing the risk of falls (Kircher et al., 2020). Therefore, their function must be known to design strength training programs for improving balance and coordination in different populations. Furthermore, the interaction between lower extremity musculature and postural control is salient when exploring how older adults react to perturbations. When faced with compounded motor tasks, such as upper limb perturbations against a fixed or sliding board, lower limb muscle recruitment is critical to maintaining balance. From research, different groups of muscles are stimulated at unique times, which indicates an intricate interwork of responses to maintain balance. Through the study of the functioning of postural muscles during these conditions, it is viable to consider how and why some strategies might be employed to enhance stability in the elderly (Lee et al., 2019). This not only contributes to the rehabilitation strategy but also to the requirement for specific training of the muscles to be able to deal with the requirements of unstable conditions to ensure enhanced quality of life for the elderly. Lastly, the functional capability of muscles in the lower limbs plays a pivotal role in successful movement and balance. Intrinsic and extrinsic foot muscles strengthening programs can significantly improve mediolateral stability, which is vital in the prevention of falls. Through findings from research, it emerges that strengthening interventions aimed at dynamic balance tasks and recruiting the abductors and adductors of the foot will lead to increased performance in a variety of activities, such as walking and cutting maneuvers. Promoting balance skills through targeted resistance and proprioceptive training not only aids mobility in the elderly but can also be used to promote enhanced athletic function. Thus, maintaining and increasing function in lower limb muscles can be applied as a preventive measure against balance trauma and promote increased independence and agility in the individual across varying age groups and physical states (Kircher et al., 2020).

Test Your Knowledge

1. What are the intrinsic muscles of the foot, and what functions do they serve?
2. Which muscles are considered extrinsic muscles of the foot, and how do they influence foot movement?

10.6. Functional Importance of Lower Limb Muscles

Learning Outcome

1. Describe the role in locomotion
2. Discuss the contribution to stability
3. Identify the impact on athletic performance

Muscles of the lower limb play a vital role in various functions required for mobility, balance, and stability of human locomotion. The lower limb muscles are categorized based on particular actions, and the main groups include the quadriceps, hamstrings, gluteal, and calf muscles. Quadriceps play a crucial role in knee extension in walking, running, and jumping, thereby promoting locomotion efficiency. On the other hand, the hamstrings aid in flexion of the knee and extension of the hip, whose primary function is postural stability against injury and sports. The gluteal muscles, like gluteus maximus, facilitate hip extension and medial rotation, significantly contributing to pelvic stability during dynamic movement. Together, these muscles provide not only functional strength but also dynamic resistance to biomechanical stresses, reinforcing the structural integrity of the lower limb with every movement. Beyond locomotion, lower limb muscles are crucial for successful balance and posture. This is well illustrated by the actions facilitated by the calf muscles, gastrocnemius and soleus, which are significant for standing, walking, and ascending. Together, these muscles generate the action of push-off in walking and running, allowing for a stable center of gravity under motion. In addition, activation of the hip flexors, such as the iliopsoas, allows for optimal alignment of the pelvis required for core stability. The functional relationship among these muscle groups entails that such equilibrium is not necessarily a static condition but rather a dynamic process and one of adaptation to internal and external disturbances. Interaction between joint stability and muscle activation influences performance and prevention of injury, such that the lower limb muscles' function is a multifaceted and vital one in different physical activities. Understanding the evolutionary history of lower limb muscles offers further insight into their functional importance. Evolutionary adaptation of locomotion has shaped the anatomical structure and function of the muscles, as reflected in the transition from quadruped to biped movement. These transitions entailed basic changes in muscle leverage and mobility of joints, which allow us to understand how the adaptations geared movement patterns toward more efficient patterns throughout various environments. Biomechanical advantages of these evolutionary developments have implications for modern human postures and movement kinematics. As human beings execute complex motor tasks, the functional coordination and dynamic versatility of muscles of the lower limb continue to play a critical role. Through the examination of these adaptive evolutions, we can appreciate the refinement subtlety of the MSK system as an excellent example of nature's optimization force in the creation of functionality within different ecological environments, supporting the continued relevance of lower limb muscles to human physical activity (Allen et al., 2017; Goswami et al., 2018).

10.6.1. Role in Locomotion

The role of the muscles in locomotion forms the core of movement mechanics, particularly of the lower limb. The muscles are associated with the bones and the joints to generate the actions required for walking, running, and jumping. The anatomy of these muscles has adapted to support many modes of motion with a tendency towards the dynamic range seen in the activity of locomotion. For instance, hip extensors possess strong architectural characteristics favorable to high contraction velocities required for quick movement. At the same time, distal muscles are specialized in the production of more force using large PCSAs. This proximo-distal pattern in muscle architecture enhances stability and effectiveness in locomotion, which is critical for balance during locomotion and energy expenditure in activities such as running or walking on uneven terrain (Cappellari et al., 2016) (Figure 10.19).

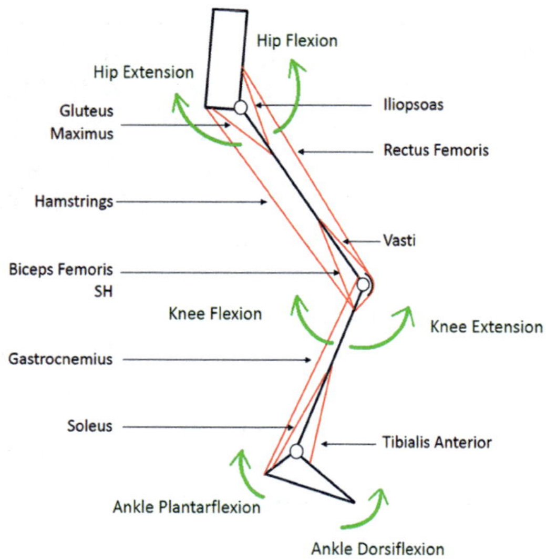

Figure 10.19. Different motions and simplified muscle groups of the lower limb.

Source: https://www.researchgate.net/figure/DIFFERENT-MOTIONS-AND-SIMPLIFIED-MUSCLE-GROUPS-OF-THE-LOWER-LIMB_fig1_305870843.

Different species have different muscle adaptations that further explain the evolutionary significance of muscle function in locomotion. For example, felids exhibit a crouched limb posture across a broad range of body size, which is consistent with their body weight support capability in executing complex movements needed for climbing and hunting. Scaling of vertebral and forelimb muscles demonstrates proportionality of muscle size to body mass, suggesting that large animals can swap relative strength of the muscle against stability. These developments evolving among different locomotory modes raise intriguing questions about how muscle architecture impacts behavior as well as ecological niches. Muscles of the quadruped and bipedal organism provide a specialized pattern of motion, which focuses on evolutionary requirements and functional loads placed on these organisms (Adams et al., 2016). Information about muscle function during walking is not merely biomechanics; it also informs clinical and research applications. It is possible to examine muscular architecture to gain an insight into potential weaknesses, particularly in those species that are predisposed to develop neuromuscular disease. The detailed study of muscle relationships and related functions finds application in the development of models for treatment and rehabilitation programs. As research advances in the realm of muscular physiology, the implications for sports performance and the prevention of injuries are vast. By realizing how complex the relationship between locomotor efficiency and muscle structure is, researchers can offer valuable information that is relevant both to veterinary medicine and human physical therapy, with these adaptations being at the forefront of biomechanical and anatomical research (Cappellari et al., 2016).

10.6.2. Contribution to Stability

The function of lower limb muscles for stability during movement and posture cannot be overstated. Muscles such as the quadriceps, hamstrings, and calf muscles work together to maintain a stable center of gravity and support during various activities. As the body's center of mass shifts, as it does when walking or running, the lower limb muscles react in a coordinated manner to resist these movements. This stabilization is essential not only for movement but also for preventing falls, particularly in the case of the elderly or balance-disordered subjects. Abdominal muscles, even positioned above the lower limb, indirectly contribute to this stability by maintaining core strength, demonstrating the interdependence between muscle groups to uphold upright posture and dynamic movement (Deering et al., 2017). Experiments have identified key factors influencing the posture stability of quiet standing and have determined the biomechanics to describe how muscles of the lower limb contribute to the function. Research on center-of-pressure excursions shows that asymmetries in loading lower limbs, notably during weight shifting, significantly influence stability. In right-handed individuals, the tendency to use a dominant side results in ground reaction forces being unequally distributed, leading to instability. This asymmetry of the limb highlights the necessity of individual muscle training because both legs must have equal strength for maximal dynamic as well as static stability. Muscle training not only enhances strength but also proprioception and therefore improves postural stability (Gutnik et al., 2008) (Figure 10.20).

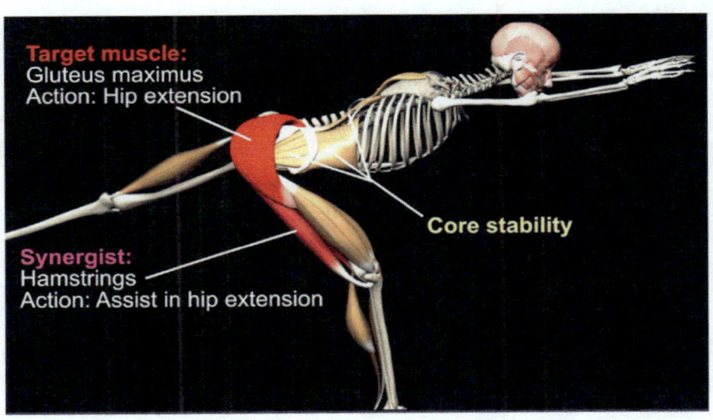

Figure 10.20. Core stability.

Source: https://external-content.duckduckgo.com/iu/?u=https%3A%2F%2Fwww.muscleandmotion.com%2Fwp-content%2Fuploads%2F2020%2F12%2FScreen-Shot-2020-12-08-at-2.16.31-PM-1024x621.png&f=1&nofb=1&ipt=b60b465011dcea6dfaa1b460e3104b40dec598b7bc9c7f954d4fd85df6ce0863.

Muscle strength and neuromuscular control have an intrinsic relationship to the contribution from muscles of the lower limb to stability. Greater strength in the quadriceps and the lower limb muscles generally suggests greater ability in maintaining coordination and alignment during movement. It is particularly significant for activities of high impact that necessitate a quick response to balance disturbances. Alongside, evidence exists of greater muscle strength being associated with decreased fatigability of the flexor muscles of the trunk, in support of the argument that more powerful lower limb muscles can provide greater overall stability. A proper alignment and strength training strategy, therefore, is not just stabilizing but also prepares people for coping with the complexity of physical action effectively and with safety (Deering et al., 2017).

10.6.3. Impact on Athletic Performance

The muscles of the lower limb are responsible for determining sporting performance in all sports and sporting activities. The muscles are employed in fundamental motor skills like running, jumping, and cutting, which are most essential in most sporting activities. The power, strength, and endurance of the lower limb muscles are the aspects on which sportsmen rely most to perform their sports optimally. For instance, sprinters exploit explosive strength to build up speed quickly, whereas distance runners exploit muscular endurance to maintain long activity. The coordination and economy of these muscles can be a significant factor in performance since those who possess better-trained lower limb musculature tend to perform better in speed, agility, and general competence. Therefore, good training strategies focus on building these physical attributes to improve competitive performance. Besides strength and resilience, recruitment and coordination of lower limb muscles are also essential in complex athletic movements. Interaction of various muscle groups, like the quadriceps, hamstrings, and calf muscles, is necessary in terms of offering stability and balance for movement. More coordination not only enables performance but also minimizes the potential for injury, as the athlete who can effectively engage and stabilize lower extremities is less apt to experience biomechanical inefficiencies that can lead to strains or sprains. Moreover, studies demonstrate that specially constructed training regimens that develop agility and proprioception can contribute to improved athletic performance. Muscle activation patterns and movement strategy-based exercises can enhance sporting performance while ensuring safety during intense effort. The influence of lower limb muscle function transcends performance; it is strongly tied to the general physical health of the athletes. Evidence suggests that repeated complaints or injuries related to these groups of muscles can lead to chronic impairment not just in performance but in the quality of life for the athletes. For instance, patients with repeated complaints following concussive events will have balance deficits reflecting impaired muscle function, which is evidenced by increased medial-lateral center of pressure displacement during activities (Cinelli et al., 2017). This puts emphasis on the importance of the athletes to look out for lower limb health because it will play a vital role in whether they can compete at elite levels or not. An athlete's success is not only a reflection of physical capacity but also their ability to have optimal muscle function within their lower limbs.

Test Your Knowledge

1. In what ways do these muscles help maintain stability during movement?
2. What is the impact of lower limb muscle strength and coordination on athletic performance?

SUMMARY

In summary, an in-depth understanding of the lower limb muscles is essential not only for use in the fields of medicine and rehabilitation but also in maximizing sports performance. Lower limb musculature permits an array of movements such as walking, running, and jumping that are all essential to human locomotion. Further, the interaction between muscle groups, tendons, and ligaments reiterates the importance of knowledge in anatomy in the identification of injuries and implementation of appropriate treatment protocols. Implications based on spinal cord injury rehabilitation studies indicate that treatment characteristics are accountable for results among patients, as evidenced by conjoint analysis (Dahlgren et al., 2008). This serves to emphasize the significance of muscular function not merely as a biological phenomenon but as a necessary aspect of therapeutic intervention. In addition, the study of lower limb muscles extends beyond functional anatomy into cognition and psychological well-being. New research is putting more focus on the relationship between motor performance and cognitive processes, particularly in cohorts such as those with Parkinson's Disease, where postural instability is a significant barrier (Agnetti et al., 2012). One of the newest approaches to rehabilitation is dance therapy, which combines mental and physical stimulation to show how certain exercises can impact both cognitive and muscle performance. This integration of studies makes the polyvalent function of the muscles of the lower limbs in integral health clear, hypothesizing that functional locomotion and strength training can amplify neuroplasticity, resulting in healthier outcomes. Lastly, the intricate interaction among the functioning of muscles in the lower limbs and integral health emphasizes the application of interdisciplinarist theories in rehabilitation and training. Combining evidence from sciences such as physiotherapy, neurology, and sports science allows one to have a greater understanding of how muscle dynamics are the basis of both physical function and intellectual health. As the discipline evolves further, further research is bound to show increasing complexity between muscular health and overall physical and mental health, meaning that optimizing lower limb function is a breaking point for enhancing quality of life. This conclusion not only supports the importance of lower limb muscles in sport and rehabilitative use but also calls for continued exploration of their functions within holistic paradigms of health.

The musculature of the lower limb plays a crucial role in locomotion, stability, and support. The significance of the major muscle groups constituting this region reflects the adaptability and intricacy required for human motion. Notably, the lower limb can be divided into several compartments from an anatomical standpoint, including the anterior, posterior, and medial thigh, as well as the leg muscles. The individual compartments house discrete sets of muscles responsible for specific movements such as hip flexion, knee extension, and foot movement. In addition, muscle interaction—through synergistic and antagonistic actions—provides the basis for smooth and coordinated movements. For instance, the quadriceps femoris group, primarily responsible for knee extension, demonstrates how muscle function is adapted to perform a specific biomechanical task in the general framework of locomotion of the lower limb. Besides, limb musculature evolution testifies to adaptations that accommodate bipedal locomotion and stability. Evolutionary study of extinct taxa, such as the sthenurine kangaroos, advises us on the biomechanics of movement impacting current anatomical structures. Sthenurine kangaroos, which were larger than the current species, exhibit morphological variations that attest to adaptations in locomotion modes, musing on the employment of bipedal gait to aid locomotion rather than the hopping characteristic of current kangaroos. This evolutionary perspective supports our understanding of lower limb musculature by explaining how muscle function has been shaped by evolutionary forces in response to environmental stimuli. Such findings validate the use of comparative anatomy in understanding current muscular capability and the role of evolutionary adaptation to lower limb function and movement patterns (Figueirido et al., 2014). Finally, the role of muscles concerning lower limb well-being cannot be overstated, especially in practice in rehabilitation and treatment of MSK disorders. Organizations like NHS Quality Improvement Scotland promote effective practice towards improving the quality of MSK health-related care. With the assessment of muscle function, strength, and coordination, healthcare professionals can formulate site-specific interventions in patients after injury. Further, an understanding of lower limb muscle anatomical and functional dynamics guides interventions applied in rehabilitation to enhance mobility, deter repeated injury, and improve overall quality of life. Thus, key points regarding the musculature of the lower limb transcend anatomical description—they encompass evolutionary significance as well as applied practice in the clinical setting with the specific aim of maximizing human movement and health (Bowers et al., 2009).

KEY TERMS FROM THIS CHAPTER

- Gluteus maximus
- Gluteus medius
- Gluteus minimus
- Iliopsoas
- Sartorius
- Quadriceps femoris
- Rectus femoris
- Vastus lateralis
- Vastus medialis
- Vastus intermedius
- Hamstrings
- Biceps femoris
- Semitendinosus
- Adductor longus
- Adductor magnus
- Gracilis

CRITICAL THINKING QUESTIONS

1. Which muscle group is primarily responsible for extending the knee?

a. Hamstrings
b. Quadriceps femoris
c. Gluteal muscles
d. Adductors

2. The hamstring muscles are located in the:

a. Front of the thigh
b. Back of the thigh
c. Calf
d. Buttocks

3. Which muscle is the largest and most superficial of the gluteal muscles?

a. Gluteus minimus
b. Gluteus Medius
c. Gluteus maximus
d. Piriformis

4. The gastrocnemius muscle is located in the:

a. Thigh
b. Hip
c. Calf
d. Foot

5. Which muscle helps in dorsiflexion of the foot (lifting the foot upward)?

a. Soleus
b. Tibialis anterior
c. Flexor digitorum longus
d. Peroneus longus

Short Answer Questions

1. What are the main anatomical regions of the lower limb, and which bones are associated with each?
2. What are the key muscles of the thigh, and how are they grouped functionally?
3. Which muscles are found in the lower leg, and what roles do they play in movement and stability?
4. Identify the main muscles of the foot and their role in balance and locomotion.
5. How do the lower limb muscles work together to support standing, walking, and running?
6. Why is the functional integrity of lower limb muscles essential for mobility and injury prevention?

Answer to Critical Thinking Questions

1. (b); 2. (b); 3. (c); 4. (c); 5. (b)

REFERENCES

1. Abbas, J. J., Crago, P. E., Kantor, C., Lan, N., et al. (1996). New control strategies for periprosthetic systems. https://core.ac.uk/download/pdf/11474899.pdf (accessed on 14th June 2025).
2. Chadwick, K. P., Regnault, S., Allen, V., & Hutchinson, J. R. (2014). Three-dimensional anatomy of the ostrich (Struthio camelus) knee joint. *PeerJ*, *2*, e706. https://doi.org/10.7717/peerj.706Adams, A., Alexander, A., Alexander, A., Alexander, A., Alexander, A., Anyonge, D., et al. (2016). The scaling of postcranial muscles in cats (*Felidae*) I: Forelimb, cervical, and thoracic muscles. https://core.ac.uk/download/159067742.pdf (accessed on 14th June 2025).
3. Aerts, P., Ayuso, M., Prims, S., Van Cruchten, S., et al. (2019). Does intrauterine crowding affect the force generating capacity and muscle composition of the piglet front limb? https://core.ac.uk/download/287940318.pdf (accessed on 14th June 2025).
4. Agnetti, V., Aiello, E., De Natale, E., Deriu, F., et al. (2012). Effects of dance therapy on balance, gait and neuro-psychological performances in patients with Parkinson's disease and postural instability. https://core.ac.uk/download/16749566.pdf (accessed on 14th June 2025).
5. Ahn, M., Burgess, M., Burggren, W., Cannatella, D., Cannatella, C., Clemente, C., Cline, T., et al. (2017). Digital dissection of the model organism *Xenopus laevis* using contrast-enhanced computed tomography. https://core.ac.uk/download/96600364.pdf (accessed on 14th June 2025).
6. Akaike, T., Belmonti, M., Birn-Jeffery, A. V., Birn-Jeffery, A. V., Bizzi, E., Capaday, C., Cavanagh, P. R., et al. (2025). How do treadmill speed and terrain visibility influence neuromuscular control of guinea fowl locomotion? https://core.ac.uk/download/36778722.pdf (accessed on 14th June 2025).
7. Allen, V., Hutchinson, J. R., Otero, A., Pol, D., & et al. (2017). Forelimb muscle and joint actions in Archosauria: Insights from *Crocodylus johnstoni* (Pseudosuchia) and *Mussaurus patagonicus* (Sauropodomorpha). https://core.ac.uk/download/141887609.pdf (accessed on 14th June 2025).
8. Anetai, Hidaka, Anetai, S., Koike, K., Kaito, T., Kumaratilake, J., et al. (2022). Gross anatomy of the gluteal and posterior thigh muscles in koalas based on their innervations. https://core.ac.uk/download/541150306.pdf (accessed on 14th June 2025).
9. Bartlam-Brooks, H. L. A., Bennitt, E., Curtin, N. A., Dewhirst, O. P., et al. (2018). Biomechanics of predator–prey arms race in lion, zebra, cheetah and impala. https://core.ac.uk/download/146489742.pdf (accessed on 14th June 2025).
10. Blottner, D., Ciciliot, S., Furlan, S., Gambara, G., et al. (2017). Gene expression profiling in slow-type calf soleus muscle of 30 days space-flown mice. https://core.ac.uk/download/84921730.pdf (accessed on 14th June 2025).
11. Boden, B. P., Chappell, D. J., Cruz, A., Dai, B., Donnelly, C. J., Ford, K. R., Frank, B., et al. (2014). A review of recent perspectives on biomechanical risk factors associated with anterior cruciate ligament injury. https://core.ac.uk/download/29841561.pdf (accessed on 14th June 2025).
12. Bowers, R., NHS Quality Improvement Scotland (Funder), & Ross, K. (2009). Best practice statement: Use of ankle-foot orthoses following stroke. https://core.ac.uk/download/9025419.pdf (accessed on 14th June 2025).

13. Buchanan, G., Ma, M., & Rea, P. M. (2014). A multimedia package for patient understanding and rehabilitation of non-contact anterior cruciate ligament injuries. https://core.ac.uk/download/16461708.pdf (accessed on 14th June 2025).

14. Burkholder, T. J., Firbas, W., Rankin, J. W., Hutchinson, J. R., Rubenson, J., & Wilson, A. M. (2016). Inferring muscle functional roles of the ostrich pelvic limb during walking and running using computer optimization. https://core.ac.uk/download/45467664.pdf (accessed on 14th June 2025).

15. Cappellari, O., Charles, J. P., Hutchinson, J. R., Spence, A. J., et al. (2016). Musculoskeletal geometry, muscle architecture and functional specializations of the mouse hindlimb. https://core.ac.uk/download/45467680.pdf (accessed on 14th June 2025).

16. Cinelli, M. E., Kalmar, J. M., Kaster, A., et al. (2017). Task-dependent modulation of cortical excitability and balance control in individuals with post-concussion syndrome. https://core.ac.uk/download/143689897.pdf (accessed on 14th June 2025).

17. Cozart, D., Hesse, D., Nichols, R., & Szymik, E. (2017). *UGA Anatomy and Physiology 1 Lab Manual* (3rd ed.). https://core.ac.uk/download/217306564.pdf (accessed on 14th June 2025).

18. Dahlgren, A., Donelly, C., Murphy, C., Mc Dowell, C. L., Rushton, D. N., Maynard, F. M., Snoek, G. J., et al. (2008). Decision for reconstructive interventions of the upper limb in individuals with tetraplegia: The effect of treatment characteristics. https://core.ac.uk/download/pdf/11479809.pdf (accessed on 14th June 2025).

19. Deering, R., Hunter, S. K., Neumann, D. A., & Pashibin, D. (2017). Muscle function and fatigability of trunk flexors in males and females. https://core.ac.uk/download/213081937.pdf (accessed on 14th June 2025).

20. Delp, S. L., Hutchinson, J. R., Rankin, J. W., et al. (2015). Musculoskeletal modelling of an ostrich (*Struthio camelus*) pelvic limb: Influence of limb orientation on muscular capacity during locomotion. https://core.ac.uk/download/36778511.pdf (accessed on 14th June 2025).

21. Esteve-Altava, B., Esteve-Altava, B., Esteve-Altava, B., Esteve-Altava, B., Villmoare, B., Rolian, C., Rolian, C., et al. (2018). First anatomical network analysis of fore- and hindlimb musculoskeletal modularity in bonobos, common chimpanzees, and humans. https://core.ac.uk/download/157769144.pdf (accessed on 14th June 2025).

22. Esteve-Altava, B., Molnar, J. L., Johnston, P., Hutchinson, J. R., & Diogo, R. (2018). Anatomical network analysis of the musculoskeletal system reveals integration loss and parcellation boost during the fins-to-limbs transition. *Evolution, 72*(3), 601–618. https://doi.org/10.1111/evo.13430 (accessed on 14th June 2025).

23. Figueirido, B., Janis, C., & Buttrill, K. (2014). Locomotion in extinct giant kangaroos: Were sthenurines hop-less monsters? https://core.ac.uk/download/pdf/30673537.pdf (accessed on 14th June 2025).

24. Goswami, A., Porto, A., Porto, A., Burrows, A. M., Esteve-Altava, B., Esteve-Altava, B., Esteve-Altava, B., et al. (2018). Primate modularity and evolution: First anatomical network analysis of primate head and neck musculoskeletal system. https://core.ac.uk/download/151211716.pdf (accessed on 14th June 2025).

25. Gutnik, B., Leaver, J., Longley, C., & Standen, C. (2008). Inferred influence of human lateral profile on limb load asymmetry during a quiet standing balance test. https://core.ac.uk/download/12525624.pdf (accessed on 14th June 2025).

26. Harris, G. F., & Slavens, B. A. (2012). *Biomechanics*. https://core.ac.uk/download/213080657.pdf (accessed on 14th June 2025).

27. Hatsopoulos, N. G., Lillicrap, T. P., Mardoum, P., et al. (2015). Temporal evolution of both premotor and motor cortical tuning properties reflect changes in limb biomechanics. https://core.ac.uk/download/213085899.pdf (accessed on 14th June 2025).

28. Henry, V., Hildebrandt, T., Hutchinson, J. R., & Panagiotopoulou, O. (2014). Regional variation in digital cushion pressure in the forefeet of horses and elephants. https://core.ac.uk/download/159067743.pdf (accessed on 14th June 2025).

29. Kircher, H. (2020). The function of the intrinsic foot muscles during turns and mediolateral shifts in balance. https://core.ac.uk/download/346453555.pdf (accessed on 14th June 2025).

30. Lee, Y. J., Liang, J. N., & Wen, Y. T. (2019). Characteristics of postural muscle activity in response to a motor-motor task in elderly. https://core.ac.uk/download/250588025.pdf (accessed on 14th June 2025).

31. Nichols, R. (2019). *UGA Laboratory Manual for Functional Human Anatomy*. https://core.ac.uk/download/287027371.pdf (accessed on 14th June 2025).

32. Ramos, V. (2015). *Introduction to Prosthetic Limbs*. https://core.ac.uk/download/58826624.pdf (accessed on 14th June 2025).

MUSCLES OF THE UPPER LIMB

11

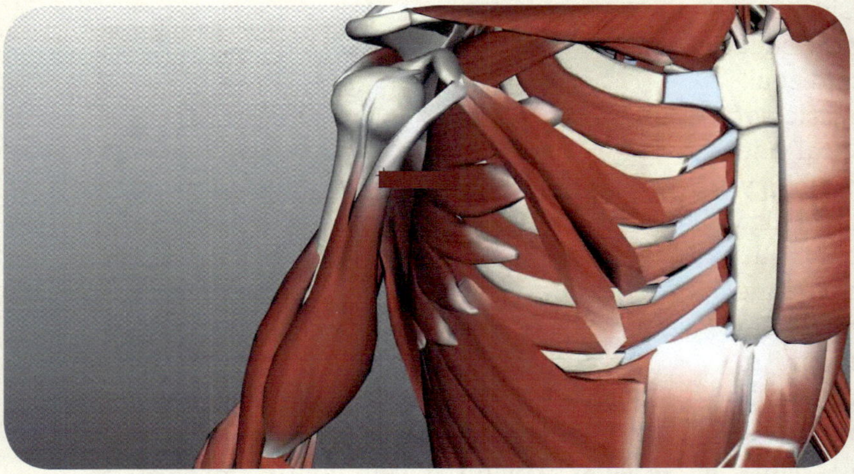

LEARNING OBJECTIVES

After studying this chapter, you will be able to:

1. Describe the anatomy of the upper limb
2. Identify the muscles of the shoulder
3. Describe the muscles of the arm
4. Identify the muscles of the forearm
5. Describe the muscles of the hand
6. Recognize common injuries and disorders

Introduction

The human upper limb is an anatomical marvel, allowing it to possess a staggering degree of motion and dexterity required to perform a broad variety of activities, from ordinary daily routines to complex athletic movements. The muscles of the upper limb play an essential part in making this mobility and strength possible. They consist of intrinsic and extrinsic muscle groups that synergize to enable such movements as flexion, extension, abduction, and adduction of the shoulder, elbow, and wrist joints. Familiarity with these muscles is critical, as they are part of functional anatomy, not to mention assessment and treatment of a variety of musculoskeletal (MSK) disorders. Therefore, the study of the MSK structure and function of the upper limb provides a foundation for subsequent studies in biomechanics, rehabilitation, and sports training, thus making it a study of interest in anatomical sciences (Cozart et al., 2017). Moreover, the complexity of muscle architecture, including the pattern of fibers of the muscle and the PCSA, has a direct impact on the functional capacity of the upper limb. These architectural characteristics influence such factors as force generation, muscle tolerance, and economy of movement. Clinicians and therapists should be aware of these correlations so that post-injury or surgical rehabilitation programs for the upper limb can be optimized. Information derived from comparative anatomy, such as the study of limb mechanics in different species, can also aid our account of human muscle function. For instance, research on locomotion in other bipedal species draws attention to evolutionary specializations that inform muscle design, and comparative observations enhance knowledge of human muscle physiology (Abourachid et al., 2014). By and large, a study of the muscles of the upper limb encompasses theoretical and practical issues in the field of human biology. This field contributes to the overall knowledge of biomechanics, comparative anatomy, and rehabilitation science. By examining the intricate interplay between anatomical structure and muscle function, scholars are better able to appreciate the adaptive processes that enable human movement. Further, the contributions to medicine and sports science are essential since with this understanding, there are improved ways of preventing injury and conditioning the body. In short, the study of upper limb muscles is where anatomy, physiology, and applied sciences meet, making its prominence both in academia as well as in practice in health and fitness (Cozart et al., 2017).

Definition of Upper Limb Muscles

The upper limb muscles are a collection of complex skeletal muscles that enable one to make wide-ranging movements, which are required to conduct daily activities and motor functions. The muscles are classified into various categories based on their anatomical location and function. For example, shoulder girdle muscles such as trapezius and deltoid play a critical role in stabilizing and facilitating movement of the shoulder joint to permit movements such as raising and rotating the arms. Similarly, arm muscles such as biceps brachii and triceps brachii are predominantly involved in flexing and extending the elbow, demonstrating the intricate relationship between muscle structure and movement. Understanding the muscles of the upper limb is at the core of the investigation of human biomechanics as well as the evolutionary adaptations seen across varying species, as varying limb and muscle configurations reflect ecological demands and lifestyle adaptation.

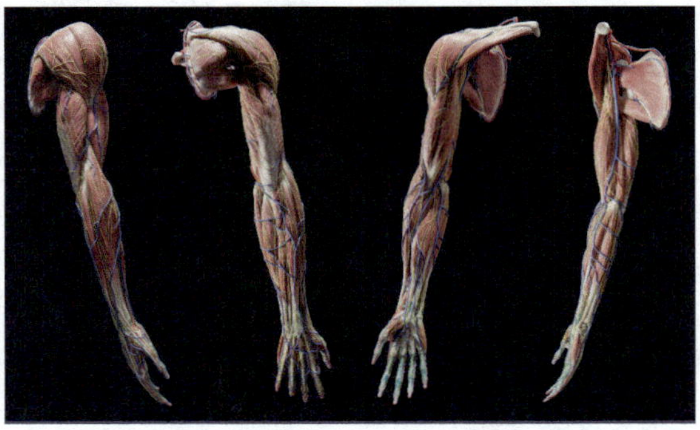

Figure 11.1. Detailed anatomical rendering of the upper limb, showing muscles, nerves, and vascular structures from multiple angles.

Source: https://external-content.duckduckgo.com/iu/?u=https%3A%2F%2Fcdnb.artstation.com%2Fp%2Fassets%2Fimages%2Fimages%2F028%2F579%2F689%2F4k%2Fneal-biggs-upperlimb-fullarm-2020-07-15-internalanatomy-a.jpg%3F1594877295&f=1&nofb=1&ipt=92e230cebd57a1f23b67d726df0b9eb8da268b84dd42bf4909e4f043c460f1ff.

Because of their intricate neuromuscular interactions that facilitate coordination and economy of movement, upper limb muscles are important for reasons beyond their simple mechanical function. Muscle and tendon distribution impacts the overall dexterity of the hand and the effectiveness of grasping tools. For example, the intrinsic muscles of the hand (interossei and lumbricals) are responsible for fine motor movements, facilitating smooth movements requiring precision. Such refinement in functionality is a demonstration of evolutionary modifications, where changes in limb morphology have impacted motor ability (Diogo et al., 2017) (Figure 11.1).

The compound nature of upper limb muscles not only contributes to human abilities but also gives rise to questions regarding the evolutionary pressures that shaped these adaptations, illustrating the reciprocity between anatomy and functional efficacy. Secondly, the study of upper limb muscles raises questions concerning the impact of several parameters, such as injury or technological advancement, on functional ability. Advances in understanding more about muscle function have led to improved rehabilitative methods and prosthetic device design that more accurately replicate natural limb movement. Evidence indicates that if factors such as neuromuscular control and muscle geometry are optimized, performance will be much improved (e.g., Bradly, 2009)). The interplay between muscle structure and functional tasks constitutes one foundation on which studies consistently aim to improve motor functions in healthy subjects and those who are injured. As scientists continue to study these relationships, the comprehension of the definition and function of upper limb muscles will continue to shape clinical practice and the creation of therapy protocols, further advancing the knowledge of human movement and adaptation.

Importance of Upper Limb Muscles in Human Movement

The muscles of the upper limb are necessary to provide a range of motions (ROMs) that are important in daily activities, sports, and labor. The complexity of these muscles makes possible gross motor functions such as lifting and throwing, and fine motor functions such as writing and dexterity manipulation. These abilities are owed in large part to the complex actions of muscle groups, like the deltoids, biceps brachii, and the forearm flexors and extensors, that act cooperatively to produce smooth, controlled movement. These muscles are critical in occupational therapy and rehabilitation, where strengthening and control improvement are vital components of rehabilitation from injury or illness affecting functionality. Last but not least, successful movement relies heavily on the power and steadiness of the upper limb muscles, which highlights their importance in human anatomy and daily life. When looking at the evolutionary history of upper limb musculature, one finds fascinating parallels with ancient locomotor transitions as established through biomechanical analysis. The evolution from quadrupedal to bipedal locomotion among archosaurs gives meaning to forelimb musculature in an adaptive sense. For instance, the MSK alterations that evolved in dinosaurian ancestors, as explained based on biomechanical modeling, illustrate how specific adaptations in muscle moment arms and joint range enhance upper limb performance. Such adaptations, apart from signifying the evolutionary pressures these animals were under, also inform us of the mechanical efficacy required in various limb postures—either to support or move about. With this understanding of the evolutionary nuances, we have a greater appreciation of the adaptability of the upper limb muscles and the implications they have for human movement today that extend so far into history (Allen et al., 2017). Also, with increasing understanding of biomechanics today, it brings to the forefront the importance of neuromechanics, as it bridges biological movement and robotic mimicry. This work points out that effective motion is the product of cooperation between physical structures and task demands, positioning upper limb muscles as adaptive components within this intricate system. Task complexity and muscle coordination correspondence represent regulations that apply within living systems as well as their robotic counterparts, promoting insight into the fundamental mechanisms of movement. This perspective upholds the significance of upper limb muscles not just for performance but also for learning and adaptation to environmental stimuli. As we wade through the complexities of human movement using experimental and theoretical lenses, it is obvious that the upper limb muscles are at the vanguard of functional and adaptive pertinence, essential for daily functioning as well as advanced robotic applications (Santello et al., 2017).

11.1. Anatomy of the Upper Limb

Learning Outcome

1. Understand the overview of the skeletal structure
2. Define major muscle groups in the upper limb
3. Explain the relationship between muscles and bones

The anatomy of the upper limb is integral to the study of its musculature and, ultimately, its function. The upper limb consists of bones, joints, and pairs of muscles that exist and interact with each other to grant elaborate movements from the level of gross motor function to very sophisticated fine motor functions.

The center of this anatomy is the shoulder girdle, the arm, the forearm, and the hand, together providing marvelous mobility and dexterity. The rotator cuff muscles, pectoral muscles, and muscles of the forearm and hand all play a crucial role in movement and stabilization. The understanding of the anatomical function and position of these muscles is also needed in areas like sports science and physical therapy, where rehabilitation and performance are the top issues. The cooperation of these structures provides the basis for upper limb function, illustrating the advanced design formulated to meet complex demands (Figure 11.2).

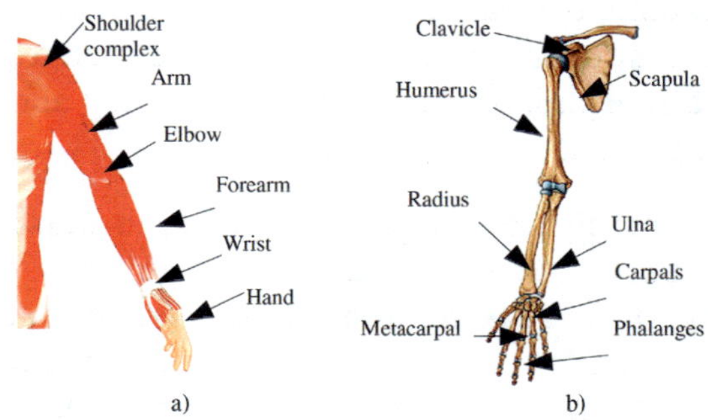

Figure 11.2. Anatomy of upper limb: (a) body segments with muscles; and (b) main bones.

Source: https://www.researchgate.net/figure/Anatomy-of-upper-limb-a-body-segments-with-muscles-b-main-bones_fig1_311099028.

Muscle architecture within the upper limb is strongly adaptive, reflecting both functional requirements and evolutionary constraints. To illustrate, the physiological cross-sectional areas (PCSA) of muscles bear important patterns of scaling that are associated with the size of the overall body stature and functional requirements. As exemplified from studies in numerous species, muscle mass and capacity for force generation can significantly differ based on size and use by the principles of allometric scaling. It has been revealed in emus and felids that muscle architecture changes influence their locomotion and movement efficiency, bearing witness to the importance of structural arrangement compared to function (Abourachid et al., 2014; Adams et al., 2016). Understanding these scaling patterns allows scientists and doctors to comprehend better how the strength and endurance of human muscles may be augmented or restored in human subjects, leading ultimately to the optimal sporting medicine and therapy practice. The delicate balance of strength and flexibility offered by the upper limb muscle group is essential to performing day-to-day activities as well as expert sporting ones. Muscles such as the biceps brachii, triceps brachii, and brachialis collaborate to allow bending and extending of the elbow, with muscles of the forearm supporting wrist and finger movements. This cooperation of muscles not only serves movements such as lifting or throwing, but also for fine motor skill-based precision movements such as typing or sculpting. These actions of antagonist and synergist muscles further show this complexity in enabling effective movement with coordination through opposing action. Additionally, as the load and angle of movement change, the muscles adapt to ensure practical function, demonstrating their role in biomechanics. Thus, understanding these interactions at a muscular level is valuable in optimizing sports performance as well as injury mechanisms in the upper limb.

11.1.1. Overview of the Skeletal Structure

The bony structure of the upper limb is a fundamental component that not only supports muscles but also ensures functional integrity in motion. The structure, from which the primary constituents consist of bones, cartilage, and ligaments, consists of the shoulder girdle, arm, forearm, wrist, and hand. The shoulder girdle, formed by the scapula and clavicle, allows for wide movement while stabilizing the upper limbs. The humerus, radius, and ulna follow, creating the arm and forearm, necessary for strength and dexterity. These are joined together by a variety of different joints, such as the shoulder, elbow, and wrist, which provide infinite movement. Understanding this skeletal structure is key to comprehending how muscular movement is coordinated in the upper limb, particularly in movements that require fine motor movement and significant strength. Additionally, the bony architecture of the limbs is an epitome of integration and modularity of bones and muscles, such that it is functionally adequate. An anatomical network analysis (AnNA) has revealed fascinating facts about how anatomical elements coexist peacefully. The study demonstrates that despite apparent structural dissimilarities, both the upper and lower limbs exhibit skeletal network similarities but with significant differences when muscular components are taken into consideration. This implies that although skeletal structure offers the structural framework necessary, bone-muscle interaction is still key to efficient limb function. Additionally, appreciation of these interrelationships has bearing on clinical practice, as any compromise in integration—like trauma or birth defects—can greatly impair mobility and requires a multidisciplinary approach to diagnosis and retraining (Figure 11.3).

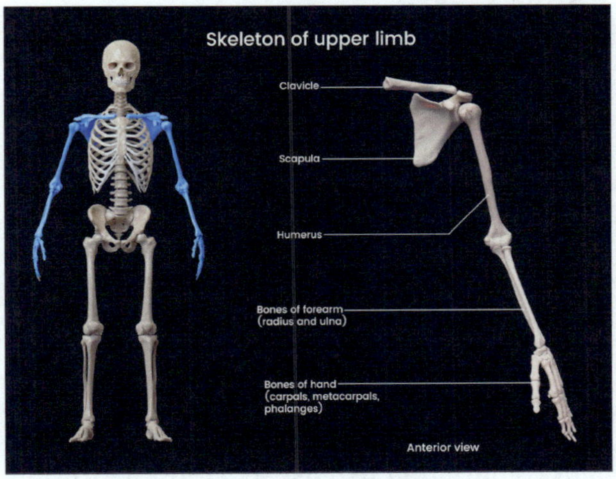

Figure 11.3. Skeleton of upper limb.

Source: https://admin.anatomy.app/Media/images/ac1538bb-1873-45cd-819e-376d6750f399_large.jpg.

Finally, the clinical importance of the upper limbs' skeletal anatomy extends beyond basic anatomy and has implications for clinical practice and decision-making in medical practice. Outcomes like the predictive salvage index (PSI) are essential when evaluating and managing limb injuries, but it begins with adults. This indicates a gap in pediatric care where special anatomical and developmental considerations must be factored into decisions, most notably in the making of informed decisions regarding amputations or reconstruction. By adjusting injury severity scores for adolescents, clinicians can better inform decision-making, ensuring effective and well-informed parent involvement. This adjustment suggests broader acceptance of the need to understand the complexity of skeletal and muscular systems as a means of improving patient outcomes across diverse populations with an emphasis on the importance of having a holistic appreciation of the complex interdependence between structure and function of the upper limb (Goswami et al., 2015; Aber et al., 2016).

11.1.2. Major Muscle Groups in the Upper Limb

The upper limb is made up of an advanced grouping of muscle groups that allow a wide range of movements required in day-to-day activities. Of the major groups of muscles, the deltoid, biceps brachii, triceps brachii, and forearm muscles play a crucial role in carrying out upper limb movements.

The deltoid on the shoulder is primarily used in arm abduction, i.e., moving the arm away from the body. This muscle is not only essential for overhead motion, but also for shoulder joint stabilization in most activities. The biceps brachii, a large muscle of the anterior arm, is significant in flexion of the elbow and supination of the forearm. Their synergistic action is the cause of the intricate motor functions associated with actions such as throwing, lifting, and reaching, and the reasons for their importance in upper limb biomechanics. In addition to the deltoid and biceps brachii, the triceps brachii is a crucial antagonist in the action of the arm. Situated at the rear of the upper arm, the triceps is utilized mainly to straighten the elbow joint, playing a counterbalancing role to the flexing action done by the biceps. Balancing the two biceps and triceps is the key to stability and function with dynamic movement (Figure 11.4).

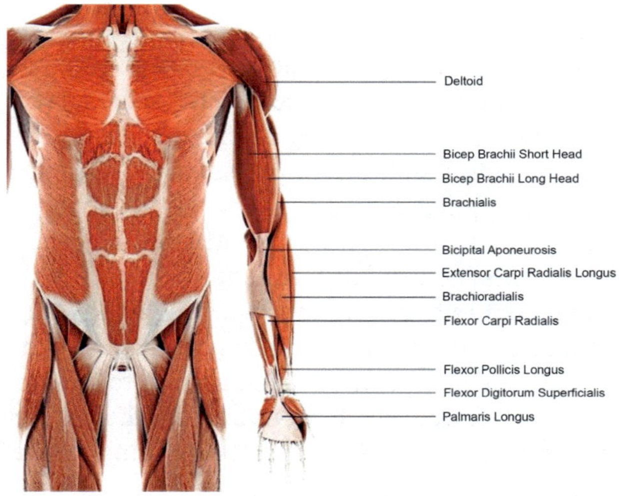

Figure 11.4. Major muscles of the upper limb.

Source: https://mblexguide.com/wp-content/uploads/2022/07/Muscles-of-the-upper-limb-anterior-e1659039477311.jpg.

Along with it, forearm extensors and flexors control finger and wrist movements, providing strength and accuracy in grip function. Through synergistic effects, these muscle groups enable upper limb function, allowing people to perform a wide range of complex tasks that require fine motor skills, strength, and coordination. An understanding of this muscle structure is critical for fields such as rehabilitation and sports medicine, in which prevention and rehabilitation of injury dominate. Furthermore, anatomical studies, such as studies of the mouse hindlimb, provide us with information that can inform our knowledge of human muscle structure and function as well. Anatomical and architectural muscle adaptations, as reported in recent literature, can have a significant impact on locomotor efficiency and stability. These findings are related to studies of the upper limb, in which the architecture of the muscle also affects the performance in tasks. The muscle structure of the upper limb, for instance, can exhibit features such as those described in biomechanical studies of other animals, e.g., emus showing complex locomotion strategy and economy of movement (Abourachid et al., 2014;

Cappellari et al., 2016). By considering these architectural specializations within different species, researchers can gain many valuable lessons regarding human musculature, further validating the significance of understanding the major muscle groups of the upper limb and their functional relevance in daily life and specialized sports activities.

11.1.3. Relationship Between Muscles and Bones

The connection of bones and muscles in the arm is a fundamental truth about human anatomy that shows the coordination of movement and strength. Muscles connect to bones via tendons, facilitating the passage of force during muscle contraction. This interacting process provides the joint articulation and results in complex movements such as raising, pushing, and turning. Muscles not only specify movement range and speed but also act to support skeletal systems, contributing to posture in the execution of a wide range of functions. Such mechanical collaboration is optimally illustrated in the forelimb, where intricate coordination of muscles is tasked with both gross and fine movements required in daily activities and sporting performances. Additional insight is given into how the evolution of features in muscle and bone has had an impact on functionality in the upper limb. Research has established that while proximal limb modules, which are crucial for power generation and stability, are very similar between various taxa, distal limb modules are very variable. For instance, the variation in muscle configuration between primate species impacts their manipulation and locomotion ability. In hominoids, as in humans, such adaptations enhance dexterity and coordination, particularly with the independent musculoskeletal (MSK) units of the thumb, differing from those of other primates. Therefore, the evolution of musculature emphasizes the importance of environmental interactions and functional needs in evolving MSK anatomy and performance criteria across species (Diogo et al., 2017). Moreover, the allometry of upper limb muscle architecture relative to body size has a strong influence on upper limb muscle and bone interaction. For example, felids accommodate a 300-fold range of body mass through a conservative MSK anatomy strategy with specializations promoting climbing, locomotion, and prey capture. Positive scaling of PCSAs of muscles of forelimbs indicates that larger-sized felines have comparatively weaker muscles compared to small animals, and there is an intriguing balance between the size of muscles and functional capability. This suggests that body weight increases do not always result in linear increases in muscle function or strength, particularly in terms of evolutionary adaptation based on behavioral change and environmental forces (Adams et al., 2016). Thus, analyzing such interactions further clarifies the integration of the skeleton and the muscles of the upper limb.

Test Your Knowledge

1. What are the key bones that make up the skeletal structure of the upper limb?
2. What are the major muscle groups found in the upper limb, and what are their primary functions?

11.2. Muscles of the Shoulder

Learning Outcome

1. Describe the anatomy of the deltoid muscle
2. Identify the rotator cuff muscles and their roles
3. Describe the pectoralis major muscle

The shoulder region contains a complex set of muscles responsible for the stability and mobility of the upper limb. Foremost among these muscles are the rotator cuff, which consists of four key muscles: the supraspinatus, infraspinatus, teres minor, and subscapularis. All these muscles together function to stabilize the glenohumeral joint, allowing for a vast array of movements of the arm without dislocation. Their combined alignment and collaboration with one another enable not only the gross movements of lifting and throwing but also fine manipulative functions, highlighting their functional importance in daily living. An appreciation of the anatomical arrangement and biomechanics of the muscles is essential to recognize common shoulder injuries and conditions that arise as a result of overuse or trauma and drastically affect an individual's quality of life. In addition to the rotator cuff, the shoulder is supported by several significant muscles, including the deltoid, pectoralis major, and trapezius. The deltoid muscle, being triangular, helps in abduction and arm flexion and functions as a primary mover for shoulder movement. The pectoralis major facilitates adduction and medial rotation of the humerus, however. The trapezius, through its extensive attachment on the spine and shoulder girdle, facilitates retraction and elevation of the shoulder, and is one of the primary muscles engaged in scapular movement. Together, these muscles constitute a dynamic system to allow free movement, which indicates the versatility of the shoulders. Besides, it is significant to understand how changes in muscle strength and function, particularly between species, may influence locomotor capacities, particularly in an evolutionary context, as explored in comparable research on varied musculature across animals (Adams et al., 2016). Coordination among these muscles is essential not just for functional motion but also for structural stability of the shoulder complex. For instance, the interaction of the deltoid and rotator cuff muscles is essential in preventing shoulder injuries among overhead athletes. Furthermore, the intricate interaction of shoulder muscles is influenced by anatomical differences and evolutionary adaptations, revealing an intriguing genetic relationship between key structures and their functions. Research on comparisons of the MSK variation across species, such as the evolutionary trend toward bipedalism from quadrupedalism, shows how shoulder muscle orientation change affects performance and biomechanical economy (Allen et al., 2017). Ultimately, this complexity emphasizes the significance of the shoulder muscular anatomy not only within human physiology but also within its evolutionary context in all taxonomic groups.

11.2.1. Deltoid Muscle and Its Functions

The deltoid muscle is a big, multi-functional upper limb structure that plays a crucial role in many movements of the shoulder. The deltoid muscle is found above the shoulder joint and is made up of three anatomical regions: the anterior, lateral, and posterior fibers, each of which plays a specific role. Anterior fibers are primarily responsible for shoulder flexion and internal rotation, but lateral fibers assist with abduction and the lifting of the arm from the body. The opposite action is shoulder extension and external rotation through the posterior fibers. This arrangement allows for a wide range of motion (ROM) required for everyday activities of reaching, lifting, and throwing, evidence of the deltoids' significant role in the biomechanics and function of the upper limb. Appreciation of the sophistication of the deltoid muscle is enhanced by recognition of its evolutionary and functional significance. Comparative studies across species provide insight into the way the architecture of the muscles dictates functionality. For example, evidence indicates that the deltoid muscle of chimpanzees possesses a greater PCSA than in humans, evidencing a greater force-generating capacity in our primate relatives that is linked with arboreal locomotion (Rodr et al., 2022) (Figure 11.5).

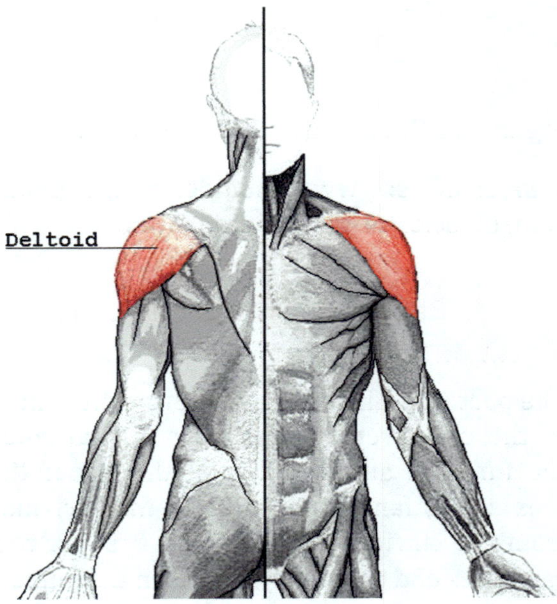

Figure 11.5. Deltoid muscle.

Source: https://upload.wikimedia.org/wikipedia/commons/9/93/Deltoideus.png.

This disparity serves to emphasize the adaptive topology of muscle associated with lifestyle demands. As such, while the two species both utilize their deltoid muscles in their upper limb movement, the specific muscular adaptation illustrates diverging evolutionary pressures necessitating unique functional demands. More recent technological developments in anatomical analysis have further served to authenticate the modularity of the deltoid muscle in the context of the upper limb. With the aid of methods like Anatomical Network Analysis (AnNA), researchers are capable of performing quantitative analysis of integration and variation of muscular and skeletal systems in different limb structures (Goswami et al., 2015). The analysis exhibits clear organizational trends in upper and lower limbs, with particular emphasis on the special adaptations of the deltoid over lower limb muscles. This research provides more understanding of how various anatomical features cooperate to achieve complex motor functions, confirming the deltoid muscle's vital role not only in single movements but also in the overall anatomy of human movement and flexing.

11.2.2. Rotator Cuff Muscles and Their Roles

The rotator cuff is a significant musculotendinous structure that stabilizes the glenohumeral joint, allowing for a wide arc of motion while guarding against dislocation of, and trauma to, the shoulder. It is composed of four individual muscles—supraspinatus, infraspinatus, teres minor, and subscapularis—and each muscle has a specific role in movement at the shoulder.

The supraspinatus primarily serves to initiate abduction of the shoulder; the infraspinatus and teres minor facilitate external rotation, and the subscapularis facilitates internal rotation. This precise coordination between the muscles not only increases the motion of the shoulder but also offers dynamic stability by placing the humeral head into the shallow glenoid cavity, with essential functions for activities from throw to lift. The biomechanical stability provided by the rotator cuff is particularly valuable in athletic and physically active environments, where injury risk is high. According to recent research, poor rotator cuff muscle strength can lead to decreased glenohumeral joint stability, significantly increasing dislocation and soft tissue injury risk, especially in contact sports (Kasslatter et al., 2025) (Figure 11.6).

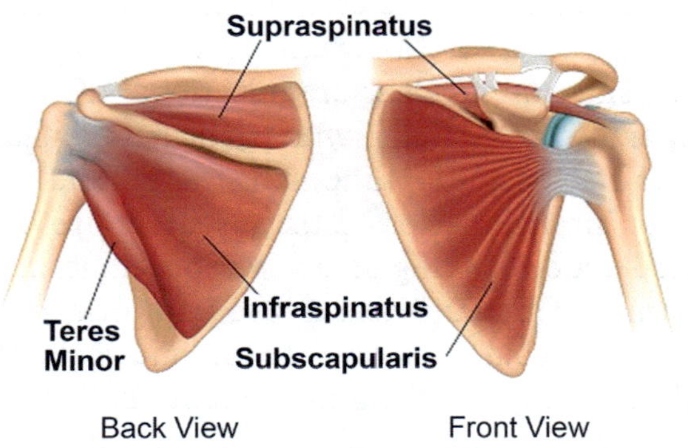

Figure 11.6. Rotator cuff muscles.

Source: https://www.shoulder-pain-explained.com/muscles-of-the-shoulder.html.

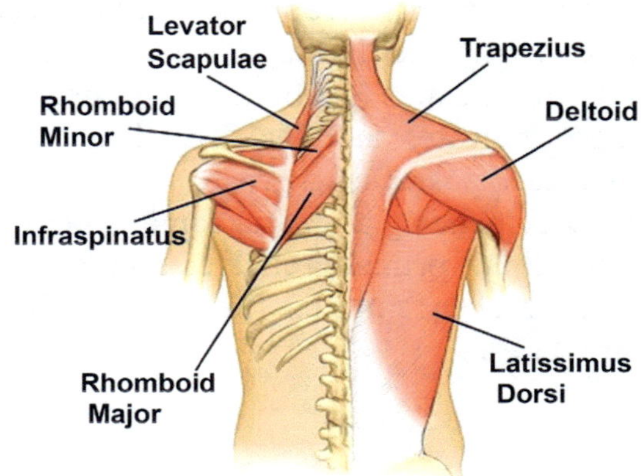

Figure 11.7. Shoulder blade muscles.

Source: https://www.shoulder-pain-explained.com/muscles-of-the-shoulder.html.

The co-activation of these muscles is responsible for maintaining joint stability under varying loads, guarding against the common shoulder problems among athletes. Evidence suggests that targeted strength training and conditioning can enhance rotator cuff function, thereby reducing the frequency of injury and enabling a more robust sports career (Trichez et al., 2024).

In addition to injury prevention, the rotator cuff also plays a fundamental role in rehabilitation programs for injuries to the shoulder. Effective rehabilitation protocols should promote strength and flexibility between the muscles of the rotator cuff to facilitate the recovery of full functional ability. Muscle-strengthening exercises in these muscles are imperative in the healing process after injury and return of the muscle-tendon interaction essential for stability of the shoulder. By understanding the specific functions and limitations of the rotator cuff, practitioners are empowered to design responsible ways to minimize the risk of injury while maximizing performance in both leisure and competitive settings. This integrated approach not only reduces the risk for future injury, but it also allows for the athletes long-term participation in bodily activities (Figure 11.7).

11.2.3. Pectoralis Major and Its Significance

The pectoralis major is a well-projection muscle of the chest region and plays a vital role in the function and mobility of the upper limb. It is a flat, fan-shaped muscle that originates from the clavicle, sternum, and first six costal cartilages and eventually inserts in the humerus. Its anatomic position and widespread size allow it to generate several movements of the upper limb, including flexion, adduction, and medial rotation of the shoulder joint. In addition to its role as a mechanical device for limb movement, the pectoralis major is also crucial for the stability of the shoulder, which is essential during dynamic activities like throwing or pushing, and therefore is vital to athletic function as well as to daily activities. In clinical practice, the pectoralis major has been of interest due to its involvement in various shoulder pathologies, particularly in sports. Muscle injury can result in severe impairments of the function of the upper limb. For instance, injury conditions such as SLAP lesions affect the timing and muscle activation, particularly of high-stress events such as tackling in rugby. Evidence has identified that players with

SLAP lesions had delayed activation times of the pectoralis major compared to uninjured players, which may influence overall shoulder stability and function. This indicates that muscle integrity is most crucial when it comes to having appropriate biomechanical function and protection of the shoulder joint from injury, and this reflects its clinical relevance in sports medicine (Bathgate et al., 2010) (Figure 11.8).

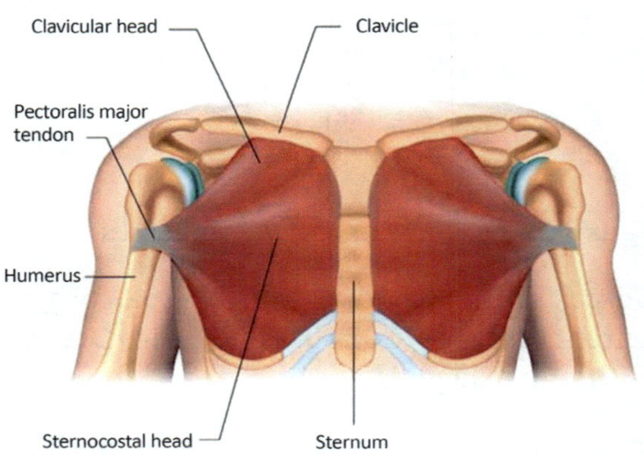

Figure 11.8. Pectoralis major muscle.

Source: https://houstonsportsortho.com/wp-content/uploads/2022/02/Pectoralis-Major.jpg.

Furthermore, further research beyond the typical anatomical dissections has elucidated the pectoralis majors complex interaction with other movement muscles. For purposes of effective rehabilitative protocols following injury to the shoulder, these dynamics need to be understood.

The muscle, as well as other rotators and scapular stabilizers, influences upper limb motion dynamics and control of posture. New imaging technologies, such as contrast-enhanced computed tomography (CT), have given new insight into the muscular anatomy of the pectoralis major, and through it, greater insight into its role within the larger MSK machine. The deeper researchers probe into these facts, the more it is reasserted that the pectoralis major plays a critical role in functional mobility and rehabilitation practice, making it a high priority for further anatomical and physiological inquiry (Ahn et al., 2017).

Test Your Knowledge

1. What are the main functions of the deltoid muscle in shoulder movement?
2. Which muscles make up the rotator cuff, and what roles do they play in shoulder stability?

11.3. Muscles of the Arm

Learning Outcome

1. Describe the anatomy of the biceps brachii and explain its functions in forearm flexion
2. Identify the triceps brachii and explain its role in forearm extension.
3. Describe the brachialis muscle

The investigation of the muscles of the arm is basic to the functional anatomy of the upper limb since they have significant roles in movements and activities. The arm is comprised mainly of biceps brachii, triceps brachii, and brachialis muscles that are all involved in flexion and extension of the elbow joint. The biceps brachii on the anterior arm is basically responsible for flexion of the elbow and supination of the forearm. The triceps brachii, however, remains stationed at the posterior aspect and executes the extension of the elbow. The muscles work in unison in dynamic movements, allowing an extensive range of functionalities in the upper limb from simple lifting to high-tech sporting movements.

Anatomically, their structure and interactions show the principles of muscular coordination in proper arm movement. Practical knowledge of arm musculature transcends single-muscle action to encompass the intricate neural and vascular networks, ensuring assistance in such movements. The brachial plexus innervate the arms musculature, and as such, nerve supply is instrumental in muscle function.

Each one of these muscles has specific innervation that not only regulates relaxation and contraction but also proprioceptive feedback on movement. Additionally, vascular supply through the brachial artery maximizes the metabolic potential of such muscles further for sustained action under effort. This interconnectedness is found to resonate with results in broader anatomical research; for instance, network analysis of anatomy highlighted differences between muscular organization in species, noting how some are specialized for particular functions (Diogo et al., 2017) (Figure 11.9).

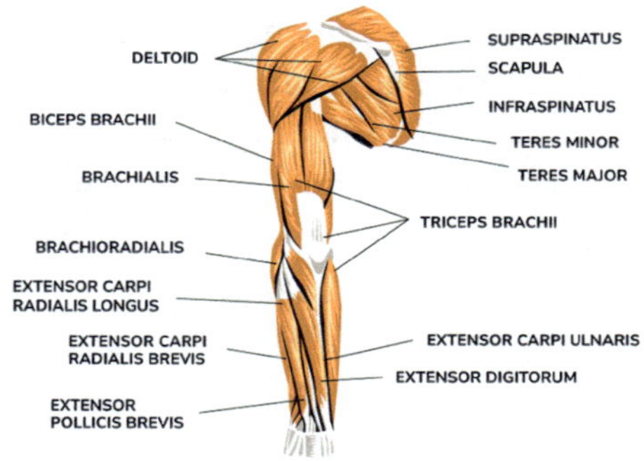

Figure 11.9. Diagram of arm muscles.

Source: https://media.geeksforgeeks.org/wp-content/uploads/20240328112244/Diagram-of-arm-muscle.png.

These findings enhance our appreciation of the evolutionary significance of arm muscle organization. Further, the anatomic adaptations of arm musculature are of profound importance in appreciating locomotion and movements over gravity. The structure of the arm muscles' form is not only critical to basic activity but also to functional adaptation observed in varying species and their evolutionary development. Studies have shown how muscles can display incredible plasticity and accommodate alternative locomotor styles that are very different from those of closely related organisms. For instance, the adaptations seen in the forelimbs of sthenurine kangaroos explain how muscle specialization determines locomotive behavior, allowing larger species to use novel modes of locomotion (Figueirido et al., 2014). Through the analysis of such differences, we may better understand how the muscles of the arm itself may also adapt to needs in the environment and what this means for human biomechanics and movement economy in contemporary environments.

11.3.1. Biceps Brachii and Its Functions

Biceps brachii is one of the large muscles of the upper arm, so well-known for its distinctive two-headed form and intricate role in arm movement. Biceps brachii, originating from the supraglenoid tubercle and the coracoid process of the scapula, attaches to the radial tuberosity of the radius. This anatomical feature allows it to function primarily as a flexor of the elbow joint, thereby making it indispensable to lifting and pulling actions, which are crucial in most daily activities and sports competitions. Additionally, its functionality during supination—the rotation out of the forearm—further enhances its utility in such actions as opening a doorknob or a screwdriver. Understanding the mechanical action of the biceps brachii enlightens us to its essential role in human motor control and the acquisition of skill. It highlights its intrinsic role in functional and athletic performance. Furthermore, the biceps brachii assists in stabilizing the shoulder joint through its connective attachments.

These attachments facilitate the correct positioning of the humeral head within the glenoid fossa, particularly during dynamic movements that combine shoulder movement with elbow flexion. The interaction of the muscle with both the forearm and shoulder girdle gives an expression of the complexity of the upper limbs' musculature. Interestingly, research has indicated that variation in the biceps brachiis PCSA can impact muscular strength and endurance of functions in the upper limbs. This is an indication of the biceps brachii's flexibility to functional loads, where individuals with increased muscle mass within this area can experience improved performance and lower risk of injury while performing heavy lifting or sport-specific movements, as evidenced in comparative analyses across populations (Figure 11.10).

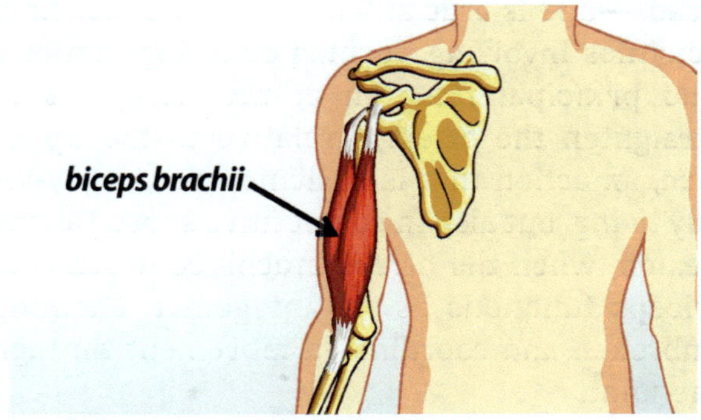

Figure 11.10. *Biceps brachii* muscle.

Source: https://study.com/cimages/videopreview/biceps-brachii-origin-insertion-function_01012922_123087.jpg.

Finally, the biceps brachii's value is not only its mechanical role; it is a valuable marker in clinical assessment of upper extremity function. Biceps brachii injuries or disease will produce noticeable deficits in arm strength and function. Diagnosis of biceps tendonitis or ruptures is significant in rehabilitation facilities since these conditions lead to appreciable impairment of activity of daily living and sporting performance. Rehabilitation training typically focuses on strengthening and flexibility exercises tailored to preserve the integrity of the synergistic muscles and the biceps brachii. In addition, understanding of the biceps brachii in the context of wider anatomical studies can be applied in describing evolutionary adaptations of MSK features in human and other animals, supporting the evidence that cooperative scaling and function of muscles, including the biceps brachii, play a significant role in terms of functional locomotion and manipulation (Goswami et al., 2015; Adams et al., 2016).

11.3.2. Triceps Brachii and Its Role in Extension

The triceps brachii, the large muscle complex at the posterior arm, is a major player in the extension of the elbow joint. It consists of three different heads—the long, lateral, and medial heads—and is crucial for nearly all upper limb activities involving pushing or lifting motions. The principal function of the triceps is to straighten the forearm relative to the upper arm, an action that is basic not just in day-to-day living, but also in competitive sport. During flexion, when the biceps brachii contracts, the triceps functions as its antagonist, enabling unbroken and coordinated movement through the joint.

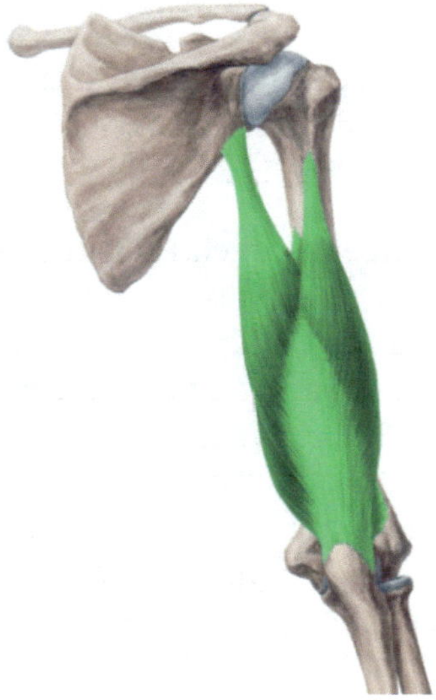

Figure 11.11. Triceps brachii muscle.

Source: https://www.kenhub.com/thumbor/HFbTJc2AayYsrOSJMmDE5axXPvs=/fit-in/800x1600/filters:watermark(/images/logo_url.png,-10,-10,0):background_color(FFFFFF):format(jpeg)/images/library/13946/aHliOOl62koJhumoZcUysg_vsBTp2iDc2_M._triceps_brachii_1.png.

This cooperative action is evidence of the importance of triceps activation in providing dynamic stability and function during strength and precision-activity performance. Apart from its role in elbow extension, the triceps brachii also assists in shoulder stabilization and arm movements. The long head of the triceps, for instance, crosses the shoulder joint and is active during shoulder extension and adduction, demonstrating that it has numerous functions. This activation of diverse muscle groups emphasizes the complex interaction that exists in upper limb biomechanics. Recent studies of muscle patterns of activation, for example, extension and flexion of the elbow, illustrate that these triceps have distinct patterns of activation which may vary based on the physical condition and level of effort of individuals. This study points out the degree to which the triceps is not only a simple extensor but also adapts its action based on evolving demands to enhance overall motor performance under different conditions (Alonso et al., 2016) (Figure 11.11). The expansion of triceps mechanism understanding has implications for therapy, particularly in the area of rehabilitation. Research shows that exercise protocols designed primarily to strengthen the triceps can make a significant difference in patients' functional outcomes after injury or surgery impairing extension of the elbow. Results of electromyogram analysis shed light on the relationship between muscle fatigue and activation patterns, and strategic recruitment of the triceps can be employed to influence recovery and mobility (Amirabdollahian et al., 2020). Consequently, a solid appreciation of the triceps brachii forms the basis for the establishment of effective rehabilitation protocols. With targeted interventions, practitioners can enhance motor control through the function of the triceps in extension, eventually contributing to the quality of life of patients with upper limb limitations.

11.3.3. Brachialis and Its Contribution to Flexion

Brachialis is a muscle of deeply located within the upper arm and is involved in flexion of the elbow. It is located beneath the biceps brachii and originates from the distal half of the anterior surface of the humerus. Its fibers insert into the coronoid process and the tuberosity of the ulna. Unlike the biceps brachii, which assists both in flexion and in supination, the brachialis is primarily tasked with flexion of the elbow joint. This particular function renders the brachialis a crucial element in movements that require power and finesse, particularly when the forearm is in pronation. Emphasis on flexion of the elbow highlights the brachialis' significance not only in everyday activities like lifting or pulling but also in sports where proper arm movement is crucial. In addition to its anatomical significance, the functional role of the brachialis during flexion of the elbow is considerable (Figure 11.12).

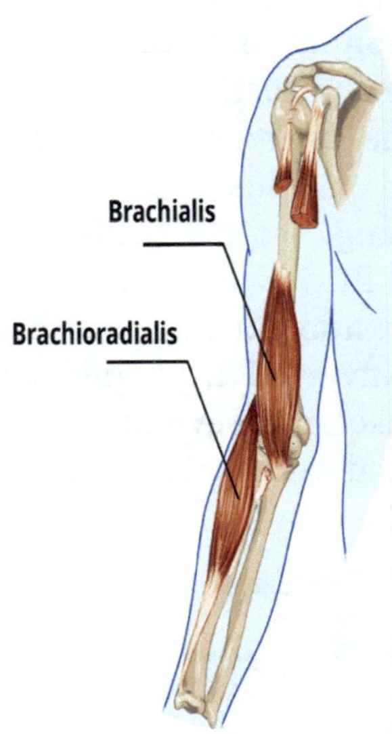

Figure 11.12. The brachialis muscle.

Source: https://upload.wikimedia.org/wikipedia/commons/thumb/3/36/1120_Muscles_that_Move_the_Forearm_Humerus_Flex_Sin.png/960px-1120_Muscles_that_Move_the_Forearm_Humerus_Flex_Sin.png.

Research has shown that in strength tasks, such as lifting heavy weights or sports, the brachialis is used to provide maximum elbow flexion force. Experiments have proven that, due to its position and attachment, the brachialis always generates tremendous amounts of force over the entire range of elbow flexion motion. This function enables effective movement mechanics, facilitating rapid and efficient arm movements that are crucial for various physical activities. Moreover, the brachialis has an important role when resistance is present in flexion, stabilizing not only the elbow joint but also contributing to general upper limb function in activities with combined actions of flexion and extension. The functional activity of the brachialis, nonetheless, is influenced by some elbow disorders, highlighting the importance of clinical recognition of its flexion role. Elbow instability or soft tissue injury around the elbow can impair the brachialis from functioning optimally. It becomes necessary to comprehend the biomechanical forces involved, as demonstrated by research on the simulation of elbow motion and its relevance to the treatment of elbow disorders, where muscle tension and flexion angle are crucial factors. The results obtained from such studies provide clinical directions toward improving treatments and recovery strategies for people with elbow disturbances. Consequently, acknowledgment of the irreplaceable function of the brachialis goes past the anatomical level; it also works to enhance clinical operations and rehabilitation strategies aimed at the restoration of arm function, consequently improving quality of life in those affected (Badre et al., 2019; Ferreira et al., 2011).

Test Your Knowledge

1. What are the primary functions of the biceps brachii muscle?
2. How does the triceps brachii contribute to the movement of the arm?

11.4. Muscles of the Forearm

Learning Outcome

1. Define flexor muscles and their functions
2. Understand the extensor muscles and their roles
3. Explain the pronator and supinator muscles

The forearm muscles are a part of the overall functioning of the upper limb, and their primary function is to generate movements of the wrist, hand, and fingers. The two anatomical groups comprising the muscles in this area are the flexors and extensors, both functioning independently in the functioning of the upper limb. The anterior compartment, which houses the flexor muscles, receives its innervation from the median and ulnar nerves, enabling diverse functions such as gripping and pinching. These muscles are also involved in crucial daily actions, which demonstrates their importance in the biomechanics of the upper limb. The posterior compartment contains extensors that extend fingers and the wrist, demonstrating another crucial aspect of forearm musculature involved in fine motor capability and gross motor function in the hand. A knowledge of this structural design is central to an appreciation of the mechanical advantages such muscles provide to the MSK system of the upper limb. In examining the functions served by the forearm muscles, a consideration of the biomechanical principles governing their action is essential. All muscle designs, including length, site of attachment, and direction of fibers, allow for certain movements and the generation of forces employable in various types of activity. For instance, the angle of the flexor carpi radialis permits wrist flexion and radial deviation to optimize doorknob turning. Furthermore, the biomechanics involved in gripping are seriously complicated insofar as several muscle groups in the forearm need to be activated simultaneously (Figure 11.13).

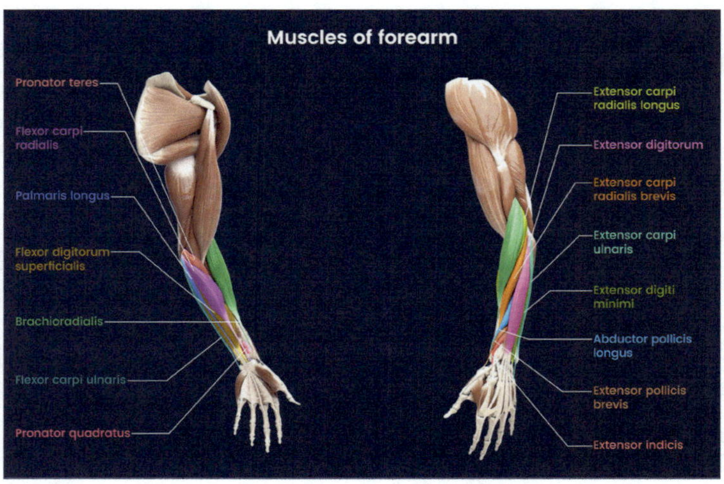

Figure 11.13. Muscles of the forearm.

Source: https://admin.anatomy.app/Media/images/1f1cc0a4-0844-412a-832d-027a83a19aa3_large.jpg.

New biomechanical modeling has uncovered more information about how these muscles interact with one another and impact limb mechanics overall, demonstrating the relationship between anatomical structure and functional capability. The implications of this dynamic relationship identify the importance of a healthy forearm musculature in preventing injury and maximizing athletic performance in upper limb dexterity-demanding events. Furthermore, all descriptions of forearm musculature must include the effects of muscular imbalances or overuse injuries. Tendonitis and carpal tunnel syndrome (CTS) most commonly occur due to repetitive effort that overloads forearm muscles, causing pain and functional deficits. Clinicians can then create efficient rehabilitation plans that restore function while reducing pain by having a thorough grasp of forearm muscle breakdown and adaptation. As Goswami et al. (2015) and Harris et al. (2012) illustrate, this increasing understanding of biomechanics and musculature forms the foundation for novel treatments and prevention. Through anatomical network exploration by methods such as Anatomical Network Analysis, insight into predisposition to injury is gained, and new biomechanical methods become part of an interdisciplinary sharing that assists in enhancing patient outcomes and recovery. Lastly, appreciation of the full functionality of the forearm muscles and their interrelatedness is essential to practitioners dedicated to facilitating maximum upper limb well-being.

11.4.1. Flexor Muscles and Their Functions

Flexor muscles play a significant role in the mobility and function of the upper limb, allowing for actions that are crucial in accomplishing daily activities. Most of the flexor muscles are located in the anterior compartment of the forearm, which allows for flexion of the fingers, wrist, and shoulder. It should be noted that the main flexor muscles include the biceps brachii, brachialis, and the flexor digitorum superficialis, among others. Upon contraction, these muscles decrease the angle between the segments they act upon, enabling the ROMs such as gripping, lifting, and manipulation. Coordination of flexor muscles is crucial in precision and strength-requiring movements, which reflects their importance to gross and fine motor skills. The biomechanics of flexor muscles also account for their adaptability to various functional demands. Evidence indicates that the specialized architecture and organization of muscle fibers allow for flexor muscles to generate considerable force while having the capability to control movement and speed. For instance, the PCSA of the muscles dictates the ability to generate force; the larger the muscles are, the larger the strength-generating ability. Furthermore, interaction between flexor muscles and tendon properties, such as elasticity, enhances their function in dynamic movement. This can be seen in studies examining locomotor behaviors across various species and suggesting that muscle effectiveness and efficiency can significantly differ depending on anatomical configurations and movement patterns (Delp et al., 2015). Further, the functional significance of flexor muscles transcends simple motion as they are essential for postural control and stabilization. Since the upper limb is engaged in complex movements, flexor muscles make a greater contribution as they are prone to co-activation with extensor muscles to counter forces applied across joints. The two-way function proves vital in maintaining joint integrity during activities such as climbing or lifting a heavy load. Also, the special scaling patterns of muscle structure in different species suggest that body size will result in adaptations in the flexor musculature so as to efficiently deal with body weight and provide dynamic movement to deal with body weight and provide dynamic movement efficiently (Adams et al., 2016). Lastly, a consideration of the flexor muscles and their consideration in terms of upper limb function proves their significant contribution to both locomotion and manipulation.

11.4.2. Extensor Muscles and Their Roles

The extensor muscles of the upper limb play a crucial role in aiding a host of movements, namely those about the extension of the wrist, forearm, and fingers. The muscles primarily include the posterior arm compartment and forearm. They are distributed along the extensor group by renowned, stout muscles like the triceps brachii, forearm extensors, and the wrist extensors.

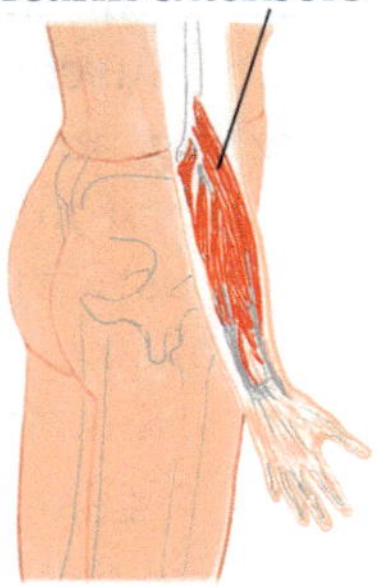

Figure 11.14. Forearm extensor muscles.

Source: https://external-content.duckduckgo.com/iu/?u=https%3A%2F%2Fimages.squarespace-cdn.com%2Fcontent%2Fv1%2F5a541e320abd04d06b3ac0b8%2F1556150661106-53Y7ANZVQOEHBZHRNXP0%2Fforearm%2Bextensors.jpg&f=1&nofb=1&ipt=c98a9d5ff9ac4bd595d2803ff826c2af908ff4daf30fddff34714377447ff81a.

The triceps brachii, for instance, is a vital muscle in extending the elbow joint to enable actions like pushing and throwing, which are essential in various sporting and daily activities. The muscle's function emphasizes the necessity of extensors in generating force and stability during extension movements, thereby ensuring limb efficiency. Understanding the individual roles of these groups of muscles puts their function into the perspective of anatomy and biomechanics, emphasizing their role in necessary motion and stability of the upper limb. In combination with the triceps brachii, the forearm extensors, including the extensor *Carpi radialis*, extensor *Carpi ulnaris*, and the extensor digitorum, help with fine motor control for sophisticated movements of the hand. These muscles enable such movements as wrist extension and extension of the fingers, necessary in the activities of grasping, releasing, and manipulating objects. Proper function of forearm extensors is crucial when engaging in activities such as playing a musical instrument, typing, or sporting activities, where precision and control are of primary importance (Figure 11.14). Along with that, injury or dysfunction to these muscles can create significant impairment in the execution of activities of daily living, an indication of their absolute significance in upper limb movement. Understanding how these groups of muscles function together in a biomechanical manner, separately as well as within the kinetic chain that culminates in upper limb performance, is of utmost significance. Furthermore, the evolutionary significance of extensor muscles is pointed out through their adaptation and evolution in various vertebrates, as it portrays the fundamental role of extensor muscles in locomotive processes. Research reveals considerable differences in actions of extensor muscles and leverages across different lineages of animals, particularly in the adaptation to a transition from quadrupedal to bipedal movement. For example, research has proved that such adaptations have an effect on the muscle moment arms and total function in the forelimbs of most organisms. The extensor muscle adaptation shows an evolutionary shift in locomotion strategies, which signals their role not only in the facilitation of movement but also in the broader field of evolutionary biology. Through examining such anatomical and functional variations, we are better equipped to make sense of how extension muscles have developed the mechanical advantages described in other species and, therefore, further our understanding of muscular layouts in an evolutionary context (Alexander et al., 2017; Allen et al., 2017).

11.4.3. Pronator and Supinator Muscles

The supinator and pronator muscles play essential roles in the action and functioning of the forearm, affecting how we perform everyday activities. The pronator teres and pronator quadratus are the principal muscles responsible for pronation, which is a movement that turns the palm backward or downward. They enable us to perform tasks like tilting liquid from a cup or screwing a screwdriver. In contrast, the supinator muscle is responsible for the supination, which is the rotation of the palm upwards or forwards. The muscle is supported by the biceps brachii in functional movements like bringing something towards the body. The anatomical location and innervation of these muscles play a major role in the interpretation of their implications in functional biomechanics, particularly if a human being's work or survival hinges on the mobility of the upper limbs. The complex co-operation of the supinator and pronator muscles is further emphasized in rehabilitation, particularly for upper extremity amputees. From studies, it has been noted that individuals who undergo such amputations are known to exhibit varied muscle activation patterns when attempting to control prosthetic limbs or experience phantom limb pains. As an example, the new patterns of muscle activation involved in prosthetic control are likely to be significantly different from those activated during voluntary limb movement, pointing to the adaptive role of the muscles in response to changes in limb availability. Experiments have confirmed that the majority of the muscle patterns used in phantom limb movement differed from anatomically normal expectations, emphasizing the need for accurate rehabilitation interventions that optimize the efficiency of muscle activation in natural and prosthetic environments (Collins et al., 2021) (Figure 11.15).

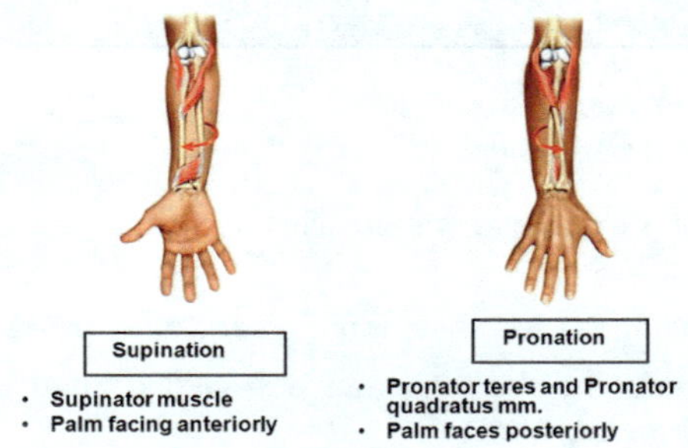

Figure 11.15. Supination and pronation of the forearm.

Source: https://external-content.duckduckgo.com/iu/?u=https%3A%2F%2Fi.pinimg.com%2Foriginals%2F2e%2F9d%2F27%2F2e9d270d66378cec9eeb3f0d9fc09e8c.jpg&f=1&nofb=1&ipt=80c55e4949e2c0c924b30165a581793be3b6798249cf9c8b1088adaa07e00f46.

Moreover, the analysis of pronator and supinator muscles is proof of the evolutionary adaptations of the musculature of limbs in various organisms. Biomechanical of locomotor transformation reveal that modifications of muscle actions, particularly in the joints of the elbow and wrist, are related to extreme transformations of postural adaptations in the archosaurian group. As the quadrupedal to bipedal transition took place within species, the mechanisms of pronation and supination evolved significantly, and this was not only a result of limb anatomy evolution but also evolving functional demands placed upon the forelimb muscles. These changes illustrate how anatomical innovations cannot be separated from the forces of evolution and moment arm kinetics at the joints, thus helping improve understanding of how muscle function allows compound behaviors in various locomotory contexts (Allen et al., 2017).

Test Your Knowledge

1. How do the extensor muscles contribute to wrist and finger movement?
2. What roles do the pronator and supinator muscles play in forearm rotation?

11.5. Muscles of the Hand

Learning Outcome

1. Discuss the intrinsic muscles and their functions
2. Explain the extrinsic muscles and their roles
3. Understand the importance of grip strength and dexterity

This intricate hand shape is supported by a diverse group of muscles that enable an unbelievable range of movement and fine actions. The muscles are categorized into two groups: extrinsic and intrinsic muscles. Extrinsic muscles originate in the forearm, where tendons extend into the hand to enable gross movements such as gripping and lifting. They are composed of the masses of flexor and extensor, allowing for extension and flexion of the fingers. In contrast, intrinsic muscles, which are entirely within the hand, provide the fine motor control required for activities involving dexterity, such as writing or playing a musical instrument. This dual-muscle arrangement is a testament to the evolutionary accommodation of the human hand, which emphasizes both power and finesse in our hand activity, contributing to various activities. Its evolutionary history directly correlates with our primate origins and divergence from others (Diogo et al., 2017). In the discussion of hand musculature's evolutionary specializations, it is necessary to investigate how anatomical integration has conditioned its functional capacity. The network analysis of the MSK components displays evident modularity among the proximal and distal components of the hand. While the proximal muscles indicate stability across multiple primate lineages, the musculature of the distal limbs shows significant variability. The reasons for variability might be due to variable loads borne by the forelimb, or coordination of separate fingers that has been optimized for higher dexterity and manipulation skills. In particular, in human beings, the intrinsic thumb muscles do not form an autonomous anatomical module, unlike other groups of primates. This modification may be caused by a shift in the functional emphasis of thumb opposition and grip that has generated the evolutionary trend differentiating humans from their primate relatives (Diogo et al., 2017) (Figure 11.16).

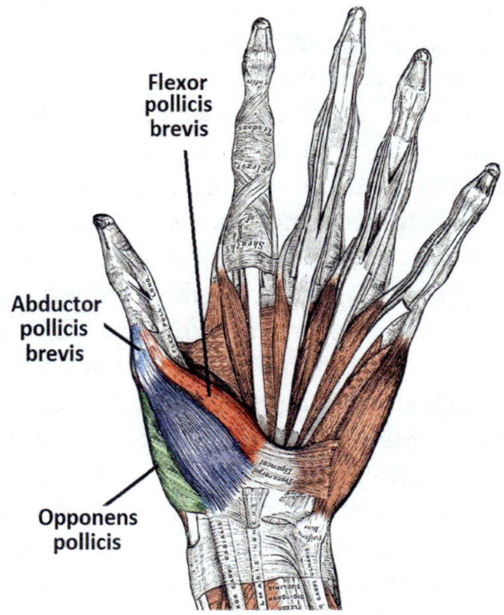

Figure 11.16. The muscles of the hand.

Source: https://teachmeanatomy.info/wp-content/uploads/Palmar-View-of-the-Thenar-Muscles-of-the-Thumb-and-Hand-Labelled-TeachMeAnatomy.jpg.

The hand musculature coordination and the limb coordination in general are a classic instance of the complexity found in human anatomy. Unlike the relative independence observed in the hindlimb, the forelimb, or the hand, has undergone radical evolutionary changes that optimize its performance for various tasks. Network analysis also accounts for how the hand's anatomical configuration renders the movements more intricate than in the rest of the primates. For instance, though the human hindlimb is as complex as that of chimpanzees, the human forelimb is comparatively , more straightforward, and implies forehand specialization with some reduction in anatomical diversity for better motor control. These findings overturn prevailing assumptions, suggesting that the anatomical intricacy of the human hand is based on an evolutionary compromise between adaptation and functional specialization and shedding light on our proficiency as dextrously talented manipulators.

11.5.1. Intrinsic Muscles and Their Functions

It is the intrinsic muscles of the upper limb that execute the complicated finger and hand joint movements required for a variety of activities in daily life. These are the muscles that originate and attach within the structure of the hand itself and include the lumbricals, the interossei, and the thenar and hypothenar muscles. By facilitating fine motor movements such as pinching and grasping, these muscles contribute dexterity and equip control for complex activities, such as playing a musical instrument or typing. According to research, the special pattern of these intrinsic muscles allows extreme flexibility with a broad ROM, and this is predominantly found to exist in the case of primate life forms, including the human species. Their anatomical variation in different species represents a testament to their evolutionary role in mediating different functions that are relevant to survival and interaction with the environment (Diogo et al., 2017). The coordination between intrinsic muscles is tightly correlated with the central nervous system's neural control mechanisms. The most prominent theory is that the premotor cortex and other cortical areas have a significant role to play in the planning and execution of movement of the limbs. Facts reveal that dorsal (PMd) as well as ventral premotor (PMv) cortices possess tuning features that are significantly involved with the biomechanical features of the intrinsic muscles. This connection suggests an active interaction among the neural representations throughout the premotor areas and motor commands generated to induce activation of these muscles. Through studies, it has been revealed that this relationship facilitates the conversion of high-level motor planning to precise muscle activation required to accomplish intricate hand movements (Hatsopoulos et al., 2015). This understanding highlights the position of the intrinsic muscles not only in function but in their representation of mental processes involved in movement.

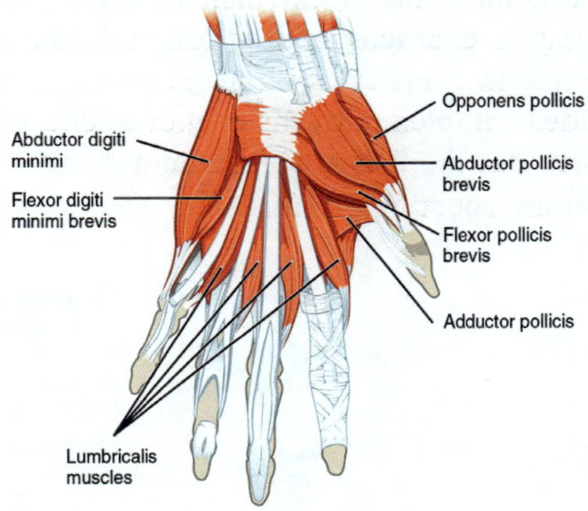

Figure 11.17. Diagrams of the intrinsic muscles of the right hand.

Source: https://radiopaedia.org/cases/intrinsic-muscles-of-the-hand-illustrations.

The functional significance of intrinsic muscles extends beyond the simplistic performance of movement; they are pivotal in enabling the gross architecture of the hand through various activities. For instance, the synergistic movement of the interossei and lumbrical muscles allows both extension and flexion of the fingers, with stability being maintained during gripping movements. The thenar and hypothenar muscles also allow opposition and fine control of the thumb and little finger, respectively, with increased grip strength and precision. Such movements are necessary in jobs that entail fine handwork, such as surgery or craftsmanship. In addition, their specific compositions and formations enable them to modify and reorganize, which means that they are capable of easily addressing novel responsibilities or injuries. This capability comes in particularly handy in the interpretation of the evolutionary changes in the functionality of hands among primates, accentuating the intrinsic muscles' roles in daily usefulness as well as broader evolutionary views (Diogo et al., 2017) (Figure 11.17).

11.5.2. Extrinsic Muscles and Their Roles

Movement of the upper limbs is predominantly governed by the extrinsic muscles that originate from structures outside the limb itself, such as the shoulder girdle or trunk. They are instrumental in generating the wide range of movement required for activities like reaching, grasping, and throwing. In contrast to intrinsic muscles, which are located deeper in the limb and primarily concerned with fine movements, extrinsic muscles provide the necessary strength for gross movement. Their anatomy is characterized by long tendons extending into the forearm and hand, which suggests their role in translating larger movements into specific actions. The extrinsic muscle coordination provides complex patterns of movement, such as in activities involving not only the placement of the arm but the use of objects in a dexterous manner, supporting their function in daily activities and many sporting events.

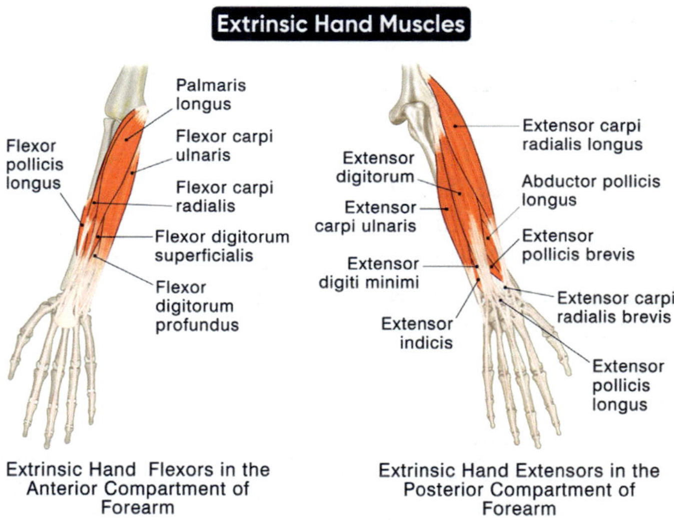

Figure 11.18. Extrinsic hand muscles.

Source: https://external-content.duckduckgo.com/iu/?u=https%3A%2F%2Fthemuscularsystem.com%2Fwp-content%2Fuploads%2F2023%2F04%2FExtrinsic-Muscles-of-the-Hand.jpg&f=1&nofb=1&ipt=f776e078c1b72f678438d159f848b8565df49f1d30ba9bceec47140cb1a1ec95.

Many of the largest extrinsic muscles of the upper limb are the pectoralis major, latissimus dorsi, and the trapezius, each with specific functions in providing shoulder and arm movement. The pectoralis major, for example, is used for adduction and internal rotation of the arm. In contrast, the latissimus dorsi is used for extension and adduction that permits movements such as pull-ups and swimming. The trapezius, being made up of its upper, middle, and lower fibers, aids in scapular motion, permitting overhead motion as well as stabilizing the shoulder for movements that involve lifting or pushing. With their complementary actions, these muscles allow for a coordinated approach to upper limb activities. The understanding of these muscles not only highlights their specific contributions but also illustrates their interaction in creating complex movements across contexts. Moreover, knowledge of the extrinsic muscles transgresses into the realm of neuromuscular control and biomechanics. Current research shows that the premotor cortex, previously thought to be a movement planner, has neural activity analogous to the biomechanics of these extrinsic muscles, revealing a more integrated system for motor control than initially supposed (Hatsopoulos et al., 2015). This highlights the significance of extrinsic muscles not just as facilitators of movement but as dynamic components that must be intelligently regulated by the nervous system when executing. Moreover, comparative anatomical network studies reveal new intricacies of MSK forelimb morphologies on hindlimb systems in the primate, revealing explicit evolutionary specializations that influence upper limb functional abilities (Esteve-Altava et al., 2018). A glimpse of the roles performed by such extrinsic muscles provides a preliminary perspective for clinical assessment as well as athletic training protocols for developing upper limb function (Figure 11.18).

11.5.3. Importance of Grip Strength and Dexterity

The value of dexterity and grip strength extends beyond simple physical function, with a considerable effect on most functions of daily living and quality of life. Grip strength is a valuable predictor of upper limb muscular function and is necessary for the execution of activities of daily living, such as holding, keyboarding, and cooking. Good grip capacity is most directly associated with hand and forearm muscle function because these areas are a complicated network of muscle and tendon tissue that generates movement and function. Grip strength tests can provide information about general health issues and, as such, are invaluable in clinical and community settings. Higher dexterity, dependent on precise coordination and control of the hand, is also needed; it allows individuals to accomplish intricate tasks, which can influence their independence and satisfaction with daily activities significantly.

Literature insists upon the exigent need for evaluation of grip strength and dexterity, particularly among individuals who are affected by neuromuscular disorders. Patients with conditions like Charcot-Marie-tooth (CMT) syndrome often report hand impairment that negatively impacts their quality of life. Their inability to carry out self-care activities is a symptom of the immense influence of compromised grip strength and dexterity. Outcomes of studies examining the relationship between hand function and quality of life often provide evidence that grip strength is highly correlated with other indicators of general health, including SF-36 scores.

This finding emphasizes the importance of regular evaluation of upper limb activities and comments on the importance of targeted interventions in enhancing hand function, thereby increasing the reported quality of life among the affected ones (Aiello et al., 2022). Furthermore, dexterity and grip strength play a key role in understanding and controlling orthopedic complications of conditions such as Morquio A syndrome. This syndrome presents with a variety of MSK deformities that can significantly impair upper and lower extremity functions. While health practitioners devise treatment plans, placing grip strength tests at the top of their priorities is not only necessary for controlling the degree of impairment but also for making effective treatment decisions. Interventions improving such physical functions can have a deciding impact on patient outcomes, leading to increased functional independence and activity participation (Bache et al., 2014). Thus, distinguishing the function of muscles in upper limb activity becomes a matter of utmost priority both in a therapeutic and a diagnostic scenario, calling for the application of informed strategies to patient care and rehabilitation.

Test Your Knowledge

1. What are the intrinsic muscles of the hand, and what functions do they perform?
2. How do the extrinsic muscles contribute to hand and finger movement?

11.6. Common Injuries and Disorders

Learning Outcome

1. Define rotator cuff injuries and their impact
2. Discuss the tendonitis in the forearm muscles
3. Identify the CTS and its effects

Recurrent disorders and injuries of the muscles of the upper limb are generally due to acute trauma, repetitive strain, or improper ergonomic utilization. Strains and sprains result from acute injury while participating in sports, falls, or lifting something in an abnormal position and cause pain, swelling, and restricted mobility in the affected part. These injuries are often incurred by athletes and laborers who work with heavy manual labor, which is why the importance of safety training and proper technique is emphasized. Moreover, long-term conditions such as tendinitis and bursitis can develop slowly through repetitive motion exercises, placing muscle and tendon tissue under overload. Not only are these conditions painful, but they also seriously compromise regular daily activity, and so preventive measures are worthwhile in recreational as well as occupational environments. Besides sports injuries, MSK disorders are most often caused by the mechanical demands of certain occupations, particularly those involving static postures for much of the working day. For instance, dentistry is an occupation where individuals tend to undergo physical strain through uncomfortable posture in performing tasks that require accuracy. Prolonged static seated postures, along with repetitive movements and posture difficulty, cause discomfort and can also lead to repetitive strain injuries (RSIs). Countermeasures for such risk involve adopting ergonomic tools that enable better posture alignment, including magnifying loupes or operating microscopes. These aids not only enhance visual accuracy but also facilitate changes in working habits that can minimize the chances of acquiring MSK disorders. Evidence based on assessment tools like the Rapid Upper Limb Assessment RULA demonstrates that the inclusion of ergonomic interventions is most appropriate for practitioners undertaking high-risk occupations (Ortiz et al., 2024). The impact of common upper limb disorders and injuries extends beyond physical disability to both psychological well-being and workplace productivity. Chronic pain or limited mobility patients may become increasingly stressed, anxious, and frustrated, leading to decreased quality of life. Moreover, the financial burden of treatment, rehabilitation, and lost workplace productivity can be high. The advances in recent medical imaging, such as the use of MRI for cervical spinal cord injury diagnosis, work to highlight the value of precise diagnostic approaches to inform robust treatment plans (Lin et al., 2025). Moreover, the knowledge of the intricate relationship between muscle damage and susceptibility to further complications remains key. Holistic management programs that encompass physical therapy, ergonomic therapy, and patient education play an essential role in promoting recovery and avoiding future injury, thereby enhancing the overall health and functioning of individuals with upper limb disorders.

11.6.1. Rotator Cuff Injuries and Their Impact

The rotator cuff, comprised of muscles and tendons that stabilize the shoulder, is susceptible to injuries that significantly influence upper limb function.

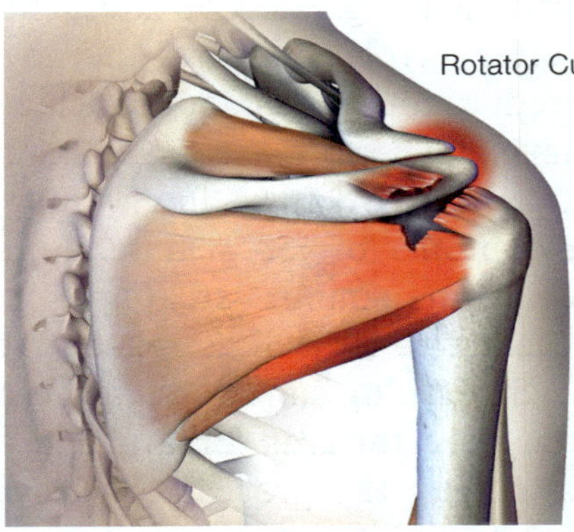

Figure 11.19. Rotator cuff injury.

Source: https://external-content.duckduckgo.com/iu/?u=https%3A%2F%2Fmedmovie.com%2F_uploads%2F2860_Rotator.jpg&f=1&nofb=1&ipt=369995d08fda680cccfe7dd77dfabeabea8faed01949c517ab5ae6bb6a3ff33f.

Tendinitis, impingement syndrome, and tears are some of the most frequent injuries in this area, typically resulting from repetitive overhead actions and trauma. Injuries of this kind impose more than just physical limitations since they also negatively affect activities of daily living, sporting performance, and the general quality of life. The patients also experience pain, weakness, and limited ROM, all of which lead to compensatory movement patterns that place additional stress on other muscles. For instance, a SLAP lesion, an injury to the cartilage in the shoulder joint, is responsible for causing muscle activation delays, as noted by a study identifying alterations in onset times of biceps and other affected muscles in injured shoulders (Bathgate et al., 2010) (Figure 11.19).

These delays can further aggravate the injury and result in chronic conditions if not taken care of immediately. Physical rehab and specific preventive measures are essential in effectively managing rotator cuff injuries. A full approach not only addresses pain and dysfunction but also focuses on strengthening the muscles around the shoulder joint. Specifically, shoulder flexibility, strength, and stability training programs play a pivotal role in minimizing injury susceptibility for sports-playing athletes. Preventive exercises such as resistance band rotations and shoulder stabilization exercises are effective in enhancing muscular endurance and minimizing rotator cuff strain (Ahonpää et al., 2024). By incorporating these exercises, athletes will be more likely to adapt to the physical demands of their sport and reduce the risk of acute injury. Additionally, having good warm-up protocols before heavy activities also conditions the rotator cuff to high usage levels, thereby ensuring long-term shoulder health. Understanding the various effects of rotator cuff injury can enhance treatment and prevention strategies. Most individuals do not pay much heed to muscle conditioning, particularly in competitive sports, where shoulder wellness is the number one priority. Sportsmen, coaches, and medical practitioners must work together in developing personalized plans that prioritize shoulder integrity. A portion of this collaborative effort must encompass not only rehabilitation drills but also education on body mechanics and injury prevention techniques. As highlighted in competitive swimmer research, strength imbalance and maximized mobility can be essential factors in the prevention of injury

(Ahonpää et al., 2024). In the end, raising awareness of the necessity of the contribution of the rotator cuffs to upper limb function is a step towards encouraging long-term athletic performance and health.

11.6.2. Tendonitis in the Forearm Muscles

This is a serious issue in the upper limb musculature study, affecting individuals who perform repetitive tasks such as typing or playing music, as well as in some sports. It is, in part, due to inflammation of tendons connecting muscles of the forearm to the bones due to overuse or stress to it.

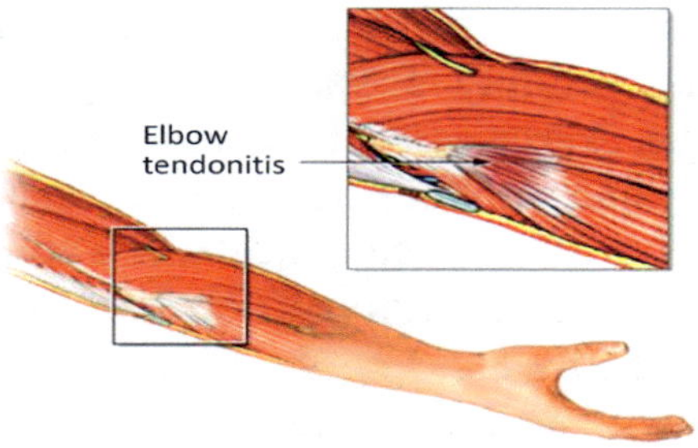

Figure 11.20. Elbow tendonitis.

Source: https://www.mountsinai.org/health-library/diseases-conditions/tendinitis.

This inflammation can lead to pain, swelling, and reduced mobility, directly impacting a person's ability to perform day-to-day activities or enjoy a hobby. If left untreated, with time, tendonitis can turn into a chronic condition, and this will result in more severe complications such as tendon rupture or degenerative change in the tendon. Hence, the early identification of the symptoms and proper management are crucial in preventing long-term disability. Individuals who engage in activities or employment that subject such key structures to repetitive stress must have a proper knowledge of tendonitis, particularly forearm musculature. Forearm tendonitis most commonly develops due to improper technique and a lack of ergonomic training. For example, musicians, particularly pianists, tend to build tendonitis because they have very fine repetitive motion in the fingers used when playing (Figure 11.20).

The importance of technique cannot be overstated, with improper postures having the potential to cause undue stress on the forearm muscles, triggering the onset of tendonitis. Research has indicated that numerous musicians who seek out medical attention for injury have overuse and misuse of playing behavior as causes for injury (Niu et al., 2020). This underlines the importance of educating individuals in good mechanics and the importance of rest stops throughout prolonged practice sessions to reduce excessive loading. Effective intervention techniques often involve physical therapy in addition to reeducation of technique to achieve a balance of maximum performance and minimum risk of injury. In addition to intervening in the acute symptoms of forearm tendonitis, an effective management strategy often employs preventative as well as rehabilitative techniques. Stretching and strengthening maneuvers targeted towards forearm muscles are essential during the process of recovery, to re-establish flexibility and create muscular balance. Occupational therapy is also helpful in modifying habits in a way that minimizes repetitive stress. Musicians, for instance, can be shown other ways of performing to interrupt the dependence on specific muscle groups, thus preventing cumulative injuries (Niu et al., 2020). An understanding of anatomical differences and susceptibility is key to the formulation of individualized recovery strategies. Not only does this holistic plan remove the agony associated with tendonitis, but it also provides one with an understanding of the grander scheme of forearm health, something that is indispensable to individuals whose daily activities or working responsibilities rely on upper arm musculature.

11.6.3. Carpal Tunnel Syndrome and Its Effects

CTS is a common entrapment neuropathy that results from the median nerve compression within the carpal tunnel, a narrow passageway in the wrist. The syndrome itself is often preceded by numbness, tingling, and weakness of the hand that can significantly impede the usual daily activities of an individual. The most frequently implicated anatomical structures are not only the median nerve but also the flexor tendons that course through the canal. This is most disproportionately affecting certain groups, particularly those with repetitive wrist movements, thereby exposing them to increased risk of symptomatic expression. The effects of CTS are more than just annoying; they can create severe limitations of hand function that result in lost productivity and compromised health status. An understanding of the etiology and symptomatology of CTS is necessary to address its impact on the upper limb muscles (Figure 11.21).

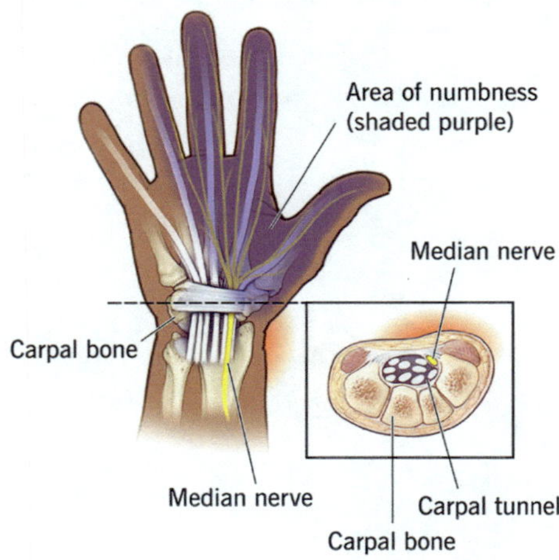

Figure 11.21. Extra pressure on the median nerve in your wrist causes carpal tunnel syndrome.

Source: https://my.clevelandclinic.org/-/scassets/images/org/health/articles/carpal-tunnel-syndrome.

Management of CTS typically involves a combination of both nonoperative and operative management, suited to the specific patient's unique scenario. Nonoperative management typically involves wrist splinting, anti-inflammatory medications, and, more recently, advanced rehabilitation techniques. For instance, a study compared the effectiveness of touchscreen-based home exercise programs with traditional paper-based programs after surgery for CTS. Results showed that the use of ReHand tablet app yielded substantial improvements in functional capacity, highlighting the importance of adaptive rehabilitation methods in recovery. This indicates the role played by technology in the evolution of traditional therapeutic procedures. In addition, timely intervention is crucial; the delay in treatment increases symptoms and complicates recovery, ultimately affecting upper limb muscle strength and dexterity. Proactive management thus becomes pivotal to stemming the long-term effects of CTS. In addition, interaction among CTS and upper limb musculature is worthy of examination, specifically concerning muscle function and neurological health. Evidence suggests that weakness of specified groups of muscles is associated with the incidence of CTS symptoms, indicating a clear relationship between neuropathy and muscular performance. A manual muscle examination with emphasis on paired muscles like the triceps and biceps revealed symptomatic limbs to have often weakness, indicative of muscular or secondary nerve entrapment involvement. The correlation is significant as it points towards the need for a thorough neurological examination in patients with upper extremity symptoms. These assessments not only enable diagnosis but also yield the information on which proper therapeutic intervention is based to restore nerve function and muscle strength. Finally, CTS's effects are multilateral, necessitating a holistic appreciation of the degree to which it affects muscular and functional integrity of the upper extremities.

Test Your Knowledge

1. What are the common causes and functional impacts of rotator cuff injuries?
2. How does tendonitis in the forearm muscles affect arm and hand movement?

SUMMARY

The intricate physiology and anatomy of the upper limb muscles play an important role not only in human movement but also in fine motor tasks and dexterity. Muscle physiology, such as muscle architecture and cross-sectional areas, informs how these muscles facilitate various activities ranging from gross locomotion to the nuances of hand movements. The approach to analysis of the mechanical properties of such muscles is similar to that of analysis in other animals, where scaling muscle to body mass reveals significant evolutionary patterns. For instance, the positive allometric scaling of emus' muscle force-generating abilities is an example of how different species evolve their muscles to meet particular biomechanical demands, which opens up the possibilities for further comparative research in human performance and muscle function (Abourachid et al., 2014). Additionally, studies on muscle architecture in different species, i.e., felids, emphasize the importance of size and functional adaptations of the upper limb. The results indicate that while greater body sizes experience increases in PCSAs of their forelimb muscles, their relative strength is observed to be decreased in comparison to lesser body sizes. This relationship represents an inferred shift in the role that these muscles play in relation to body size and locomotor capability. Having an appreciation of these scaling patterns gives valuable insights into the driving forces of muscle evolution and can have relevance in human upper limb evolution and adaptation. To engage with this comparative window, scientists can better appreciate the complexity that surrounds muscular adaptations within other taxa, which in turn assists our appreciation of human biomechanics (Adams et al., 2016). In total, knowledge of the muscles of the upper limb must be put into a general evolutionary context wherein anatomical and functional factors both apply. What this serves to do is highlight not just adaptation in human musculature but also physiological principles that underlie muscle function generally. The results of the research on emus and felids contribute to the understanding of muscle performance and adaptation in humans, with possible clinical relevance in rehabilitation and sports medicine. Lastly, understanding how muscular efficiency, anatomical variability, and functional ability relate to each other gives a holistic appreciation of the muscles of the upper limb and how they play a pivotal role both in everyday activities and specialized motions. This growing understanding of musculature can also drive research in numerous fields, ranging from evolutionary research to biomechanics, and further our comprehension of human anatomy and the consequences (Abourachid et al., 2014; Adams et al., 2016).

Upper limb muscles play a pivotal role in generating a broad range of movements that are necessary for daily functions. The key muscle groups include deltoids, biceps brachii, triceps brachii, and rotator cuff muscles, all of which generate different types of movements such as flexion, extension, and rotation. These muscles not only have the job of moving the arm and the shoulder but also of stabilizing the joint so that accurate movement can be made in intricate maneuvers. It is crucial to have good knowledge of these muscles, particularly in clinics where ROM evaluation is called for. As discussed in a comparative study of human pose estimation models for the assessment of upper limb ROM, such direct knowledge of the functionality of the muscles impacts measurement accuracy and rehabilitation outcomes, emphasizing the importance of accurate anatomical information in practical measurements (Moreira et al., 2024). Prevention of RSIs of the upper limb is a prominent area of research, given the priority to which these muscle groups are subjected within today's work environments. A scoping review detailing numerous strategies employed to prevent RSIs among computer users surfaced, with a focus on ergonomic interventions, breaks, and individual worksite adjustments. Ergonomic equipment proved helpful in minimizing the risk of harm, particularly in rich countries, whereas strategies deviated widely in various economic environments. In general, the effectiveness of these measures relies on a clear understanding of muscle function, with targeted intervention being essential for MSK health. This points to the interdisciplinary scope of muscle anatomy and its practical application in the prevention of muscle overuse disorders (Alita et al., 2024). Despite advances in technology and interventions for assessing the functionality of the upper limb, measurement accuracy and reliability remain challenges. From studies, it has been clear that while HPE models are promising rapid assessment tools, image quality and weather also play a significant role in influencing outcomes. For example, MoveNet Thunder INT16 model demonstrated improved performance for some shoulder movements but its deficiency in elbow examination indicates the ongoing advancement of these technologies. Clinicians must be cautious when relying solely on automatic systems for ROM measurement, as the comprehensive evaluation of muscle function occasionally requires the expertise of seasoned professionals to provide context and make necessary adjustments. This close regard for both technological and anatomical considerations is the key to successful practice in the prevention and treatment of upper limb injury.

KEY TERMS FROM THIS CHAPTER

- Deltoid
- Infraspinatus
- Subscapularis
- Biceps brachii
- Triceps brachii
- Pronator teres
- Flexor carpi ulnaris
- Extensor carpi ulnaris
- Supraspinatus
- Teres minor
- Teres major
- Brachialis
- Anconeus
- Flexor carpi radialis
- Flexor digitorum superficialis
- Extensor digitorum

CRITICAL THINKING QUESTIONS

1. **Which muscle is the primary mover for flexion of the elbow?**
   a. Triceps brachii
   b. Biceps brachii
   c. Deltoid
   d. Brachialis
2. **The deltoid muscle is responsible for:**
   a. Extension of the wrist
   b. Abduction of the shoulder
   c. Flexion of the fingers
   d. Rotation of the forearm
3. **Which muscle group is primarily responsible for extension of the forearm at the elbow?**
   a. Biceps brachii
   b. Triceps brachii
   c. Brachioradialis
   d. Flexor carpi
4. **The rotator cuff muscles help to:**
   a. Flex the elbow
   b. Stabilize the shoulder joint
   c. Extend the wrist
   d. Abduct the fingers
5. **Which muscle is located on the anterior surface of the forearm and helps in wrist flexion?**
   a. Flexor carpi radialis
   b. Extensor digitorum
   c. Brachialis
   d. Supinator

Short Answer Questions

1. What are the central anatomical regions of the upper limb and their key bones?
2. Which muscles make up the anterior and posterior compartments of the arm, and what are their roles?
3. Describe the general functions of the forearm muscles.
4. What are the key muscles of the hand involved in fine motor skills?
5. List two common injuries or disorders that affect the muscles of the upper limb.
6. How do upper limb muscles contribute to coordinated movement and daily activities?

Answer to Critical Thinking Questions

1. (b); 2. (b); 3. (b); 4. (b); 5. (a)

REFERENCES

1. Aber, R. (2016). Improving health literacy: Parental medical decisions regarding lower extremity amputations. https://core.ac.uk/download/84402968.pdf (accessed on 14th June 2025).
2. Lamas, L. P., Main, R. P., & Hutchinson, J. R. (2014). Ontogenetic scaling patterns and functional anatomy of the pelvic limb musculature in emus (Dromaius novaehollandiae). *PeerJ*, *2*, e716. https://doi.org/10.7717/peerj.716Adams, A., Alexander, A., Anyonge, D., et al. (2016). The scaling of postcranial muscles in cats (*Felidae*) I: Forelimb, cervical, and thoracic muscles. https://core.ac.uk/download/159067742.pdf (accessed on 14th June 2025).
3. Ahn, M., Burgess, M., Burggren, W., Cannatella, D., Cannatella, C., Clemente, C., Cline, T., et al. (2017). Digital dissection of the model organism *Xenopus laevis* using contrast-enhanced computed tomography. https://core.ac.uk/download/96600364.pdf (accessed on 14th June 2025).
4. Ahonpää, A. M. (2024). The prevention of the most common shoulder injuries in competitive swimming: A narrative literature review. https://core.ac.uk/download/638724828.pdf (accessed on 14th June 2025).
5. Aiello, A., Cotellessa, F., Grandis, M., Lagostina, G., et al. (2022). Quality of life and upper limb disability in Charcot-Marie-Tooth disease: A pilot study. https://core.ac.uk/download/590397433.pdf (accessed on 14th June 2025).
6. Alexander, R., Biewener, A., Biewener, C., Bishop, A., Brainerd, E., Charles, J., et al. (2017). Gearing effects of the patella (knee extensor muscle sesamoid) of the helmeted guineafowl during terrestrial locomotion. https://core.ac.uk/download/141439106.pdf (accessed on 14th June 2025).
7. Alfieri, F. M., Battistella, L. R., Bernardo, W. M., Correia, W. S., et al. (2013). Cumulative trauma disorders in upper limbs: Rehabilitation. https://core.ac.uk/download/268364468.pdf (accessed on 14th June 2025).
8. Alicea, B. J. (2009). Range-based techniques for discovering optimality and analyzing scaling relationships in neuromechanical systems. https://core.ac.uk/download/pdf/288557.pdf (accessed on 14th June 2025).
9. Allen, V., Hutchinson, J. R., Otero, A., Pol, D., et al. (2017). Forelimb muscle and joint actions in Archosauria: Insights from *Crocodylus johnstoni* (Pseudosuchia) and *Mussaurus patagonicus* (Sauropodomorpha). https://core.ac.uk/download/141887609.pdf (accessed on 14th June 2025).
10. Alonso López, J. F., Jordanic, M., Mañanas Villanueva, M. Á., Rojas Martínez, M., et al. (2016). Prediction of isometric motor tasks and effort levels based on high-density EMG in patients with incomplete spinal cord injury. https://core.ac.uk/download/87651829.pdf (accessed on 14th June 2025).
11. Amirabdollahian, F., Steuber, V., & Thacham-Poyil, A. (2020). Influence of muscle fatigue on electromyogram-kinematic correlation during robot-assisted upper limb training. https://core.ac.uk/download/288394226.pdf (accessed on 14th June 2025).
12. Bache, C. E., Harmatz, P. R., Jester, A., Mackenzie, W. G., et al. (2014). Orthopedic management of the extremities in patients with Morquio A syndrome. https://core.ac.uk/download/323062594.pdf (accessed on 14th June 2025).

13. Badre, A. (2019). Radial head stability in anterior Monteggia injuries: An *in vitro* biomechanical study. https://core.ac.uk/download/215391998.pdf (accessed on 14th June 2025).

14. Bathgate, A., Burkhart, A., Cresswell, A., Miller, A. L., Wilson, B. D., Morgan, C. D., Rolf, C., et al. (2010). Does a SLAP lesion affect shoulder muscle recruitment as measured by EMG activity during a rugby tackle? https://core.ac.uk/download/1664813.pdf (accessed on 14th June 2025).

15. Blanquero, J., Cortés Vega, M. D., García-Frasquet, M. Á., Nieto Díaz de los Bernardos, M., et al. (2019). Exercises using a touchscreen tablet application improved functional ability more than an exercise program prescribed on paper in people after surgical carpal tunnel release: A randomized trial. https://core.ac.uk/download/225123836.pdf (accessed on 14th June 2025).

16. Cappellari, O., Charles, J. P., Hutchinson, J. R., Spence, A. J., et al. (2016). Musculoskeletal geometry, muscle architecture and functional specializations of the mouse hindlimb. https://core.ac.uk/download/45467680.pdf (accessed on 14th June 2025).

17. Casado Rodríguez, A., de Diego, M., Gómez, M., Pastor, J., et al. (2022). Anatomical and molecular analyses of the deltoid muscle in chimpanzees (*Pan troglodytes*) and modern humans (*Homo sapiens*): Similarities and differences due to the uses of the upper extremity. http://diposit.ub.edu/dspace/bitstream/2445/190882/1/723431.pdf (accessed on 14th June 2025).

18. Collins, K. (2021). Muscle activity in upper extremity amputees. https://core.ac.uk/download/401538398.pdf (accessed on 14th June 2025).

19. Cozart, D., Hesse, D., Nichols, R., Szymik, J., et al. (2017). *UGA Anatomy and Physiology 1 Lab Manual* (3rd ed.). https://core.ac.uk/download/217306564.pdf (accessed on 14th June 2025).

20. de Waal, A., Killian, A., Gagela, A., Baartzes, J., de Klerk, S. (2024). Therapeutic approaches for the prevention of upper limb repetitive strain injuries in work-related computer use: A scoping review. *Journal of Occupational Rehabilitation, 35*, 234–267. https://www.semanticscholar.org/paper/83ff335150237bb9bbc6af6d7357967a7fd6cc33 (accessed on 14th June 2025).

21. Delp, S. L., Hutchinson, J. R., Rankin, J. W., Rosenbluth, K. H., et al. (2015). Musculoskeletal modelling of an ostrich (*Struthio camelus*) pelvic limb: Influence of limb orientation on muscular capacity during locomotion. https://core.ac.uk/download/36778511.pdf (accessed on 14th June 2025).

22. Diogo, R., Esteve-Altava, B., Molnar, J., Rolian, C., et al. (2017). Comparison of musculoskeletal networks of the primate forelimb. https://core.ac.uk/download/141439115.pdf (accessed on 14th June 2025).

23. Esteve-Altava, B., Esteve-Altava, B., Esteve-Altava, B., Esteve-Altava, B., Villmoare, B., Rolian, C., Rolian, C., et al. (2018). First anatomical network analysis of fore- and hindlimb musculoskeletal modularity in bonobos, common chimpanzees, and humans. https://core.ac.uk/download/157769144.pdf (accessed on 14th June 2025).

24. Ferreira, L. M. (2011). Development of an active elbow motion simulator and coordinate systems to evaluate kinematics in multiple positions. https://core.ac.uk/download/61660605.pdf (accessed on 14th June 2025).

25. Figueirido, B., Janis, C., & Buttrill, K. (2014). Locomotion in extinct giant kangaroos: Were sthenurines hop-less monsters? https://core.ac.uk/download/pdf/30673537.pdf (accessed

on 14th June 2025).

26. Goswami, A., Porto, A., Porto, A., Leroi, A. M., Esteve-Altava, B., et al. (2015). Anatomical network comparison of human upper and lower, newborn and adult, and normal and abnormal limbs, with notes on development, pathology and limb serial homology vs. homoplasy. https://core.ac.uk/download/36779022.pdf (accessed on 14th June 2025).
27. Harris, G. F., & Slavens, B. A. (2012). *Biomechanics*. https://core.ac.uk/download/213080657.pdf (accessed on 14th June 2025).
28. Hatsopoulos, N. G., Lillicrap, T. P., Mardoum, P., Suminski, A., et al. (2015). Temporal evolution of both premotor and motor cortical tuning properties reflect changes in limb biomechanics. https://core.ac.uk/download/213085899.pdf (accessed on 14th June 2025).
29. Jepsen, J. R. (2014). Can testing of six individual muscles represent a screening approach to upper limb neuropathic conditions? https://core.ac.uk/download/pdf/50696309.pdf (accessed on 14th June 2025).
30. Kasslatter, F. (2025). Preventative strategies for shoulder dislocation in ice-hockey players: Educational booklet for the Red Bull Ice Hockey Academy. https://core.ac.uk/download/638726265.pdf (accessed on 14th June 2025).
31. Lin, F., Wang, K., Lai, M., Wu, Y., Chen, C., Wang, Y., & Wang, R. (2025). Multicenter study on predicting postoperative upper limb muscle strength improvement in cervical spinal cord injury patients using radiomics and deep learning. *Scientific Reports, 15*. https://www.semanticscholar.org/paper/6d20efbb3cdd939e14a6b2055783f45514599230 (accessed on 14th June 2025).
32. Moreira, R., Teixeira, S., Fialho, R., Miranda, A., Lima, L. D. B., Carvalho, M. B., Alves, A. B., et al. (2024). Validity analysis of monocular human pose estimation models interfaced with a mobile application for assessing upper limb range of motion. *Sensors (Basel, Switzerland), 24*. https://www.semanticscholar.org/paper/e58bf01c32c5b58164d6af2cf0bfd83b8da1a78d (accessed on 14th June 2025).
33. Niu, R. (2020). Types and causes of physiological injury in piano playing, with emphasis on piano pedagogy in China. https://core.ac.uk/download/328100066.pdf (accessed on 14th June 2025).
34. Ortiz, H. J. C., & Adorno, C. G. (2024). Rapid upper limb assessment (RULA) and Rodger's muscle fatigue analysis (RMFA) of dentists using optical microscope, loupes, or no magnification during endodontic access: A pilot study. *Journal of Clinical Advances in Dentistry*. https://www.semanticscholar.org/paper/a81e07247db86fb2c10486ca2b9711fdd7c585eb (accessed on 14th June 2025).
35. Santello, M., & Valero-Cuevas, F. J. (2017). On neuromechanical approaches for the study of biological grasp and manipulation. http://arxiv.org/abs/1710.08557 (accessed on 14th June 2025).
36. Trichez Júnior, A. N. (2024). Changes in contact mechanics of the glenohumeral joint in the presence of osseous defects: A numerical study. https://core.ac.uk/download/654368137.pdf (accessed on 14th June 2025).

INDEX

C

D

E